# Varicose Veins and Related Disorders

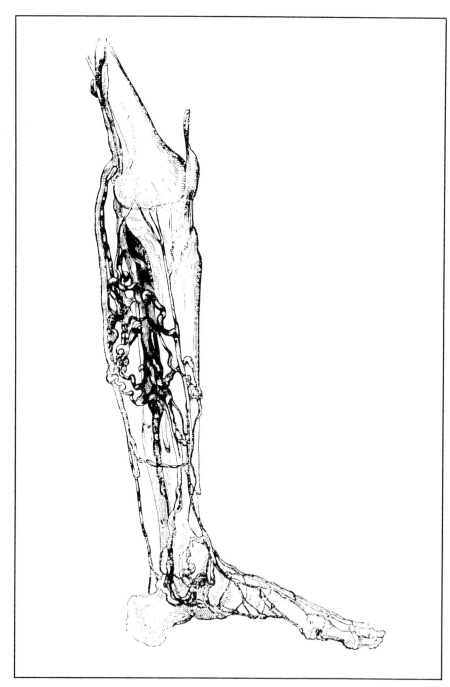

*Early Victorian view of varicose veins. (Woodcut by Bagg. In* Elements of Surgery. *By Robert Liston, Surgeon to North London Hospital, Professor of Clinical Surgery. Published by Longman, Orme, Brown, Green and Longmans, London, 1840.) (Reproduced by courtesy of the Royal Society of Medicine, London.)*

    *This illustration of short saphenous varicose veins shows a clear understanding of their arrangement, in keeping with our own 150 years later (compare with Figure 4.22(a)), including communication with the deep veins. The failure of valves was clearly recognized in Liston's writings and in the same year he refers to* 'the current of blood in either direction' *in the* 'saphena vein', *so it is probable that he realized a circuit of downflow in the system of varicose veins could occur (see also Historical note, page 561).*

# Varicose Veins and Related Disorders

**David J. Tibbs** MA, MS, FRCS
*Honorary Consulting Surgeon, John Radcliffe Hospital, Oxford*

Radiology by **E.W.L. Fletcher** MA, MB, BCh., FRCR
*Consultant Radiologist, John Radcliffe Hospital, Oxford; Lecturer in University of Oxford; Fellow of Green College, Oxford*

## With contributions by

Terence J. Ryan DM, FRCP
*Consultant Dermatologist, Department of Dermatology, Slade Hospital and University of Oxford*

Tarik F. Massoud MB, BCh., BAO, FRCR
*Senior Registrar, Department of Radiology, Radcliffe Infirmary and John Radcliffe Hospital, Oxford*

and

Basil J. Shepstone MA, DPhil., MD, DSc., FRCR
*Consultant Radiologist, Department of Radiology, Radcliffe Infirmary and John Radcliffe Hospital, Oxford*

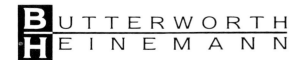

Butterworth-Heinemann Ltd
Linacre House, Jordan Hill, Oxford OX2 8DP

 PART OF REED INTERNATIONAL BOOKS

OXFORD   LONDON   BOSTON
MUNICH   NEW DELHI   SINGAPORE   SYDNEY
TOKYO   TORONTO   WELLINGTON

First published 1992

© Butterworth-Heinemann Ltd 1992

**British Library Cataloguing in Publication Data**
Tibbs, David J.
  Varicose Veins and Related Disorders
  I. Title
  616.14

ISBN 0 7506 1032 8


**Library of Congress Cataloguing in Publication Data**
Tibbs, David J.
  Varicose veins and related disorders/David J. Tibbs;
  radiology by E. W. L. Fletcher;
  with contributions by Terence J. Ryan,
  Tarik F. Massoud and Basil J. Shepstone.
  p. cm.
  Includes bibliographical references and index.
  ISBN 0 7506 1032 8
  1. Varicose veins. 2. Varicose veins – Surgery. 3. Veins – Diseases. I. Title.
  [DNLM: 1. Varicose Veins. 2. Veins – physiopathology. WG 600 T552v]
  RC695.T53 1992                                        92–19243
  616.1′4–dc20                                          CIP


Printed and bound in Great Britain by
Butler & Tanner Ltd, Frome and London

# Contents

# Foreword

This is certainly a book which will provide all the information one is ever likely to need about varicose veins, ranging from clinical presentation to diagnosis and management. David Tibbs has drawn on a wealth of personal experience in this area as well as the extensive literature on different aspects of the subject, which tends to be a Cinderella of surgery. Nowhere else does so much information about venous disorders exist between the two covers of one book. Commencing with the distinction between the abnormal and the normal, the author moves through descriptions of the patterns of abnormality to more specific problems such as superficial vein incompetence and the post-thrombotic syndrome, but has not neglected the more unusual venous problems such as congenital venous disorders. The management of these various venous disorders by surgical and non-surgical means is discussed extensively. There are excellent contributions on the use of functional phlebography in venous disorders of the lower limb by Dr E. W. Fletcher and alternative methods for imagining veins are described by Drs Shepstone and Massoud. The investigation of venous disorders using the directional Doppler flowmeter to define both simple and more complex venous problems

is dealt with in detail by the author who has developed the use of these diagnostic tools to a level of some considerable sophistication.

This is the most comprehensive but still readable book on venous problems that I have had the pleasure of reading. It calls on the vast experience of one of the pioneer vascular surgeons in the UK as well as the work of others. David Tibbs' interest in varicose veins and related problems grew steadily during his career in vascular surgery, primarily because he felt that there was so much to learn about what are very common problems, but still relatively neglected by the surgeon. This will be a book that should serve all surgeons, vascular or otherwise, who deal with varicose veins as it is a goldmine of information and it will provide a splendid source of information for the diagnosis and management of both the simple and complicated problems associated with veins.

*Peter J. Morris*
*Nuffield Professor of Surgery*
*Chairman of Department of Surgery*
*John Radcliffe Hospital, Oxford*

# Preface

This book was conceived 15 years ago at a time when varicose vein surgery had changed little over the previous 20 years but during which arterial surgery had been transformed. Great enthusiasm was channelled into exploiting the new arterial techniques and, on the venous side, thromboembolism was studied intensively, but treatment of the commonplace venous disorders in the lower limbs was regarded as a routine matter suitable for delegation to the least experienced member of the surgical team. Discussion centred around perforators or the virtues of sclerotherapy, but little progress was made in understanding more fully the fundamental failures in veins, how to diagnose them and to find the best methods of treatment. Arterial surgeons, repeatedly exposing the long saphenous vein for use as arterial bypass grafts, had soon found that some well-entrenched beliefs about saphenous incompetence were not correct and the thought grew that careful study of the veins would be rewarded with a rich harvest. It was clear that the venous system, especially in its manifestations of abnormality, differed greatly from the arterial system, and the recently acquired knowledge on arteries was of no help with veins. A levelling off in the rate of new attainments in arterial surgery gave impetus to the feeling that it was time to take a fresh and critical look at the venous disorders, and to re-examine the rather confused existing beliefs. At this stage, the directional Doppler velocimeter made a timely appearance with its ability to give an extraordinary insight into patterns of flow in superficial and deep veins in the lower limbs. Soon after this the main restrictions of phlebography, reaction to contrast medium and the severe limits imposed by radiation dosage, were lifted by the introduction of low osmolar contrast media and the advent of the electronic image intensifier. The new understanding that these innovations opened out gave origin to our book. It is a product of the pooled ideas and work of a surgeon (D.J.T.) and a radiologist (E.W.L.F.); its text, apart from two chapters by invited authors, has been written by the surgeon, with the essential contribution by the radiologist expressed in the numerous functional phlebograms and varicograms appearing throughout the book. From first acquaintance with the directional Doppler flowmeter, the surgeon-author, an arterial surgeon since the pioneering mid-1950s, progressively turned towards the search for an accurate understanding of venous disorders in the lower limbs, based on the incontrovertible evidence that flowmetry and functional phlebography could provide. At an early stage a decision was made to publish eventually the findings and conclusions as a book; to this end much relevant material was collected and stored but the pressures of clinical work often caused this to be fragmentary so that meaningful statistical analysis has not been possible.

Meanwhile, other surgeons in Britain had also decided that it was time for venous surgery to have its turn and from this sprang the Venous Forum of the Royal Society of Medicine, a discussion group where surgeons, dermatologists, radiologists, nurses and any other interested groups could exchange views. An early benefit from this was the quarterly journal *Phlebology*, which has proved of inestimable value in promoting interest and scientific study. Continental Europe, particularly France, was well ahead of the UK in this and already had a thriving organization for venous conferences – Union de Phlebologie – and the journal *Phlebologie*. Strong international bonds, including USA, Japan and many other nations, have been established, each country sharing conferences with the others. In this way the mood has changed and it is realized that venous problems are full of interest, requiring special skills and individual thought, all matched by an ever expanding range of diagnostic technology. The simple Doppler flowmeter which opened the doors to an era of advancement now has its modern counterpart in imaging by ultrasound with velocity of flow measurable at any designated point and the direction of flow coded in colour. It is not hard to foresee the development of a computerized, three-dimensional display of the entire venous system in the limb of a patient exercising in the upright position, that is, the position in which problems of venous return against gravity become apparent.

The recent surge of interest in veins has not brought

any unexpected revelations. Everything in the new understanding has been said before but now conflicting beliefs have given way to secure knowledge in many areas. The outstanding change has been the acquisition of an ability to demonstrate the basic manifestations of venous disorder and from this stems accurate, logical treatment. Opportunities stand waiting; surgery has always made its most rapid advances when pathogenesis by structural failure has been identified so that technical ingenuity can be turned towards finding a method of repair; now that it is known what features the diagnostic machines should be looking for, engineers can be urged to develop a further generation that will far excel the present one; for those who enjoy the search for basic knowledge the areas upon which future studies should concentrate have been defined.

It is hoped that our book illustrates how the special investigations can take diagnosis well beyond the limits of clinical examination alone. Many cases are presented and care has been taken to ensure the accuracy for each patient; all are true life examples. The views expressed are consistent with our experience and reflect the trends shown in numerous studies from all over the world. The present understanding is explained, and the opinions of international authorities are discussed, as the basis for practical guidance to surgeon, physician or nurse. The book is not intended to be read from cover to cover but rather to be dipped into, and each chapter is designed to stand alone without having to cross-refer endlessly. For similar reasons numerous coded abbreviations are avoided since they can cause tedious searches for their meaning. Perhaps it should also be explained that the direction of venous flow is described throughout the book as 'upwards' or 'downwards' because so often it is the gravitational relationship that matters rather than the anatomical and, moreover, since virtually all meaningful tests are carried out with the patient upright it is the simplest and most revealing way of expressing direction of flow.

All phlebography was carried out by Wattie Fletcher, usually with myself making 'helpful' suggestions alongside; in this way attention was directed to the aspects that clinical examination had indicated were most important. This book would not have been possible without Wattie's tireless efforts and patience to obtain direct visualization on the image intensifier screen and static recordings on film, all annotated immediately afterwards. At the time of writing it looks as though it may not be too long before functional phlebography and varicography become superseded by colour-coded ultrasound imaging. But perhaps our efforts will help by showing the sort of phenomena that should be looked for. Patterns of abnormal venous flow have emerged showing an extraordinary fluidity that resembles electronics, with flow and counterflow in circuits that are within yet other circuits. Functional phlebography still has much to offer and in many respects is superior to the best of ultrasonography, but we are in a transition period where one method can complement the other, until the time eventually comes when ultrasonography is capable of excelling in all respects. Because we both believe in minimizing dosage of even low osmolar contrast medium, many of our X-ray pictures are faint. These are sufficient when the films are seen by transmitted light on the viewing screen, but do not photograph well. The cost and effort to enhance each frame for reproduction as prints would be prohibitive and we can only apologize for weak outlines; however, it is hoped that the many composite pictures, some backed by line diagrams, will compensate for this.

Inevitably, in assembling the book, a great deal of invaluable support has been freely given by many colleagues and my grateful thanks are due to Professor Peter Morris, a splendid leader of the Oxford surgical team, for giving inspiration and support from the very start, Terence Ryan, Tarik Massoud and Basil Shepstone for the sections they have written and also to David Lindsell for his advice on aspects of ultrasound. The line illustrations come from many sources, some prepared many years ago by Fay McLarty and Audrey Arnot, and special thanks are due to Sylvia Barker, whose drawings appear in many chapters, and to Gillian Lee for the excellent series on surgical technique. Many photographs are the author's own hurried efforts but the better ones are by David Floyd who showed great skill at every step of producing a picture. There are so many other people upon whom I have been dependent, for example Jim Webb, Orthotist, from whom I learnt much, and the Ward, Vein Clinic and Technical Staff, Heather Wood, Vivienne Denton, Phyl Gardner, Peggy Wilson, Pat Franklin and Mary McDougall, Secretaries Cathy Hitchman and Jane Carlo, and many others, who were so supportive and encouraging when something new was to be introduced. It has been a great pleasure and stimulus to learn from one's colleagues, at venous conferences and by visits, so many new ideas, but then, from student days onwards this has been one of the joys of medicine and a debt that can only be repaid to the next generation by passing on the best of what has been learnt from others and through one's own experience – by a book perhaps? As always, the patients have been a wonderful help, showing forebearance when I have kept them waiting or wished to take a photograph, and even saying with kindly interest, 'I hear you are writing a book, doctor', and to them, too, I can only say thank you. The publishers Butterworth-Heinemann amalgamated during the run in to publication, but a brief delay was more than compensated for by the excellence of the newly formed team who soon steered the book to completion; it has been a pleasure to work with Charles Fry, Deena Burgess, Chris Jarvis, and, with grateful appreciation for all her painstaking reading, Pat Croucher. Not least, my fond gratitude to my wife, Marie, who sustained me throughout; she has been marvellous.

*David J. Tibbs*

# I

# The normal and the abnormal

The essential function of veins is to return blood from the peripheral capillary beds to the heart. Veins are constructed to allow flow in one direction only and this is ensured by their numerous delicate valves. With remarkable simplicity of design, each portion of valved vein is capable of acting as a pumping unit so that the normal venous system is not only a unidirectional duct system but one liberally supplied with pumping units each capable of urging blood towards the heart against gravity in the upright position (Figure 1.1). Return against gravity is an essential requirement and most venous problems are related to some form of failure in this due to inadequacy of valve function, or to obstruction of flow in major veins. This is the essence of understanding venous disorders. The forces creating or opposing purposeful movement of venous blood will be considered first.

## Venous flow

### Direction of venous flow

Venous blood is removed from the limbs by flow towards the heart and, if this is insufficient, excess blood accumulates within the veins causing a potentially damaging rise in venous pressure (venous hypertension). Flow in veins towards the periphery, counter to the normal direction, caused by some form of valve failure, can only diminish the overall return of blood from the limb and, if sufficiently large, create an abnormal state. Such retrograde flow is nearly always determined by gravity.

*Some definitions*

*Flow:* Movement sustained without reversal for an appreciable time. In the direction of the heart this is desirable and normal but directed towards the periphery it is undesirable and abnormal.
*Surge:* Movement first in one direction and then back again and failing to achieve purposeful flow towards the heart.

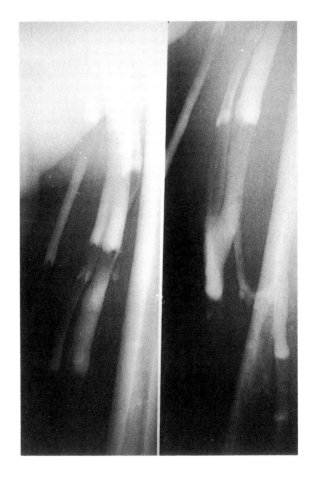

**Figure 1.1** *Valves in superficial and deep veins visualized during functional phlebography. These views were obtained by rapid repositioning from vertical to horizontal and back again (the swill test). Valves are seen resisting return of opacified blood that had moved upwards during this manoeuvre. A common variant of normal, a double femoral vein, is present*

*Reflux:* A return against the natural direction of flow governed by valves.

*Retrograde flow:* Flow away from the heart against the direction allowed by valves. Such flow is usually determined by gravity.

*Flow rate:* The speed or velocity of flow. The amount or volume may be negligible or considerable, depending upon the effective lumen of the vein concerned.

*Flow volume:* The volume moved by flow. The accompanying rate of flow may be low or high depending on the effective lumen.

*Retrograde circuit:* Describes a retrograde flow of blood which returns, in effect, to its starting point but by a different route. Thus, blood pumped from below the calf muscles up deep veins to the common femoral vein may spill over and down a retrograde circuit in the superficial veins to re-enter the deep veins in the lower leg.

*Incompetent valve:* A valve not fulfilling its role satisfactorily, that is, it is failing to prevent blood returning in the direction from which it has come. The valve cusps do not meet adequately and leakage occurs, especially in the upright position when gravitational pull is maximal and the vein is fully distended. The term is a relative one since minimal leaks may have insignificant effect on overall valve function and indeed this may vary with the distension of the vein which is influenced by such circumstances as pressure within it and the venous tone determined by temperature.

*Some synonyms:* Long saphenous vein, also known as internal or great saphenous vein. Short saphenous vein, also know as external, lesser or small saphenous vein.

*Factors creating flow in veins of the limbs*

Flow only occurs when there is a pressure gradient and three main factors may cause this:

- Gravity
- Venous pumping
- Arterial inflow

There are several other factors, of brief duration, but nevertheless of significance to the lower limbs:

- Abdominal pressure
- Thoracic pressure
- Elastic recoil and muscular contraction in vein wall

In addition various other factors which can affect flow will be considered under:

- Extraneous factors

**Gravity** Fluid, such as blood, will always take any opportunity it can to flow by gravity to a lower level. The pressure behind such flow depends on the difference in height between the two levels; the speed and volume of the flow will depend on this pressure and the calibre of the vessels connecting the two levels. Within a closed but distensible system, flow will continue until the lower level has filled to capacity and the pressure equalizes. When a person with normal valves changes from a standing position to lying with the feet elevated above horizontal, the venous blood from the limb runs back freely to the central abdominal and thoracic veins by gravity, in the direction allowed by valves. On standing again, the valves act immediately to prevent the blood from returning (Figure 1.2), but if the valves leak, blood flows down the limb until all the veins are completely filled. Thus gravity in the elevated limb gives perfect venous return flow but when standing is a force that opposes venous return and has to be overcome and resisted by a well-valved pumping mechanism.

Gravity is an ever-present force against which the limb's venous system is designed to compete in the upright position. If the valves fail, it is gravity that causes any blood that has been shifted upwards to fall back again and this has various effects. In the superficial veins it may cause visible tortuosity (varicose veins) but, much more damaging, the reflux of blood through superficial or deep veins may cause the rapid build up of an uninterrupted column of blood to the heart with consequent high venous pressure at the ankle. But yet the same force, so malign in the upright position, can be used as a powerful therapeutic measure promoting venous return if the limb is elevated so that the foot is above horizontal and gravity is creating flow in the direction of the heart.

*The influence of gravity in the activation of venous disorders and the methods by which its effects can be removed or reversed are fundamental to understanding and treating venous problems in the lower limbs.*

In the upright position any imperfection in the valves will be exploited by gravity to create retrograde flow. Most venous disorders are comparatively harmless in the horizontal limb and only when the upright position is assumed does gravity exert its influence so that the adverse features become fully evident.

**Figure 1.2** *Composite phlebograms demonstrating the effect on deep vein valves in the lower limb of rapid repositioning from vertical to horizontal and then back again (the swill test).*

*(a) Passive filling of the deep veins with the patient upright and standing still. The valve cusps are swept back by the slow upward drift of venous blood and do not show except for a few below the knee (see page 3).*

*(b) Immediately after repositioning from horizontal to vertical position. Valves are shown throughout the limb each supporting a column of blood trying to return down the limb by gravity. The popliteal and superficial femoral veins show fewer valves than normal and some cusps demonstrated appear to be poorly formed and incompetent. The overall impression in the tibial and peroneal region is of numerous effective valves. Renewed venous filling will cause a slow upward movement to recommence and will open the valve cusps again so that they cease to be visible (see page 3)*

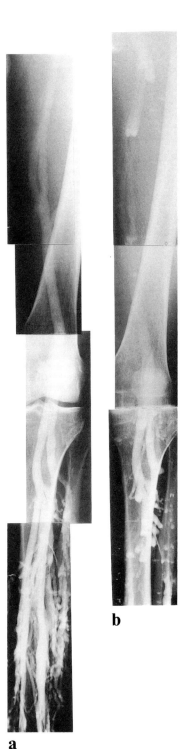

**a**

**Figure 1.2**

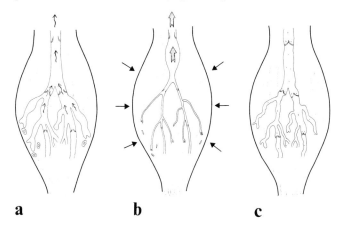

**Venous pumping** Only the peripheral pumping mechanism (musculovenous pump) can cause full venous flow against gravity. This forceful pumping action is brought about when multiple veins are compressed by contraction of surrounding skeletal muscle (Figure 1.3). The valves direct the blood heartwards and prevent it from falling back again. Thus, by this simple arrangement, the harder the muscles work, the more vigorously is the massive flow of blood generated by this activity returned towards the heart. Gravitational opposition is easily overcome by this mechanism which is essential in preventing accumulation of blood and development of a sustained high venous pressure in the lower limb (Figure 1.4).

**a**                    **b**                    **c**

**Figure 1.3**    *Diagrams of the musculovenous pumping mechanism in calf muscles.*

*(a)  The veins and venous sinuses are filled with blood.*

*(b)  On contraction of the surrounding muscles the blood is forced upwards by compression of the veins.*

*(c)  Valves prevent the blood from returning so the veins are slack and ready to be filled again with venous blood (also see Figure 1.24)*

**Figure 1.4**    *Normal variation of venous pressure in the leg with exercise. This is a tracing from photoplethysmography in a normal subject and closely follows changes in venous pressure. The patient was sitting in a legs down position and during five exercise movements the pressure fell to a low level but over the next 37 seconds gradually returned to its original level as the veins refilled and a continuous column of blood, uninterrupted by valves, built up again*

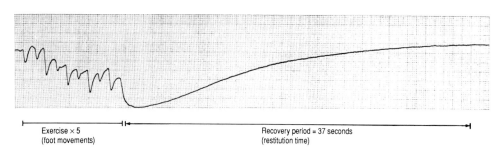

Exercise × 5
(foot movements)

Recovery period = 37 seconds
(restitution time)

Sensor 5 cm above ankle, antero-medially

*The venous pumping mechanism is fundamental to normal venous return against gravity and if it is damaged by thrombosis, or if it is overwhelmed by heavy retrograde flow in superficial or deep veins, then the resulting venous hypertension will cause some of the worst manifestations of venous disorder.*

**Arterial inflow** Inflow of blood at arterial pressure and crossing the capillary bed to enter the peripheral veins is, of course, the normal source of blood from which venous flow arises. In the elevated limb this blood flows back to the heart by gravity, through undistended veins and independent of valves or pumping mechanisms. In the standing subject, and in the absence of any muscle contraction, arterial inflow to the limb will steadily fill the veins to maximal capacity at full venous pressure to form a continuous column of blood from the foot up to the level of the heart. Further entry of arterial blood now causes a slow upward movement in the column as a passive flow, driven only by pressure from the arterial side. Although this is tolerated over short periods the accompanying sustained high venous pressure is undesirable and normally soon relieved by muscular contraction pumping blood upwards with immediate, temporary reduction in venous pressure. Even the slight muscle contractions involved in maintaining balance are sufficient to create appreciable active upward flow. In the dependent limb passive venous return caused by arterial inflow alone leaves it in a state of continuous venous congestion with pressure at the ankle related to the degree of dependency. Thus falling asleep in a chair, without any muscle movement, will cause prolonged raising of the venous pressure with formation of oedema, and the same may be seen in paralysed limbs given insufficient care.

*Passive venous return against gravity, without muscle contraction, but driven by arterial inflow alone, is no more than venous overflow and is insufficient to maintain a healthy limb in the dependent position.*

**Abdominal pressure** During coughing, straining and various other muscular efforts there is considerable increase in abdominal pressure. This may be sharp and brief, or sustained at various levels for appreciable time. This force can only tend to push blood out of the abdominal cavity and down the limbs so that for its duration it will oppose venous return from the limb. If there is a full normal complement of valves it will not, however, cause any significant retrograde movement of venous blood. If valves are incompetent or deficient in number, then a considerable retrograde surge will occur down the affected veins, perhaps as a strong cough impulse or as a steady streaming back for several seconds during straining. The valves in the external iliac and common femoral veins will prevent this happening and similarly the long saphenous vein is guarded by a valve in its uppermost part, but an appreciable number of people do not have

these valves, or the valves may have become incompetent. Strong retrograde impulses from the abdominal cavity must put considerable stress upon the valves that first withstand them and this may be an important factor in valve failure.

*Intermittent abdominal pressure, particularly when there is an inborn deficiency of iliac, femoral and saphenous valves, can exert a brief but damaging influence that will help to create and aggravate venous disorders.*

Raised abdominal pressure can only oppose venous return from the lower limbs and relaxation of abdominal pressure can only offer a cessation of resistance rather than any suction effect.

**Thoracic pressure** The upward flow in, say, the femoral vein is influenced slightly by thoracic movement and is most evident in the supine position. Thus breathing gives a gentle undulation in flow as the column of blood in the inferior vena cava ebbs and flows with each movement. Indrawing, as if to take an inward breath, against a closed glottis produces a decided upward movement by causing a marked negative pressure in the thoracic cavity; probably this is due to a lessening in pressure in the vena cava but possibly it is one of the few examples of venous flow caused by suction as blood is drawn towards negative pressure in the chest.

Raised thoracic pressure, as in coughing or blowing, can certainly create retrograde flow in the limb with incompetent valves but here it is difficult to distinguish from the effects of the accompanying raised abdominal pressure. However, as an example, a clarinet player recently seen, described how her varicose veins distended when she commenced to play and deflated again as she ceased.

**Elastic recoil and muscular contraction of vein wall** Elastic recoil in distended veins will cause brief flow until the distension has been reduced. It will initiate flow earlier than would otherwise occur when resistance to venous return drops, as in a change of posture. Muscular contraction and relaxation is under autonomic and chemical control and will vary, for example, with temperature and circulating hormones or vasoconstrictors (Sharpey-Schafer, 1961). In venous disorders these properties of the vein walls may be greatly reduced and, in some, may be a principal cause of the disorder (see Chapter 7).

**Extraneous factors** External pressure on the limb compresses veins and, given effective valves, will initiate a burst of upward flow. Pressure to the underside of the foot by body weight does, of course, drive blood upwards at each step and this is perhaps the only occasion on which gravity actually helps upward movement of blood within the veins! The foot, however, is a well-recognized pumping mechanism (Gardner and Fox, 1989) and, as with other forms of external compression, no more than one variety of venous pumping.

No doubt there are other extraneous factors that can

cause flow. Centrifugal force, as might be encountered by aeronauts or astronauts, clearly can cause a strong and prolonged pull affecting venous flow in one direction or the other, in much the same way as gravity. This is an important but specialized field and other authorities must be consulted. Atmospheric decompression selectively applied to a limb could well affect flow by causing movement of blood into the limb but seems a most unlikely circumstance that need not be considered here.

From the above description it will be seen that the undesirable state of sustained venous filling to capacity and the accompanying high venous pressure can only be relieved by, either, elevation of the limb so that the blood flows away by gravity, or, by the peripheral force-pump being brought into action by muscular contraction. The pumping mechanism is of paramount importance and is considered further later in this chapter.

## Normal anatomy and physiology: some aspects of abnormality

The overall anatomy of the veins in the lower limbs is illustrated in Figure 1.5, but certain points do require emphasis. The traditional division into superficial and deep veins remains as fundamental as ever because each is vulnerable to its own range of disorders and consequent manifestations. The communicating or perforatoring veins are essential to normal function but there is much debate about their role in the abnormal states and this topic will be returned to later in this chapter and Chapter 11.

### Superficial veins

The superficial veins lie in subcutaneous tissues outside the deep fascia except in their final approach to join a deep vein and are arranged in two intercommunicating systems based on the long and the short saphenous veins. Nearly all other surface veins drain into them but there is widespread alternative drainage through the perforating or communicating veins into the deep veins. Normally superficial veins are liberally supplied with valves but these vary considerably in number and quality, with corresponding variation in their robustness and efficiency. The long saphenous vein (Figure 1.5(b)1, (c)1) terminates in the common femoral vein by passing through a well-defined aperture (fossa ovalis) in the deep fascia immediately overlying it. The short saphenous vein usually takes a less direct approach and runs for some inches immediately beneath the deep fascia of the calf before plunging more deeply to join the popliteal vein within the popliteal fossa (Figure 1.5(b)2). Again, there is an oblique aperture in the deep fascia where the vein enters it but this varies in level from mid-calf up to the popliteal fossa itself so that there is considerable variation

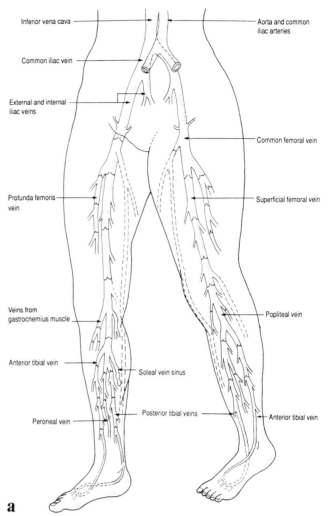

**Figure 1.5** *Venous anatomy in the lower limbs.*
*(a) The principal deep veins. The innumerable branch veins and those lying within muscle are omitted but some idea of their complexity may be gathered from the many phlebograms illustrating this book. The tibial and peroneal veins are usually paired veins uniting in their upper parts (and see page 6).*

in the distance of subfascial course it may run. Within the fossa there is again variation in the level at which it may join the popliteal vein (Figures 1.5(c), 4.22, 4.23, 4.24, 5.9, 5.11(d)) and in the branches its receives (see Chapter 20). The foot has a particularly free interchange between superficial and deep veins (Figure 1.5(d)). The details of venous anatomy seen at surgical operations are illustrated in Chapter 20, together with some of the more important variations.

### Deep veins

The massive venous return from the muscles during exercise is handled by the veins lying within the deep fascia. These deep veins may be classified into those more concerned with collecting and conducting than with pumping, and those within the muscles specifically 'designed' as pumping units. The principle named conducting

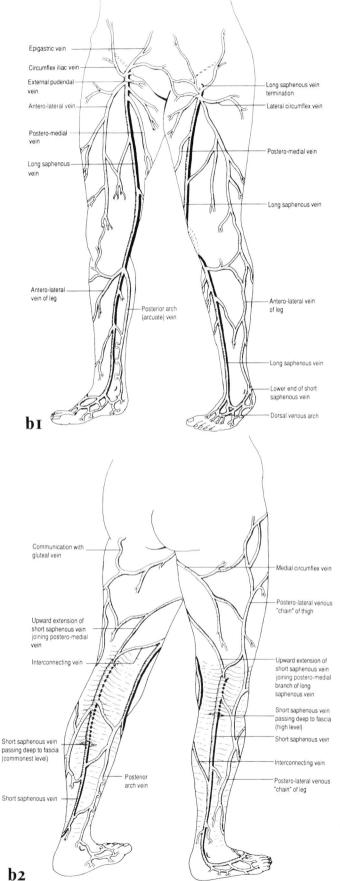

b1

b2

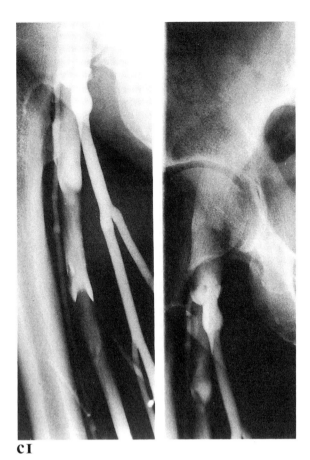

c1

**Figure 1.5** *(continued) (b) The principal superficial veins. The network of innumerable small interconnecting veins and many lesser veins are omitted but they may become active participants in venous disorders and, for example, undergo considerable enlargement. A few perforating veins are indicated as representative of these numerous and widespread communications between superficial and deep veins (see also Figures 11.1, 11.5).*

*(c) Phlebograms of saphenous terminations.*
   *1. Two views of a typical long saphenous termination. This is relatively constant but can occasionally join at a lower level, or rarely as a double vein.*
   *2. A normal short saphenous vein joining the popliteal vein at the most usual level, opposite the femoral condyles.*
   *3. An incompetent short saphenous terminating at normal level.*
   *4. Termination of incompetent short saphenous vein near mid-shaft of femur.*
   *5. An incompetent short saphenous vein joining the popliteal vein at usual level but sending an upward extension to join the profunda femoris vein; a common variant of this is an upward extension running subcutaneously and posteriorly to join the long saphenous vein. An upward extension of this sort often becomes an important collateral vein in post-thrombotic deep vein occlusion.*

*(d) Arrangement of superficial and deep veins in the foot with multiple interconnections between them. The deep veins are joined by venous sinuses from the plantar muscles which, together with the whole complex of veins under the foot, form an important pumping mechanism*

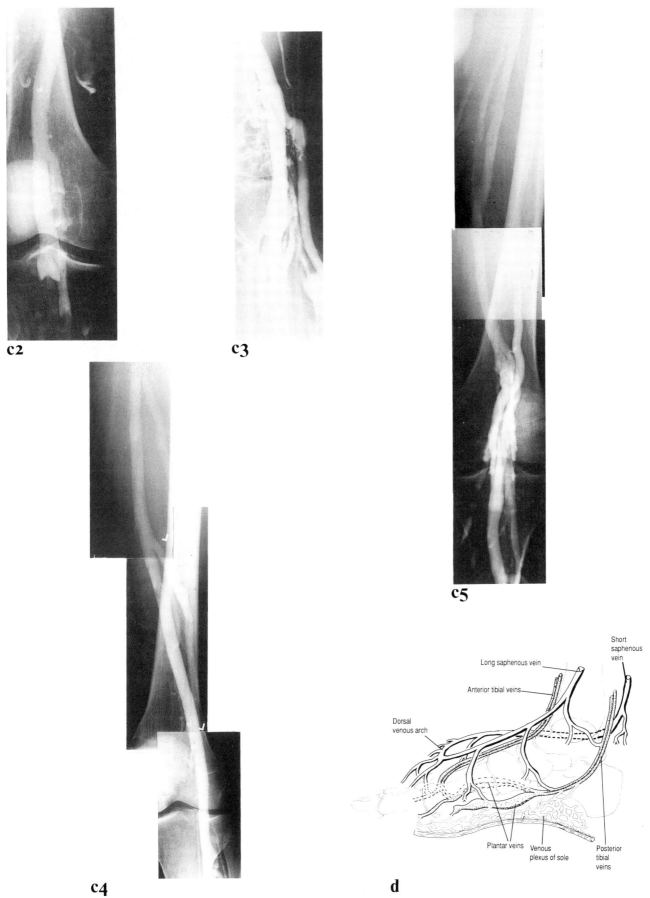

**c2**

**c3**

**c4**

**c5**

d

Long saphenous vein

Short saphenous vein

Anterior tibial veins

Dorsal venous arch

Plantar veins

Venous plexus of sole

Posterior tibial veins

**Figure 1.5** *(continued)*

veins are illustrated in Figure 1.6(a), (b). Below the knee these veins are usually double channels (Figure 1.6(c)) with each pair corresponding with the three main arteries, the anterior and posterior tibial and the peroneal. At knee level they become a single channel so that damage or occlusion to them may cause severe problems of venous return. Whereas superficial veins may be sacrificed with relative impunity this is certainly not true of the conducting deep veins which must always be treated with great respect. This is especially true of the popliteal, common femoral and iliac veins where there is no satisfactory alternative channel of venous return and they are virtually venous 'bottlenecks'. Loss of these veins may leave only lesser deep veins and superficial veins to act as collateral channels and it is in these circumstances that some of the most intractable and disabling problems arise. One of the most commonly practised vein operations, flush ligation at the termination of the long saphenous vein, takes the surgeon in close proximity to the common femoral vein so that there should be a constant awareness of the irreplaceable role of the deep veins.

## Occlusion of deep veins and the formation of collateral veins

If a principal deep vein is occluded by thrombosis or injury, venous return is forced to follow other channels, either lesser and possibly inadequate neighbouring deep veins, or overlying superficial veins which may become clearly visible. These channels of alternative flow, substituting as best they can, are referred to as collateral veins. Such veins are based on one or more existing veins which respond to the increase in flow and pressure within them by enlarging considerably. According to the

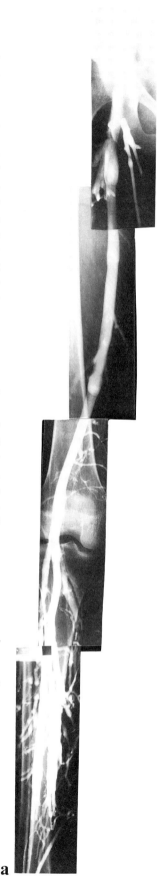
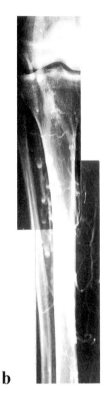
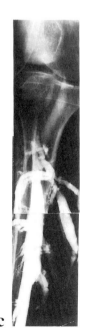

**Figure 1.6** *The principal conducting veins illustrated by phlebogram.*

*(a) Below the knee paired tibial and peroneal veins can be seen together with a few muscular branches. The venous 'bottle-necks' formed by the popliteal, common femoral and iliac veins are evident. Only the commencement of the profunda femoris is shown but this forms a large system of veins in the thigh capable of acting as collaterals. The superficial veins, not seen, become important collateral channels if the venous bottle-necks are obstructed or severely deformed by thrombosis or injury.*

*(b) The same patient taken after the swill test to show valves below the knee. The distribution is normal with a good valve in the popliteal vein and in the short saphenous vein alongside; numerous valves are seen down tibial and peroneal veins. Two perforating veins run between the posterolateral (arcuate) branch of the long saphenous vein and posterior tibial vein.*

*(c) Lateral views in a different patient showing paired anterior tibial veins uniting to form a single vein joining the popliteal vein. A large sinus within the soleal muscle is also shown and is but one of these numerous pumping chambers*

a

b

c

relationship with the damaged deep vein, flow in them may be in the natural direction allowed by valves, or counter to the valves, in which case tortuosity will develop in the veins in addition to enlargement (Figure 1.7). This latter variety of veins is often referred to as secondary varicose veins to distinguish them from primary (or simple) varicose veins where the initiating defect (valve failure) is in the vein itself.

## Generation of new veins (neovascularization)

There is considerable evidence that veins may also develop from newly grown vessels that form during the repair processes around a damaged vein (Glass, 1987). These new channels lack the shape and structure of normal veins and are without valves. The stimulus to their formation and orientation of flow is determined by the pressure gradient between veins below the obstruction and above it. A similar development is seen in one variety of recurrent varicose veins after saphenous ligation (Figure 1.8; see Chapter 5).

## Deep veins in muscles

It is the units within the muscles that provide the main pumping force in the limb. These veins are an essential part of the pumping mechanism removing a large volume of blood from contracting muscle and, of course, return-

ing blood against gravity. They are highly specialized veins arranged as sinuses to form numerous pump chambers emptying into conducting veins (Figures 1.6(c), 1.9). Each chamber is ideally adapted for its purpose, surrounded by muscle, with a large capacity and thin walled to allow filling with minimal resistance when the muscle

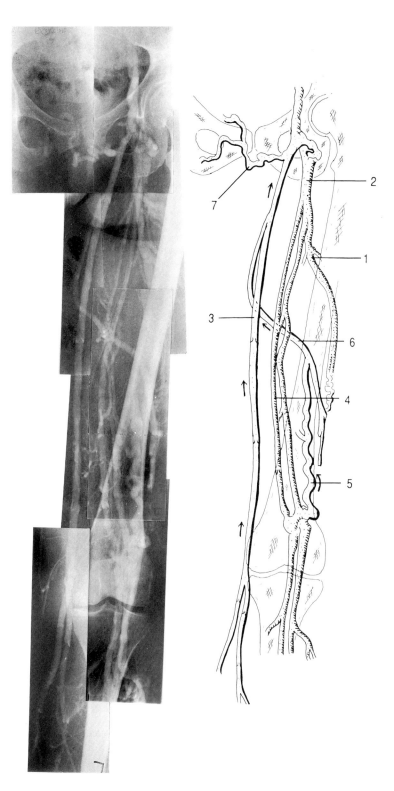

**Figure 1.7** *Composite phlebogram from mid-leg up to the pelvis taken 2 years after extensive deep vein thrombosis in the lower left limb. It shows the following features: popliteal and femoral veins have failed to fill; the profunda femoris vein ( 1 ) is open but it runs into a deformed common femoral ( 2 ) and attenuated external iliac vein; the common iliac vein could not be visualized; the extensive obstruction to the deep veins has caused strong preferential flow up the long saphenous vein ( 3 ) and through some lesser veins following the course of the deep veins ( 4 ); the short saphenous vein is acting as a collateral and a tortuous upward extension of this ( 5 ) connects with the profunda femoris and also with a posterolateral branch of the long saphenous vein which curves round the back of the thigh to join the saphenous vein in the upper thigh ( 6 ); because the common iliac vein is occluded the uppermost branches of the long saphenous vein are being forced to act as collaterals with the development of varicosities running across the pubis ( 7 ); most of the superficial veins acting as collaterals in the limb are flowing in their natural direction and do not show tortuosity; the upward extension of the short saphenous does however show tortuosity; the pubic varicosities are enlarged veins which should normally be flowing towards the common femoral vein but are now being forced to accept flow against their natural direction and hence show tortuosity*

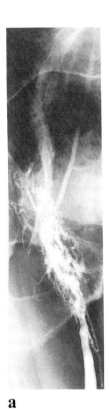 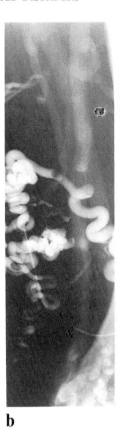

**a**                    **b**

**Figure 1.8**  *Generation of new vessels (neovascularization), facilitated and orientated by pressure difference between two parts of a vein interrupted by surgical ligation and division.*

*(a)  Ten years after long saphenous high ligation without stripping. A leash of vessels has formed between site of ligation and intact, but still incompetent, saphenous vein.*

*(b)  Similar connection at site of short saphenous ligation by a knot of slender, coiled veins to newly developed varicose veins*

is relaxed.  Inflow comes from venules draining muscle capillaries, from cross-connections with neighbouring 'pump chambers' and deep veins, and also, by perforators, from the superficial veins.  The outlet, unlike the multiple small inlets, is large and runs directly into ample-sized collecting veins running from each muscle to join the major deep veins in the direction of the heart.  These distinctive units within the muscles provide by far the most effective pumping force in the limb and only they can shift the great volume of blood required by contracting muscle.  It is a remarkable mechanism; immediately after each contraction the pump chambers stand empty ready to be primed again by inflow from the muscle or any neighbouring source, including the superficial veins (Figure 1.24).  Indeed, during studies by functional phlebography the impression is gained that removal of blood from the superficial veins of the leg is in large part by perforators to the muscle pumps rather than direct entry into the main conducting veins.

A further example of the numerous pumping sinuses

within the muscles is illustrated by venogram in Figure 1.9.  Those within the soleus and gastrocnemius muscles are particularly large and capable of giving a high volume output appropriate to the size and work required of these muscles.  Loss of activity in these muscles, as may be caused by painful ulceration and the fibrotic changes of venous stasis at the ankle, deprives the limb of its most powerful pumping mechanism which will in its turn aggravate the venous stasis further.  These venous sinuses may be of significance in the initiation of deep vein thrombosis, and exercise to prevent stagnation within them is an important precaution against this.  The complexities of the deep veins will be considered further in Chapters 9 and 10.

## Perforating or communicating veins

These veins form a direct communication, through the deep fascia, between the superficial and the deep veins (Figure 1.10(a)–(e)), including the muscle sinuses just described above (Figure 1.10(c)).  There are numerous

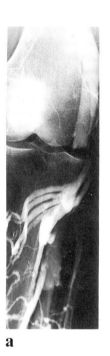 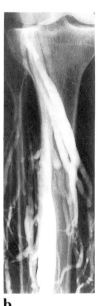 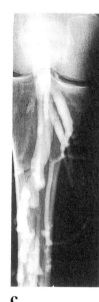

**a**              **b**              **c**

**Figure 1.9**  *The large pumping units provided by venous sinuses (pumping chambers) within gastrocnemius and soleus muscles.*

*(a)  A group of gastrocnemius sinuses running into a conducting vein (lateral gastrocnemius) emptying into the popliteal vein.*

*(b)  Medial gastrocnemius sinuses running upwards to join a conducting vein running into popliteal vein. Note the interconnections evident in the lower half of the picture.*

*(c)  Gastrocnemius and soleal sinuses. The gastrocnemius sinuses are longer and narrower than the capacious soleal ones.*

*(and see page 11)*

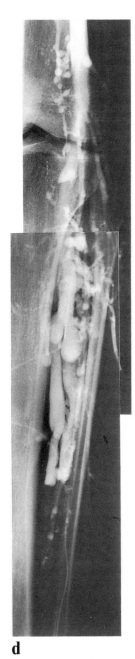

**d**

*(d) Soleal sinuses running into conducting veins which join tibial veins*

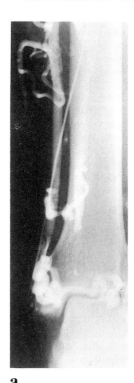

**a**

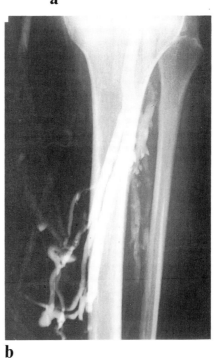

**b**

such perforators and only some are illustrated in Figure 11.5. Many studies have emphasized that these veins have effective valves which only allow inward flow from superficial to deep veins. Failure of these valves has been blamed for a variety of venous problems and debate still centres around their role in the causation of these states. The perforating veins are far more numerous than many surgical descriptions admit, perhaps around 100 on each side, and they have the important function of allowing equalization of pressure in either direction. This can readily occur by flow inwardly from superficial to deep but in theory the reverse should be prevented by the valves. However, in practice, pressure between deep and

**Figure 1.10** *Perforating or communicating veins.*

*(a) Near the ankle, running from the long saphenous vein through the deep fascia and into the posterior tibial vein. This example was seen in massive long saphenous incompetence with flow down this vein and into the tibial veins through this perforating vein which is enlarged and valveless, capable of giving flow in either direction.*

*(b) Easy communication via perforators between the posterior branch of the long saphenous vein and tibial veins.*

*(and see page 12)*

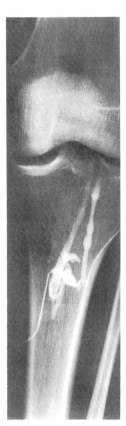
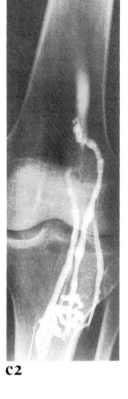
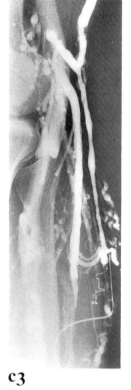
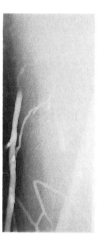
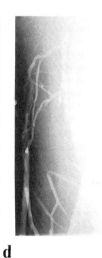

c1    c2    c3    d

**Figure 1.10** *(continued) (c) Phases of filling of gastrocnemius vein from overlying varicosities:*

> *1, 2. Patient in horizontal position. Medium enters a medial gastrocnemius sinus and the short saphenous vein simultaneously.*
>
> *3. Lateral view to give more detail of the paired perforating veins from superficial, through deep fascia, to the gastrocnemius veins. This is not necessarily abnormal as flow here is in the normal inward direction.*

*(d) Two phases in filling of perforating veins running between saphenous vein and femoral vein in mid-thigh. Patient is horizontal and flow in both pictures is in the normal inward direction, but in a vertical position outward flow could not be demonstrated, presumably because of functioning valves; a double femoral vein is present (normal variant).*

*(e) A mid-thigh perforator between superficial varicosities and the femoral vein and in corresponding position to previous illustration (d). Here, however, substantial flow outwards was demonstrated when patient was in the vertical position, in keeping with incompetence; varicosities can be seen in the superficial veins*

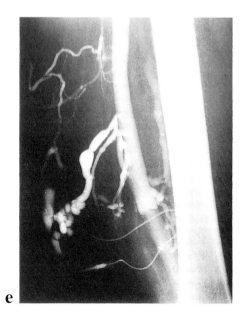

e

superficial veins can rapidly adjust in either direction in normal limbs. It seems that although a number of perforators are effectively guarded by valves, others are not, and it is best to regard the perforators collectively as a mechanism for interchange of blood in either direction to equalize pressures between superficial and deep veins. Certainly in the normal there are safeguards against the high pressures generated by muscle contraction being directly transferred to the superficial veins. The valves in perforators are important in this but perhaps equally important is the anatomical disposition of fascia around muscles which closes off perforators at the moment of contraction. Perforators are implicated in many venous disorders and a constant question is whether the perforator is the primary cause or merely incidentally involved in a more widespread process. This is discussed in Chapter 11.

*Note:* The term communicating vein is also used to describe veins communicating between superficial veins. In 1981 May proposed that it should be confined to this use but, unless specified, it is still widely used to describe a communication between superficial and deep veins, that is, a perforator.

## Structure of veins

Veins are thin-walled, elastic, collapsible tubes and not 'pipes' of fixed capacity. The ability of veins to collapse gives them a variable capacity of considerable range and is a necessary feature allowing veins to empty completely on compression so that they are ready to refill as a prelude to the next pumping action. The property of easy collapse means that suction and siphon effects in the limbs can scarcely occur and the veins act collectively as a force pump but never as a suction pump. Within the chest a weak suction is possible and in the intracranial sinuses a degree of siphonage may occur but these are not processes influencing the lower limbs. By contrast, raised abdominal pressure will oppose and attempt to reverse venous flow but this is immediately resisted by the valves.

*Note:* Some authorities (Bourne, 1986) report finding a slight negative pressure in the veins of an elevated limb and explain this by the dumb-bell cross-sectional configuration adopted by a collapsed vein. This gives two minute lumens at each edge of a flattened tube, possibly capable of giving a detectable suction effect in a cannulated vein and a weak siphonage effect in high elevation.

Veins in full distension are much broader than the corresponding arteries so that to carry the same volume of blood the speed of flow is far less than that in arteries; in the resting limb, when the arterial input is minimal, venous flow becomes very slow, almost to the point of cessation, for quite long periods and, no doubt, is then at its most vulnerable to venous thrombosis.

## Venous tone

An additional factor in venous capacity is the venous tone provided by the circular muscular and elastic layers in the vein walls. Changes in this cause a considerable variation in the maximal capacity a vein can expand up to at that moment. This is influenced by the autonomic system, local and circulating vasoconstrictors, hormones and the venous pressure (Sharpey-Schafer, 1961). The increased pressure caused by the upright position is resisted by a reflex increase in venous tone. The capacity of veins is used as a variable reservoir in the regulation of the total blood volume.

## Variations in venous tone in superficial veins

Distension of superficial veins is under the control of the autonomic system, as part of regulation of body temperature, but it is also influenced by posture, circulating vasoconstrictors and hormones, especially in pregnancy. The prominence of veins may vary from one hour to the next and the competence of valves that are less than perfect may diminish with the degree of distension. External temperature has considerable effect on the state of the superficial veins so that they expand or contract according to whether the body is trying to loose or conserve heat. Even varicose veins share in this variability so that it is quite easy to underrate the patient's state if seen in cold conditions. Apprehension will, in similar fashion, contract the veins and, when injecting veins, the first warning of an impending faint may be their virtual disappearance. Superficial veins act to some extent as a reservoir of venous blood and in states of reduced blood volume will contract down and this may occasionally affect the practical management of venous disorders.

## Endothelium and fibrinolysin

The endothelium lining the veins has the property of forming fibrinolysin which disperses any clot formed within them (Todd, 1959). Without this they would be vulnerable to intravenous clotting during long periods when the pump is not being used. This fibrinolytic mechanism is enhanced by muscle activity.

## Valves and valve failure

### Valves

The valves are bicuspid (Figure 1.11(a)) with gossamer-thin, highly flexible cusps. These are exceedingly strong for such delicate looking structures but nevertheless easily damaged and rendered ineffective if involved in the organization of thrombus on its surface. There is considerable variation in the number and quality of valves

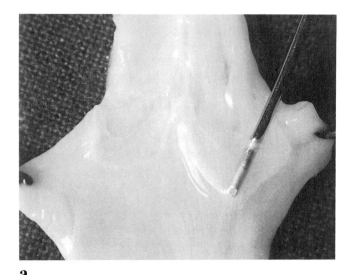

**a**

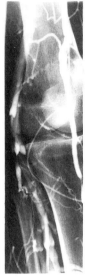

**d**

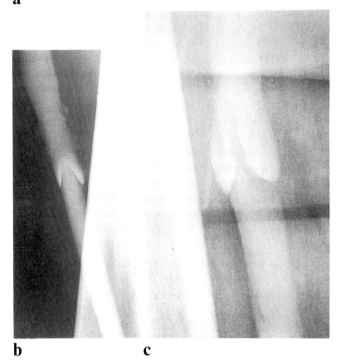

**b**        **c**

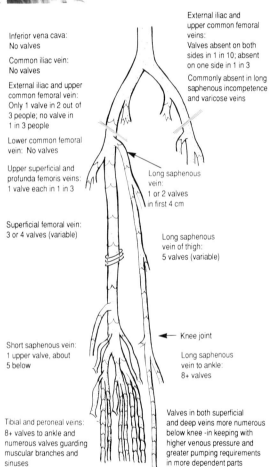

Inferior vena cava:
No valves

Common iliac vein:
No valves

External iliac and upper
common femoral vein:
Only 1 valve in 2 out of
3 people; no valve in
1 in 3 people

Lower common femoral
vein: No valves

Upper superficial and
profunda femoris veins:
1 valve each in 1 in 3

Superficial femoral vein:
3 or 4 valves (variable)

Short saphenous vein:
1 upper valve, about
5 below

Tibial and peroneal veins:
8+ valves to ankle and
numerous valves guarding
muscular branches and
sinuses

External iliac and
upper common femoral
veins:
Valves absent on both
sides in 1 in 10; absent
on one side in 1 in 3

Commonly absent in long
saphenous incompetence
and varicose veins

Long saphenous
vein:
1 or 2 valves
in first 4 cm

Long saphenous
vein of thigh:
5 valves (variable)

Knee joint

Long saphenous
vein to ankle:
8+ valves

Valves in both superficial
and deep veins more numerous
below knee -in keeping with
higher venous pressure and
greater pumping requirements
in more dependent parts

**e**

**Figure 1.11** *Valves and valve cusps.*

*(a) Valve within an opened long saphenous vein to show the paired cusps typical of valves in superficial and deep veins. They are gossamer thin and highly flexible but yet very strong. This particular valve was incompetent and it may be relevant that the cusps appear unequal in size.*

*(b) A normal valve in the femoral vein. The two cusps are partly opened by upflow but on downflow closed completely without any leakage. There are many similar valves through the major deep veins.*

*(c) At first sight this appears a normal bicuspid valve in the femoral vein but under the image intensifier it could be seen that its cusps failed to meet and it leaked heavily; moreover it was the only valve present in the popliteal, femoral or iliac veins and there was a marked lack of valves below the knee; venous stasis with ulceration was present at the ankle. Phlebographic demonstration of cusps does not necessarily indicate adequate valve function.*

*(d) Lateral view of patient shown in Figure 1.6(a), (b) showing a good valve in popliteal deep vein and a valve guarding the uppermost short saphenous vein; further valves can just be seen at the commencement of the tibial veins.*

*(e) Diagram summarizing distribution of valves in the lower limb; all figures are rounded off to indicate approximate frequency of occurrence but there is considerable variation in the positioning and number of valves within the normal range. Inborn deficiency of valves does occur and may be associated with serious disorders of venous pumping against gravity*

(Figure 1.11(b), (c)) seen in the normal; incomplete formation of cusps to give only partial function in a valve is not uncommon and especially so in the clinically abnormal states. Valves are not found in the common iliac veins, the venae cavae, hepatic, renal, uterine or umbilical veins, nor within the portal system or in pulmonary, cerebral and spinal cord veins; very small veins, less than 2 mm diameter, do not contain valves (Johnston and Whillis, 1938; Boileau Grant, 1947). The characteristic arrangement of valves guarding the outlets of major branches joining the deep veins is illustrated by a phlebogram of the short saphenous at popliteal level in Figure 1.11(d); similar valves are positioned near the termination of the long saphenous vein. The distribution of valves in the veins of the lower limbs is indicated in Figure 1.11(e); this illustration uses information gathered from Dodd and Cockett's excellent account (1976) and from our own experience with 150 functional phlebograms; see also Basmajian (1952), May (1979), Lea Thomas (1982) and Kistner (1978).

Venous disorders have a significant proportion of patients lacking the usual number of valves, apparently due to an inborn deficiency (see Chapter 7), and valves may be absent in congenital venous abnormalities (see Chapter 12); thrombosis in deep veins will damage valves and render them ineffective even if the lumen remains open. This may occur, on a small scale, as a subclinical event or as a clinically obvious episode, with corresponding damage to the pumping mechanism.

## The manifestations of valve failure

### In superficial veins

Leaking valves in the superficial veins are commonplace. This leakage varies from a small, slow one that produces no symptoms or outward evidence and is only detectable by instruments such as the ultrasonic flowmeter, to a massive escape that causes obvious local and widespread secondary effects. This produces two local effects of importance, one due to turbulence below a leaking valve causing a saccule to develop and the other caused by heavy reversed flow in a branch vein which responds by progressive enlargement and tortuosity.

### Saccules below valves

These are most obvious in the long and short saphenous veins. A jet of blood escaping downwards between leaking cusps produces strong turbulence and consequent sideways thrust; eventually the wall of the vein in the vicinity may yield to produce a substantial bulge or saccule (Figure 1.12). This is a similar phenomenon to the post-stenotic dilatation described by Holman (1954a, b, 1955) in the formation of an aneurysm below aortic coarctation and other forms of arterial stenosis. The best known

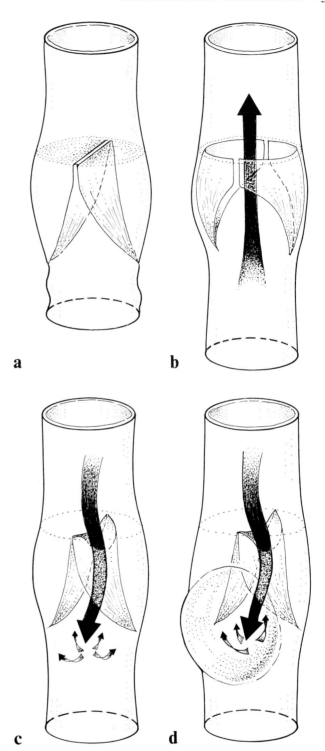

**Figure 1.12**  *Diagrams to illustrate formation of a saccule below leaking valve cusps.*

*(a)  Cusps of a competent valve closed and resisting reflux into slack vein beneath it.*

*(b)  Cusps swept into fully opened position by upward flow.*

*(c)  Incompetent valve with jet of blood passing through leaking cusps and causing turbulence beneath them.*

*(d)  Sideways thrust due to turbulence may eventually cause formation of a saccule below cusps*

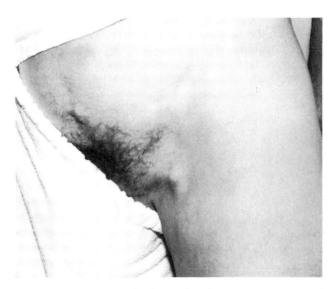

**Figure 1.13**   *Photograph of typical saphena varix at upper end of long saphenous vein. There was a palpable thrill on coughing and on first standing. Gross incompetence in the saphenous vein, with large varicosities on the calf, were present, with a tapwave easily transmitted to saphena varix. Note: the bulge just above pubes is a small incisional hernia in an old cystostomy scar and in these circumstances a diagnostic pitfall*

**Figure 1.14**   *Saccules on the long saphenous vein.*

*(a)  1. Functional venogram showing retrograde flow down long saphenous vein outlining a saccule just above mid-thigh.
2. Enlarged view of saccule to show vortex of turbulent flow outlined by opaque medium.*

*(b)  Photograph of similar saccule distended with saline; this specimen was taken from a saphenous vein 2.5 cm below its termination proved, by syringe flushing before its surgical removal, to have no competent valves.*

*(c)  The same saccule opened to show two well-formed cusps raised on probes with the opening of the saccule immediately beneath them.*
*(and see page 17)*

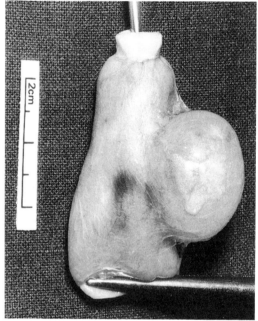

**b**

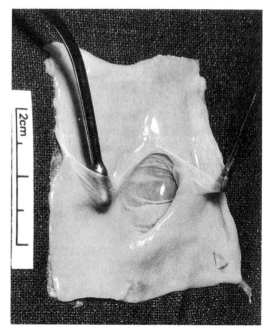

**c**

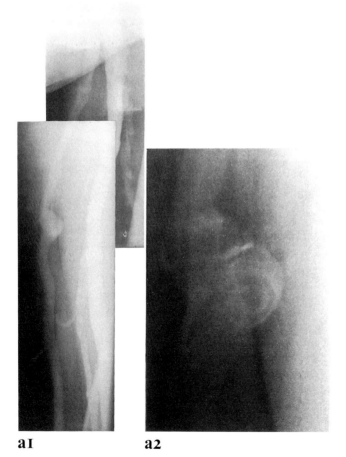

**a1**          **a2**

*(d) Further view of interior to show unequal size of cusps, possibly a reason for their incompetence.*

*(e) Although a saccule usually lies below the valve cusps this is not invariably so as this saccule taken from the same saphenous vein in mid-thigh shows. The mouth lies mainly within a large cusp which may have been prolapsing beneath the other much smaller cusp.*

*(f) Two further examples, before and after opening, taken from different patients.*

*1, 2. A typical single saccule below the cusps.*
*3, 4. A double saccule lying beneath the cusps.*

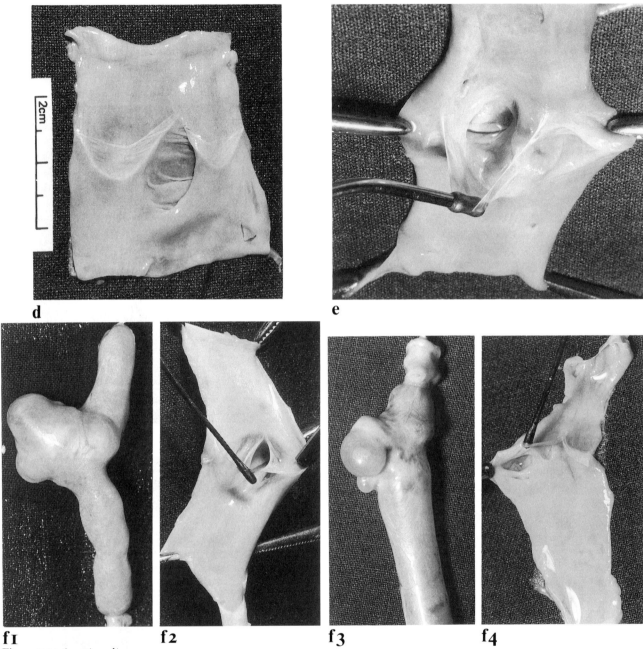

d

e

f1          f2          f3          f4

**Figure 1.14** *(continued)*

example is the saphena varix which occurs below the uppermost valve of the long saphenous vein (Figure 1.13), but similar saccules quite frequently develop at any level in the thigh portion of this vein (Figure 1.14(a)–(f)). All show the same feature of a visible or palpable bulge on the vein which, on coughing, or when the patient first stands, give a marked thrill, easily palpable, audible to stethoscope and characteristic on Doppler flowmetry.

However, by no means all incompetent saphenous valves develop a saccule but when one is present it provides immediate identification of a heavily incompetent valve and, by inference, incompetence of valves above and below this. In this way saccules on a saphenous vein are the hallmark of substantial incompetence and retrograde flow in that vein – a most important physical sign (Figure 1.15).

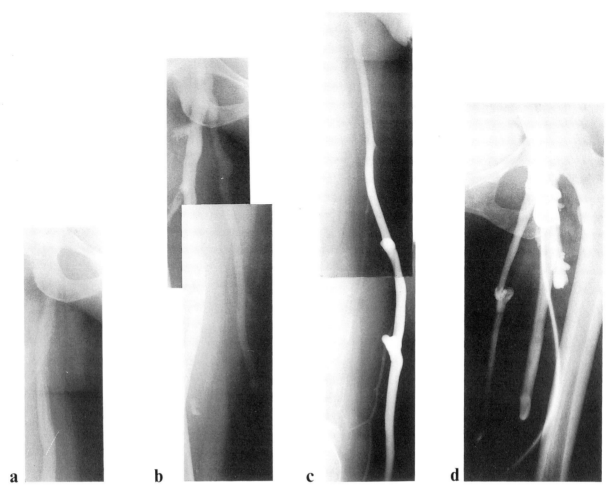

a          b          c          d

**Figure 1.15** *Incompetent valves in long saphenous vein allowing reversed flow. Phlebograms taken in upright position.*

*(a) Passive flow up femoral vein with patient standing still.*

*(b) After two exercise movements flow can be seen spilling over from common femoral vein and down the long saphenous vein.*

*(c) A later stage of filling; the long saphenous vein shows at least three saccules in the portion visualized as a clear hallmark of valvular incompetence. It has not however developed the tortuosity so commonly found in its branches.*

*(d) A descending phlebogram showing sacculation in upper long saphenous vein. The cusps of the associated valve can be well seen. (Courtesy of S. G. Darke and R. Sutton)*

It is as well that a saphenous vein so often declares its incompetence in this way because it is too robust a vein to develop another characteristic sign of incompetence, tortuosity, so frequently seen in its branches. True tortuosity is seldom seen in the long or short saphenous veins but is common in their branch veins.

*Note:* The question is inevitably asked whether the development of a saccule is a primary weakness in the vein wall and is the cause of a valve leaking, or, the leak comes first and eventually causes a saccule to form as a secondary event. The fact that incompetent valves are commonly seen without any associated saccule and that it is rare to see a venous saccule that is not close to a valve, points to the saccule being a secondary phenomenon rather than a primary weakness. However, it is possible that both factors act together, at least in some cases.

### Reverse flow and tortuosity

If valves become incompetent then reverse flow will occur when the patient is upright and moving. The saphenous veins respond to this turbulent flow by overall enlargement but are usually too strong walled to develop the tortuosity shown in the less substantial branch veins. These expand so much, both in width and in length, that the vein is forced into numerous folds upon itself in order to accommodate the massive increase in length, giving the tortuosity that characterizes varicose veins (Figure 1.16(a)). Every degree and variety of this may be encountered, derived from moderate-sized branches down to insignificant veins that have enlarged at least tenfold (Figure 1.16(b)–(h)).

**Figure 1.16**   *The development of tortuosity.*

*(a)*  *1. Original state of the vein.*
*2. Reversed flow causes the vein to enlarge in width and length so that tortuosity appears.*
*3. The process progresses with continuing enlargement and increasing turbulence at the bends.*
*4. A fully developed varicosity with saccule formation at the outer aspect of a bend. This is seldom very evident until the vein is straightened.*

*Various phlebograms illustrating tortuosity follow:*

*(b)  A varicosity arising from long saphenous vein near knee and meandering down inner aspect of leg. Note the flow into a gastrocnemius venous sinus.*

*(c)  A massive long saphenous vein at knee level gives off a varicose anterior lateral branch; just beneath this a large varicosity continues down the inner leg (only showing faintly) and near the ankle divides into a lateral branch, which sends its flow into anterior tibial deep veins, and a large branch continuing onto the foot.*

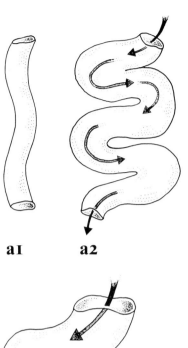

**aI**     **a2**

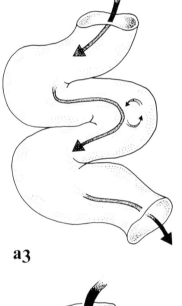

**a3**

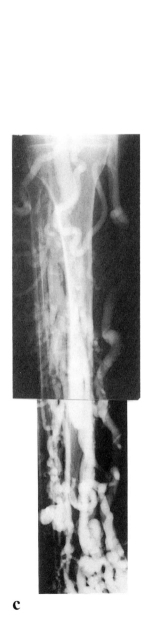

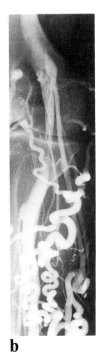

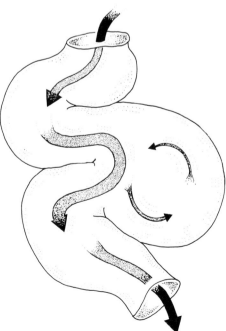

**b**          **c**          **a4**

*(d)   Tortuous superficial veins on the calf arising from the short saphenous vein. Notice how the saphenous vein, although heavily incompetent, is too robust to show tortuosity; the varicose veins are flowing into underlying tibial deep veins.*

*(e)   In spite of the massive varicosities this long saphenous vein gives to the front of the leg it does not show tortuosity.*

*(f)   A large varicosity on the lower posterior thigh taking crossflow from the uppermost short saphenous to the long saphenous vein and down a large varicosity arising from it.*

*(g)   Recurrent varicosities from a stump of long saphenous vein following inadequate surgery. These had appeared within 2 years and no varicose veins had been present at this level before. They are likely to have been formed by dilatation of side branches surviving the operation.*

*(h)   A tightly coiled varicosity arising as a recurrence after short saphenous ligation, in similar fashion to (g).*

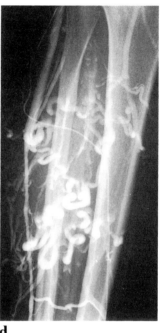

**d**

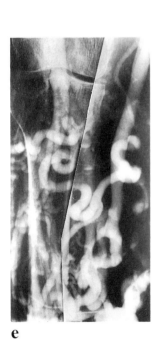

**e**

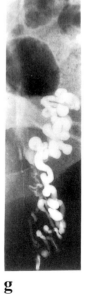

**f**          **g**

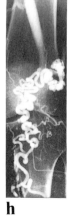

**h**

**Figure 1.16** *(continued)*

*(i)  1. A distended, tortuous vein seen clinically, or outlined by X-ray, may not show obvious saccules on it but yet when removed and straightened they appear. Why should this be? 2–6. If two pieces of string are arranged to form two parallel half-circles, one with a radius twice that of the other, then the circumference of the outer one is twice that of the inner one. If the 'bend' is undone and an attempt made to straighten the strings, the shorter one is pulled tight but the longer string forms a considerable outward bulge. This is exactly what happens when a tortuous vein is straightend during dissection or after its removal, as shown in 3 and 4. However, the non-sacculated portions of vein contract down to give the appearance shown in 5. If the vein is laid out on gauze it will adopt the form shown in 6, with very obvious pseudosaccules along its length. Perhaps concealed sacculation might be a better term – see comment in text*

i1

i2

**Figure 1.16** *(continued)*

i3

i4

i5

i6

*Pseudosacculation in tortuous veins*

Multiple small pseudosaccules often develop, each placed on the outer aspect of a bend, greatly increasing the varicose effect. These are only seen clearly in veins that have been removed and laid out. In some respects they are a surgical artefact only apparent when a tortuous vein is straightened by the surgeon, hence the qualification – 'pseudo'. The diagrams in Figure 1.16(i)1–6 clarify why this should be.

Is this sacculation really 'pseudo', that is, an incidental formation secondary to the bending back of the vein upon itself and only revealed when it is straightened, or, does the saccule form from a localized weakness and by its shape cause acute angulation of the vein? The latter seems probable and perhaps the author should have used the expression 'disguised' or 'concealed' sacculation.

The walls of these saccules become very thinned, fragile and often quite strongly adherent to their surroundings, especially the underside of the skin. This may be due to a reaction to degenerative changes in the wall of the pseudosaccule, which has lost its muscle layer and shows

fragmentation of collagen and elastic fibres. The neighbouring non-sacculated portion of vein may have a more normal structure and retain the ability to contract down. A saccule may collapse when empty but has little power to contract on its own and when disconnected from incompetent downflow is unable to return to normal so that it may persist ready to distend fully again if ever a new source of incompetence connects with it. The same is often true of an overstretched vein involved in the varicose process, valvular competence within it may never be regained and it remains a potential pathway of incompetence. This has an important bearing upon treatment because varicose veins not removed surgically or obliterated by sclerotherapy tend to persist and take any opportunity to renew incompetent downflow as 'recurrent' varicosities.

The changes of tortuosity and pseudosacculation may occur apparently in any vein that becomes part of a pattern of reversed, gravitational downflow. This may be in a regular branch vein or in a series of insignificant veins that have become linked to form a pathway of downward incompetence. Such small veins may enlarge into a tortuous, sacculated vessel, one centimetre or more across, with walls too fragile to dissect surgically; other varicosities, derived from more robust veins, are quite strong and easily handled at surgery but all are liable to break with unexpected ease. Varicosities not only tend to become adherent to the skin but eventually may cause the overlying skin to become so thin that it breaks with minor trauma and haemorrhage occurs.

The presence of reversed flow, against the natural direction, i.e. against the valves, is easily confirmed by the Doppler flowmeter and it is interesting to consider whether varicose veins occurring elsewhere in the body also indicate reverse flow. Clearly this is likely to be so in the enlarged superficial veins acting as collaterals past occluded deep veins such as the iliac (Figure 1.17) or

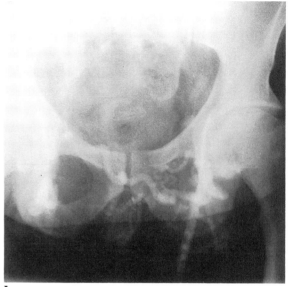

**b1**

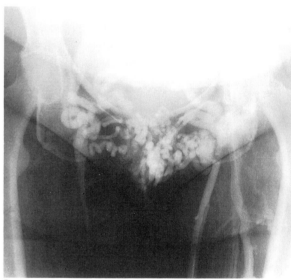

**b2**

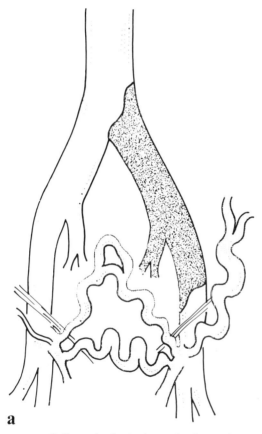

**a**

**Figure 1.17** *Collateral veins in deep vein obstruction.*

*(a) Diagram of left iliac occlusion and associated collateral veins; pubic and pelvic veins take flow to the opposite side. These veins show enlargement and tortuosity because they are being forced to accept reversed flow.*

*(b) 1. Phlebogram of left iliac and femoral vein occlusion due to thrombosis 5 years previously. Enlarged pubic veins take flow across to the right side. The left long saphenous vein is acting as a collateral and shows preferential upflow indicating that there is resistance to flow in the femoral vein.*
*2. Another patient with left iliac vein occlusion and extensive collateral flow crossing to the other side where the right long saphenous vein is incompetent and shows downflow (see also Chapter 5)*

axillary (Figure 1.18) veins, and the Doppler flowmeter readily confirms this. Again, oesophageal varicosities are likely to be the same phenomenon (Figure 1.19) and portal phlebography shows this to be so. Another striking example is the varicocele and here Doppler flowmetry shows heavy venous flow in the standing patient (Figure 1.20); phlebography through a catheter into the testicular vein confirms massive flow down, through the varicocele and out via cremasteric veins into pelvic veins (Figures 1.21, 1.22(a)) which are valved (Figure 1.22(b)) and are thus effective pumps able to set up the pressure difference necessary for flow. A corresponding state of ovarian vein incompetence (Figure 5.11(g)) can occur in women and is described in Chapter 5.

Varicose veins are due to more than a passive stretching of the veins by loss of protective valves. They are the result of a dynamic process and the response to the hydraulic force of turbulent (reversed) flow within them.

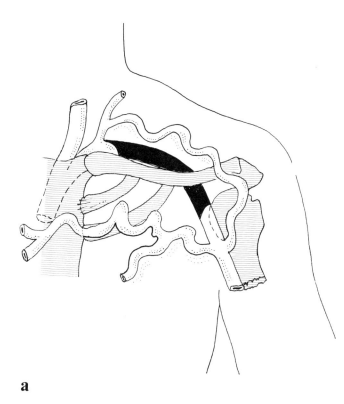

a

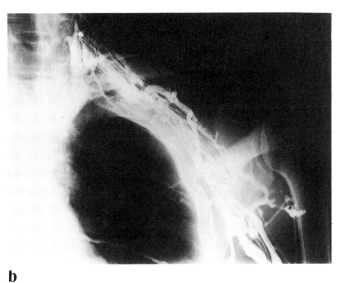

b

**Figure 1.18** *Collateral veins in axillosubclavian vein obstruction.*

*(a) Axillary vein occlusion with tortuous superficial veins on the front of the shoulder acting as collaterals.*

*(b) Phlebogram of collateral vein formation around left axillary vein occluded by thrombosis*

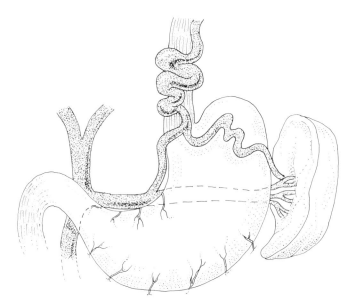

**Figure 1.19** *Oesophageal varicosities caused by reversed flow from veins of the portal system to oesophageal and thoracic veins*

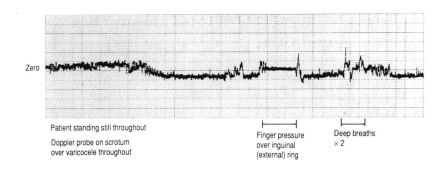

Zero

Patient standing still throughout

Doppler probe on scrotum over varicocele throughout

Finger pressure over inguinal (external) ring

Deep breaths ×2

**Figure 1.20** *Doppler flowmeter tracings showing substantial flow through a varicocele when the patient stands and accentuated by breathing. It is not possible to determine direction of flow because of the extreme tortuosity and coiling of the veins within the varicocele. For this reason the tracings show abrupt apparent changes in direction in flow due to slight movement of the probe (and see page 24)*

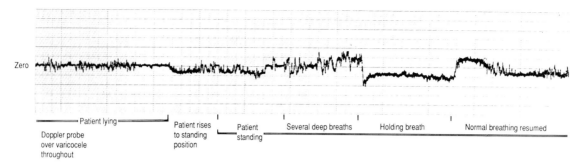

Zero

Patient lying

Doppler probe over varicocele throughout

Patient rises to standing position

Patient standing

Several deep breaths

Holding breath

Normal breathing resumed

**Figure 1.20** *(continued)*

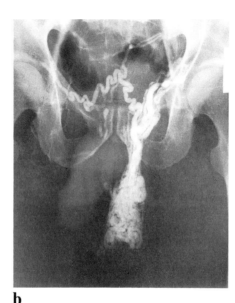

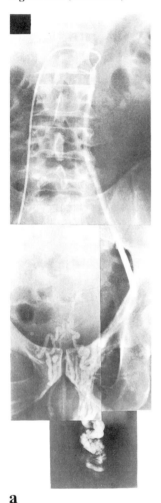

b

a

**Figure 1.21** *Flow pathways in a varicocele.*

*(a) Typical left varicocele outlined by transfemoral vein catheterization to upper end of left testicular vein, with patient tilted 45 degrees head upwards.*

*(b) The same varicocele outlined during surgical operation by direct cannulation of the testicular vein in the inguinal canal. Contrast flows without resistance through the varicocele and out by cremasteric vein to the external iliac vein and via pubic branches across to the opposite side*

In most circumstances tortuous or varicose veins denote reversed flow and this applies not only in the lower limb but wherever encountered in the body. This will often be in superficial veins acting as collaterals but only if they are being forced to accept flow counter to their natural direction. Collateral flow is not necessarily against the natural direction, for example, the upward collateral flow past deep vein occlusion in mid-thigh (Figure 1.23). Here the veins enlarge but seldom become tortuous; those that do can be shown to be part of a complex flow pattern and to have at least an intermittent component of reversed flow (see Chapter 10). Those collaterals, such as

pubic veins in iliac occlusion (Figures 1.7, 1.17(b)) or around axillary thrombosis, with heavy reversed flow, do become tortuous and this is considered further in Chapters 8 and 9. The guiding rule that *tortuous veins denote substantial reversed flow* is of importance in the recognition and understanding of venous disorders of the lower limbs and indeed elsewhere.

*Note:* Etymology of 'varix'. The words varices, varicose and varicosity are derived from the Latin word, *varix*, meaning a dilated vein, and probably taken from varus, meaning bent (some authorities give, a pimple or a

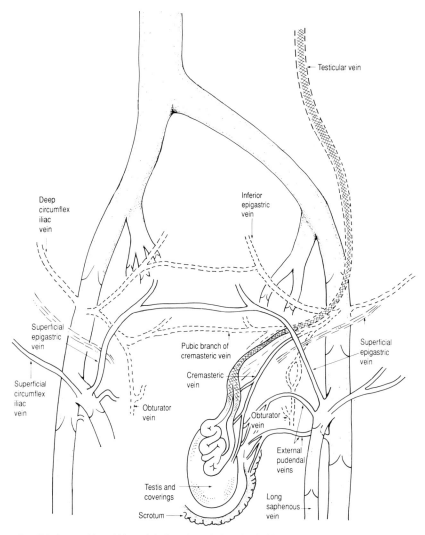

Deep circumflex iliac vein

Inferior epigastric vein

Testicular vein

Superficial epigastric vein

Superficial circumflex iliac vein

Pubic branch of cremasteric vein

Cremasteric vein

Superficial epigastric vein

Obturator vein

Obturator vein

External pudendal veins

Testis and coverings

Scrotum

Long saphenous vein

Note: Veins from vas deferens joining vesical veins, and scrotal to internal pudendal veins, are omitted. Almost any branch vein can anastomose with opposite side.

**a**

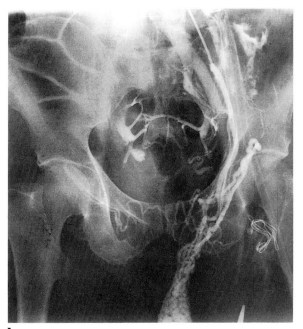

**b**

**Figure 1.22** *Creation of the pressure difference necessary for flow through a varicocele.*

*(a) Diagram of venous connections between the testicular veins and the pelvic veins.*

*(b) A peroperative phlebogram by direct cannulation in another example of varicocele to show easy flow into pelvic veins of both sides. Valves can be seen clearly in branches of the internal iliac veins. These valves create the pressure differential that causes flow down a valveless testicular vein and through its branches to areas of reduced pressure in the pelvic veins. This heavy reversed flow causes enlargement of testicular veins to form a varicocele*

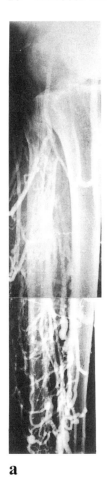

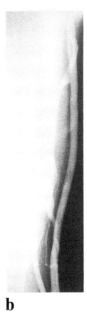

b

a

**Figure 1.23** *Post-thrombotic occlusion of popliteal and femoral veins.*

*(a) This phlebogram shows failure to fill the popliteal vein, with preferential upflow in the superficial veins which lead to the long saphenous vein.*

*(b) Separate view of long saphenous vein at the level of the knee and lower thigh showing strong preferential upflow in it because it is acting as a collateral. In spite of the heavy flow there is no suggestion of tortuosity in either the branches or the long saphenous vein because flow is in their natural direction (see also Figure 1.17(b)).*

*(c) Doppler flowmeter tracing from the same patient showing upward flow in the long saphenous vein accentuated by exercise.*

*(d) Photoplethysmographs in limited bilateral post-thrombotic occlusion (right side more marked) showing pressure changes near the ankle with exercise; patient sitting with legs down. The angle of descent is shallow compared with the excursion at each movement and the pressure rapidly reverts to full resting level within 10 seconds. Temporary occlusion of right superficial veins does not improve this abnormally rapid return to full pressure*

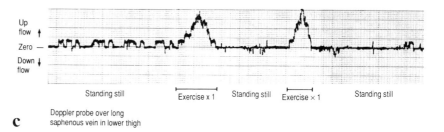

c

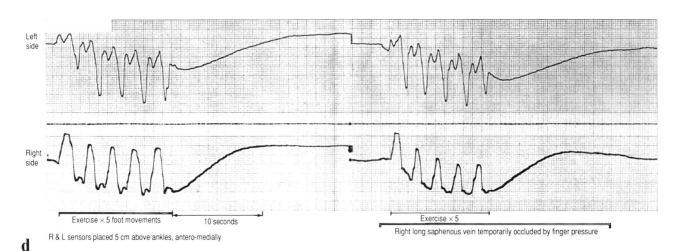

d

blotch), or less likely, vermis, that is, worm like . Medical dictionaries in defining varicose veins use such terms as dilated or enlarged and, in addition, knotted, tortuous or twisted. It is these latter terms that describe the most distinctive visible feature of a varicose vein, its tortuosity.

## Musculovenous pumping

### The normal venous pumping mechanism

Any pump, whether naturally occurring or man made, will require adequate ducts, effective valves and some form of compression. Thus, a venous pump unit consists of a vein with an adequate, undeformed lumen, at least one, but preferably two, effective valves, and intermittent compression of the vein provided by contraction of surrounding muscles. Numerous such units are spread through the lower limbs and referred to collectively as the musculovenous pump, but this term is often used to refer to the important complex of such units grouped within the calf muscles. The specialized pumping chambers, or sinuses, within muscles are referred to in more detail earlier in this chapter. Compression may be applied in other ways to give effective pumping, for example, body weight on the underside of the foot (Pegum and Fegan, 1967; Gardner and Fox, 1986, 1989) or squeezing the calf by hand pressure. Changes in posture will also give a 'pumping' effect, for example, if the limb is elevated and then put down again, the blood that has run centrally will be held there by the valves. However, muscular contraction is by far the most important means for promoting venous flow against the influence of gravity. Each muscle has its own set of units.

## Priming the pump

Immediately after any form of pumping the veins of the pumping mechanism become slack and the pressure minimal. In this state there is no resistance to blood re-entering to prime the pump once more (Figure 1.24),

normally by arterial inflow across the capillary beds or from neighbouring veins. If defective valves are present, reflux of blood previously pumped to a higher level will occur with a corresponding loss in effective action by the pump.

## The poor pumping capability of superficial veins

A distinction must be made between deep and superficial vein pumping capability. Superficial veins do not possess specific pumping chambers and, because they lie outside the deep fascia, are not surrounded by muscle so that without any regular compressing force their ability to pump is very weak in comparison to the deep veins. They are, nevertheless, well endowed with valves which are of course essential when the patient is upright to prevent spillage via them from deep veins to an area of slack veins below a pumping mechanism. This is in fact the essential failure that occurs in superficial vein incompetence (Figure 1.25) and will be referred to in detail in Chapter 4. The short saphenous vein for the upper part of its course shares a strong fascial compartment with muscles and is compressed when they contract so that an appreciable pumping action is set up within it. By contrast, the long saphenous vein lies outside the main fascial layers throughout its course and at most is ensheathed in a thin layer which may exert sufficient compression with movement of underlying muscles to give a weak pumping action; this is however a variable feature and usually most

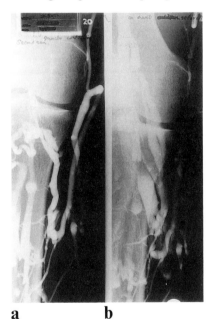

**a    b**

**Figure 1.24**  *Functional phlebograms of veins in calf region during and after contraction.*

*(a)  Taken whilst patient contracts calf muscle by rising on toes.*

*(b)  Picture taken immediately after relaxing down again. In the first picture no blood can be seen in the gastrocnemius or soleal sinuses but after relaxation these pumping chambers rapidly fill with opacified blood which appears to come, to a large extent, from the superficial veins which have now ceased to be visible*

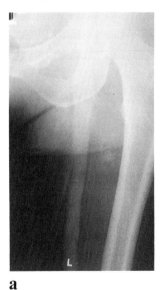 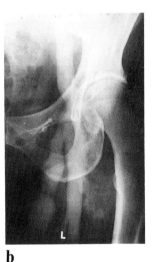

**a    b**

**Figure 1.25**  *Valve failure allowing gravitational retrograde flow in superficial veins and the essential cause of simple varicosities. Phlebogram of spillover from a common femoral vein and down the long saphenous vein following exercise.*

*(a)  Patient upright and standing still with passive outlining of the femoral vein.*

*(b)  After calf muscle contraction by rising on toes and relaxing down again, blood spills down the saphenous vein to low pressure areas created in lower leg and foot by exercise*

superficial veins, including the long saphenous, do not contribute to upward movement of blood in the upright position. A slow passive upward drift may occur in superficial and deep veins when the patient has been standing still for some minutes, not by any pumping, but as a result of all veins being filled to capacity by arterial inflow with a slow upward venous overflow.

## Problems caused by the upright position

It has already been pointed out that when the patient is horizontal, or especially if the limb is elevated above the horizontal, blood will run towards the heart in both superficial and deep veins without the need for a pumping mechanism, which brings us back to the thought that it is the upright position that causes problems. Of course, when upright, any form of external compression of the veins, superficial or deep, for example, squeezing with the hand, will cause upward flow and this includes pressure on the underside of the foot. The effect of pumping is not only to return blood towards the heart but also to cause an intermittent reduction in venous pressure peripherally;

by facilitating flow across the capillary bed this forestalls development of high intracapillary pressure and the accompanying excess exudate which in the long term causes the changes of venous hypertension (see Chapter 6).

## Reasons for inadequacy in venous pumping

There are two basic reasons for the musculovenous pumping mechanism proving inadequate so that venous hypertension, and ultimately ulceration, may occur: it may be overwhelmed by abnormal superficial downflow or it may fail to meet normal pumping requirements.

### Overwhelming the musculovenous pump

Blood may cascade down incompetent superficial veins in such large quantity that the main pumping mechanism is overwhelmed and venous pressure remains unrelieved in the upright and exercising state (Figure 1.26). This sustained pressure has similar undesirable consequences to failure of the musculovenous pump itself and this is considered further in Chapter 6.

### Failure of the musculovenous pump

A massive failure of the main pumping mechanism may arise after the deep veins and valves have been damaged by extensive thrombosis, or, because the patient has been born with too few, and perhaps insufficiently strong, valves in the deep veins. This can vary in severity but reduces the effectiveness of venous return against gravity

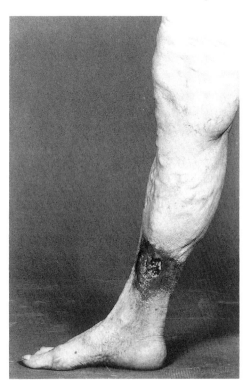

**a**

**Figure 1.26**  *Overwhelming of the musculovenous pump.*

*(a) Severe venotensive change, with ulceration caused by massive gravitational retrograde flow down long saphenous vein overwhelming the pumping mechanism when patient is upright.*

*(b) Photoplethysmograph tracing showing very little reduction in pressure and brief recovery time following exercise in sitting position. In the second tracing the long saphenous vein has been occluded by fingertip pressure only, in lower thigh. This has brought about a dramatic improvement in the ability of the pump to reduce venous pressure; there has been a full drop in venous pressure in response to exercise and this is maintained for 20 seconds. Surgical removal of the long saphenous vein gave a good result with rapid healing of the ulcer even though the patient remained up and about*

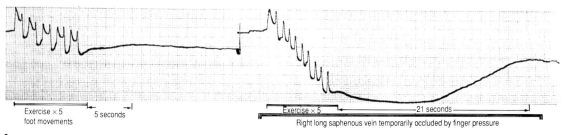

Exercise × 5 foot movements    5 seconds      Exercise × 5    21 seconds

Right long saphenous vein temporarily occluded by finger pressure

**b**

from the lower part of the limb in response to exercise so that pressure may remain high without relief (Figure 1.23(d)). The resulting venous hypertension eventually causes a series of changes, often called lipodermatosclerosis, and typified by oedema, fibrosis, pigmentation, eczema and ulceration. These disabling changes will be considered more fully in Chapters 7–9 and their treatment is a very important aspect of the surgeon's work with venous disorders. Although they may also arise from incompetence in the superficial veins the most severe forms come from failure in the deep vein pump and this emphasizes the essential role of the pumping mechanism.

## References

Basmajian, J. V. (1952) The distribution of valves in the femoral, external iliac and common iliac veins and their relationship to varicose veins. *Surgery, Gynecology and Obstetrics*, **95**, 537–542

Boileau Grant, J. C. (1947) *An Atlas of Anatomy*, Ballière, Tindall and Cox, London

Bourne, I. H. J. (1986) An investigation of the function of apparently flat and empty superficial veins observed in the leg of a patient undergoing treatment by vertical leg drainage. In *Phlebology 85* (eds D. Negus and G. Jantet), John Libbey, London, pp. 282–284

Dodd, H. and Cockett, F. B. (1976) *The Pathology and Surgery of the Veins of the Lower Limbs*, Churchill Livingstone, Edinburgh

Gardner, A. M. N. and Fox, R. H. (1986) The return of blood to the heart against the force of gravity. In *Phlebology 85* (eds D. Negus and G. Jantet), John Libbey, London, pp. 65–67

Gardner, A. M. N. and Fox, R. H. (1989) *The Return of Blood to the Heart: venous pumps in health and disease*, John Libbey, London

Glass, G. M. (1987) Neovascularization in recurrence of the varicose great saphenous vein following transection. *Phlebology*, **2**, 81–91

Holman, E. (1954a) The obscure physiology of poststenotic dilatation: its relation to the development of aneurysms. *Journal of Thoracic Surgery*, **28**, 109

Holman, E. (1954b) 'On circumscribed dilation of an artery immediately distal to a partially occluding band': poststenotic dilatation. *Surgery*, **36**, 3–24

Holman, E. and Peniston, W. (1955) Hydrodynamic factors in the production of aneurysms. *American Journal of Surgery*, **90**, 200–209 (and accompanying discussion by Longmire W.P. Jr)

Johnston, T. B. and Whillis, J. (eds) (1938) *Gray's Anatomy*, Longmans Green, London

Kistner, R. L. (1978) Transvenous repair of the incompent femoral valve. In *Venous Problems* (eds J. J. Bergan and J. S. T. Yan), Year Book Medical Publishers, Chicago

Lea Thomas, M. (1982) *Phlebography of the Lower Limb*, Churchill Livingstone, Edinburgh

May, R. (1979) *Surgery of the Veins and the Pelvis*, W. B. Saunders, Philadelphia; Georg Thieme, Stuttgart

Sharpey-Schafer, E. P. (1961) Venous tone. *British Medical Journal*, **2**, 1589–1595

Todd, A. S. (1959) The histological localisation of fibrinogen activator. *Journal of Pathology and Bacteriology*, **78**, 281

## Bibliography

Cheatle, T. R., McMullin, G. M. and Scurr, J. H. (1991) Deep vein reflux is reduced by compression of the foot venous plexus. *Phlebology*, **6**, 75–77

Cockett, F. B. (1991) Venous valves: history up to the present day. *Phlebology*, **6**, 63–73

Daseler, E. H., Anson, B. J., Reimann, A. F. and Beaton, L. E. (1946) The saphenous tributaries and related structures in relation to the technique of high ligation. *Surgery, Gynecology and Obstetrics*, **82**, 53–63

Hamblin, T. J. (1990) Endothelins. *British Medical Journal*, **301**, 568

Holman, E. (1955) The development of arterial aneurysms. *Surgery, Gynecology and Obstetrics*, **100**, 599–611

Komori, K., Okadome, K. and Sugimachi, K. (1991) Endothelium-derived relaxing factor and vein grafts. *British Journal of Surgery*, **78**, 1027–1030

Laverick, M. D., McGivern, R. C., Crone, M. D. and Mollan, R. A. B. (1990) A comparison of the effects of electrical calf muscle stimulation and the venous foot pump on venous blood flow in the lower leg. *Phlebology*, **5**, 285–290

Pegum, J. M. and Fegan, W. G. (1967) Physiology of venous return from the foot. *Cardiovascular Research*, **1**, 249

# 2

# Recognizing the abnormal: clinical examination and the special tests

The borderline between the normal and the abnormal is often vague and there is considerable overlap between the two. Normality is not easy to define because many aspects are instinctively recognized and it is perhaps more helpful to state those features which may deceive both patient and doctor, either to cause unnecessary alarm, or, to underrate a significant abnormality.

## Judging the normal

### Variation with individual build

Normal veins should not be unduly prominent but there is no standard for this. In the very thin patient, veins will inevitably show clearly and may cause worry just because they appear to stand out more than in other people. In addition, some people do have very much larger veins than average which, if not concealed in subcutaneous fat, may appear unnaturally large. Not infrequently, assurance of normality has to be given to such patients but, if the physician is uncertain, it is easy enough to examine these large veins for positive evidence of abnormality by such tests as Trendelenburg's or by use of the Doppler flowmeter and photoplethysmograph.

The reverse may happen and grossly abnormal veins, especially varicosities, may be underrated in the obese patient where the size and extent of the veins is almost completely masked by surrounding fat so that only the 'tip of the iceberg' shows. This pitfall is very real if inspection alone is relied upon and it is only by palpation and the tapwave test that the true state can be recognized; these are skills that must be developed by anyone seriously interested in venous problems.

### Variation in the same individual

A number of factors may cause variation over a short interval in the same patient. Assessing the veins when the patient has taken the morning off for the consultation and arrives fresh and rested, perhaps on a cold day and midway between menstrual periods, is certain to minimize any defects, much to the chagrin of the patient who knows just how bad the veins can be. Certainly veins tire with prolonged standing so that as the day wears on they yield to the venous pressure and enlarge progressively; with a night's rest they recover and may be disarmingly inconspicuous and, indeed, leaking valves may have temporarily recovered good function. This is not a rare phenomenon and every surgeon knows the discomfiture of finding that the varicose veins of a patient in hospital for surgery have almost disappeared and can scarcely be identified for preoperative marking! The superficial veins are very susceptible to temperature and hormones. Thus a hot bath causes maximal dilatation, as the patient sees in the mirror, and so will hot weather or heavy physical exertion; conversely cold may contract the veins to the point of disappearance. Apprehension is another factor causing constriction of subcutaneous veins which may make venepuncture unexpectedly difficult and indeed may herald an impending faint when sclerotherapy is being carried out. Hormonal influence just before menstruation has a considerable effect in maximizing veins and, of course, pregnancy has a profound effect in relaxing veins, added to by the haemodynamic effects of the pregnant uterus.

## The patient's outlook

The physician will inevitably be influenced by the patient's own appraisal which may underrate or overrate the importance of venous changes. The patient may fail to heed or understand the significance and deterioration typical of venous disorder and may need strong persuasion to take effective action to prevent a steady decline into venotensive changes and ulceration. In contrast, many patients are worried most by the cosmestic aspects and a small defect may be greatly exaggerated in their minds and centered upon some feature which is within the accepted range of normality, such as venules on the thigh in middle age, or a mild tendency to acrocyanosis.

Thus various factors conspire to deceive the doctor into underrating or, less often, overrating the patient's complaint. The direct question 'Am I seeing your veins at their worst?' will often give guidance whether the patient should be given a further examination some other time in the hope of catching the veins at their most obvious.

## Recognizing and assessing the abnormal

Here we are seeking positive evidence of the abnormal. There is no better device for this purpose than the clinical examiner's own sensory skills and ability to interpret the physical signs that have been elicited; at times special instruments will be needed to gather additional information but often a good clinical examination is sufficient to produce the right answer. The background of the patient's general health, including the medical history and any current medication, is clearly of importance but it would be tedious to consider all the possibilities here and only those strictly of relevance will be referred to.

### Clinical history

The patient's actual reasons for seeking advice must be clearly elicited. Many patients are diffident because it is the appearance that worries them and will need drawing out upon accompanying symptoms such as discomfort or skin irritation. All patients with a possible venous disorder should be asked about circumstances which may have been associated with deep vein thrombosis in the past. For example, was pregnancy ever associated with a 'white leg of pregnancy', have they suffered an accident leading to a major fracture or ever had a prolonged illness? Have they at any time had severe swelling of a limb or have they ever been on long-term anticoagulants? This sort of question may reveal strong evidence of iliac or femoral vein thrombosis many years before, often regarded as of no relevance by the patient. Because disfiguring varicosities are present, even on the opposite side, these may well be blamed for discomfort that is most unlikely to arise from the veins, and to treat them without understanding the true origin of the symptoms would be most unwise. For instance, intermittent claudication due to arterial disease is quite often at first attributed to the obvious defect of large varicose veins; pain referred from the spine, arthritis in hip or knee and even gross neurological disorder may be overlooked by too ready an acceptance of ugly but relatively harmless varicose veins as the cause for pain or disability. If the symptoms are not in keeping with the veins then careful thought must be given to a more likely origin and, at least, the patient must be warned that treating the veins may not relieve the discomfort complained of. Some of the reasons for seeking advice in the presence of a venous disorder are:

1. Unsightly appearance.
2. Tired or heavy leg(s) at the end of the day; restless limbs.
3. Nocturnal cramps.
4. Discomfort, which may be severe, in the vicinity of enlarged veins; it is usually more marked as menstruation approaches.
5. Fear of future deterioration in moderate varicose veins.
6. Fear of having inherited the 'same veins' suffered by an elderly parent.
7. Skin irritation or active eczema.
8. Skin changes with threatened or actual ulceration, which may be painful.
9. Fear of, or actual, haemorrhage.
10. Phlebitis, as a single or recurring episode.
11. Swelling of the limb.

The patient may not have realized that skin changes are the direct result of the venous state and may even be surprised when asked to expose both limbs fully. Nevertheless this must be insisted upon for the veins usually speak eloquently for themselves when uncovered and if there is any hint of a previous deep vein thrombosis then at some stage the examination must include inspection of the groin and lower abdomen in the standing position to look for tell-tale varicosities at that level (see Chapters 8–10).

### Physical examination

The patient must be examined in the position in which problems of venous return arise, that is to say, upright. Even when the venous condition is not bilateral, comparison between the two sides is always necessary as an obvious difference between them may well be the best evidence of abnormality. The effect of exercise (i.e. activating the musculovenous pump) must be observed in various ways during the examination. Good lighting is essential and the use of an additional artificial source to give oblique illumination is most valuable to accentuate by 'shadowing' any small prominences.

#### Inspection

This must cover from foot to groin (and often the pubes and lower abdomen). The features to be looked for are:

1. Undue prominence and changes in the overall pattern of the superficial veins.
2. Tortuosity of veins (varicose veins), so often caused by gravitational, reversed downflow.
3. Saccule formation usually showing as an isolated, rounded bulge on the inner thigh (often best detected

by touch) and signifying an ineffective valve in the saphenous vein with downflow through it.

4. Skin changes, particularly pigmentation, eczema and ulceration. These may be the result of venous hypertension (stasis) caused by a defective musculo-pump or massive downflow in incompetent superficial veins, or both.

5. Venous flares, showing as obvious blue-black venules branching in the skin, especially near the ankle and inner side of the foot, and denoting overstressed superficial veins, often with venous hypertension. Intradermal venules at higher levels may signify underlying incompetent superficial veins or be the 'spider' or 'thread' veins which appear in the middle years of life (see Chapters 4 and 19).

6. Swelling may well have a venous origin, particularly if unilateral, but this should not be too readily assumed and causes such as infection, lymphoedema, hanging leg out of bed to relieve ischaemic rest pain (see Chapter 17), or, when both limbs are affected, a generalized oedema due to heart or renal disease must be considered.

*Palpation*

This is an important aspect of the examination because palpation and associated tests can detect some of the best clues in the diagnosis of the underlying state. Running the fingers gently across the skin is a good way of detecting enlarged veins concealed in subcutaneous fat, or in conditions of poor light, or on the far side of the limb; the prominence of the veins under the fingers is also the most sensitive way of gauging changes in their tension before and after the performance of the exercise tests. The following signs may be elicited:

1. Tortuosity and sacculation in the unseen vein is often detectable by touch; it denotes reversed flow down these veins.

2. Warmth over a vein in comparison with neighbouring skin, and indicating active flow through the vein of blood at true body temperature; this usually signifies abnormal reversed flow from deep to superficial veins due to incompetent superficial valves.

3. Cough impulse at any level indicates that no effective valve is present between the abdomen and the examining fingers.

4. Thrill, on first standing, on exercising or on coughing represents turbulence caused by a jet of blood coming through a leaking valve; any saccule may give this sign because they so often lie below an incompetent valve and the best example of this is the saphena varix. However, it is not uncommon for a leaking valve to produce a thrill without a saccule being present. This will be loudly heard through a stethoscope.

5. Changed texture of tissue, especially near the ankle, which may feel thickened and firm, indicating underlying fibrosis as part of the manifestations of venous hypertension (stasis).

6. Pitting oedema, which may or may not be due to venous abnormality.

7. Venous hollows and grooves when the veins are emptied by high elevation of the limb above the hori-

Included with palpation are two special procedures essential to correct diagnosis:

**I. Mapping out the superficial veins by tapwave** (Chevrier's or Schwartz's test) An elastic tube filled with fluid under slight tension will readily transmit a wave along its length if it is sharply compressed or tapped. This can only be properly applied to veins in a patient who has been standing still for at least 30 seconds to ensure that the veins are well filled with a continuous column of blood (Figure 2.1(a)). If the fingers of one hand tap or compress sharply over the vein, the other hand can detect the tapwave travelling along the vein at some distance and this gives a very characteristic signal to the receiving fingers (Figure 2.1(b)). This is an important skill to acquire because not only does it allow continuity of the veins to be mapped out but veins not otherwise detectable can be located and traced along their course. In this fashion interconnection of varicosities can be shown and whether they connect with either long or short saphenous veins, or, the presence of an enlarged but concealed saphenous vein detected; failure to detect this is perhaps the most common fault in everyday examination of veins. In the obese patient the method can act as a very impressive 'radar'.

Transmission of a tapwave does not, of course, necessarily indicate that the vein is abnormal; indeed, this test has long been used by arterial surgeons to confirm the presence of a satisfactory saphenous vein for use as an arterial substitute. However, the quality of the tapwave received usually gives a clear impression of the size of the underlying vessel and whether it is unnaturally enlarged and therefore likely to be abnormal. The larger the vein the more obvious the response but this depends on the site and method of generating the tapwave and, as regards method, a sharp compression is much more effective in a very large vein than a tap with the fingers, and vice versa.

This test should be strictly confined to the detection and mapping out of veins as it is not a satisfactory indicator of valve function. It may be used in either upward or downward directions but, certainly, a tapwave, in the standing patient, travelling upwards in the natural direction of flow cannot give any information upon the valves; a tapwave travelling downwards, against the valves, may be suppressed by their presence and this may have some significance but, apart from this, it does not give a reliable indication of their state. Strong transmission against the valves does not indicate with any certainty that they are incompetent because in a vein, well filled by standing for

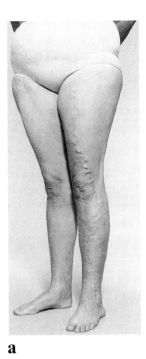 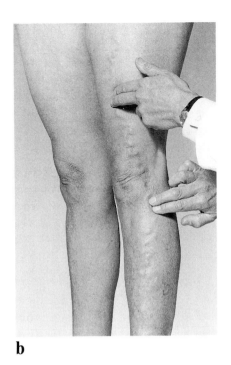

**a**       **b**

**Figure 2.1** *Mapping out veins by the tapwave technique.*

*(a) The patient stands still for 30 seconds so that the veins to be examined are well filled throughout the limb. In the patient illustrated, a varicosity winds its way from the upper thigh down to the foot.*

*(b) Here a tapwave is being sent from just below the knee to mid-thigh. The tapwave is generated by, either, a light tap with two fingers, or, if the vein is large, a sharp compression. The fingers of the upper hand are lightly placed over the vein to detect the characteristic sensation of a tapwave travelling along it. This can be used to locate a vein that is not visible or palpable. It also demonstrates that there is continuity in the vein between these two points. The direction of signal can be reversed if the upper hand sets up the tapwave and is received by the lower hand, but it is more difficult to do this against the soft background of the thigh as compared with the firm upper leg. The process may be continued up and down the vein to give a complete understanding of its course and connections. This method is not reliable in judging the competence of valves, which must be assessed by other means*

30 seconds, the valve cusps may all be fully opened by the slow upward drift of blood and, therefore, fail to interrupt a downward-travelling tapwave.

The process of mapping out is an essential preliminary and it is valuable to put a few ink marks along the line of the principal veins to help in carrying out the next step, which is the all-important selective occlusion (Trendelenburg) test.

**II. Selective superficial vein occlusion (Trendelenburg) test – the KEY TEST** This test is the key that will reliably distinguish between the commonplace, curable state of simple superficial vein incompetence and the difficult deep vein problem that will not respond to surgery and indeed may be made worse by it. A surgeon is most unwise to remove a saphenous vein unless satisfactory control of varicosities with the selective occlusion (Trendelenburg) test is obtained. This not only proves the diagnosis of superficial vein incompetence, but also confirms accurate identification of the pathway of incompetence upon which the operation should be based. Failure to control enlarged veins points strongly towards either incorrect indentification of a pathway of simple incompetence, or that this is not the correct diagnosis; in both cases further investigation is required before any decision for surgery is made.

The test depends upon the temporary occlusion of a superficial vein suspected of incompetence in order to demonstrate that, by preventing downflow in it when the patient first stands, the varicosities arising from it do not fill. Using a rubber tourniquet is not a satisfactory method of occlusion. It is not easy to apply at a pressure that will occlude the superficial veins without affecting the deep veins (Figure 2.2). Thus it may either fail to control the surface veins or it will congest the deep veins

and in both cases will give a false-negative result; if put on excessively tightly it can shut off both superficial and deep veins and conceal a state of massive incompetence in the deep veins. A carefully applied, narrow width pneumatic tourniquet might meet these criticisms but still fails in another important respect because it does not selectively compress a suspected pathway of incompetence in the way that fingers can. Our recommendation is that the veins are mapped out and marked so that the selective occlusion test can be performed with one or more fingers, or a thumb, accurately applied over the suspected pathway of incompetence. If two pathways are

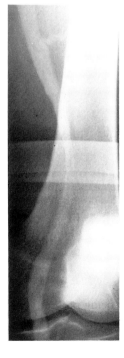

**Figure 2.2** *A venous 'tourniquet' should not be used in any of the clinical tests because it is likely to compress the deep veins and give misleading results. In this phlebogram a rubber band has been applied to the lower thigh with no more pressure than was considered necessary to occlude the long saphenous vein but, as can be seen, the underlying deep vein is displaced and narrowed. The use of fingers to give selective compression over a likely pathway of incompetence, mapped out by tapwave, does not have this disadvantage and is more informative because it confirms the location of the vein at fault*

suspected it is usually possible to compress each in turn and then both together.

The selective superficial vein occlusion (Trendelenburg) test is performed in the following way:

1. With the patient laid flat on a couch the limb is elevated to empty the veins (Figures 2.3(a), 2.4(a)).
2. The fingers are placed over the suspected pathway of incompetence and maintained firmly in place whilst the patient stands (this manoeuvre requires practice) (Figures 2.3(a),(b), 2.4(b),(c)).

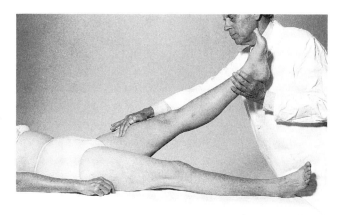

a

**Figure 2.3** *Selective superficial vein occlusion (Trendelenburg) test. Perthes' test.*

*(a) With the patient horizontal, the limb to be examined is elevated to empty the veins and two fingers placed over the suspected pathway of incompetence, that is, the upper part of the varicose vein shown in Figure 2.1.*

*(b) The patient now stands whilst pressure is maintained over the vein. The varicosities are watched for 10–15 seconds and in the illustration there has been no filling of the varicose vein which is only evident as grooving in the subcutaneous fat.*

*(c) Control of the vein is now released. Within 2 or 3 seconds a wave of distension travels down the length of the limb and the varicose vein fills completely.*

*(d)–(f) Selective occlusion (Trendelenburg) test with exercise carried out whilst the varicose vein is controlled by finger compression.*

*(d) The varicosities are well controlled in the standing patient.*

*(e) The patient exercises three times by rising up on the toes; barely detectable filling has occurred and the veins remain essentially collapsed; venous grooving is still present and would be easily recognizable by palpation with the examiner's left hand.*

*(f) Ten seconds later control of the varicosity is released and within 3 seconds the varicose vein fills throughout its length. This test has demonstrated that exercise causes no appreciable outward pumping into the leg varicosities and that they fill only from the pathway of incompetence in the thigh (see page 35).*

*(g)–(i) Perthes' test to demonstrate emptying of varicose veins when the pathway of incompetence is temporarily blocked in its upper part and exercise carried out (see page 35).*

*(g) The patient stands still for 30 seconds so that the varicose vein fills throughout its length. Finger compression is then applied to its upper part.*

*(h) With compression maintained, the patient exercises three times by rising on the toes and down again, relaxing fully between each movement. In response to this the outline of the varicosities softens and the upper few inches can only be recognized as a venous groove; palpation by the examiner's left hand below this would find the varicosities to be less prominent and to have appreciably softened to the touch.*

*(i) The controlling fingers are now removed and the varicose vein promptly fills over its full length, its outline hardens as it tenses up again and on palpation it feels firm with full prominence restored. This test has demonstrated that when filling from above is prevented, the varicose vein is partially emptied by exercise, confirming that there is no outward pumping in the leg and the pathway of incompetence has been correctly identified*

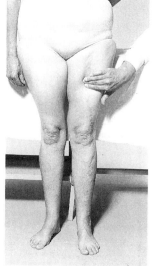
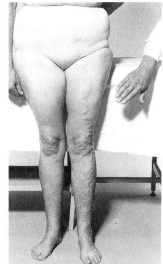

b      c

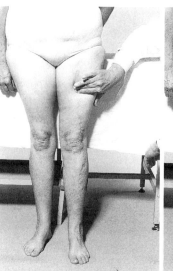
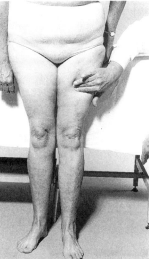

d      e

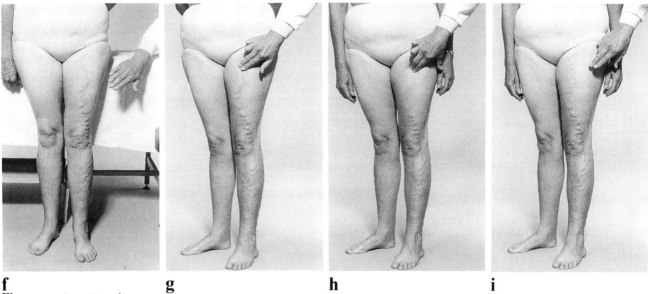

**f**          **g**                    **h**                    **i**

**Figure 2.3** *(continued)*

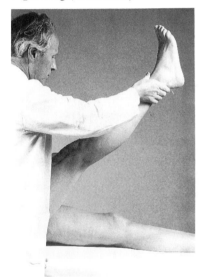

**a**

**Figure 2.4**    *A further example of selective occlusion (Trendelenburg) test.*

*(a) With the patient horizontal the limb is elevated and fingers placed over the suspected pathway of incompetence, in this case, the long saphenous vein.*

*(b) Whilst control over the vein is maintained the patient is asked to stand.*

*(c) There is no filling of the veins after 15 seconds. The right hand is used to give counter pressure and also to control a branch varicosity running across the knee.*

*(d) On release of control the leg varicosities fill within 1 or 2 seconds. The test is positive and incompetence in the long saphenous vein and its branches has been demonstrated*

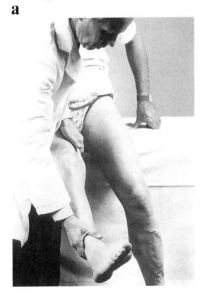

**b**

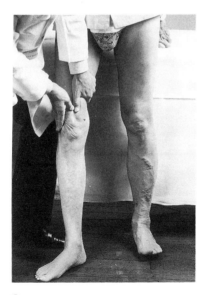

**c**

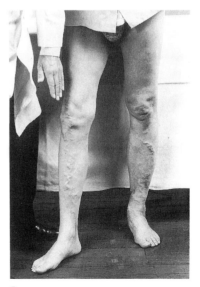

**d**

3. Observe the varicose veins and wait 15 seconds (Figures 2.3(b), 2.4(c), 2.5(a), 2.6(a), 2.7(a)). If there is no significant filling of the veins the fingers are released. Prompt filling of the veins from above confirms incompetence of valves in the superficial veins just released (Figures 2.3(c), 2.4(d), 2.5(b), 2.6(b), 2.7(b)). This can often be seen to ripple down the limb as a travelling wave of filling. The patient may be exercised before releasing the fingers to demonstrate that no outward pumping occurs and this gives very complete proof of filling of the varicose veins only from above (Figures 2.3(d),(e), 2.8(a)).

4. If the fingers fail to control filling of the veins then either the test is being incorrectly applied or there is a probability of deep vein problems and very careful further evaluation is needed.

*Note:* Localized pressure by fingers controlling, say, a saphenous vein identifies precisely the pathway of incompetence and is greatly to be preferred to the application of rubber tubes which may well disturb deep vein function and give false results.

Slow-filling varicosities may cause difficulties in interpretation. This may be inherent or be due to contraction of superficial veins because the patient is cold or apprehensive, or is a response to manipulation of the veins. This difficulty may appear as the examination proceeds so that veins which were well filled when first seen now stubbornly refuse to enlarge up again. If 10 seconds after release of the controlling fingers the varicose veins have not fully distended again the test cannot be regarded as valid. Slow-filling varicosities, whether this is their usual state or brought on by venous constriction, renders the test impractical. It can be repeated after a short interval, ensuring the patient is warm, and carefully timing the refilling times without and with control of the venous pathway. If the difference remains unconvincing then the test has to be abandoned and reliance put on examination with directional Doppler flowmetry (see later). Such veins usually tend to be small and can respond well to sclerotherapy.

**Perthes' test – a valuable backup** Although this further test is not always easy to be sure about, it often gives an undoubtedly positive result which is of great value in simple superficial incompetence in two ways: it confirms that the pathway of incompetence has been correctly identified and provides positive evidence that the deep vein pumping mechanism is working satisfactorily. It depends on the ability of musculovenous pumping to reduce deep and superficial venous pressure with exercise. The pressure in superficial veins, and hence their tension and prominence, closely follows that of the deep veins because of the rapid interchange of blood between them. Normally, superficial veins slacken in response to exercise but if excessive leakage down an incompetent superficial vein fills varicosities as quickly as they empty into deep

veins, then this will not happen. However, temporary blockage of the leaking vein, usually a saphenous vein, may briefly restore the normal response to exercise thus giving good evidence of its adverse influence. This complements the selective occlusion (Trendelenburg) test but does not replace it.

Perthes' test may be carried out as follows:

In the standing position, the patient exercises three times by rising on the toes and the varicosities are checked to confirm that this does not cause any detectable deflation in them. Leakage down superficial veins is then temporarily prevented by finger pressure over the suspected pathway of incompetence and the sequence of exercise repeated (Figure 2.3(g)–(i), 2.8(c)–(e)). If the varicose veins now partially deflate, this gives valuable confirmation of incompetence in the suspected vein and of a good musculovenous pump. Deflation is judged by visible and palpable changes in the varicosities. These may be seen to soften or reduce in outline, often with partial disappearance of the uppermost veins previously visible, and to harden up again on release of the compressing fingers (Figures 2.3(h),(i), 2.8(d),(e)). Palpable change depends on judging the tension in veins by touch, either by pressing gently upon it, or by stroking a finger across its surface to gauge its prominence, which varies according to the pressure within it; the latter is the more sensitive method of judging by touch whether or not deflation has occurred and this is all that is required. In effect, the elasticity of the vein walls is being used as a spring against which the pressure within is estimated. It must not be expected that varicose veins will collapse and virtually disappear; the change in them reflects an appreciable fall of venous pressure in the underlying deep veins but the residual pressure is usually sufficient to cause some persisting distension, moreover, varicose veins tend to lack the venous tone required for complete emptying in the upright position.

## Special examinations: the role of instruments and radiology

In the majority of patients a straightforward clinical examination, as outlined above, is sufficient to reach a diagnosis and to act upon it. Usually selective saphenous occlusion (Trendelenburg's test) provides the positive evidence for a decision but there is a sizeable minority of patients in whom the evidence is equivocal or it is clear that a real problem exists which requires more detailed investigation. The decision to tell a patient that there is no cure, and that only measures to limit the condition are available, is an important one and requires backing with all possible evidence. This can be provided by a variety of special investigations but the most practical ones available are: directional Doppler flowmetry; venous

**Figure 2.5**    *A further example of selective occlusion (Trendelenburg) test applied to incompetence in the left long saphenous vein.*

*(a) Control has been maintained for 15 seconds and the varicosities are not evident.*

*(b) On release of control, a wave of distension travels down the limb, an enlarged saphenous vein fills rapidly with large varicose veins appearing within 2 or 3 seconds*

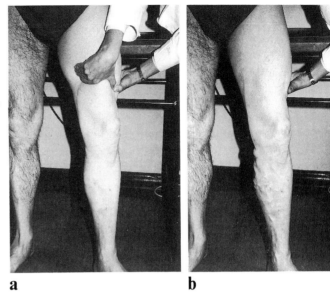

**a**          **b**

**Figure 2.6**    *Control of a massive thigh varicosity by selective occlusion (Trendelenburg) test. This varicosity arose from the anterolateral branch of the uppermost long saphenous vein and formed a pathway of incompetence bypassing a single competent valve in the upper part of the saphenous vein. In the lower thigh it re-entered the saphenous vein down which the incompetence continued to the leg.*

*(a) Selective occlusion, by finger compression over the upper part of the thigh varicose vein, demonstrates complete control of the varicosities in the thigh and leg.*

*(b) On release of control, the varicose veins in the thigh spring into prominence together with leg varicosities. Varicose veins bypassing a functioning saphenous valve in this fashion are not uncommon in the thigh (see Chapter 4)*

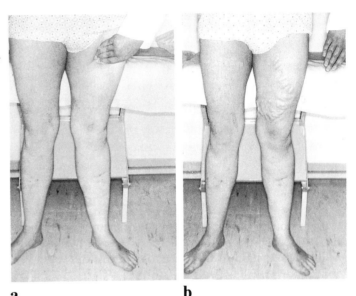

**a**          **b**

**Figure 2.7**    *Selective occlusion (Trendelenburg) test applied to the short saphenous vein.*

*(a)  Mapping out has shown a strong tapwave between calf varicosities and the short saphenous vein. The limb has been elevated to empty the veins and a finger compresses the short saphenous vein whilst the patient stands. After 15 seconds there is no sign of filling of the varicosities.*

*(b)  After release of short saphenous compression the calf varicosities rapidly distend with a wave of downward filling*

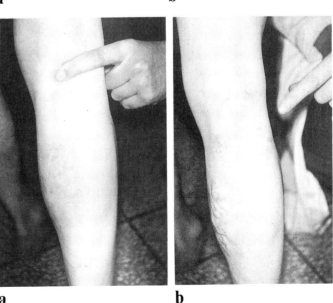

**a**          **b**

**Figure 2.8** *Exercise during selective occlusion (Trendelenburg), followed by Perthes' test, in a case of right long saphenous incompetence.*

*(a) Whilst compression of the long saphenous vein in the lower thigh is maintained the patient has been exercised three times by rising on the toes and it can be seen that this has caused only very slight filling of the varicosities in the leg.*

*(b) On release of control the varicosities rapidly fill. Filling comes from above and there is no evidence of outward pumping in the leg*

*(c) After the patient has been standing for 30 seconds the long saphenous vein is compressed by fingers in the lower thigh.*

*(d) Compression is maintained and after three exercise movements there is significant softening in the outline and feel of the varicosities; in this illustration the examiner's right hand can be freed to do this.*

*(e) On release of control, the varicosities' outline sharpens again and they become firm and prominent to the touch*

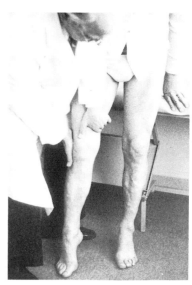

a

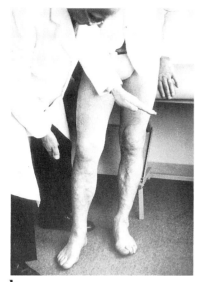

b

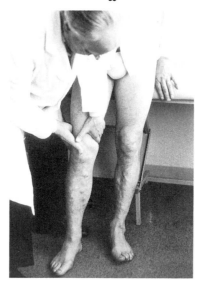

c

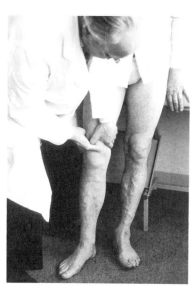

d

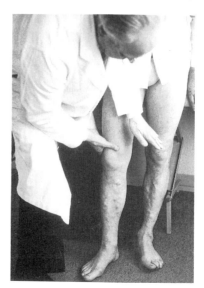

e

pressure and venous volume changes (plethysmography) with exercise or during maximal venous outflow; imaging by functional phlebography or ultrasonography. The role of these investigations will now be considered (see also Chapters 23 and 24).

### The directional Doppler flowmeter

The simplest and most informative use of the directional Doppler flowmeter is to apply it to the superficial veins (Figure 2.9). It is of course measuring the direction and velocity of flow but there is a great deal to be learnt from this. Flow will always be from an area of higher pressure to one of lower pressure and thus the direction and duration of a pressure gradient is indicated by the Doppler signal. Heavy downflow in a superficial vein after exercise indicates simple incompetence due to flow from above a pumping mechanism to below it (see Chapter 4) and incidentally gives indication of a functioning musculovenous pump. Conversely strong flow upwards in the superficial veins indicates the likelihood that these veins are acting as collaterals past deformed or obstructed deep veins. The great value of the Doppler flowmeter used in this way is that it can give rapid positive identification of either a simple superficial incompetence or, by contrast, deep vein impairment. The details of the technique in using this instrument are given in detail in Chapter 24 and the findings in the various disorders are clarified in the appropriate sections.

### Direct pressure measurement

This requires the insertion of a needle or cannula into a superficial vein of the foot where the pressure equalizes so quickly with the deep veins that it can be regarded as fully representative of them. Normally, with exercise in the upright position, the pressure drops by 50 mmHg and returns to the normal of about 110 mmHg after 25 seconds or more. In any form of extensive valve failure, either superficial or deep, not only is the fall in pressure much less but the recovery time to full standing pressure is much shorter. If the defect is in a superficial vein, temporary occlusion of this will bring about a clear lengthening, approaching normal, in the recovery time. This is diagnostically and prognostically of great value. Correspondingly, if failure of any manipulation of superficial veins fails to lengthen the recovery time it is likely that the fault lies in the deep rather than the superficial veins. However this method does require venepuncture and for this reason one of the non-invasive alternative methods is to be preferred.

### Indirect or non-invasive pressure estimation

There are various methods giving measurements that closely parallel the actual venous pressures and will accurately mirror the deep vein pressure changes, especially recovery time.

**Figure 2.9** *Using the directional Doppler flowmeter (Sonacaid BV.381).*

*(a),(b) A flat-headed probe is placed over an incompetent long saphenous vein in the lower thigh and the direction and velocity of flow recorded in response to various manipulations, including squeezing the calf, exercise by rising on the toes and repeating this whilst the saphenous vein above the probe is occluded by finger pressure, and raising the foot slightly off the couch with the knee straight. The response to these and various other manoeuvres in the different venous disorders are considered in the relevant chapters and in Chapter 24. The tracing from the patient in the photograph is shown; note the downflow responses typical of saphenous incompetence*

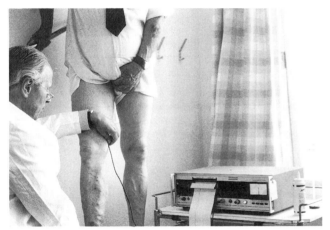

**a**

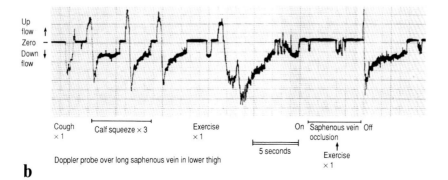

**b**

**Plethysmography, or measuring volume changes, in the foot and ankle region** The volume varies with venous distension which in its turn runs parallel with deep vein pressure. The displacement methods tend to be rather ponderous for everyday use but Nicolaides, Christopoulos and Vasdekis (1989) report satisfactory results using an air chamber made of polyvinyl chloride film and enclosing the leg up to the knee. For most purposes a strain gauge around the foot or leg gives a sufficiently accurate representation of the volume changes and is simple in use (see also Chapter 24).

**Photoplethysmography (PPG) (Figure 2.10)** The number of red cells lying in a portion of skin is photoelectrically estimated by this method. It is in effect estimating the degree of the congestion or distension of the skin capillary bed and this in its turn runs parallel with the venous pressure. In a way, the elasticity of the capillary bed is being used as a 'spring' against which venous pressure is being assessed. The method cannot measure true pressure as such and is limited to observing changes representing venous pressure and the time taken for these to occur, but it is quick and easy to use and certainly gives a reliable indication of recovery time of venous pressure following the drop caused by exercise. An improved response to exercise whilst a superficial vein in the thigh or calf is temporarily compressed will confirm gross superficial incompetence satisfactorily and predict the improvement in performance that is likely to follow surgical removal of these veins (see Chapter 24). It is a valuable adjunct that will readily identify a defective venous pumping mechanism (short recovery time) and, in cases of actual or threatened ulceration, give positive evidence (recovery time reverts to normal when the saphenous vein at fault is occluded) that simple saphenous vein incompetence is the cause. However, this method is not reliable in identifying the less severe venous disorders when recovery time is near normal and a negative result cannot be regarded as excluding superficial incompetence; the result is only of value when an improvement in recovery time of 5 seconds or more is obtained and is repeatable (see Chapter 24).

**Figure 2.10** *Use of the photoplethysmograph.*

*(a) The patient sits on a couch with the limbs completely relaxed and free from the floor. Probes are applied symmetrically over lower legs anteriorly. Infrared light emitted from a cold diode source in each probe is reflected back by the red cells in the underlying capillary bed to a photoelectric sensor and the signal is proportionate to the number of red cells present. It estimates the amount of filling in the capillaries which, in fact, run parallel with venous pressure in the leg so that any change in this is immediately apparent. The speed of recovery after a fall in venous pressure caused by exercise is recorded and then repeated with the saphenous vein occluded. In this way inadequacy of the venous pumping mechanism, and whether this is due to an incompetent saphenous vein, may be determined (see Chapter 4).*

*(b) Two photoplethysmograms from the same limb are shown. The upper one shows an abnormally brief recovery or refilling time of 6 seconds; in the lower tracing an incompetent saphenous vein has been temporarily occluded and the recovery time reverts to a full normal, well in excess of 20 seconds. This is typical of severe incompetence*

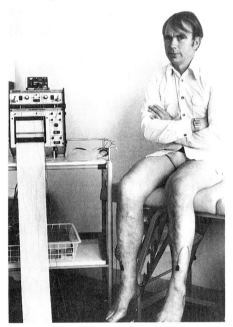

**a**

Without saphenous occlusion

6 seconds

Long saphenous vein occluded by finger pressure throughout

35 seconds

**b**

*Maximum venous outflow*

In this method the 'volume' of a limb is estimated by a strain gauge before and after deliberate venous congestion with a pneumatic cuff which is abruptly released. The rate of shrinkage of the limb 'volume' is slowed in states of deep vein obstruction and this non-invasive method can give clear recognition of this state (see also Chapter 24). However, in our own experience it may fail quite frequently to recognize the well-compensated deep vein obstruction and its use in a busy clinic is not encouraged; the other methods will have given warning of possible venous outlet problems with equal reliability and if more detailed information is required then it is best to turn to phlebography.

*Functional phlebography (venography) aided by image intensifier*

This method (Figure 2.11) studies the veins radiographically with the patient in the position where problems arise, that is, upright. No constricting bands or tubes should be used and the intention is to visualize the veins performing in as natural a manner as possible. The image intensifier runs up and down the leg observing the direction of flow, the outlines and the valve state of the deep veins; function can be gauged by exercising the patient by rising on the toes. Static films are exposed as required. This method can demonstrate long saphenous incompetence with flow *down* the varicosities, *in* through perforators and *up* the deep veins only to recycle, in part, down the long saphenous vein again (retrograde circuit).

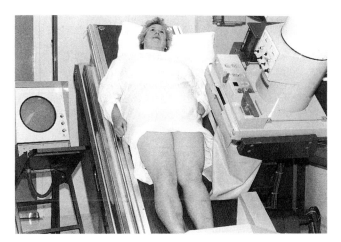

**Figure 2.11** *Functional phlebography being carried out. The patient is on a tilting X-ray table and a butterfly needle will be inserted into calf varicosities. The procedure is monitored by an image intensifier throughout and static films can be taken as desired. Most of the examination is carried out with the patient in a near vertical position, exercising as required. Artificial constriction by any form of tourniquet is avoided unless there is a specific reason. The intention is to study venous function, in an upright position, with the least possible disturbance to the usual pattern of events. This technique is described more fully in Chapter 22*

Alternatively it may show blood travelling preferentially up a long saphenous vein, which is acting as a collateral, past a deep vein deformed by an old thrombosis. By rapid change from vertical to horizontal and back again to outline valves (swill test), it may show all veins, superficial and deep, widely open but valveless. An occluded iliac vein will fail to fill and show tortuous pelvic collateral veins nearby. The procedure takes perhaps 25 minutes as an outpatient and does not unduly disturb the patient. The surgeon-investigator should be present to collaborate with the radiologist and in this way an accurate assessment of the pattern of disorder can be made. It is the nearest we have at the moment to a 'court of appeal' and very valuable when other methods leave doubts about the diagnosis and the role of surgery (see Chapter 22). Numerous studies by functional phlebography are used in the illustrations throughout this book.

*Ultrasonography*

Scanned, pulsed beam ultrasound can be used to give an image on a video display unit to show tissue interfaces and movement. It may be used to display structures in any desired plane from horizontal cross-cuts to longitudinal sections and show clear images of vein walls and valves, their movements and the direction and speed of blood flow within them. The latter can either be shown by special markers (Duplex) (Figure 2.12) or with the direction of flow represented by colour (Triplex or colour flow imaging – see Colour Plate 24). In this way the function of veins and the competence of valves, otherwise inaccessible, may be given prolonged and repeated study. Anatomy of importance to the surgeon, such as the short saphenous termination, can be displayed without recourse to phlebography. Blood clot in deep veins is easily recognized by altered flow and immobile walls. It is ideal for close scrutiny of a limited area of vein but not very suitable for more widespread display but it can be used to study venous function within a limb by measuring flow volumes in key veins such as the popliteal vein. However, it is capable of considerable further development and may increasingly displace phlebography (see Chapters 22 and 23).

**Bibliography**

Bergan, J. J. and Yao, J. S. T. (1991) *Venous Disorders*, Saunders, Philadelphia

Coleridge Smith, P. (1990) Noninvasive venous investigation. *Vascular Medicine Review*, **1**, 139–166

McMullin, G. M., Coleridge Smith, P. D. and Scurr, J. H. (1991) A study of tourniquets in the investigation of venous insufficiency. *Phlebology*, **6**, 133–139

Nicolaides, A., Christopoulos, D. and Vasdekis, S. (1989) Progress in the investigation of chronic venous insufficiency. *Annals of Surgery*, **3**, 278–292.

Nicolaides, A. N. and Sumner, D. S. (1991) *Investigation of Patients with Deep Vein Thrombosis and Chronic Venous Insufficiency*, Med-Orion Publishing Co, London

Scott, H. J., Coleridge Smith, P. D., McMullin, G. M. and Scurr, J. H. (1990) Venous disease: investigation and treatment, fact or fiction? *Annals of the Royal College of Surgeons of England*, **72**, 188–192

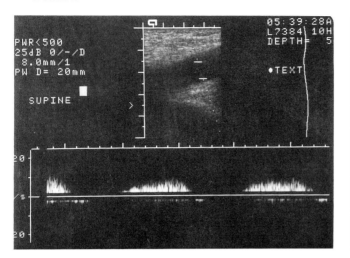

**a**

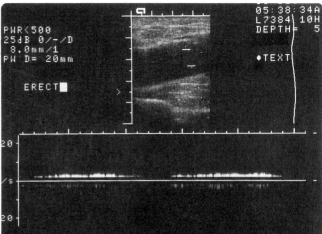

**b**

**Figure 2.12**   *Imaging of a vein and measurement of flow velocity by duplex ultrasonography. Two frames are shown from a pulsed, ultrasound scanner using a phased array of transducers (Acuson 128) with a pulsed beam Doppler velocimetry facility. This has no moving parts and gives a rectangular image, unlike the other form of scanner, the rotating beam, which gives a wedge-shaped image. Structures lying beneath the probe are shown on the screen alongside a vertical scale giving the depth from skin surface in 0.5 cm divisions. Where flow in blood vessels is to be studied, a gate of variable width, indicated by two parallel cursors, may be positioned within the vessel and set to define the width to be sampled; the angle of the Doppler ultrasonic beam is shown by an interrupted line. The direction and speed of flow are shown in the lower part of the frame; vertical graticules represent velocity in centimetres per second, a time scale runs horizontally in seconds; signals above the base line indicate flow away from the probe and, below the baseline, towards the probe; when both are present simultaneously this indicates turbulence or poor positioning of the probe.*

*(a) Right common femoral vein with patient supine without movement. The vein outline is clear and the Doppler signal shows intermittent flow away from the probe (towards the heart), in*

*phase with respiration; a maximum velocity of flow of 8 cm per second is reached and there is no significant downflow. The gate measuring flow has been adjusted across the vein lumen at 8.0 mm width, with its centre 20 mm deep and the mean velocity of flow is taken from within this gate.*

*(b) The same vein with the patient in the erect posture without movement and the instrument settings unchanged. As might be expected the vein width has increased by over 25% and this increased capacity has reduced the velocity of flow to 4 cm per second (cross-sectional area has been doubled and therefore the same volume of flow is conducted at half the speed).*

*These pictures were obtained during examination for suspected deep vein thrombus. Phasic flow was recorded wherever sampled in the vein lumen and this, together with the easy distension of the vein, gave clear indication that thrombus was not present. Used in similar fashion, colour coded scanning (see Colour Plate 24), showing flow across the full width of vein with great clarity, and easy compressibility on external pressure, is even more effective in giving rapid recognition of the vein state. (By courtesy of Dr D. R. M. Lindsell, John Radcliffe Hospital, Oxford)*

# 3

# The patterns of abnormality: an overall view

In this chapter an overall view of the main venous disorders is given to put the basic patterns of abnormality into perspective. The groups described are based on the findings over 10 years in approximately 900 patients seen in a vein clinic (Radcliffe Infirmary and John Radcliffe Hospital, Oxford, UK) and investigated by the methods referred to in this book. Aspects of this have been published previously (Tibbs and Fletcher, 1983) and the simple classification of the basic disorders used then has continued to serve well. The percentage proportions given for each group are only an approximation since it is difficult to avoid an element of selection, but they give a reasonable indication of the frequency of occurrence to be expected.

## The retrograde circuit of superficial vein incompetence: simple or primary varicose veins

This is by far the largest group containing over 80% of new patients attending the vein clinic. It includes most varicose veins and the complications arising from them, and is a major cause for venous hypertension and venous ulceration. The essential characteristic is lack of effective

valves in a chain of superficial veins so that reversed flow is possible and this allows a retrograde circuit of gravitational downflow to occur on exercise in the upright position (Figure 3.1). This circuit has four components:

- *The source,* through which blood spills over from a deep vein at high level into superficial veins (commonly the upper end of a saphenous vein).
- *The pathway of incompetence* in the superficial veins, down which the blood falls (usually a saphenous vein and its branches).
- *The re-entry points through* which the blood flows back into deep veins at low level (one or more perforating veins), beneath a pumping mechanism.
- *The return pathway* (formed by the deep veins and the musculovenous pumping mechanism) returns the blood to its starting point where some may be recycled downwards once more.

Two forces drive this circuit; gravity causes superficial downflow and musculovenous pumping creates upflow in the deep veins. On rising from horizontal to vertical posture, a single episode of downflow occurs by gravitational downflow into empty veins at low level, but

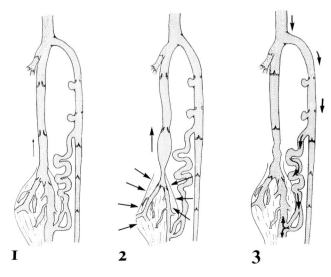

**I**       **2**       **3**

**Figure 3.1** *Simple (or primary) incompetence in superficial veins. After muscle contraction has partially emptied the deep veins at low level, blood spills over from deep veins at a higher level to fall down incompetent superficial veins to enter the deep veins just emptied, setting up a retrograde circuit of superficial incompetence; this is only operative when the patient is upright and moving. It is the turbulent reversed downflow that causes varicosis in the branch veins. A typical long saphenous incompetence with varicose veins is illustrated; the saphenous veins are not always involved and other veins may act as source or pathway of incompetence.*
*1. Standing still*
*2. On contraction of leg muscles*
*3. Immediately after muscle contraction*

the circuit is only fully activated by the musculovenous pumps. Thus, in the upright position, on muscular contraction blood is pumped upwards and causes the deep veins at low level to become slack, giving opportunity for superficial downflow to enter them through perforating veins. With the next contraction this blood is pumped up the deep veins, so making room for further superficial flow to enter when the muscle relaxes again; as the downflow occurs more blood spills over from the source to replenish the pathway of incompetence from the deep veins at high level. This process is endlessly repeated as the patient walks, with continuous turbulent flow down the superficial pathway of incompetence. Gravitational downflow to the foot may also occur when it is first raised off the ground and this is an important factor in patients with varicose veins running to the foot; this and other subtleties of the retrograde circuit are discussed in Chapter 4.

This retrograde circuit is undesirable and has two main effects:

1. The reverse flow causes the superficial veins to become tortuous, that is, to form varicose veins, and it is a continuing process with progressive enlargement over the years; there is a great variety in the detail and pattern of this.
2. If the volume of downflow is sufficiently large it can overwhelm the deep vein pumping mechanism and create venous hypertension; about 45% of new patients attending a clinic with venotensive changes and ulceration are suffering from this.

This is the essential phenomenon behind commonplace varicose veins and is described in more detail in Chapters 4 and 5; the varicose veins are the most obvious clinical expression of this abnormal state of flow. Diagnosis depends on demonstrating the downflow in the incompetent veins that follows rising from a horizontal to a vertical position or, when upright, on exercise or raising the foot off the ground. This downflow is shown by the clinical tests, use of a directional Doppler flowmeter or, if necessary, by other supporting investigations referred to in Chapter 2.

In a significant proportion of this group phlebography reveals a marked deficiency in valves in both the superficial and deep veins. This probably reflects an inborn variation in the number and quality of valves, and also in the robustness of the vein walls which support the cusps. Inherited deficiency in the strength and number of valves is probably a determining factor in the occurrence of valvular incompetence in both superficial and deep veins, and may well account for differences found in the capability of the pumping mechanisms of patients. There appears to be a spectrum of valve deficiency, at one end affecting only the superficial veins, but along the spectrum the deep veins increasingly share in this so that at the far end there is a gross overall deficiency in both superficial and deep vein valves; corresponding with this is an increasing likelihood of venotensive change and ulceration. Towards the far end, the spectrum merges with the most extreme category, the valveless syndrome, described below.

## Note upon perforators in superficial vein incompetence

In simple superficial vein incompetence, the perforating veins are not usually primarily at fault and, although an essential part of a retrograde circuit, flow through them is inwards, in the natural direction allowed by their valves. They are playing their normal role, although greatly exaggerated by the unimpeded downflow from the superficial veins. The perforators here are incidentally involved but in some patients they enlarge considerably and allow a component of perforator outflow so that there is a surge, first outwards on muscle contraction and then, on relaxation, predominantly inwards as the superficial veins empty downwards into the now slack deep veins (see Chapter 11). Usually the outward surge is not of great significance but at the far end of the spectrum of severity referred to above it can become an important factor to be taken into account during surgery; it is a constant feature of the valveless syndrome.

## Valveless syndrome

This small group (8%) appears to be an extension of the previous group and indeed there is a broad band of patients who could be placed in either group. These patients are characterized by severe venous stasis without any history of preceding deep vein thrombosis. Phlebography shows the deep veins to be widely open, undeformed (i.e. no suggestion of previous thrombosis) and with few, if any, normal valves in the principal deep and superficial veins. All veins tend to be oversized and in some patients may be massive as though there is an inherent weakness in the vein walls. There is much reason to believe that this syndrome of deficient valves and oversized veins is inborn, but diffuse damage by a process of 'silent' thrombosis cannot be totally excluded. It may be apparent from an early age or appear later in life, possibly because a reduced number of valves, poorly supported by weak veins, succumb to wear and tear. The valveless state results in a severely impaired pumping mechanism and blood tends to surge back and forth with each muscle contraction (Figure 3.2), with little effective upward movement so that severe venous hypertension occurs with progressive tissue change and eventual ulceration. There is a large component of superficial incompetence here but the dominant factor is the absence of an effective deep vein pump and removal of incompetent superficial veins is not sufficient to cure the condition.

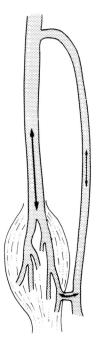

**Figure 3.2** *The valveless state. The patient has an inborn deficiency of valves in both superficial and deep veins so that muscle contraction causes a surge without purposeful movement and is ineffective in returning blood against gravity. Sustained venous hypertension when the patient is upright is inevitable and will be expressed by pigmentation, thickening of superficial tissues (lipodermatosclerosis) and a strong tendency to ulceration*

The perforators play an adverse role in allowing surge outwards between deep and superficial veins but the main defect is widespread lack of deep valves essential for effective pumping (see Chapter 7).

## Impaired deep veins: post-thrombotic or postphlebitic syndrome

Here the term 'impaired' is used to convey that the deep veins and their valves have been damaged by some process, almost always thrombosis. This results in severe damage to the pumping mechanism and the patients present with some aspect of venous hypertension, often severe ulceration, and usually with a clear story of deep vein thrombosis in pregnancy, or following a major fracture in the lower limbs. Over 6% of all venous disorders fall in this group and around 50% of all new cases with venotensive changes and ulceration have this cause; indeed, the majority of severe and intractable venous problems come from this group.

On phlebography the deep veins show varying degrees of deformity, or actual occlusion, with collateral channels formed from greatly enlarged lesser deep veins. In addition, venous return from the lower part of the limb travels preferentially up through superficial veins, par-

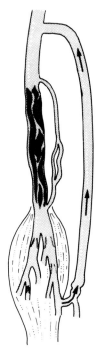

**Figure 3.3** *Deep vein impairment is usually caused by a previous deep vein thrombosis which has caused deformity and obstruction to deep veins. The superficial veins are forced to act as collaterals so that they conduct an upward flow which is accentuated by exercise (muscle contraction). This causes the superficial veins involved to enlarge but if this is in their natural direction of flow they do not become tortuous (varicose). Depending on the severity of deep vein damage, venous hypertension occurs when the patient is upright with all the venostatic consequences referred to in Figure 3.2. The problem is compounded by accompanying destruction of many valves in veins that have recanalized, and by unnaturally enlarged collateral veins in deep and superficial layers losing all valve function*

ticularly the saphenous veins (Figure 3.3). These veins are clearly acting as collaterals past impaired deep veins which are resisting upward flow so that an alternative pathway through the superficial veins proves easier to follow. This has diagnostic importance and an unsatisfactory selective vein occlusion (Trendelenburg) test should alert the clinician to the possibility of upward flow in the long saphenous vein caused by obstructed deep veins. Such flow is readily confirmed by directional Doppler flowmeter and, in this case, functional phlebography will be required to complete the diagnosis.

The other fundamental feature in the post-thrombotic limb is the widespread loss of effective valves in the deep veins with corresponding damage to the pumping mechanism; any upward movement is quickly lost by blood falling back again through valveless deep veins. In addition, collateral veins may become so enlarged that the unnaturally distended channels lack any competent valves. Thus, not only is musculovenous pumping resisted by deformed deep veins but its effectiveness is reduced by inability of the valves to retain any upward movement.

Moreover, blood pumped out collaterally to the superficial veins transfers pressure to the surface layers and skin which are so vulnerable to venous hypertension. These are the aspects that conspire to make an extensive impaired deep vein (post-thrombotic) syndrome so formidable (see Chapters 8 and 9).

### Note on perforating veins in post-thrombotic syndrome

In this condition the perforators certainly can pump blood outwards as part of a compensatory collateral mechanism and this is a useful role that may be best left undisturbed. The term 'incompetent perforator' is too often loosely used and it should always be qualified by the reason for its incompetence. The controversial role of the perforator in the various venous disorders is discussed in Chapter 11.

### Obstructed venous outlet syndrome (iliac vein occlusion)

This is again the result of old deep vein thrombosis but one which has caused permanent occlusion in a venous 'bottleneck', such as a common iliac or popliteal vein, where venous return from the limb is channelled through one major vein and alternative return is only by lesser veins. The best example occurs with occlusion of a common iliac vein (an incidence of 2% but appreciably higher if those patients with accompanying post-thrombotic damage lower in the limb are included); it also occurs in the axillary vein where thrombosis causes similar manifestations in the upper limb. In iliac vein occlusion tortuous collateral veins develop across the pubic region (Figure 3.4), the lower abdomen and within the pelvis. There is a strong tendency for oedema in the affected limb due to the venous pressure being raised by the restricted outlet. The original thrombosis often involves the femoral and popliteal deep veins, so that there is, in addition, severe deep vein impairment throughout the limb. Thus, in its most benign form obstructed venous outlet may bring little more inconvenience than mild oedema but others may suffer the much more severe manifestations of iliofemoral post-thrombotic syndrome (see Chapters 8 and 9).

### Mixed and complex states

In this book the term 'mixed' is used to describe states of superficial incompetence where there are either multiple sources and/or the source is in the opposite limb. 'Complex' is used where two or more of the groups described above exist together, for example, superficial incompetence and deep vein impairment co-exist (Tibbs, 1986).

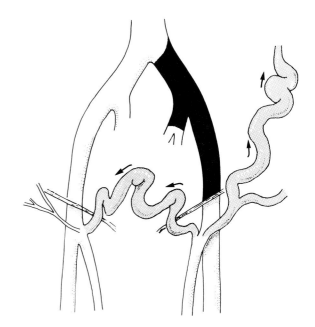

**Figure 3.4** *Obstructed venous outlet syndrome. The best example of this is post-thrombotic occlusion of the iliac veins, illustrated here. Superficial veins in the groin are forced to act as collaterals which are often seen as varicosities crossing the pubic region, where their flow is counter to the natural direction. Resistance to venous return if the collateral outlet is not adequate causes a strong tendency to oedema in the limb and this may be the predominant symptom. However, the deep veins below the inguinal ligament have often been involved in the original thrombosis so that the features of deep vein impairment in the limb are present as well and this combination can cause severe manifestations*

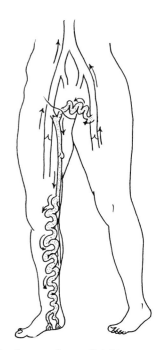

**Figure 3.5** *A mixed state of superficial incompetence where the source is in the opposite limb. In this example, long saphenous incompetence in the right limb arises from the uppermost branches of the long saphenous vein, persisting after inadequate surgery, on the left side*

It is certainly possible for varicose veins to arise from the opposite limb as crossover incompetence (Figure 3.5), or for superficial vein incompetence to set up typical retrograde circuits below deep vein impairment (Figure 3.6); indeed, combined mixed and complex states can

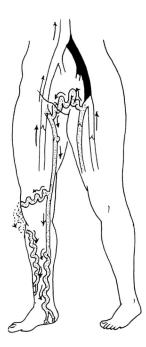

**Figure 3.7** *Mixed and complex patterns may be combined, as in this example, where pubic varicosities caused by iliac vein obstruction on the left side are the origin of simple long saphenous incompetence and varicosities in the right limb*

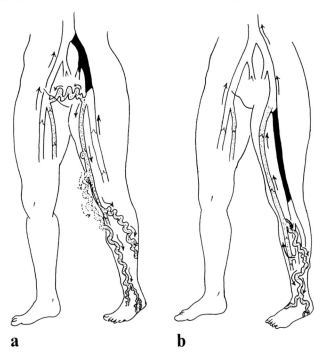

**a**    **b**

**Figure 3.6** *(a) A complex pattern of venous abnormality with typical long saphenous vein incompetence below obstructed iliac deep veins on the left side.*

*(b) Localized examples of superficial incompetence can occur below popliteal and femoral vein obstruction*

occur with crossover incompetence to the right limb arising from the left limb which itself has iliac vein occlusion (Figure 3.7) and, sometimes, with left long saphenous incompetence as well. Thus, the groups described in the sections above are by no means sharply defined and various combinations are not rare. They are the basic components of venous disorder and convenient for descriptive purposes but it must not be taken that every patient fits neatly into one or the other. Mixed and complex states are described in Chapters 5 and 10.

## Congenital venous malformations including the Klippel–Trenaunay syndrome

A wide range of failure in normal development of veins may occur (less than 3% of venous patients, if trivial lesions are excluded), varying from a minor capillary blemish to a massive replacement of deep veins by cavernous haemangioma. Many of the complications are those of the acquired disorders outlined above, including venous hypertension and ulceration, arising from inadequacies in valve mechanisms, but the distinctive feature

is the development of abnormal vascular tissue and connections, such as angiomas and arteriovenous fistulas. Anatomical variants may occur, for example, the persistence of a sciatic vein taking over from the femoral vein, and this may be relatively harmless in itself, but it may be combined with other developmental errors of major significance to the venous function of the limb. In some of these patients these changes are associated with abnormal growth in the neighbouring bones, particularly overgrowth in their length, and the combination of venous abnormality with overlengthening of the limb is known as Klippel–Trenaunay's syndrome. Errors in development of the lymphatic system may accompany the venous ones. These matters are considered in more detail in Chapter 12.

## Other venous conditions

The overall view given in this chapter does not include a number of conditions which are described in their appropriate chapters, notably:

- Acute and subacute deep venous thrombosis
- Injury to veins
- Arteriovenous fistula
- Combined arterial and venous states, especially ischaemia
- Obstruction to deep veins by external pressure
- Oedema of venous origin

## Comment

The basic patterns of venous disorder and the underlying defects have been outlined here but there is great variation in the extent and complexity from case to case; moreover, it is not unusual for two or more of the states described to be present in the same limb. Each patient, indeed each limb, is individual, and in many the condition is far from straightforward. Each deserves careful study and analytical thought if the right diagnosis and form of management are to be decided upon. Some indication of this is given in the chapters that follow.

## References

Tibbs, D. J. (1986) The intriguing problem of varicose veins. *Internal Angiology*, **4**, 289–295

Tibbs, D. J. and Fletcher, E. W. L. (1983) Direction of flow in the superficial veins as a guide to venous disorders in the lower limbs. *Surgery*, **93**, 758–767

# 4

# Valvular incompetence in the superficial veins: simple (primary) varicose veins

Valvular incompetence in the superficial veins is by far the largest group in the venous disorders and its effects vary from a trivial blemish to a severe venous stasis with ulceration and serious disability. Because the basic fault is in the superficial veins, which can usually be removed without harm, most patients can be cured, or at least improved, by a procedure adequately removing or sclerosing the defective veins. This is the area in which the surgeon can achieve most and where a full understanding will be of the greatest value.

*Note on terminology:* Varicose veins are the most obvious manifestation in this condition but they are not always present and there are other causes for varicosities than valvular incompetence in the superficial veins. Varicose veins from this cause are often referred to as 'primary' in order to distinguish them from those which have developed as a secondary or compensatory phenomenon due to underlying, defective deep veins, particularly post-thrombotic occlusion. The term 'primary' is not ideal because the varicose state, tortuosity, of the veins is likely to be secondary to a primary defect in their valves; however, as the valves are an integral part of the veins, perhaps the term 'primary' is permissible. The term 'simple' varicose veins is frequently used in this book as an alternative to 'primary', both designating varicosities associated solely with defective or absent valves in the superficial veins and not related to any deep vein disorder. The term 'simple' is used to imply a single fault, valvular incompetence, with all the other changes developing from this. This state does not always occur on its own and mixed states where primary and secondary varicosities co-exist are not rare; these are considered in Chapter 10.

## General considerations

Everything that is said in this Chapter applies to the upright patient, exercising intermittently (external compression of the leg activates upward pumping in the same way as exercise and is often used to simulate this in diagnostic procedures such as Doppler flowmeter examination); in these circumstances, if superficial valves are defective, gravitational downflow is possible from a higher level to a lower level and into slack veins below a venous pumping mechanism. It is important to realize that in normal superficial veins, including the long saphenous vein, there is little or no upward movement with exercise in the upright position. This is easily demonstrated with a directional Doppler flowmeter used upon normal subjects. With exercise and the accompanying reduction in deep vein pressure, the valves in the principal superficial veins separate the blood into segments each tending to empty by perforating veins into the neighbouring deep veins (Figure 1.1), but there is no purposeful movement along the length of the vein. If defective valves allowing gravitational downflow are present, exercise is followed by strong downward movement and this is the basic characteristic found in all simple (primary) varicose veins (Bjordal, 1977, 1986; Tibbs and Fletcher, 1983; Tibbs, 1986). This useless circuit of blood in the veins, spilling over from a deep vein at high level and falling down to enter deep veins at low level, is referred to in this book as a retrograde circuit (Figure 4.1). There is a great variation in the rate and volume of flow, and distance over which such a circuit may run. It may occur on a miniature scale, perhaps from above one valve to just beneath it, or it may be of considerable size, with many branches, running the full length of the limb from the groin to the underside of the foot; this may be of such magnitude that it overwhelms the efforts by the pumping mechanism to reduce venous pressure in the leg so that sustained, unrelieved hypertension occurs. The retrograde circuit is of fundamental importance in understanding simple varicose veins and will now be defined in more detail.

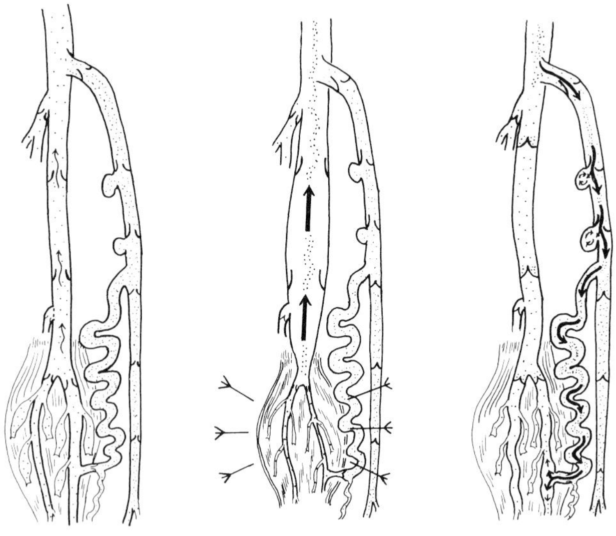

**Figure 4.1** *The retrograde venous circuit.*

*1. Deep and superficial veins after the patient has been standing still for 30 seconds. All veins are well filled and there is only a slow upward drift of flow mainly in the deep veins.*
*2. At the moment of calf muscle contraction, deep veins are compressed and valves direct the blood upwards.*
*3. On muscle relaxation the deep veins in the leg are slack, at low pressure, and ready to receive any inward flow. Above this level, valves prevent return flow in the deep veins; however, the superficial valves are incompetent so that downward flow occurs to the low pressure area beneath the muscles. This flow is continuously replenished from the deep vein at the upper end and runs, via perforators, to deep veins at a lower level until these are filled again and pressures equalize. A wide variety of retrograde circuits operated by upward pumping in deep veins and consequent gravitational downflow in incompetent superficial veins may occur and are characteristic of simple (primary) varicose veins; the one illustrated is based on the long saphenous system*

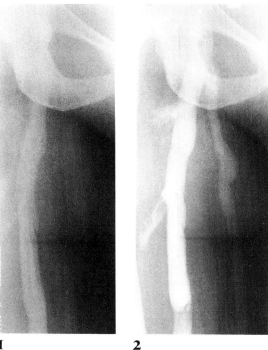

**1**      **2**      **3**

**Figure 4.2** *The source of downflow in a retrograde circuit. The example shown here by functional phlebography is at the upper end of the long saphenous vein.*

*1. Whilst the patient stands still, opaque medium injected into a superficial vein on the calf has filled the deep veins and ascended to the groin, but has not entered the saphenous vein.*
*2. Immediately after two exercise movements. Opacified blood can be seen spilling down the long saphenous vein; the concentration of opaque medium in the deep veins has increased because blood from lower levels has been pumped upwards, thus creating slack veins towards which the superficial downflow moves. The long saphenous vein shows obvious enlargement and two saccules, in keeping with its incompetent state*

**I**      **2**

## Haemodynamics of valve failure in the superficial veins: the retrograde circuit

The retrograde circuit of gravitational downflow will have the following components:

### The source of downflow

This will be from a deep vein at higher level in the limb, spilling over by a vein that has no effective valves and running to the superficial veins (Figure 4.2). This spillover is equivalent to a leak from a pipe in which fluid is being pumped upwards from below and the escaping fluid falls back to the level from which it started. In the case of incompetent superficial veins the blood spilling over from the deep vein will tend to fall down to any area of lower pressure. The commonest source is the uppermost end, the termination, of a long or short saphenous vein, but there are many other possible sources provided by perforating veins with defective valves or even veins running down the thigh from the pelvis. In the case of the long saphenous vein not only will its own valves be incompetent but the valve usually present in the femoral or iliac vein, guarding the saphenous termination, is often missing (Dodd and Cockett, 1976).

### The pathway of incompetence

This term describes the incompetent superficial veins down which retrograde flow occurs. It will run from the source, described above, for a variable distance down the limb to enter the deep veins below a pumping mechanism (Figures 4.3, 4.4(a)). Every time the pumping mechanism causes the deep veins in its vicinity to become slack and at low pressure, flow down the pathway of incompetence

occurs until the deep veins are filled to capacity and the pressures equalize (Figure 4.4(b)–(d)). With each movement that actuates the pump this cycle of events is repeated yet again. The pathway of incompetence will always run from above a pumping mechanism to veins below it; the classical example is an incompetent long saphenous vein running from the groin and via one or more of its branches to the lower leg, that is to say,

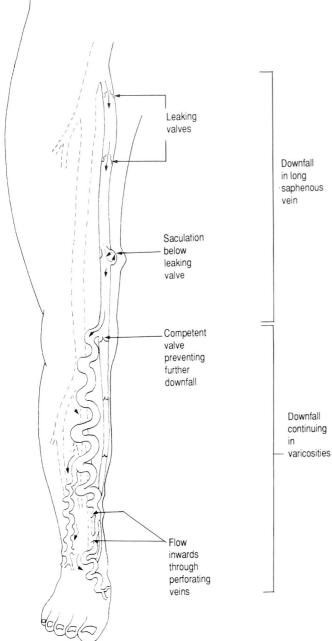

**Figure 4.3** *Diagram to show the features of a major pathway of incompetence in the long saphenous system. The thigh portion of the long saphenous vein is enlarged, the valves are incompetent and beneath one valve a saccule is present. At knee level, incompetence is continued down a large branch which shows gross tortuosity; competent valves are present in the long saphenous vein below the knee and prevent downflow in this. The varicose branch breaks into branches which terminate by entering perforators in the lower leg. Innumerable variations of this basic pattern occur*

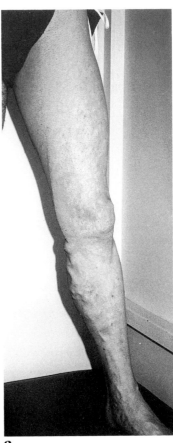

a

**Figure 4.4** *Clinical findings and special investigations in a long saphenous retrograde circuit of incompetence.*

*(a) Clinical photograph of simple (primary) varicose veins to show a typical retrograde circuit based on the long saphenous vein. This vein can be seen in the lower half of the thigh but was palpable up to the groin. It shows obvious enlargement but no saccules are visible. A large varicosity is given off from it at knee level and meanders down the inner aspect of the leg breaking into several branches running across the front to the outer aspect and others to the inner side and ankle region where they will join perforating veins. On the foot, the lower part of the saphenous vein is seen giving off further varicosities running to the underside. It is clear from this that the long saphenous vein is incompetent throughout its length and the pathway of incompetence is formed by the long saphenous vein from groin to foot and also by one large varicosity breaking into multiple tributaries. Note how there are no skin changes except for the dilated venules and it appears that the pumping mechanism is able to cope adequately with a considerable retrograde flow of blood. Selective saphenous occlusion gave complete control of all varicosities and reduction in prominence with Perthes test.*

*(Figure 4.4 continued on page 52)*

**Figure 4.4** *(continued)*

*(b) Tracing from a directional Doppler flowmeter placed over the long saphenous vein of a similar patient just above the knee. It shows a downsurge on coughing, downflow following squeezing the calf or by rising on the toes (calf muscle contraction); blocking the saphenous vein above the probe prevents the downflow in response to exercise until the vein is released.*

*(c) Photoplethysmogram representing changes in venous pressure in the lower leg of the same patient in response to exercise, without and with temporary occlusion of the long saphenous vein on the affected side; the right side gives the normal drop in pressure in response to exercise and a recovery (or restitution) time of over 16 seconds before full venous pressure is restored; on the affected side the recovery period is 14 seconds but when downflow in the long saphenous vein is prevented by compression in the lower thigh this improves to over 19 seconds.*

*(d) Doppler tracing from a patient with a slender varicosity giving prolonged flow over 16 seconds or more*

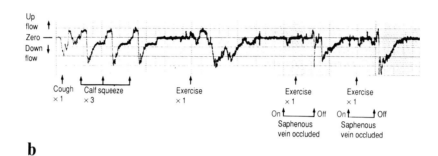

**b**

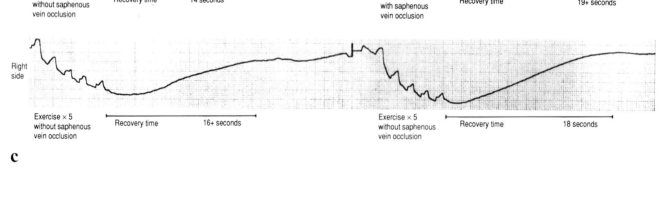

**c**

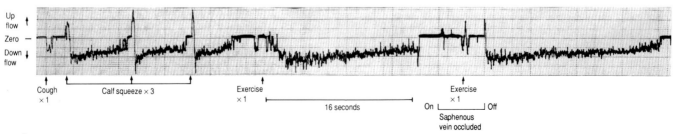

**d**

beneath the calf muscle pumping mechanism (Figure 4.5); it may continue from here downwards to the underside of another pumping mechanism, the foot (Tibbs and Fletcher, 1983; Gardner and Fox, 1986, 1989). There is much variation in the details of this in size, extent and complexity; although a saphenous vein is most commonly at fault it is not necessarily involved and in this case the pathway is formed from a succession of lesser veins. It may even occur on a miniature scale with a single valve creating the pressure difference necessary for gravitational downflow in a small retrograde circuit from

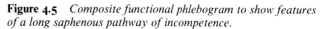

**Figure 4.5** *Composite functional phlebogram to show features of a long saphenous pathway of incompetence.*

*1. The upper thigh immediately after two exercise movements, showing opacified blood from the femoral vein flowing down the saphenous vein.*

*2. Lower two-thirds of the limb. The saphenous vein is only faintly outlined at knee level but just below this gives off two large varicose branches; one of these (posterior arcuate vein) runs to the inner side and its tributaries disperse via perforators into deep veins there; the other crosses over to disperse into the anterior tibial vein and its muscular branches. The opaque medium for this phlebogram was injected into the calf varicosity; with the patient standing still, it has entered the deep veins of the leg and ascended passively up to the femoral vein in the groin. It is only after exercise that downward movement in the long saphenous vein has occurred to cause the spillover shown in 1*

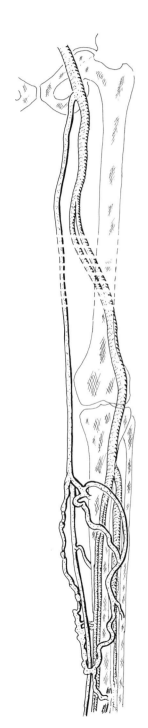

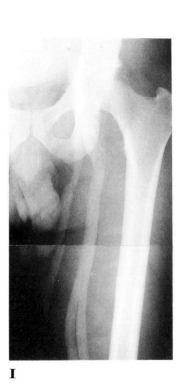

**1**

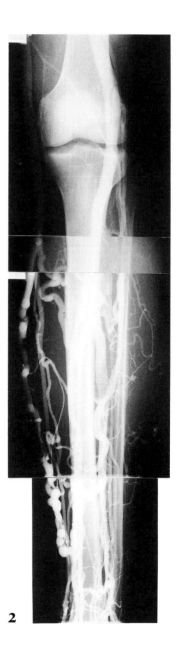

**2**

above the valve to below it. A pressure difference of this sort can be created by change in the limb from horizontal to vertical, by muscular contraction or brief external pressure and, in the case of the pelvic veins, by respiratory movements (Milliken *et al.*, 1986). In clinical practice a major retrograde circuit is of course the most obtrusive but a minor one, otherwise insignificant in its effect, may be of cosmetic importance and awareness of this possibility will help in deciding upon treatment.

The concept of a pathway of incompetence, often made up of a series of veins joining together rather than one single vein, is essential in the treatment of varicose veins. Treatment may be inadequate if the pathway is not accurately mapped out (see Chapter 2) over its full length and effectively removed. Leaving portions of the pathway intact is the commonest cause of residual or recurrent varicose veins (see Chapter 5). If only the upper end is interrupted, the valveless pathway remains as a large open conduit directly communicating with the low pressure areas beneath the pumping mechanisms and constantly inviting any vein at higher level (and higher potential pressure) to leak flow down it. It can form a low pressure zone running the length of the limb and creating a pressure difference which all too easily attracts renewed flow from the deep veins in the upper part of the limb.

The ever-repeated rushes of turbulent, reversed flow (downflow) in an active pathway create the typical local manifestations of superficial valve incompetence and these are:

1. Enlargement, a form of hypertrophy, of all the veins concerned.
2. A saphenous vein may develop saccules caused by turbulence beneath leaking valves but it is usually too strong to develop tortuosity.
3. The branch veins and other lesser veins enlarge in width and length and thus become tortuous or varicose. Varicose veins themselves are, of course, very much part of the pathway of incompetence which in its lower parts may divide into several tributaries, rather like the delta of a river, each dispersing to one or more perforators at different levels.

Because the stimulus is repeated frequently without remission the veins involved show progressive hypertrophy and increasing tortuosity. Some varicosities reach impressive dimensions but many eventually appear to stabilize and remain unchanged for years as though a balance has been achieved between the rate of downflow and the pump's ability to shift this.

### The destination – a zone of slack veins in the vicinity of a pumping mechanism

The pumping mechanisms which propel venous blood up the deep veins towards the heart, against gravity, lie in the main conducting veins and in numerous venous sinuses within the muscles. Normally blood from the superficial veins runs by multiple perforating veins into these deep veins where muscular contraction compresses the deep vein 'pumping chambers' to force the blood in the direction allowed by the valves, upwards, towards the heart. Valves prevent return of this blood so that after muscular contraction the deep veins in this vicinity are virtually empty and normally remain slack, at low pressure, for up to 20 or 30 seconds whilst they refill across the capillary beds. It is during this interval that a pathway of incompetence can empty its contents by gravitational downflow through perforators and into the deep veins. This will continue until all the deep veins are filled to capacity and pressure within them rises sharply to resist further inflow from the superficial veins. Flow down the pathway of incompetence will then cease until further muscular contraction empties the deep veins again to allow another burst of flow down the pathway. There are several points to emphasize here:

1. The source of flow can provide an unending flow down the pathway and, depending upon the magnitude of incompetence, may be anything from a prolonged trickle to a massive downrush. A distinction must be made between velocity of downflow and the volume per second delivered. A fast, thin stream may deliver little but a slow, broad stream can deliver large amounts quite quickly (a Doppler 'flowmeter' records velocity of flow only – not volume).
2. If a substantial volume is rapidly delivered, the deep vein pressure lowered by muscular contraction rises again at unnatural speed so that the intervals of reduced pressure become briefer and hypertension more prolonged. In severe cases the downrush may be so great that venous hypertension is continuous because of the pump's inability to meet the demands put upon it (Figure 4.6). As will be explained later, there is a considerable individual variation in the effectiveness of musculovenous pumping mechanisms. One poorly endowed with valves will be overwhelmed more easily than a strongly effective pump which may be able to cope with the burden of a massive pathway of incompetence.
3. The other factor is, of course, the speed and volume of downflow in the pathway; even with large varicose veins there may be several pairs of valve cusps with sufficient function to restrain the speed and volume of downflow. This is a common finding on opening a saphenous vein removed at surgery where incompetence has been unequivocally demonstrated by syringe testing (see later). In this way, the source of flow may be unending but the maximal volume of flow down incompetent veins bears little relationship to their external diameter and may in fact be quite restricted. This, of course, gives the pump much better

**Figure 4.6** *Downflow in a retrograde circuit overwhelming the musculovenous pump. This patient had severe venous stasis with ulceration just above the right ankle.*

*(a) Doppler flowmeter tracing from the right long saphenous vein in the lower thigh shows all the features of incompetence, a marked downward surge on coughing, downflow after squeezing the calf and after exercise, and downflow temporarily prevented by occlusion of the saphenous vein.*

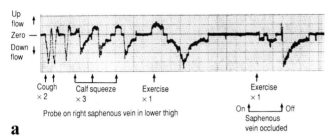

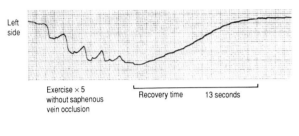

*(b) Photoplethysmography in the same patient. On the left side a satisfactory fall in venous pressure is shown in response to exercise, with a somewhat shortened recovery time of 13 seconds. On the right side, however, there is a poor response and recovery time is brief at about 8 seconds. Repeating this whilst maintaining firm finger pressure over the long saphenous vein on the right side gives immediate improvement in the size of the response and in prolongation of the recovery time which reverts to normal at 23 seconds. Compare this unequivocal improvement when the saphenous vein is blocked with the marginal improvement shown in Figure 4.4(c) in a patient with near normal recovery time and no venous stasis, and in whom the musculovenous pump was fully capable of coping with the superficial vein downflow. Venous stasis is evidence of the pump's inability to cope and this is confirmed by a short recovery time on photoplethysmography; the role of the long saphenous vein is confirmed by the obvious improvement with occlusion of this vein*

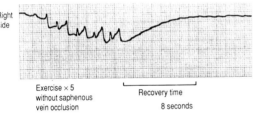

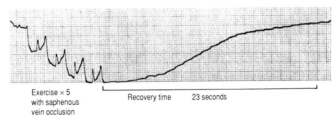

**a**

**b**

opportunity to manage and explains why massive varicosities do not invariably overwhelm the pump.

### The return pathway

The circuit is completed by venous blood being pumped towards the heart up the deep veins and as it reaches the 'source' a proportion will spill over to be recycled down the retrograde circuit yet again (Figure 4.5). This depends upon having an effective and undamaged set of valves throughout the deep veins, including those guarding the muscular pumping chambers.

To a large extent the development of simple varicose veins is dependent upon an effective deep vein pumping mechanism and a return pathway clearing the way for downflow in the superficial veins. Simple varicose veins are not merely the result of static distension but are a dynamic phenomenon caused by the forceful thrust of turbulent downflow, and in this the deep veins play an indirect but essential part.

### Factors limiting the speed and volume of downflow: relationship to venous hypertension (stasis)

The severity of venous manifestations is strongly related to the volume of downflow in the pathway of incompetence. It is of value to consider the various factors that can modify this because many are the basis for important principles in treatment. The following factors will govern the volume of blood per second that can be delivered down a pathway of incompetence:

1. The head of pressure at which flow is delivered through the source must influence the speed of delivery and this will depend upon the height of the column of blood above this level (hydrostatic pressure). This, however, is an oversimplification as one or more valves may interrupt the column; perhaps it can be said that the peak pressures will be equivalent to the height between source and heart but the presence of valves will restrict the duration of full pressure and of flow from above the source; in this way valves can limit the rate of delivery. Posture, of course, will have a profound effect upon the head of pressure. This will

be maximal when upright and dwindle progessively to zero as the horizontal position is assumed so that posture is a crucial limiting factor. Other factors affecting the head of pressure are: increased abdominal pressure, as in coughing, which can cause a sharp rise that is limited by any intervening valves; the rate of upflow from below, which will influence pressure at the source and, for instance, a rapid forceful upflow during exercise in the upright position will ensure it is maximal regardless of valves above the source.

In this book the expression 'spillover' has been used frequently to describe the outflow from the source falling down the pathway of incompetence but it is not entirely appropriate in other respects. 'Leak' is probably a more accurate term in view of the column of blood above it.

2. The overall size and capacity of the veins forming a pathway of incompetence, including the source; this varies with venous tone and can change quite quickly with alterations in external temperature.

3. Constrictions within these veins, caused by scarring from old phlebitis or sclerotherapy, or by valve cusps of appreciable size. The latter, although heavily incompetent, are fully capable of impeding downflow; they may be associated with saccules and deformity of the lumen, so that turbulence will further delay flow. Thus, there is usually a limit to the speed of delivery that is possible down a pathway of incompetence. In most patients it is well within the ability of the pump to deal with the maximal downflow, but in others it can so exceed the pump's ability that the venous pressure remains high without relief.

4. The vigour of downflow in the retrograde circuit depends on the rate at which blood is shifted upwards by musculovenous pumping. Flow down the pathway of incompetence is regulated by the state of filling in the deep veins; when they are slack and the pressure is low, it will be maximal, but as they fill the pressure in them will rise until they are filled to capacity and then, with venous pressure at high level, further inflow will be resisted and will cease. Thus, if a standing patient is inactive, with only occasional use of the musculovenous pump, venous pressure will be sustained at an undesirably high level, even though there is little flow down the incompetent superficial veins; a defective pump will have a similar effect by giving reduced opportunity for inflow.

Vigorous walking may promote maximal volume of downflow but usually a good pump will outstrip this and succeed in reducing venous tension. This gives rise to a curious conflict; active walking, so often encouraged in venous conditions, will be beneficial in avoiding venous hypertension and stasis, but will give yet further stimulus to enlargement of varicosities by augmenting the turbulent downflow (assuming elastic support is not being used). It seems most unlikely that active walking will benefit large varicose veins, as is widely believed, rather the reverse, but it can help to forestall the damaging state of venous hypertension which they might otherwise cause.

(*Comment upon hypertrophy of incompetent superficial veins:* The author has been impressed by the number of successful athletes or enthusiastic walkers who may generate unusually large varicosities without any tendency to venotensive changes. Their limbs are in good condition but, unilaterally, there is a massive bunch of varicosities arising from a single pathway of long or short saphenous incompetence, easily controlled by finger compression. One explanation is that the unusual amount of lower limb activity has caused more than average hypertrophy in a pathway of incompetence by prolonged periods of maximal downflow within it. Presumably the musculovenous pump is robust and often the athlete concerned has accepted the varicosities for some years, fearing any interference that might conceivably upset his success. Moreover, these veins seem to reach a large size and then stabilize with little further enlargement.)

5. The volume delivered down incompetent superficial veins is determined by the musculovenous pump activity, but it is limited by the maximal downflow possible in the superficial veins. This means that even a substantial volume of downflow may not ever cause venous stasis by exceeding the capacity of the pump. However, a modest downflow does not exclude the possibility of unrelieved hypertension. With an inactive or weak pump, predisposed to venous hypertension, superficial downflow will be small but these are the very circumstances where any downflow, further handicapping the pump's precarious state, is least desirable; with a poor pump, even a small downflow can nullify its efforts.

Two opposite circumstances, or a combination of the both, will cause flow down a retrograde circuit to be decisive in causing venous hypertension:
 (a) A downflow volume so massive that it overwhelms even the strongest of pumps.
 (b) A weak or inactive pump easily overwhelmed by even a small volume of downflow.
 (c) A combination of the above factors, that is, a comparatively weak pump and a moderately high potential volume of downflow.

6. At the actual moment of muscle contraction flow down a pathway of incompetence leading to these muscles will cease. However, if a varicosity runs to the underside of the foot (pump), downflow in it will start as soon as the foot is raised off the ground and cease when it is replaced. In a pathway running down both to muscle pumps of the leg and to the underside of the foot, the foot component may dominate during such exercises as 'rising on the toes' to give a misleading impression of downflow into contracting muscles.

7. Any form of sustained external compression, for example, an elastic stocking, can reduce or prevent superficial downflow and bring relief to an over-burdened pumping mechanism, an important principle in treatment.

## Some aspects of the pumping mechanism in simple superficial vein incompetence

The 'musculovenous pump' referred to above is not a single unit. It is composed of innumerable units with each small group of muscle fibres having its own pumping unit, often with a perforating vein running directly into it. Thus, minor retrograde circuits based on small muscle groups can give a localized set of varicosities. The possibilities in size and distribution are endless, which is in accord with the findings in clinical practice; virtually any muscle group can be the destination of flow in incompetent superficial veins. The foot pump is somewhat different, being partly operated by plantar muscles but mostly by pressure on the large venous complex on the underside of the foot; blood will flow down into it when the foot is raised but will be forcibly returned upwards when it is replaced to the ground. This mechanism may enlarge greatly in superficial vein incompetence or in any case where venous hypertension is present, such as post-thrombotic syndrome, because of massive expansion in the complex of veins under the foot. These veins can form a significant venous pool that shifts back and forth, greatly handicapping efficiency in return of venous blood from the lower part of the limb. This is a form of failure in a particular venous pumping mechanism, the foot, that has not received the attention it deserves until recently.

### The importance of venous pooling in the foot

If a pathway of incompetence extends to the foot, an appreciable quantity of blood runs down and is sequestered in the foot every time it is raised (Figures 4.7, 4.8) and this diverts blood at the very moment that it should be available to the pumping mechanisms of the leg (Tibbs and Fletcher, 1983). Moreover, when the foot is replaced to the ground, the venous pool under the foot is ejected upwards via both superficial and deep veins to veins of the lower leg which are already well filled by downflow from incompetent superficial veins (Figure 4.8(b),(d)). When the venous pool in the foot is large this forceful surge of blood will cause a peak of excessive venous pressure, certainly shared by the superficial veins in the lower leg. These momentary peaks may be far above the usual maximal pressure (hypertension) of a column of blood from foot to heart level (Figure 4.9). When endlessly repeated as the patient moves about, they may be very damaging if superimposed on a sustained hypertension and it is possible that they are a decisive factor

in the occurrence of ulceration. Elimination of this component is an important aspect of treatment in venous stasis and threatened ulceration (lipo(dermato)sclerosis) and this may be achieved in two ways:

1. Appropriate surgery removing the pathway of incompetence, with particular attention paid to varicosities crossing the ankle to the foot.
2. Use of elastic support with a firm foot piece capable of preventing filling of the venous pool in the foot. However, inelastic containment by a paste bandage applied when the leg is in high elevation, as used in the treatment of venous ulcers, will be more effective.

### Assessing the venous foot pool in superficial incompetence

The degree of venous pooling in the foot can be gauged by the amount of downflow in the pathway of incompetence in response to raising the foot off the ground for 20 seconds whilst standing. This is best done with the knee straight and by tilting the pelvis so that there is no accompanying contraction of muscles in the limb. The flow is assessed by a directional Doppler flowmeter with its probe over an appropriate vein or varicosity in the lower thigh or upper leg (Figure 4.8(b)). A heavy or prolonged downflow will indicate a sizeable pooling in the foot, and an obvious upsurge on replacing the foot will confirm that this is a significant factor that should be eliminated if possible. It is a valuable addition to the routine when using a Doppler flowmeter and will often draw attention to varicosities running across the foot.

### Valves in simple incompetence

Incompetence in the superficial valves arises either because the patient has too few valves or the valves are weak and give way, or both. During the course of several hundred operations the author has carried out a syringe test down the long saphenous vein (Figure 4.10) just before stripping it to confirm that there was no resistance, that is, the valves were leaking heavily; this was often accompanied by a visible bulge in the varicosities and showing the correct pathway of incompetence had been identified. Immediately after stripping (usually from groin to upper calf) the vein was opened and its interior scrutinized. In about one-third either no valve could be seen or, at most, one or two vestigial-looking valves were present, strongly suggesting an inborn deficiency in the number and quality of valves. In the remainder, between two and six valves with an apparently well-formed pair of cusps were found; single cusps were occasionally seen. Visual inspection in an opened vein cannot judge how well the cusps meet but the previous syringe test had, of course, established that the valves offered no resistance to full delivery by the syringe. Thus it seems probable

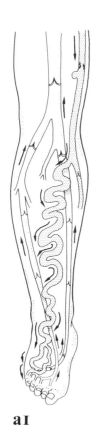

**a**

**a1**

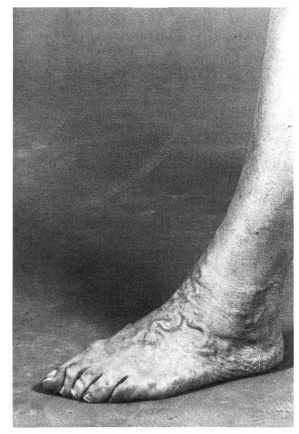

**a2**

**Figure 4.7** *The pathway of incompetence extending to the foot.*

*(a) 1. Varicosities arising from the long saphenous vein often extend across the ankle to form a leash of tributaries running round the side of the foot to a plexus of enlarged veins on its underside. Such varicosities may arise at any level from the groin downwards, or even from pelvic veins via internal pudendal varicosities. The short saphenous vein commonly gives off varicosities to the foot, usually running on the outer aspect of the ankle.*
*2. Typical foot varicosities arising from the long saphenous vein.*

*(b) Perforating leg veins, previously a point of inflow from long saphenous incompetence, may become a source of downflow to the foot after surgical removal of the incompetent veins above this level; less frequently perforator outflow from leg to foot is an independent 'primary' phenomenon. In deep vein impairment found in post-thrombotic syndrome, circuits of simple incompetence to the foot arising from superficial veins acting as collaterals are quite commonly present, giving rise to a complex pattern of venous disorder*

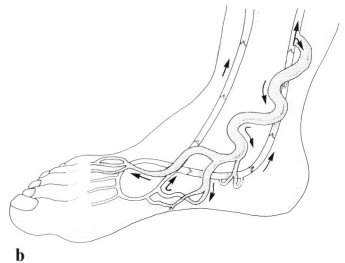

**b**

that the patient had been born with a full complement of valves but these had yielded to stress in some fashion to become incompetent. Often the cusps looked so normal that it seemed likely that the weakness was in the vein wall supporting the cusps so that they had become unduly separated and no longer able to meet accurately. Many valves were associated with a saccule lying beneath them (Figures 1.12–1.15), with considerable deformity and intimal thickening, and in these it was evident that the cusps could not meet effectively; accompanying this the

vein was often grossly oversized, in keeping with a wall unable to support the valve ring and cusps adequately (Rose, 1986; Thulesius, Gjores and Berlin, 1986; Clarke *et al.*, 1989; Psaila and Melhuish, 1989). It is difficult to decide whether the unnatural width of the vein was the cause of the valve incompetence or a secondary effect (Ludbrook, 1963) from the turbulent flow (Fegan and Kline, 1972) caused by valve failure. Perhaps most likely is that one circumstance encourages the other so that a vicious cycle is set up.

**Figure 4.8**  *Varicose veins running to the foot.*

*(a) Clinical photograph of long saphenous incompetence giving rise to a large varicosity running to the foot; venous stasis with ulceration is present.*

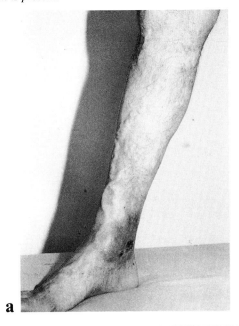

*(b) Directional Doppler flowmeter tracings in the same patient:*
*1. With probe over the long saphenous vein in the lower thigh showing the typical features of incompetence; raising the foot causes saphenous downflow with an upsurge on putting it to the ground again.*
*2. With probe placed over the varicosity just above the ankle and on the foot whilst it is is being raised up and down. Each time the foot is replaced to the ground there is a strong upward flow over some seconds, indicating a considerable transference of blood upwards.*

*(c) Photoplethysmogram in the same patient. Right side showing recovery time markedly improved by temporary occlusion of the long saphenous vein at thigh level; left side showing normal response and recovery time with exercise.*

Note: *During this examination the foot plexus is not affected because the patient is sitting with his feet clear of the ground; this may explain why the photoplethysmograph changes are less than would be expected in the presence of ulceration and are not fully representative. Also of relevance, this patient declined surgery so that treatment was given by compression sclerotherapy to the varicose vein running to the foot; this successfully obliterated it and the ulcer healed, even though the long saphenous vein itself was not closed off, suggesting that the foot vein was the determining factor in ulceration here.*

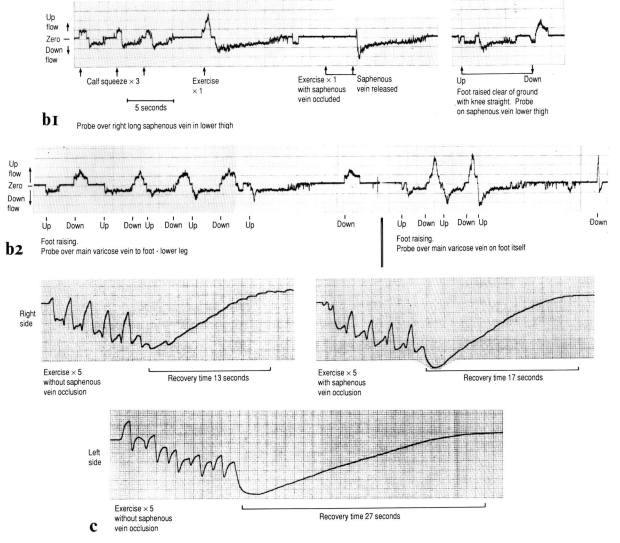

**a**

**b1**

Up flow — Zero — Down flow

Calf squeeze × 3     Exercise × 1     Exercise × 1 with saphenous vein occluded     Saphenous vein released

5 seconds

Up     Down
Foot raised clear of ground with knee straight. Probe on saphenous vein lower thigh

Probe over right long saphenous vein in lower thigh

**b2**

Up flow — Zero — Down flow

Up  Down  Up  Down  Up  Down  Up  Down  Up     Down     Up  Down  Up  Down  Up     Down

Foot raising.
Probe over main varicose vein to foot - lower leg

Foot raising.
Probe over main varicose vein on foot itself

**c**

Right side

Exercise × 5 without saphenous vein occlusion     Recovery time 13 seconds

Exercise × 5 with saphenous vein occlusion     Recovery time 17 seconds

Left side

Exercise × 5 without saphenous vein occlusion     Recovery time 27 seconds

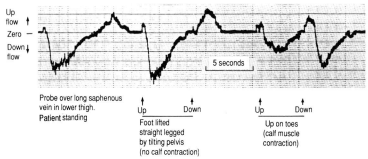

**d1**

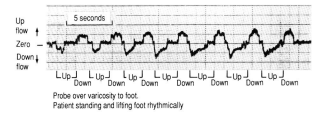

**d2**

**Figure 4.8** *(continued)*
*(d) Further studies in a similar patient. With a Doppler probe:*
  *1. Over the long saphenous vein in the thigh, showing the considerable downflow caused by raising the foot off the ground and the upsurge at thigh level when it is replaced again.*
  *2. With the probe over a large varicosity leading to the foot the tracing shows almost equal components of downflow and upward surge when the foot is raised up and down from the ground. At this level the pattern is one of heavy surge rather than predominantly downward flow. Each upsurge will be accompanied by a sharp increase in pressure at ankle level before this is dissipated up the length of the limb*

Thus, it is possible to recognize that some patients are born with too few valves, whilst a larger group have an adequate number of valves which eventually break down; these categories are not sharply separated as all gradations between the two extremes are found. However, it is reasonable to conclude that underdevelopment of superficial valves, in number and in quality, can be a decisive factor in the causation of incompetence; moreover, phlebography suggests that in some patients there is an accompanying deficiency in deep vein valves, possibly causing a weak pumping mechanism unable to cope with heavy downflow in superficial incompetence (Tibbs and Fletcher, 1983, and see Figure 4.17 and Chapters 6 and 7). A separate factor is that well-developed valves in adequate number commonly acquire incompetence and here the vein wall may be at fault. As regards the inbetween group, it is not rare to find only a single, sacculated valve in an otherwise valveless saphenous vein and perhaps the patient with a low valve count is at particular risk because the breakdown of the few valves that are present may occur more readily and have greater significance than in the limb well endowed with valves.

**Figure 4.9** *Diagrams illustrating the shift of venous blood that occurs when a patient with a large venous plexus under the foot is walking. The likely accompanying venous pressures in the 'ulcer area' just above the ankle are also indicated.*

*1. Patient has been standing still for 30 seconds with weight fully on foot; all veins are filled except those under the foot.*
*2, 3. Patient rising onto the forefoot so that venous plexus on its underside starts to fill as the heel lifts. The accompanying contraction of muscles in the leg causes emptying of its deep veins, first in the lower part, and then in the upper part.*
*4. The foot is now clear of the ground and the foot venous plexus rapidly fills. The leg deep veins, previously emptied, are slack and ready to accept inflow from any source. Venous pressure is rising quickly by inflow crossing the capillary beds, but mainly by downflow in leg varicosities.*

*5. The heel returns to the ground and compression of the foot veins commences. A strong upward surge in both superficial and deep veins starts, and pressure rises rapidly.*
*6. Full body weight is now resting upon the plantigrade foot and the contents of the foot plexus have been forcibly ejected upwards to cause a sharp rise in venous pressure within the deep and superficial veins of the lower leg. The respite from full venous pressure has been small and brief. An effective support – either elastic or inelastic – to the foot can prevent this undesirable accumulation of blood under the foot whenever it is raised, but the surgical removal, or obliteration by sclerotherapy, of the varicosity delivering the downrush of venous blood can be curative*

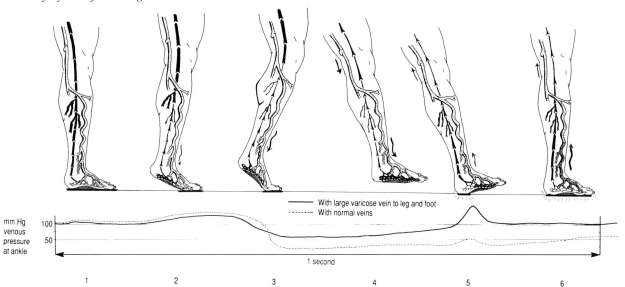

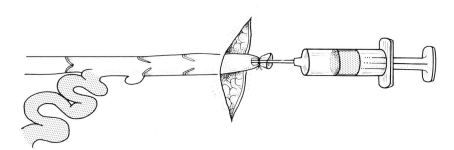

**Figure 4.10** *The syringe test carried out during surgery to confirm incompetence in a vein before removing it. A cannula has been inserted into the divided upper end of the long saphenous vein to allow normal saline from a 20 ml syringe to be sent down the vein. If fully competent valves are present there will be an immediate resistance, but if the valves are incompetent, or absent, there will be no resistance and, in many cases, saccules or varicosities may be seen to bulge as the syringe empties. This gives immediate confirmation that the pathway of incompetence has been correctly identified. Partial resistance indicates valves which are leaking but capable of delaying flow and here the test is best viewed as being indecisive. Care must be taken to ensure that the tip of the cannula is not in the cusp of a high-level valve as this would give a false impression of resistance*

## Clinical aspects of superficial vein incompetence – varicose veins and saccules

### Occurrence and predisposing factors

Many more women are seen with varicose veins than men but this does not accurately reflect the true incidence because women whose veins are clearly visible will seek advice more readily than men whose veins are hidden from sight. Probably men have an inherent weakness as commonly as women but are not exposed to the same stresses of hormonal changes, particulary pregnancy, so that the incidence in men appearing for treatment is about one-third of that in women.

The family history given by so many patients suggests strongly that valvular weakness leading to varicose veins is inherited (Ludbrook and Beale, 1962; Dodd and Cockett, 1976; Gundersen, 1977). This is further supported by the comparatively frequent appearance of varicose veins in young people of both sexes in their early teens or even younger (Widmer, Mall and Martin; 1977; Belcaro, 1986; Quaile and Rowland, 1986; Schultz-Ehrenburg and Weindorf, 1986). It seems that men and women are endowed either with robust valves that will stand up to all the stresses of life, or, with valves (and vein walls) that are weak in varying degree and will fail accordingly. Incidence by ethnic group (whether inherited or influenced by life-style) is more problematical; the traditional view is that varicose veins are much more prevalent in European than in African, Middle Eastern or Asiatic people (Lorenzi et al., 1986), but Thulesius, Gjores and Berlin (1986) have some reservations on this because many series are based upon attendance at hospital rather than the actual occurrence within the population.

The findings of the extensive Basle Studies between 1959 and 1978 (Widmer et al., 1981, 1986) are well worth summarizing here. These were carried out on 'apparently healthy employees of the Basle chemical industry', with a maximal number of 6329 subjects, 77% men and 23% women, with slight variation in these proportions over the period of the study. This study does include people with enlarged veins due to deep vein impairment but these would form only a small percentage of an active workforce; age at the outset varied from 15 to 64 years but many were seen again when 10 years older. It was found that 55% of all leg complaints were related to varicose veins; the other 45% had a variety of other conditions, mainly arterial, orthopaedic, rheumatic or neurological. Fifty-six per cent of men aged between 25 and 75 years had 'varicosities of all types and degree' but not necessarily of medical importance, 9% had varicose veins of medical significance and a further 3% had 'pathological varicosity'. It was estimated that of the general population in Switzerland, 1 in 50 adults (2.0%) had medically significant venous problems and 1 in 17 (5.9%)

had potential venous problems for the future. Of young adults 0.5% had medically significant venous disease but the corresponding figure in the oldest patients was 9%. Factors giving increased risk of developing venous changes were found to be:

1. *Age.* In the older patient minor varicose veins were six times, and 'trunk' (major) varicosities ten times, more likely to be found than in the young patient.
2. *Hereditary.* 'Trunk' varicose veins were 2.4 times more common when a definite family history of varicosities was given.
3. *Overweight.* 'Trunk' varicose veins were 1.9 times more common in overweight subjects.
4. *Pregnancy.* 'Trunk' varicose veins were 1.6 times more common in women who had been pregnant (but an element of selection diminishing this figure is admitted by nature of employment).
5. *Use of the contraceptive pill.* No significant relationship was found.
6. *Incidence in men and women.* Minor varicose blemishes were 1.5 times more common in women but no great difference was found in the incidence of major varicose veins in the two sexes. However, 3 times more women appeared for treatment.

The authors make a firm distinction between 'venous disorder' of no medical importance and 'venous disease' of definite medical significance.

A report on the incidence of varicose veins in Ireland (Henry and Corless, 1989) gives rather different findings with 13% of adults having varicose veins, women outnumbering men by 3 : 1 and 70% of sufferers over the age of 45 years; those with standing employment and women with many pregnancies showing a higher incidence than average for their age.

Without doubt a most potent stress is pregnancy, in part due to the relaxing effect of hormones on the vein wall, rendering valves incompetent, often for the first time, and partly the physical and haemodynamic effects of the gravid uterus. The effects of pregnancy are reversible but often recovery is only partial and from then on the veins deteriorate gradually over the years, a process accelerated by further pregnancy. However, the influence of the hormones is not confined to pregnancy because at each menstruation the same effects occur in some degree. No doubt there are other stresses, such as prolonged standing, which may determine breakdown or not. Once established, further enlargement is encouraged by exercise and the inevitable downflow this brings, so that the process become self-perpetuating.

### Symptoms

Varicose veins are unsightly and the patient's thoughts may be dominated by concern over their appearance rather than their possible significance. Many will experience an aching or burning discomfort after standing for a while or towards the end of the day; this is worse at period time and may be sufficient to cause the patient to seek advice. The discomfort bears little relationship to the size of the varicosities and often lesser varicosities, superficially placed and of recent appearance, seem to cause the most discomfort. It is difficult to evaluate the psychological upset of a disfiguring condition in these patients but there is no doubt that often the discomfort is very real and can be quite distressing. By contrast, many patients with massive varicosities deny any symptoms and even after successful surgery abolishing the veins will not admit to any improvement in comfort. Another reason why it is so difficult to assess the pain factor is that any discomfort in the limb is understandably blamed on the clearly visible defect of the veins. The possibility of another explanation must never be overlooked but in the absence of any other abnormality it is reasonable to accept the varicose veins as the cause if the discomfort is in their vicinity and has the usual provoking factors of standing and, in women, menstruation. In cases of real doubt a trial of elastic support up to the knee (elasticated tubular stockinette, such as Tubigrip Size D, used as a double layer, or SSB D/E, is very suitable for a temporary requirement of this sort) may give such definite relief that the cause is confirmed.

Many patients do worry about the significance, however, and will compare what lies ahead with the 'dreadful state' endured by their mother (or father) in their later years and a major fear is of severe ulceration even though there is no immediate threat of this. Some patients may be heading towards this but it is by no means inevitable and, in any case, should be preventable. Lifelong massive varicose veins do not necessarily lead to ulceration even if this was so in a parent. As we shall see later on, varicose veins on their own are insufficient to cause ulceration but usually need the added factor of poorly valved or impaired deep veins for this to occur. Assessing the future is an important aspect upon which advice must given in these patients; deterioration is usually slow and even 10 years may show little real change, but once skin changes have appeared ulceration may not be far away. Pruritus or eczema in the vicinity of varicose veins is a common early warning of venotensive skin changes.

Saccules on a saphenous vein, usually in the thigh, are not often noticed by the patients and appear to give little in the way of symptoms. However, a saphena varix (Figure 4.13) at the upper end of the long saphenous vein may be so large that it is noticed by the patient and may be mistaken occasionally for a hernia. Substantial long saphenous incompetence will almost invariably accompany a saphena varix. The complications of varicose veins and associated venous stasis will cause a range of symptoms which are considered in Chapter 6; these include superficial phlebitis, haemorrhage, venous stasis or lipodermatosclerosis and ulceration.

## Clinical examination

The recognition of venous abnormality has already been considered in Chapter 2 and it is sufficient here to summarize the sequence of examination.

The patient is interviewed sitting and a clear understanding of the patient's symptoms obtained so that their relevance to any venous changes may be assessed. It is important to enquire about possible deep vein thrombosis in the past (prolonged swelling, hospitalization or use of anticoagulants), particularly around the time of pregnancy or following major fractures to the lower limbs. The patient is then examined standing on a raised platform of some sort; a strengthened examination couch, with hand-holds on the wall alongside, is very suitable for this purpose.

Inspection of all aspects of the lower limbs must be carried out looking for: (1) the presence and pattern of tortuous veins, including those extending over the foot (Figures 4.14 and 4.15): (2) venous flares (Figure 4.16(a)–(c)) over foot and ankle, indicating stressed veins – the elderly are particularly prone to this change; (3) intradermal venules or spider veins on thigh or leg (Figure 4.16 (d)), these often portray an underlying superficial vein incompetence and must be distinguished from the similar blemishes of middle age without obvious cause (see Chapter 19); (4) any visible sacculations; (5) any evidence of complications such as skin changes, scratch marks, eczema, ulceration or threatened haemorrhage.

Palpation by light touch will often detect enlarged veins and saccules that are not visible; it will also recognize areas of unusual warmth over incompetent veins due to the retrograde flow of blood at true body temperature. Impulse upon coughing denotes absence of functioning valves between abdomen and the examining fingers.

Mapping the veins by use of the tapwave test is essential so that a complete understanding of the arrangement and interconnection of the veins is built up. This may take several minutes but without it varicosities may be incorrectly assumed to arise from the short saphenous vein instead of the long and vice versa. It is also invaluable in detecting an enlarged but concealed long saphenous vein; this is of great importance when skin changes are present. Enlargement of the short saphenous vein in the popliteal fossa is best detected by palpation with the knee relaxed and continuity with varicose veins is confirmed by tapwave. A selective occlusion (Trendelenburg) test must be carried out to the suspected pathway of incompetence that has been mapped out; this is the key test that will give absolute confirmation of incompetence in superficial veins or give warning that this may not be the diagnosis. An unsatisfactory test makes it obligatory that further

**Figure 4.11** *Massive varicosis in the long saphenous system.*

*(a)* *1. A 48-year-old man with a massive varicose vein arising from long saphenous vein in mid-thigh and ramifying over leg and foot; a small ulcer behind the medial malleolus had recently healed with prolonged elevation.*

*2. The same limb 6 months after surgery by flush saphenofemoral ligation, stripping of the saphenous vein down to mid-thigh and removal of the main varicosities by stripping and multiple dissection down to the foot. The skin at the ankle is now healthy and all significant veins have gone (and see (a)6).*

*3, 4. The uppermost bend on the main thigh varicosity distended after removal to show sacculation and apparent weakening of the wall. The same vein is also shown after it has been laid open; the irregular interior and mouths of saccules are obvious and two inadequate cusps can be faintly seen in the lower part. This process in a branch vein is somewhat different from the saccule below valves found in the saphenous vein itself and suggests an inherent loss of integrity in the wall structure. See Chapter 1 and Figure 1.16 on whether this is a primary defect or secondary to stress from valve failure.*

*5. Preoperative Doppler flowmetry and photoplethysmography. The directional Doppler recordings show characteristic downflow after calf squeezing and exercise. The lower two tracings are of simultaneous recordings from Doppler flowmeter with the probe over the saphenous vein in the lower thigh and a*

*photoplethysmograph with the sensor over the lower leg. Here, a variant of the usual tests has been used; the limb has been swung from a downward position up to 45 degrees elevation and then returned vertically downwards. This has been done twice, first without any occlusion to the long saphenous vein and the second time with occlusion by finger pressure in the thigh. Without occlusion, the Doppler flowmeter shows strong flow towards the groin as the leg is elevated and this is accompanied by marked venous emptying shown on the plethysmogram. When the leg is swung down again to the vertical position, the Doppler flowmeter shows strong downward flow dwindling away over 10 seconds; in parallel with this the plethysmogram shows venous refilling over the same time. When the manoeuvre is repeated with the saphenous vein occluded, only slight Doppler movement occurs because the vein is blocked; with elevation the plethysmogram shows venous emptying as before but when the leg is swung down to the vertical position venous refilling takes more than 25 seconds, that is, it has reverted to normal. This and other similar manoeuvres gave conclusive evidence that massive incompetence in the long saphenous vein was the cause for venous hypertension and ulceration at the ankle. In these circumstances surgery removing the long saphenous vein is strongly indicated (and see page 65).*

*6. Postoperative photoplethysmogram, 6 months later. This has returned to normal recovery time (and see (a)2) (and see page 65).*

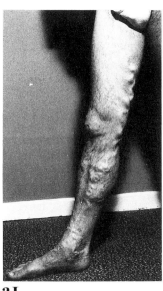

**a1**

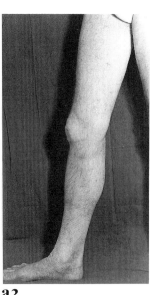

**a2**

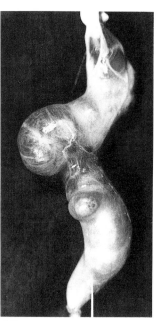

**a3**

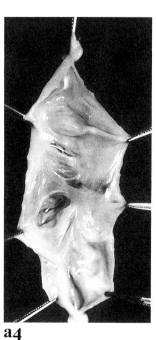

**a4**

```
Up
flow
Zero
Down
flow

   Cough   Calf squeeze   Exercise        Exercise              Exercise
   × 1        × 3          × 1             × 1                    × 1
                                                           On ⌐──────┐ Off
Doppler probe on long saphenous vein in lower thigh         Long saphenous
                                                           vein occluded
```

**a5**

**a** *(continued)*

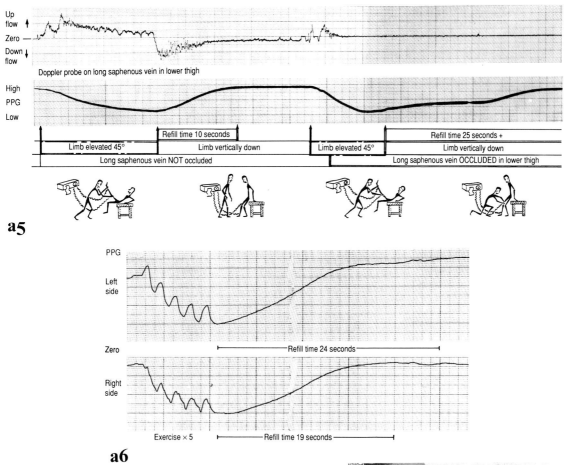

**a5**

**a6**

**Figure 4.11** *(continued)*

*(b) A 35-year-old man more worried by appearance than discomfort. The thigh portion of the long saphenous vein forms the first part of a pathway of incompetence and is seen to be very enlarged with at least two saccules on it. The second part of the pathway is formed from a large varicosity arising from the saphenous vein at knee level and breaking into tributaries down the leg, which run variously to perforators on its inner and antero-lateral aspects. Further varicosities run to the foot. All these veins were easily controlled by fingertip compression of the saphenous vein in the thigh; characteristic Doppler flowmeter downflow was shown after exercise. In spite of the large veins and many intradermal venules there was no skin pigmentation or threat of ulceration near the ankle which suggests that the musculovenous pumping mechanism is strong and fully able to deal with the burden of superficial vein downflow. This was confirmed by photoplethysmography at near normal level*

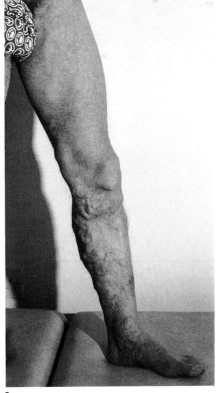

**b**

examination by the special investigations should be carried out before surgery can be decided upon.

Perthes' test can often give clear support to the diagnosis of superficial incompetence with the additional information that the deep veins and the musculovenous pump are in good order. In neither this test nor in Trendelenburg's test should any form of tourniquet be used as this can give misleading results (Bjordal, 1977; Tibbs and Fletcher, 1983; Tibbs 1986). It is a good routine to use the Doppler flowmeter on all patients, to confirm the clinical findings, even though this is perhaps not strictly necessary; quite often this gives additional information and it does ensure complete familiarity with this valuable diagnostic tool.

In most cases with varicosities this system of examination will give a positive diagnosis upon which a decision for treatment can be made without further diagnostic examination. However, it is a good time, with all the facts fresh in mind, to plan the details of any surgical operation required and this should be recorded clearly in the notes at this stage so that only confirmation and marking out is needed immediately before operation. In other cases the special diagnostic tests will be needed.

### Special diagnostic investigation

The special investigations are summarized below.

The simplest non-invasive general test is by the directional Doppler flowmeter applied to the superficial veins (Tibbs and Fletcher, 1983; Hubner and Schultz-Erhenburg, 1986; Sakaguchi et al., 1986; Mitchell and Darke, 1987). The standing patient is exercised with the flowmeter lightly applied over the suspected pathway of incompetence, either a saphenous vein or a varicose vein. A characteristic pattern of downflow is diagnostic of a retrograde circuit of superficial incompetence; upflow, accentuated by exercise, is almost diagnostic of impaired deep veins; a surge up and down suggests an overall absence of valves. The response to raising the foot, with knee straight, will give an indication of any significant venous pooling in the foot. Use of the Doppler is described in Chapter 24.

The photoplethysmograph is useful but usually only decisive when venous stasis is present. A normal recovery time after exercise indicates either a normal venous state or superficial varicosities (backed by a good deep vein pump) not sufficient to cause any serious imbalance in the venous state of the limb. An abnormally short recovery time is in keeping with either massive superficial incompetence or deep vein problems, such as valve deficiency or impairment by previous deep vein thrombosis. If finger occlusion of a suspected pathway of superficial incompetence, (but not with a tourniquet) restores a near normal recovery time then this is clear confirmation of this diagnosis. Failure to change the short recovery time by any manipulation points strongly to

deep vein problems and a phlebogram may be necessary to make a proper diagnosis. Photoplethysmography is described in Chapter 24.

Functional phlebography is not usually necessary in states of uncomplicated varicosities but may be needed to outline a short saphenous termination or to locate the precise origin of recurrent varicosities in order to plan an operation. When varicosites are complicated by venotensive changes and ulceration, then phlebography is valuable to confirm or exclude a concealed long saphenous incompetence which should respond to surgery. This will be considered presently. During phlebology, the characteristic features of superficial incompetence to be looked for in response to exercise in the upright position are: downflow in superficial veins and in through perforators to the deep veins; with exercise the opaque medium travels up the deep veins but spills over at a high level into the superficial veins to be recycled down them once more. This last phenomenon is a hallmark of the condition and gives clear support to the likely benefits of surgical removal of the incompetent veins. The technique of this valuable investigation is described in detail in Chapter 22.

## Incompetence in the long saphenous system: the typical configuration

### The incompetent long saphenous vein: saccule formation

The commonest cause for varicosities is incompetence in the long saphenous vein and its branches (Figures 4.3–4.5, 4.11). This vein forms the first part of a pathway of incompetence. The long saphenous vein itself is usually (Figure 4.12) too robust to respond to the reversed flow within it by developing tortuosity and, beyond enlargement, may show little obvious change. However, it does often develop a saccule immediately below one or more of the leaking valves and these are usually readily palpable in the standing patient and often clearly visible. The saphena varix is a saccule of this sort situated in the uppermost part of the long saphenous vein and, presumably, given its own name because of the distinctive bulge it causes in the groin (Figure 4.13). Absence of any detectable saccule tells us little, but the presence of even one is absolute evidence of substantial leakage in the underlying valve and, by implication, also in valves above and below it; in other words the existence of a retrograde circuit based on that vein.

### The varicose veins

Usually the second part of the pathway of incompetence is formed by one or more major branches of the saphenous vein taking off at any level (Figures 4.4, 4.11

**Figure 4.12**  *The long saphenous vein seldom shows tortuosity in its thigh portion although it occasionally does so below the knee. However, an example is shown of marked tortuosity in a man of 28 years who first developed enlarged veins for which medical advice was sought at the age of 8 years (a). At operation it was found that each tortuosity corresponded to a large saccule on the outer angle of a bend and valve remnants were present above these. It seems that some form of congenital weakness leading to early valve failure and sacculation was present; no other vascular abnormality was found and the limb was the same length as the opposite side. In all other respects this was a typical long saphenous incompetence with large varicosities arising from it, at and below the knee, and early skin changes were present near the ankle. The Doppler flowmeter tracing is typical of simple long saphenous incompetence with a substantial foot component (b). Appropriate surgery gave a good result*

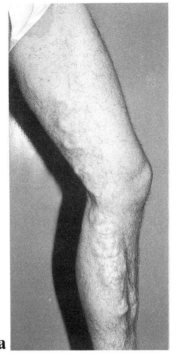
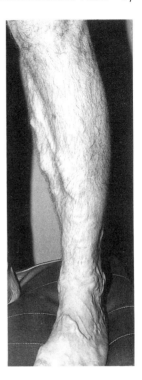

**a**

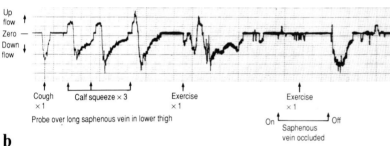
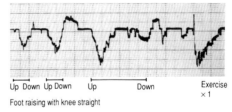

**b**

**Figure 4.13**  *(a) A saphena varix in the left groin (1) with the usual accompanying gross incompetence in the long saphenous vein and varicosities down the limb (2 – see page 68). The saphena varix gave a strong cough impulse with a typical thrill; the tapwave test showed clear intercommunication between the varix and the varicose veins in the leg. A large varicosity can be seen running from the upper calf, across the front of the leg, breaking into tributaries running into anterolateral perforating veins and across the outer aspect of the ankle and foot to its underside. Skin changes with threatened ulceration were present over this varicosity in the lower outer leg; complete control of all varicose veins by finger-tip compression of the saphenous vein was easily achieved and in all respects this was a typical simple long saphenous incompetence. The Doppler tracings are also shown (b) (see page 68). Surgery, with stripping of the long saphenous vein to the upper calf and detailed removal of the large varicosities in the leg, gave a good result*

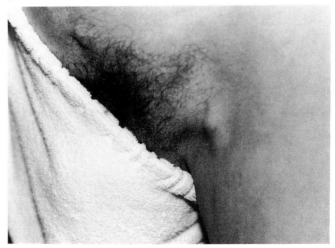

**a1**

**Figure 4.13** *(continued)*

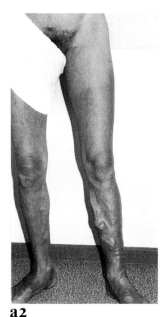

**a2**

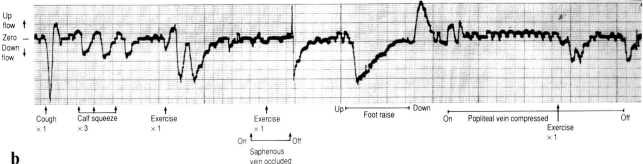

**b**

and 4.14) and winding down to one of the muscle groups in the front or back of the leg (Figure 4.15), to the deep veins of the lower leg or across the ankle (Figures 4.7, 4.8 and 4.16) to the underside of the foot. Almost any combination of this distribution can be encountered and it often breaks into many small tributaries before merging with perforators taking the flow into the deep veins. Intradermal venules in the vicinity may become greatly distended to give rise to venous flares, a sure sign of venous stress, especially marked below the ankle and inner foot. The general pattern of long saphenous incompetence is summarized in Figure 4.3 and the many variants on this are described in Chapter 5. Composite functional phlebograms of long saphenous incompetence are shown in Figures 4.5 and 4.17.

## Concealed or 'straight-through' incompetence

Less frequently there may be no intervening branches between the saphenous vein and the perforating vein inlets so that massive incompetence exists without varicosities and gives a 'concealed' form of incompetence; this is an important diagnostic pitfall as it may well be the cause of venous hypertension and ulceration (Figures 4.18–4.20).

**Figure 4.14** *Perforator surge and special investigations in long saphenous incompetence (see page 69).*

*(a) Long saphenous vein incompetence with a large varicosity taking off in the thigh and running a tortuous course down to the lower third of the leg where it breaks into various tributaries; pigmentation with threatened ulceration was present. The upper part of the long saphenous vein was grossly incompetent and the varicosity arose from this in the lower thigh. There was no suggestion of an incompetent perforator in this vicinity and its origin is in keeping with the great majority of varicosities arising at this level in the thigh. In the lower third of the leg an enlarged perforating vein was present (confirmed at surgery) underlying the bulge seen in the photograph.*

*(b) Doppler flow, however, amply confirmed that the predominant flow in this perforator was inward but that there was a component of outward flow at the moment of muscle contraction, giving an initial surge outwards immediately followed by prolonged inward flow on muscle relaxation. The upflow induced artificially by popliteal compression is commonly found in long saphenous incompetence. The major defect is incompetence in the long saphenous vein and its varicose branch, and removal of this pathway of incompetence is essential in treatment. However, the enlarged perforator should also be removed since otherwise its outward surge would become dominant and tend to maintain any surviving varicosities in the leg and give retrograde flow to the foot.*

*(c) Photoplethysmogram of this patient is also shown. Appropriate surgery gave a good result*

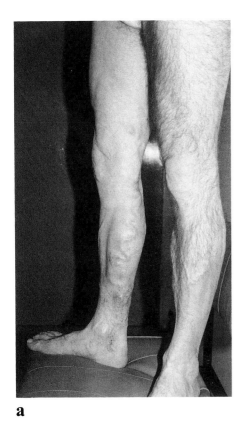

**a**

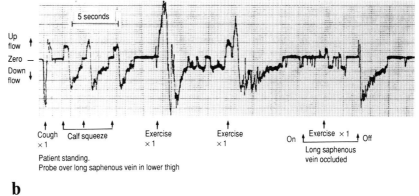

Up flow ↑
Zero —
Down flow ↓

5 seconds

Cough
× 1

Calf squeeze

Exercise
× 1

Exercise
× 1

On   Exercise × 1   Off

Patient standing.
Probe over long saphenous vein in lower thigh

Long saphenous
vein occluded

**b**

Up flow ↑
Zero —
Down flow ↓

5 seconds

Foot
raised

Foot
down

On

Small
exercise × 1

Full
exercise × 1

Off

Popliteal compression

**b** *(continued)*

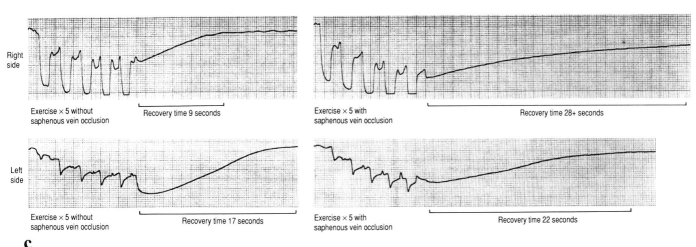

Right
side

Exercise × 5 without
saphenous vein occlusion

Recovery time 9 seconds

Exercise × 5 with
saphenous vein occlusion

Recovery time 28+ seconds

Left
side

Exercise × 5 without
saphenous vein occlusion

Recovery time 17 seconds

Exercise × 5 with
saphenous vein occlusion

Recovery time 22 seconds

**c**

**Figure 4.14** *(continued)*

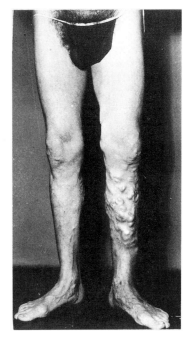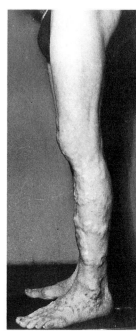

**Figure 4.15** *Massive long saphenous incompetence extending onto the foot. A saccule is visible in the lower thigh giving rise to slight tortuosity, and below this, a massive leash of varicosities arises and runs across the front of the leg to disperse into tributaries running to anterolateral, soleal and posterior tibial muscles, and also down to the lateral aspect of the foot (Mr S. Rose's case)*

**Figure 4.16** *Superficial incompetence and venous flares on the foot and ankle.*

*(a) 1, 2. Patient aged 53 with a large varicosity arising from long saphenous vein in the mid-thigh and giving off branches to lower leg and foot. An area of pigmentation and*

*induration is present on the mid-calf; a flare of venules overlies varicosities of the foot.*
*3. Doppler flowmetry shows downflow typical of saphenous incompetence and on photoplethysmography a recovery period of 5 seconds improves to 12 seconds with selective saphenous occlusion (and see page 71).*

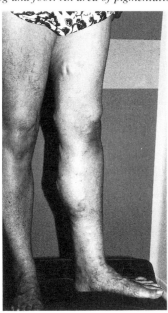

**a1**

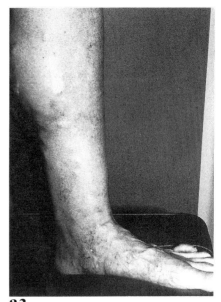

**a2**

**a3**

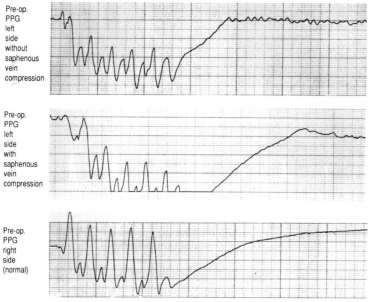

Pre-op.
PPG
left
side
without
saphenous
vein
compression

Pre-op.
PPG
left
side
with
saphenous
vein
compression

Pre-op.
PPG
right
side
(normal)

**a3** *(continued)*

*4. Surgery gave a good result and 6 months later photoplethysmography is normal at over 20 seconds.*

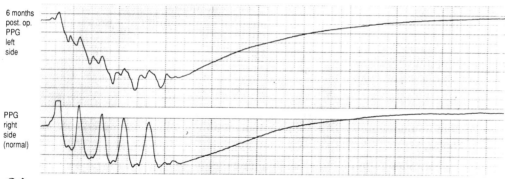

6 months
post. op.
PPG
left
side

PPG
right
side
(normal)

**a4**

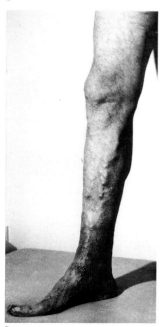

**b1**

**Figure 4.16** *(continued)*

*(b) 1. Patient aged 74 years with gross incompetence of the long saphenous vein which runs down to the lower leg before giving off varicose veins; it is associated with a marked flare of distended venules on ankle and foot.*

*(Figure 4.16 continued on page 72)*

*2. Photoplethysmogram confirms moderate hypertension with a recovery period of 10 seconds which improves to 25 seconds with selective saphenous occlusion; surgery gave a correspondingly good result.*

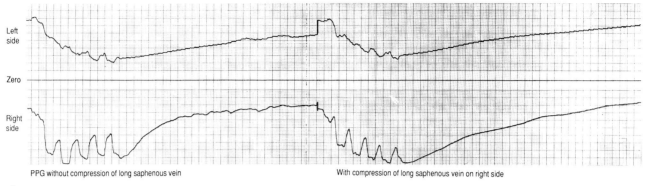

**b2**

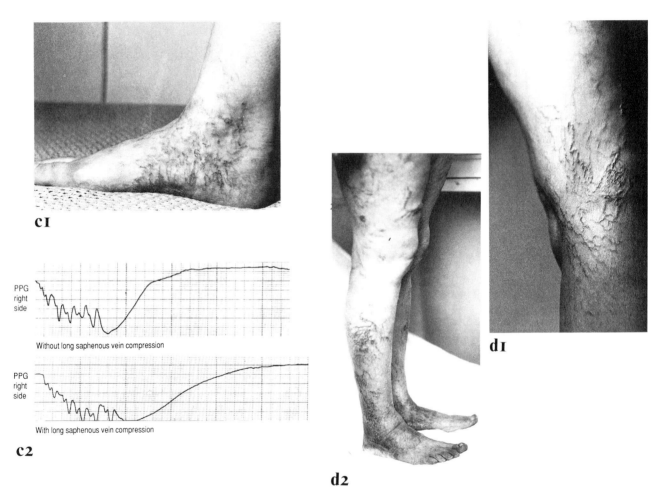

**c1**

**c2**

**d1**

**d2**

**Figure 4.16** *continued)*

*(c) This female, aged 58, complained of the flare of veins on the foot illustrated (1) and a feeling of heaviness. An enlarged long saphenous vein was palpable and Doppler flowmetry confirmed substantial incompetence; photoplethysmography (2) improved from under 10 seconds to over 15 with selective saphenous compression. The patient wished to have no more than local sclerotherapy which gave a considerable improvement but is likely to deteriorate again because the underlying fault of saphenous incompetence has not been properly eliminated.*

*(d) 1,2. Examples of extensive intradermal venules due to underlying superficial vein incompetence. Treatment by sclerotherapy to venules and underlying veins gave a good result*

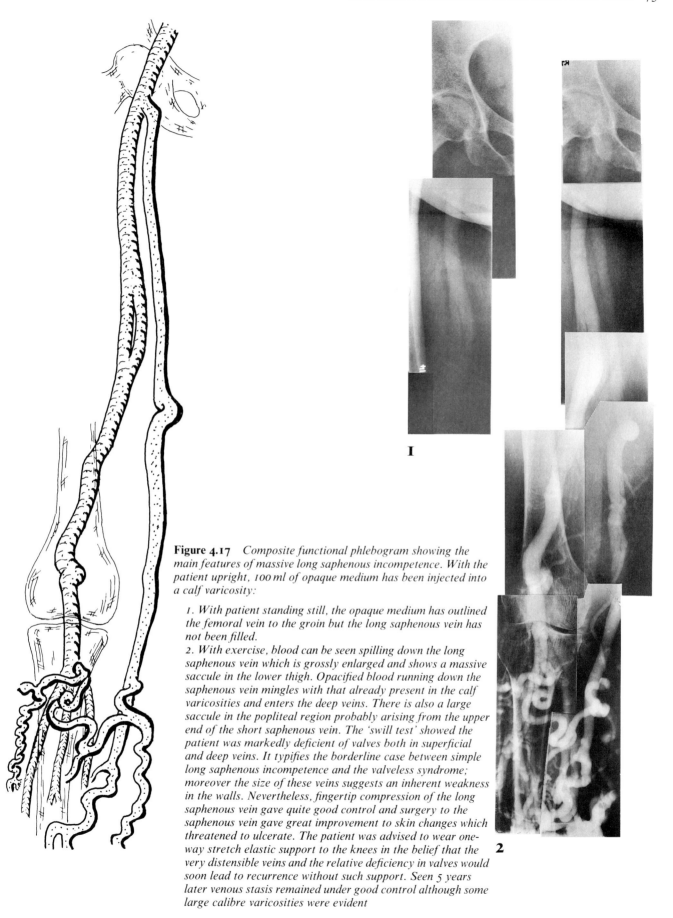

**Figure 4.17**    *Composite functional phlebogram showing the main features of massive long saphenous incompetence. With the patient upright, 100 ml of opaque medium has been injected into a calf varicosity:*

*1. With patient standing still, the opaque medium has outlined the femoral vein to the groin but the long saphenous vein has not been filled.*

*2. With exercise, blood can be seen spilling down the long saphenous vein which is grossly enlarged and shows a massive saccule in the lower thigh. Opacified blood running down the saphenous vein mingles with that already present in the calf varicosities and enters the deep veins. There is also a large saccule in the popliteal region probably arising from the upper end of the short saphenous vein. The 'swill test' showed the patient was markedly deficient of valves both in superficial and deep veins. It typifies the borderline case between simple long saphenous incompetence and the valveless syndrome; moreover the size of these veins suggests an inherent weakness in the walls. Nevertheless, fingertip compression of the long saphenous vein gave quite good control and surgery to the saphenous vein gave great improvement to skin changes which threatened to ulcerate. The patient was advised to wear one-way stretch elastic support to the knees in the belief that the very distensible veins and the relative deficiency in valves would soon lead to recurrence without such support. Seen 5 years later venous stasis remained under good control although some large calibre varicosities were evident*

**Figure 4.18** *Diagrams to illustrate the difference between:*

*(a) The usual pattern of long saphenous incompetence in which varicosities are clearly visible as the lower part of the pathway of incompetence.*

*(b) The concealed or 'straight-through' variety in which the long saphenous vein empties by retrograde flow directly into perforating veins without any intervening varicosities. This is a common cause of venous stasis and ulceration with only minimal or no varicosities being visible*

**Figure 4.19** *Clinical photographs of concealed or 'straight-through' incompetence. All three patients are relatively slim so that superficial veins are easily seen.*

*(a) A prominent long saphenous vein is present below the knee with little evidence of varicose veins. Pigmentation and two crusted ulcers are present near the ankle. Clinical tests and special investigations confirmed heavy downflow in the long saphenous vein typical of simple incompetence, and surgery removing this gave a good result.*

*(b) A similar patient in whom only one comparatively small varicose vein at the knee can be seen even though venous stasis with pigmentation and threatened ulcer is present at the ankle. Testing by tapwave detected an enlarged long saphenous vein up to the groin and finger occlusion of this in the thigh controlled the single varicosity; Doppler flowmetry showed the typical downward flow of simple incompetence.*

*(c) An example of comparatively concealed incompetence. The long saphenous vein can be seen from the lower thigh downwards but the only varicose veins evident are a slender one meandering from the groin to the knee and another running across the inner ankle to the foot. All tests confirmed heavy incompetence in the saphenous vein itself with subsidiary incompetence in the thigh and foot varicosities. Venostatic changes were present but healed after surgery removing the saphenous vein*

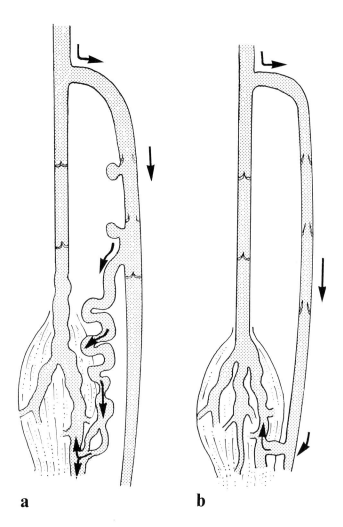

a             b

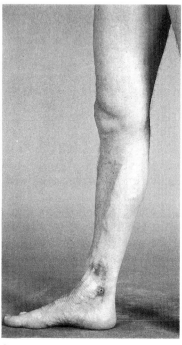
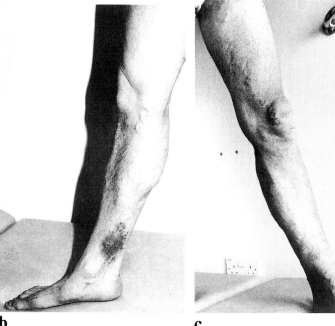

a         b         c

**Figure 4.20** *Concealed incompetence of the long saphenous vein.*

*(a)* 1, 2. *This patient, a female of 62 years, was worried by purple areas of severe venous congestion on ankle and foot. All superficial veins showed easily because the patient was thin, but on the affected (right) side the long saphenous vein and its branches to the foot showed obvious enlargement but no tortuosity.*

*3. Doppler tracing from long saphenous vein in upper leg shows downflow after exercise characteristic of simple incompetence.*

*4. Directional Doppler tracing and photoplethysmogram obtained simultaneously in concealed long saphenous incompetence. Photoplethysmogram carried out simultaneously shows that recovery of venous pressure mirrors the decline of saphenous downflow as the pressures' differences creating flow equalize. The photoplethysmogram shows a brief recovery period at 8 seconds but temporary occlusion of the saphenous vein causes it to revert to a normal value, with the absence of downflow. Appropriate removal of this vein relieved the patient's symptoms and the skin discolouration disappeared (see page 76).*

*(b)* 1. *Patient aged 58 with a history of two attacks of superficial phlebitis some years previously now has discomfort and marked tendency for swelling of the right foot and ankle. No varicose veins were evident but pigmented venotensive change and threatened ulceration were present; the long saphenous vein was easily detectable with the tapwave test.*

*2. Doppler flowmetry confirms substantial incompetence in the saphenous vein. Photoplethysmography shows recovery period is shortened to 7 seconds but improves to 14 seconds with selective long saphenous compression. Appropriate surgery gave a good result (see page 76)*

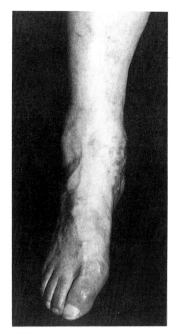

**a1**

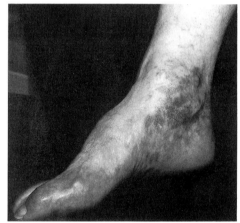

**a2**

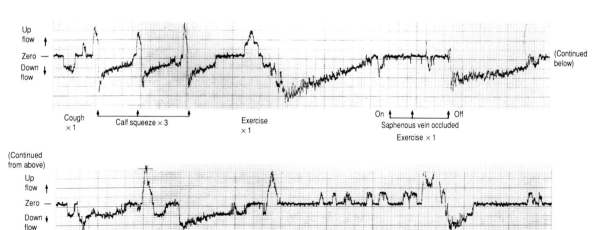

**a3**

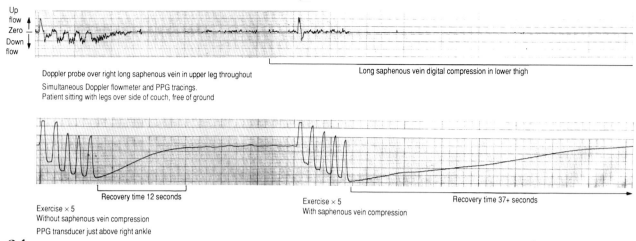

Up flow

Zero

Down flow

Doppler probe over right long saphenous vein in upper leg throughout

Simultaneous Doppler flowmeter and PPG tracings.
Patient sitting with legs over side of couch, free of ground

Long saphenous vein digital compression in lower thigh

Recovery time 12 seconds

Exercise × 5
Without saphenous vein compression

PPG transducer just above right ankle

Exercise × 5
With saphenous vein compression

Recovery time 37+ seconds

**a4**

**Figure 4.20** *(continued)*

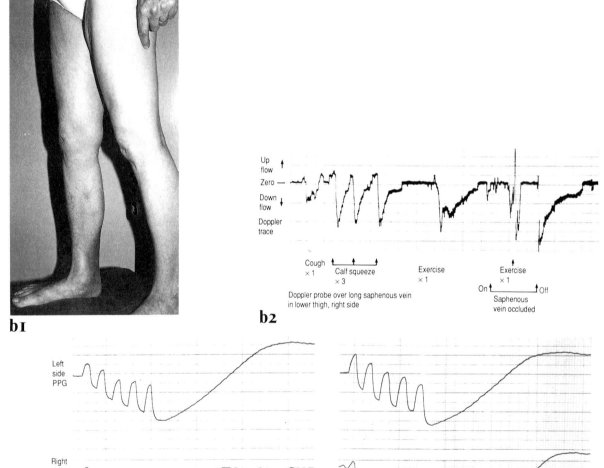

Up flow

Zero

Down flow

Doppler trace

Cough × 1

Calf squeeze × 3

Exercise × 1

Exercise × 1

On          Off

Saphenous vein occluded

Doppler probe over long saphenous vein
in lower thigh, right side

**b1**

**b2**

Left side PPG

Right side PPG

Recovery time 7 seconds

PPG sensors over lower left and right
legs, carried out simultaneously

Recovery time 14 seconds

Right long saphenous vein occluded by finger pressure in lower thigh

**b2**

**Figure 4.20** *(continued)*

**Figure 4.21** *Variations in the pathway of incompetence.*

*(a) Diagram of the bypassing phenomenon commonly seen in the thigh. A varicosity arising from the upper part of the long saphenous vein bypasses a functioning valve in it and rejoins the otherwise incompetent saphenous vein at a lower level. Thus the first part of the pathway of incompetence is formed by a varicosity instead of the long saphenous vein itself. Many variations of this may be encountered at all levels in the limb and, as in the diagram, the varicosity may wander in an upward direction for a short distance to give apparently contradictory direction of flow. In the example shown, control of the lower part of the long saphenous and the varicosities arising from it would be given by temporary compression of the thigh varicosity, but compression of the upper half of the saphenous vein would not do so. Moreover, a Doppler flowmeter would not find retrograde downflow in the upper saphenous vein but would do so in the varicosity, in the saphenous vein in lower thigh and its varicose branch on the leg.*

*(b) A clinical example of the bypassing phenomenon illustrated in (a).*

*1. After emptying the veins by elevation of the limb, pressure has been applied over a thigh varicosity and the patient asked to stand. After 20 seconds there is still no evidence of varicose veins in thigh or leg.*

*2. Upon removing compression, a large varicosity immediately appeared and could be seen to fill rapidly in a downward direction, followed by appearance of enlarged veins and varicosities in the leg. The thigh varicosity breaks into at least two tributaries in its lower part before joining the saphenous vein. Surgery confirmed that the thigh varicosity arose from the anterolateral branch of the uppermost saphenous vein and that a syringe test applied to this met no resistance and caused the varicosity to bulge, but when applied to the saphenous vein itself encountered full resistance by a valve in the upper third of the thigh. Dissection confirmed that the lower tributaries of the varicosity did indeed rejoin the saphenous vein and a syringe test at this level met no resistance and caused the leg varicosities to bulge. Appropriate surgery removing the thigh varicosity and the incompetent lower portion of the saphenous vein gave a good result*

## Variations in the pathway of incompetence

The concept of a pathway of incompetence, whether overt with obvious varicosities or concealed without varicosities, is essential to proper understanding of varicose veins and venous stasis. It is the basic component that is always present in some form, underlying all the other variable manifestations, and its accurate indentification is the key to successful treatment. The pathway of incompetence, with any saccules along it and the varicosities in its lower part, is only fully evident and active when the patient is standing and exercising. It runs from above a pumping

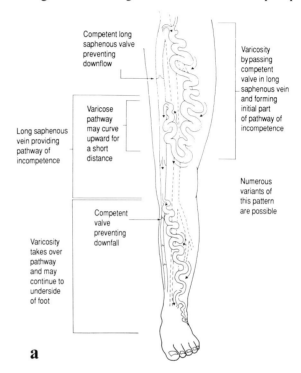

Competent long saphenous valve preventing downflow

Varicosity bypassing competent valve in long saphenous vein and forming initial part of pathway of incompetence

Long saphenous vein providing pathway of incompetence

Varicose pathway may curve upward for a short distance

Numerous variants of this pattern are possible

Competent valve preventing downfall

Varicosity takes over pathway and may continue to underside of foot

**a**

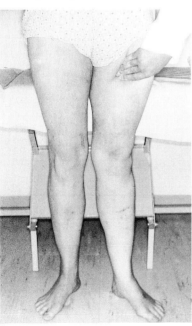

**b1**

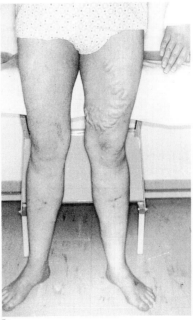

**b2**

mechanism to below it, typically from upper thigh to lower leg, but often follows unexpected routes (Hubner and Schultz-Ehrenburg, 1986; Tibbs, 1986) dictated by any local pressure differences which in turn depend upon such factors as partial function in a valve nearby. Thus, it is not uncommon to find a thigh varicosity meandering outwards from the long saphenous vein, and even upwards for a short distance, before running back into the saphenous vein from which it arose (Figure 4.21). The explanation here is that the varicosity is bypassing a surviving valve in the saphenous vein that is still able to impede downflow and create a pressure difference above and below it. The varicosity has been established on any convenient veins that will convey flow from the higher pressure above the valve to the lower pressure below it even if this involves an upward meander by whatever pathway offers least resistance. The whole process is determined by any veins locally able to allow flow between areas of pressure differences and this may have no anatomical pattern because varicosities so often evolve from the vast network of lesser unnamed veins. Many variations of this sort are encountered at all levels and the most characteristic ones are described in Chapter 5.

## Incompetence of the short saphenous system

The long saphenous system just described typifies the features of superficial vein incompetence, for here they are seen most clearly. The short saphenous system becomes incompetent almost as frequently and varicose veins from this cause are commonplace; all the same principles apply (Figure 4.22(a)) and need not be repeated. The visible pattern of varicosities is characteristically behind the knee and on the back of the calf, but position alone cannot be relied upon to establish the origin of the varicosities (Figure 4.22(b)–(f)). Palpation of the enlarged short saphenous vein behind the semiflexed knee has already been referred to as a valuable pointer. Mapping between calf veins and the short saphenous behind the knee is usually easy and convincing. Intercommunication between long and short systems frequently occurs and long saphenous varicosities often wind round to the back of the calf, so that it cannot be assumed that a varicosity here is short saphenous; this is one of the common causes of unsuccessful results to surgery. The only safe method is to demonstrate by the tapwave test direct continuity of the veins with one system or the other and then to prove this by undoubted control of the varicosities by localized finger pressure over that saphenous vein. More ingenuity in diagnosis is required when varicosities are fed from both systems and this is considered in Chapter 5. Mapping out will alert the examiner to this possibility and compression over long or short saphenous veins individually will fail to control the varicosities, but simultaneous compresssion over both veins will do so.

Surgery should never be employed without a convincing demonstration that temporary occlusion of the suspect vein gives prolonged control of the varicosities and this is especially true in the calf region. A cough impulse over the short saphenous vein implies that there is a wide and valveless deep vein above that point and is not a good augury for the long-term outcome of any surgical procedure.

The directional Doppler flowmeter is valuable for mapping out and thus confirming continuity of varicosities with the short saphenous vein (but do not overlook the possibility of intercommunication between the two systems). Confusion may arise between signals from the underlying popliteal vein and the saphenous vein but valve failure in the two veins may be distinguished by blocking the short saphenous below the transducer which temporarily eliminates the saphenous component. It is usually simplest to place the Doppler over the varicosities at a lower level to avoid this confusion, and then demonstrate that compression of the short saphenous vein causes cessation of flow down them.

Compared with the long saphenous termination there are added factors that make the short saphenous termination more difficult for diagnostician and surgeon:

1. There is much greater variation in the level of termination and in its connections, and these are more inaccessible for diagnosis.
2. Veins from the gastrocnemius muscles, which often include a lateral or medial gastrocnemius vein (or both), may join its terminal portion, so that a high ligation of the short saphenous vein is not possible without also ligating a large muscle vein. Providing there is no evidence of incompetence in this vein, and if there are no other branches joining the final portion, it is permissible to preserve the gastrocnemius vein by ligating the saphenous beneath this level. Ligation of a major muscle branch should not be resorted to unless there is good evidence of incompetence in it, but it must be admitted that no lasting harm appears to arise from depriving the muscle of even a large vein; presumably re-routing occurs readily.
3. Gastrocnemius branches entering the short saphenous may share incompetence with it and lack effective valves so that a pathway of incompetence is formed down the vein, through a venous sinus in the muscle and out through a perforating vein to a superficial set of varicosities. On calf muscle contraction, this type of 'perforator' may pump blood outwards at some pressure and ligation of its upper end concurrently with high saphenous ligation should be carried out (Hobbs, 1988). This condition is considered further in Chapter 11.
4. Surgery is more difficult and offers more danger, partly because of the variable anatomy referred to above but also because of the closeness and variable relationship

**Figure 4.22** *Incompetence in the short saphenous vein.*

*(a)* 1. *Typical configuration of incompetence shown in a composite phlebogram of a short saphenous vein. Its junction with the popliteal vein is the source and the main part of the vein is the pathway of incompetence as far as mid-calf where it emerges through the deep fascia; here a large varicose branch continues the pathway which disperses by further branches, through perforators, into the deep veins.*
2. *Typical Doppler flowmeter tracing from an incompetent short saphenous vein which shows similar features to a long saphenous incompetence; foot raising, with the knee straight, often produces downflow when contraction of calf muscles may not (see page 80).*

*(b)* 1–4. *Short saphenous incompetence encircling the upper calf in a female patient, aged 28 years, a keen athlete, with discomfort and unsightly varicose veins. The varicosities arise from the short saphenous vein, palpable and confirmed by tapwave test; the anterior varicose vein joins the long saphenous vein in the upper calf. Doppler flowmetry showed the typical downflow of incompetence in the short saphenous vein, around the leg in its varicose branches and down the long saphenous vein below the point of connection; above this point there was slight flow upwards with exercise. A large short saphenous varicosity extends posteriorly down to the ankle.*
5. *Functional phlebogram (lateral) showing short saphenous vein joining popliteal vein at the most common level; the upper part of the saphenous vein shows three saccules, one close to its termination and confirming its incompetence. The 'necklace' of varicose veins is shown, the larger set is that running on the outer and anterior aspects.*
6. *Composite oblique functional phlebogram. This confirms the flow patterns found by Doppler flowmetry, including entry and flow down the long saphenous to re-enter deep veins by a perforator in the lower leg (see pages 80 and 81).*

*(c)* *Varicosities on the posteromedial aspect of the calf. These could well arise from either long or short saphenous veins, or from both. In this example an enlarged short saphenous vein could be felt behind the knee, a strong tapwave was present showing undoubted continuity between the varicose veins and the short saphenous vein, but not with the long saphenous; control of varicosities was only possible by short saphenous compression; Doppler flowmetry confirmed substantial downflow after exercise or foot raising only in the short saphenous vein and appropriate surgery to this vein gave a good result (see page 81).*

*(d)* *Short saphenous incompetence with a bypassing phenomenon. A varicosity can be seen arising from the short saphenous vein behind the knee and meandering down to rejoin its lower part 5 cm above the ankle. At this point an area of venous stasis and threatened ulceration is present. The opposite leg shows a rather similar state and it is quite common for varicosities to show symmetry in this fashion (see page 81).*

*(e)* *The anteromedial aspect of the knee and upper leg in another patient. Moderate sized varicosities can be seen winding from the vicinity of the long saphenous vein at knee level down to the front of the leg. At one point a vein is covered with only the thinnest layer of skin and is capable of bleeding with minor trauma. These varicosities could easily be assumed to have long saphenous origin but in fact arise from the uppermost part of the short saphenous vein as was proved by tapwave, control by finger pressure over the short saphenous and Doppler flowmeter studies; syringe testing at operation gave further confirmation and appropriate surgery gave a good result. (See page 81; Figure 4.22(f) is on page 82.)*

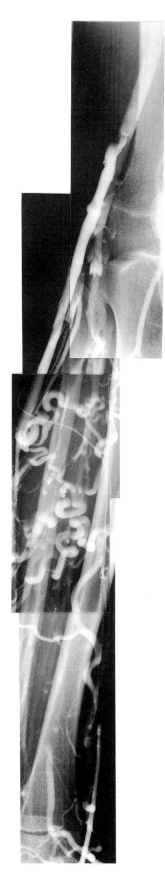

**a** I

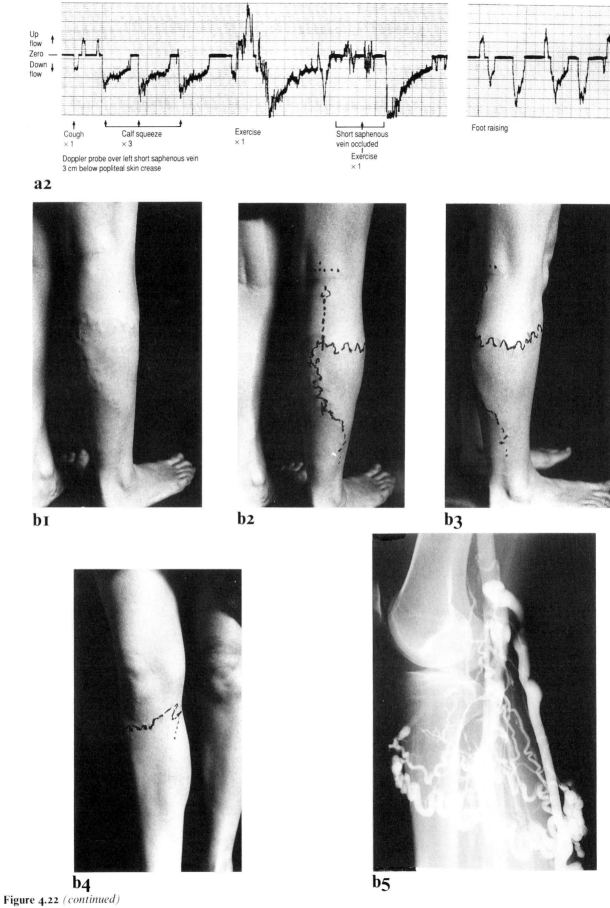

**Figure 4.22** *(continued)*

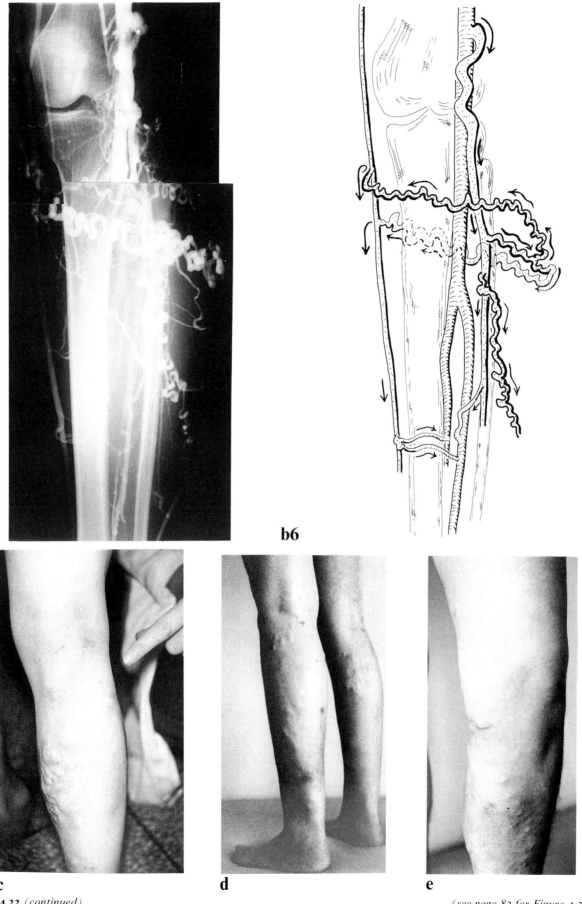

**b6**

c

d

e

**Figure 4.22** *(continued)*

*(see page 82 for Figure 4.22(f))*

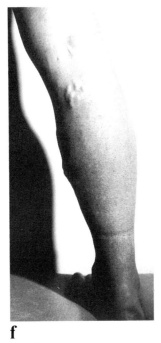

**f**

**Figure 4.22** *(continued)*

*(f) Varicose veins arising from short saphenous vein at high level, and penetrating the fascia to emerge in the upper calf; from here they wind round the inner aspect to long saphenous territory. Note the imprint of sock suggesting mild oedema in the lower leg*

with anatomical structures of major importance, notably the medial and lateral popliteal nerves, and the popliteal artery and vein; large fragile branch veins in a confined space can prove troublesome. High ligation of the short saphenous vein is not suitable for an inexperienced surgeon.

Many of the uncertainties referred to above are avoided by a phlebogram (Figures 4.23, 4.24) or ultrasonography beforehand. This is best carried out as an outpatient

procedure, a day or two beforehand, so that functional venography may be performed as well as an 'upward trace' to reveal anatomy. A preliminary phlebogram on the operating table (Hobbs, 1980; Corcos, Peruzzi and Romeo, 1987) is more limited in its information and the opaque medium, taking the least line of resistance, does not always show anatomy, such as an upward extension to join the long saphenous system, satisfactorily (see Chapter 22). When interpreting the phlebograms it is easy to confuse gastrocnemius veins with the short saphenous itself and care is required here. Recently Duplex and colour flow ultrasonography (discussed in Chapters 23 and 24, and see Figure 2.12 and Colour Plate 24) have been shown to be an excellent non-invasive alternative to phlebology in demonstrating the short saphenous termination (Hobbs, 1988; Nicoliades, Christopoulos and Vasdekis, 1989).

**Figure 4.23** *Unexpected changes and variations in the termination of the short saphenous vein. Variations in the arrangement of branches and in the level of termination are often encountered. In addition unexpected abnormalites may be found and it is advisable for the surgeon to be forewarned of these by phlebography beforehand. These phlebograms above were taken 48 hours before surgery by outpatient attendance. Opaque medium was injected directly into a convenient varicosity on the back of the calf with the patient face down and in a position of slight head up-tilt. Views were taken at various phases of filling and at three angles of rotation. These show clearly unexpected tortuosity in the final portion of short saphenous vein which does however join the deep vein at normal level. An upward extension of the short saphenous vein can be seen and it is advisable that this should be found and ligated at surgery. The tortuous portion is composed of two sacculations which are not fully distended in the phlebogram because the patient is near horizontal. Such sacculations are likely to be fragile, as was indeed the case. It was most helpful for the surgeon to be aware of these possible difficulties and to know that a normal deep vein lay beyond this so that dissection could be continued until this was reached*

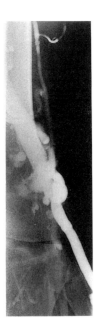
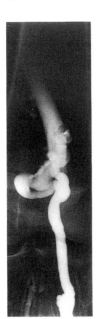
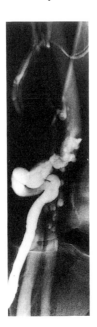
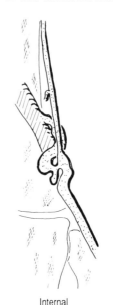
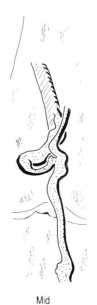
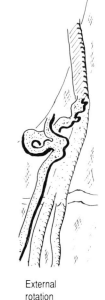

Internal rotation          Mid rotation          External rotation

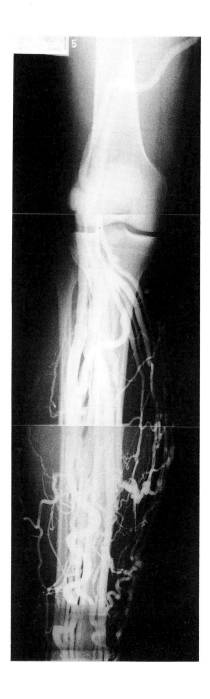
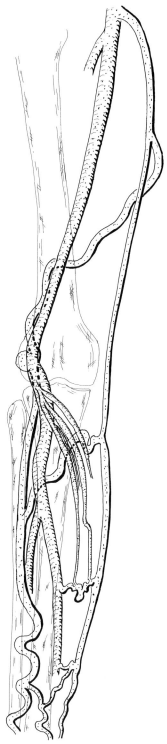

**Figure 4.24**    *A composite phlebogram obtained through a mid-calf varicosity in a man aged 30 with prominent calf veins and marked venotensive changes. This shows an enlarged, tortuous short saphenous vein in the lower leg giving off varicose branches from which the deep veins have filled. In the upper calf the short saphenous is relatively straight and lies just to the inner aspect of the fibula; a large varicose connection runs obliquely from mid short saphenous to join the long saphenous vein in the upper calf. Gastrocnemius veins have filled from calf varicosities but appear normal. A large saccule arises from the short saphenous vein close to its termination and the popliteal vein can be identified. An upward extension of the short saphenous overlies the deep vein and runs across the back of the lower thigh where it is in continuity with the posterolateral branch of the long saphenous vein. Undoubtedly the short saphenous vein is incompetent as shown by its large size, the saccule in its upper part and the tortuosity and varicose branches in the lower part. From this phlebogram it is not possible to decide whether the upward extension is incompetent but at operation it was removed by a stripper passed up from the popliteal fossa. Attempts to display valves during phlebography showed very few and there appeared to be a marked overall deficiency in both deep and superficial veins. The other limb showed a similar lack of valves and in view of this the patient was advised to wear knee-length one-way-stretch stockings as a long-term measure*

Anatomical variants in the upper termination of the short saphenous vein are quite common and include: upward extension to join the profunda femoris or long saphenous veins; connection upwards by a single incompetent pathway to connect with pudendal and pelvic veins; other forms of interconnection between long and short saphenous veins; gastrocnemius branches, sometimes incompetent, joining the terminal short saphenous vein. These are described in Chapter 5 and also Chapters 1, 20 and 22. An awareness of these possibilities is necessary during clinical examination because they may account for unusual varicosities on the back of the thigh and again this is considered in Chapter 5.

## The principles of treatment in superficial vein incompetence

The characteristic features of superficial incompetence and varicose veins arising from this have been described above and this is a good stage at which to state how this understanding can be used logically in treatment. The essential principle of curative treatment is quite simple – *the pathway of incompetence must be obliterated as completely as possible, either by surgical removal or by sclerotherapy.* This must include the source at the upper end (usually, but not always, the termination of a long or short saphenous vein), the main pathway of incompetence (often a saphenous vein), and the main varicose veins arising from it. Enlarged perforators may be incompetent and capable of outward leakage, so that they can become the source of a persisting pattern of varicose veins or continuing hypertension; if this is thought possible the procedure should include shutting off these veins. In most circumstances the success of the operation will depend upon the completeness with which the procedure is carried out. It is evident that the surgeon's efforts must be directed towards a correctly identified pathway of incompetence but this has many possible patterns. There is no standard pattern and, for example, interconnection between long and short saphenous systems may be present, or the varicosities may have more than one potential source of filling, or even deep vein impairment may co-exist with superficial varicosities. These and other circumstances may lead to failure in treatment if they are not recognized. In the next chapter various patterns of superficial incompetence are considered in relation to the requirements of treatment. The detailed aspects of treatment are described in Chapters 18–20.

## References

Belcaro, G. V. (1986) Sapheno-femoral incompetence in young asymptomatic subjects with a family history of varices of the lower limbs. In: *Phlebology 85* (eds D. Negus and G. Jantet), John Libbey, London, pp. 30–32

Bjordal, R. I. (1977) Haemodynamic studies of varicose veins and the post-thrombotic syndrome. In *The Treatment of Venous Disorders* (ed. J. T. Hobbs), MTP, Lancaster, pp. 37–53

Bjordal, R. I. (1986) The clinical role of dilated perforating veins in varicose disease. In *Phlebology 85* (eds D. Negus and G. Jantet), John Libbey, London, pp. 42–44

Clarke, H., Smith, S. R. G., Vasdekis, S. N., Hobbs, J. T. and Nicolaides, A. N. (1989) Role of venous elasticity in the development of varicose veins. *British Journal of Surgery*, **76**, 577–580

Corcos, L., Peruzzi, G. and Romeo, V. (1987) Intraoperative phlebography of the short saphenous vein. *Phlebology*, **2**, 241–248

Dodd, H. and Cockett, F. B. (1976) *The Pathology and Surgery of the Veins of the Lower Limbs*. Edinburgh, Churchill Livingstone

Fegan, W. G. and Kline, A. L. (1972) The cause of varicosity in superficial veins of the lower limb. *British Journal of Surgery*, **59**, 798–801

Gardner, A. M. N. and Fox, R. H. (1989) The return of blood to the heart against the force of gravity. In *Phlebology 85* (eds D. Negus and G. Jantet), John Libbey, London, pp. 65–67

Gardner, A. M. N, and Fox, R. H. (1989) *The Return of Blood to the Heart*, John Libbey, London

Gundersen, J. (1977) Hereditary factors in varicose veins. In *The Treatment of Venous Disorders* (ed. J. T. Hobbs), MTP, Lancaster, pp. 13–17

Henry, M. and Corless, C. (1989) The incidence of varicose veins in Ireland. *Phlebology*, **4**, 133–137

Hobbs, J. T. (1978) Per-operative phlebography to ensure accurate sapheno-popliteal ligation. *British Medical Journal*, **2**, 1578

Hobbs, J. T. (1988) The enigma of the gastrocnemius vein. *Phlebology*, **3**, 19–30

Hubner, H. J. and Schultz-Ehrenburg, U. (1986) Simple and hidden atypical refluxes of the leg veins. In *Phlebology 85* (eds D. Negus and G. Jantet), John Libbey, London, pp. 58–60

Lorenzi, G., Bavera, P., Cipolat, L. and Carlesi, R. (1986) The prevalence of primary varicose veins among worker of a metal and steel factory. In *Phlebology 85* (eds D. Negus and G. Jantet), John Libbey, London, pp. 18–21

Ludbrook, J. (1963) Valvular defect in primary varicose veins. Cause or effect? *Lancet*, **2**, 1289–1292

Ludbrook, J. and Beale, G. (1962) Femoral venous valves in relation to varicose veins. *Lancet*, **1**, 79–81

Milliken, J. C., Dinn, E., O'Connor, R. and Greene D. (1986) A simple Doppler technique for the rapid diagnosis of significant sapheno-femoral reflux. *Phlebology*, **1**, 125–128

Mitchell, D. C. and Darke, S. G. (1987) The assessment of primary varicose veins by Doppler ultrasound – the role of sapheno-popliteal incompetence and the short saphenous systems in calf varicosities. *European Journal of Vascular Surgery*, **1**, 113–115

Nicolaides, A., Christopoulos, D. and Vasdekis, S. (1989) Progress in the investigation of chronic venous insufficiency. *Annals of Vascular Surgery*, **3**, 278–292

Psaila, J. V. and Melhuish, J. (1989) Viscoelastic properties and collagen content of the long saphenous vein in normal and varicose veins. *British Journal of Surgery*, **76**, 37–40

Quaile, A. and Rowland, F. H. (1986) A retrospective study of the epidemiology and treatment of varicose veins. In *Phlebology 85* (eds D. Negus and G. Jantet), John Libbey, London, pp. 33–37

Rose, S. (1986) The aetiology of varicose veins. In *Phlebology 85* (eds D. Negus and G. Jantet), John Libbey, London, pp. 6–8

Sakaguchi, S., Koyano, K., Hishiki, S. and Takihara, M. (1986) A modified stripping operation for varicose veins of the legs based on Doppler flowmetric findings. In *Phlebology 85* (eds D. Negus and G. Jantet), John Libbey, London, pp. 206–208

Schultz-Ehrenburg, U. and Weindorf, N. (1986) Prospective epidemiological study on the development of varicosis in German grammar schools (Bochum study I). In *Phlebology 85* (eds D. Negus and G. Jantet), John Libbey, London, pp. 22–25

Thulesius, O., Gjores, J. E. and Berlin, E. (1986) Valvular function and venous distensibility. In *Phlebology 85* (eds D. Negus and G. Jantet), John Libbey, London, pp. 26–29

Tibbs, D. J. (1986) The intriguing problem of varicose veins. *International Angiology*, **5**, 289–295

Tibbs, D. J. and Fletcher, E. W. L. (1983) Direction of flow in superficial veins as a guide to venous disorders in the lower limbs. *Surgery*, **93**, 758–767

Vasdekis, S. N., Clarke, G. H, Hobbs, J. T. and Nicoliades, A. N. (1985) Evaluation of non-invasive and invasive methods in the assessment of short saphenous vein termination. *British Journal of Surgery*, **78**, 929–932

Widmer, L. K., Mall, Th. and Martin, H. (1977) Epidemiology and sociomedical importance of peripheral venous disease. In *The Treatment of Venous Disorders* (ed. J. T. Hobb), MTP, Lancaster, pp. 3–12

Widmer, L. K., Stahelin, H. B., Nissen, C. and da Silva, A. (1987) *Venen-, Arterien- Krankheiten, koronare Herzkrankheit bei Berufstatigen*, Huber, Bern

Widmer, L. K., Zemp, E., Delley, A. and Biland. L. (1986) Varicosity: prevalence and medical importance. In *Phlebology 85* (eds D. Negus and G. Jantet), John Libbey, London, pp. 87–90

## Bibliography

Bruce Campbell, W. (1990) Varicose veins. *British Medical Journal*, **300**, 763–764

McPheeters, H. O. (1929) Varicose veins – the circulation and direction of the venous flow. *Surgery, Obstetrics and Gynecology*, **VXLIX**, 29–33

Obitsu, Y., Ishimaru, S., Furukawa, F. and Yoshihama, I. (1990) Histopathological studies of the valves of varicose veins. *Phlebology*, **5**, 245–254

Sutton, R. and Darke, S. G. (1986) Stripping the long saphenous vein: peroperative retrograde saphenography in patients with and without venous ulceration. *British Journal of Surgery*, **73**, 305–307

Thulesius, O., Al-Douary, Eklof, B. *et al.* (1986) Incidence of venous disease in Kuwait (1984). In *Phlebology 85* (eds D. Negus and G. Jantet), John Libbey, London, pp. 38–40

# 5

# Superficial vein incompetence: further considerations

In many respects varicose veins are random developments, depending on distribution and quality of valves. This is superimposed upon a structure of somewhat variable superficial vein anatomy to give the great variety of patterns of varicose veins that may be seen. Certain patterns predominate and these have been illustrated in the last chapter, although a warning has been given upon the overlapping of territories that often occurs and the interconnection between the long and short saphenous systems. Nevertheless, although many confusing patterns are seen, only unravelled by patient mapping out, there are a number of characteristic patterns to which the eye should be attuned.

In the last chapter the concept of a pathway of incompetence allowing gravitational downflow giving rise to varicose veins has been discussed. Such a retrograde circuit is based on a source of outflow from deep veins at high level to feed the pathway of incompetence with unlimited downflow. The source and pathway considered in the last chapter were one or other of the saphenous veins with varicosities arising from it, but other veins may provide the primary source of downflow and main pathway of incompetence. Such variants are quite common and this chapter will describe the most important of those occurring in untreated states and in the disturbed anatomy of superficial veins following surgery. The success of surgery, and sclerotherapy, is determined by the accurate recognition of the pathway and the design of operation that is based on this. Recognition will depend not only on visible patterns of veins, illustrated here, but, even more so, on mapping out by touch and tapwave (see Chapter 2), confirmation by clinical tests, especially the selective occlusion (Trendelenburg) test by localized compression with fingers, and use of the Doppler flowmeter (Goren and Yellin, 1990). The more important reasons for failure in treatment, arising from shortcomings in the initial assessment, will be considered in the second part of the chapter.

## Varicosities on the anterior and lateral aspects of the thigh

Varicose veins arising on the inner aspect of the thigh usually arise directly from the long saphenous vein or a major branch of it (Figure 5.1). Varicosities seen on the front or outer aspect of the upper or mid thigh are most likely to arise from one of the uppermost tributaries of the long saphenous, usually the superficial circumflex iliac vein. However, there are a number of anatomical variations in the terminal veins and a common variety is a large antero-lateral (accessory saphenous) branch, often sharing a common stem with the circumflex iliac and running down the front of the thigh to break into clearly visible varicosities in the mid-thigh (Figures 5.2 (right limb), 5.3–5.5). From here the varicosities may run laterally to wind round the outer side of the thigh, knee and down the leg to end here, or by running to the underside of the foot; other varicosities may run from mid-thigh anteromedially over the knee and calf where they may rejoin the long saphenous vein, perhaps as part of the bypassing mechanism referred to in Chapter 4, or terminate independently through various perforators on the leg or underside of the foot. One pattern of bypassing mechanism is illustrated by diagram in Figure 5.2 (left limb), and by a clinical example in Figure 5.6, where a lateral accessory saphenous vein divides on the front of the thigh to give a varicosity winding down to enter the long saphenous vein in lower thigh below a competent valve and is the source of long saphenous incompetence beneath this, with the varicosities arising from it. Another branch may continue down the outer side of the thigh and leg as previously described. These patterns are quite common but easily missed so that they persist after surgery if a special effort has not been made to remove them. Treatment by sclerotherapy will usually succeed in closing off these meandering varicosities but often fails to obliterate the source, that is, a lateral accessory saphenous vein, so that the pattern of varicosities re-emerges within a year or two. However, if the varicosities

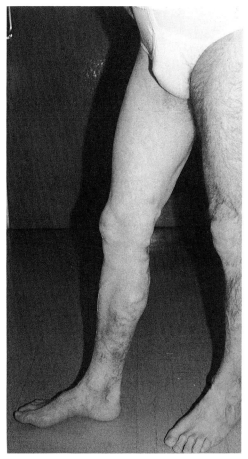

**a1**

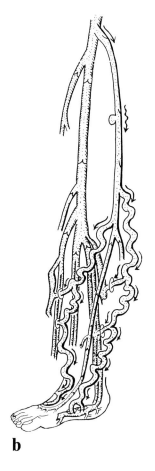

**b**

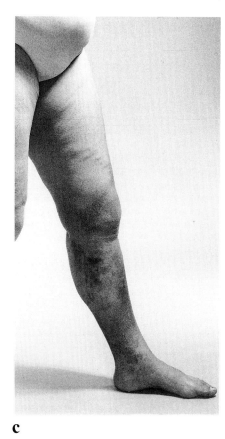

**c**

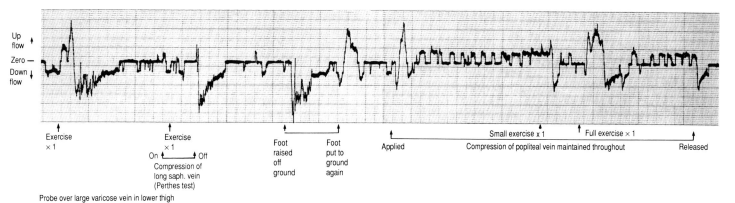

**a2**

**Figure 5.1** *Varicosities arising on the inner aspect of the thigh.*

*(a)* *1. Varicosities formed from a branch of the long saphenous vein in mid-thigh and running posterolaterally to the ankle where pronounced venotensive skin change (venous stasis) is present. Selective Trendelenburg's test completely controlled these veins.*
*2. Directional Doppler tracing from the same varicosity just above the knee, showing characteristic downflow after exercise and upflow only on popliteal compression.*

*(b)* *Schematic diagram illustrating a similar pattern of varicosities and direction of flow in upright exercising patient.*

*(c)* *An example of a varicose vein arising from long saphenous vein in mid-thigh and running anteriorly across it*

**Figure 5.2**    *Diagram of varicosities seen on the front of the thigh.*
Right limb. *An incompetent anterolateral branch from the termination of the long saphenous vein runs down the front to the mid-thigh where it becomes visible as varicosities crossing the outer aspect of the knee and running down the leg to the foot; another branch commonly seen runs down towards the inner thigh and knee, and down the leg.*
Left limb. *Again, an anterolateral branch is incompetent and gives rise to varicose branches in the mid-thigh; one of these runs back into the long saphenous vein, thus bypassing a fully competent valve in its upper part and feeding incompetent flow into the long saphenous vein below this level. At operation, a syringe test to the long saphenous vein (see Figure 5.7) will show resistance corresponding to the functioning valve, but the same test to the anterolateral branch offers no resistance and may cause bulging varicosities arising from the long saphenous vein below the knee, as well as those on the thigh*

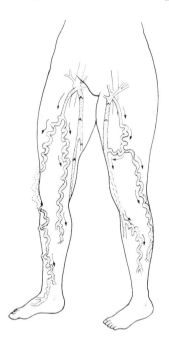

**Figure 5.3**    *Two views of a large varicose vein arising from the anterolateral branch at the termination of the long saphenous vein. The saphenous vein itself did not show any other evidence of incompetence. This corresponds to the varicosities in the right limb of Figure 5.2. (By permission of Mr S. Rose)*

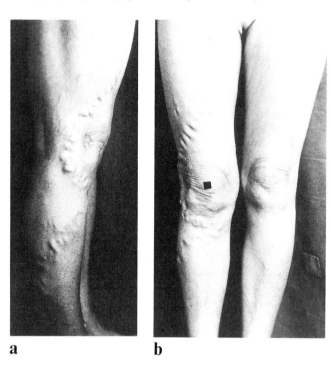

**a**                    **b**

**Figure 5.4**    *Varicosity arising from the anterolateral branch of the long saphenous vein in the groin and running the full length of the limb down to the ankle where there are early venotensive changes*

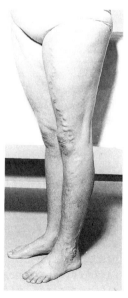

**Figure 5.5**  *(a)  Multiple branching of varicosities in the left thigh arising from the anterolateral branch of the long saphenous vein. Two branches run medially where one joined the long saphenous vein down which the pathway of incompetence was continued. Two laterally running branches merge to form a varicosity running down the outer side of the leg to a pigmented area of venotensive change in its lower part.*

*(b)  The same patient 5 weeks later after surgery removing the varicosities through multiple incisions*

**Figure 5.6**  *An example of an anterolateral branch varicosity which runs from the uppermost long saphenous down to rejoin the long saphenous vein in the lower thigh. This varicose vein bypassed a competent valve, proved by syringe testing at operation, in the upper part of the long saphenous vein. The pathway of incompetence was continued down the saphenous vein from the point at which the varicosity joined it and further varicosities were given off from this in the calf. Selective Trendelenburg's test controlling this massive varicose vein in the thigh is illustrated in Figure 4.21*

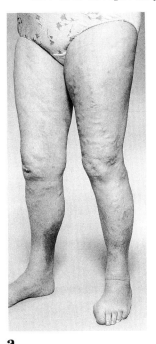 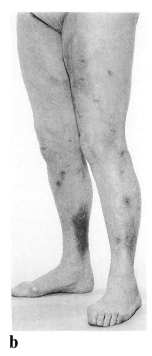

**a**   **b**

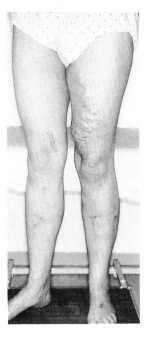

are not too massive a worthwhile result lasting some years may be achieved by a single set of injections.

*Note on treatment*

In the right limb depicted in Figure 5.2, surgical treatment should include flush ligation of the saphenous termination, together with all the terminal branches, stripping of the lateral accessory saphenous vein and removal, as extensively as possible, of the varicose pathway of incompetence down the limb by multiple dissections or avulsions. However, the right long saphenous vein itself may be fully competent and this can be demonstrated by retrograde flushing with a syringe (Figure 5.7.); if there is complete resistance to syringing, and a similar test to the lateral accessory has fully explained the origin to the varicosities, then the long saphenous vein need not be stripped. However, in the left limb of Figure 5.2 the circumstances are somewhat different and whilst the long saphenous in its upper part need not necessarily be stripped (although it often will be), this should be carried out to the incompetent portion below the entry of the bypassing varicosity and down to the point of take off of any calf varicosities from the saphenous vein; the laterally

running thigh varicosities should of course be removed as far as possible, as described for the right side.

If these thigh varicosities meandering down the length of the limb are not removed at the time of surgery, they are very likely to remain open and clearly visible, although less prominent. Not only is the patient disappointed but the veins are likely to acquire some new source of filling which gives increasing flow down them so they enlarge steadily. Sclerotherapy is usually effective in forestalling this but should be regarded as an occasional 'back-up' treatment for incomplete surgery rather than a routine policy used to economize on surgical time.

**Varicosities on the posterior aspect of the thigh**

The most commonly found varicosity on the back of the thigh arises from the long saphenous vein itself or from its posteromedial branch (Figure 5.8(a) right limb). These varicosities take a variable course down to the calf and may even continue to the foot; many will remain on the posteromedial aspect and perhaps mingle with other long saphenous varicosities; others will descend on the posterior calf where they may be mistaken for short saphenous varicosities and indeed there is often

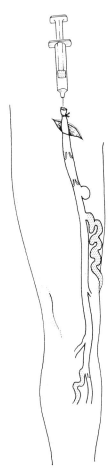

intercommunication with the short saphenous system; another variant is to cross the back of the thigh to form varicosities on the outer side of the limb often linking with varicose veins running from the uppermost saphenous branches in the groin on the anterolateral aspect as described in the previous section.

Another pattern of varicosity is one which arises at a high level from an uppermost branch of the long saphenous vein, usually the superficial external pudendal vein, to run posteriorly round the uppermost thigh, crossing over its back to the outer aspect to run down the leg or to the foot (Figure 5.8(b) (right limb)). Again, this pattern may link with anterolateral varicosities from the groin.

**Figure 5.7** *The syringe test for assessing competence of valves during surgical operation. Here a 20 ml syringe containing normal saline has been connected to the open end of a divided long saphenous vein and steady pressure is applied to see if the valves offer any resistance to retrograde flushing. In the illustration, valves are present but they are grossly incompetent so that there is no resistance and the varicose veins in the thigh and in the upper leg bulge slightly as the syringe is emptied. Such a clear demonstration of incompetence in a vein confirms that it is the pathway of incompetence and that it is correct to strip it. By contrast, full resistance indicates that the valves are competent so that the vein is not at fault and need not necessarily be stripped; it is likely that the pathway is in another vein and this must be located and removed; the anterolateral branch, or a variant of it, is most likely to be at fault but this may connect into a long saphenous vein incompetent in its lower part so that, after all, it requires removing (see Figures 5.2, 5.6).*

Note: *In practice, the cannula need not be tied into the vein; holding between finger and thumb will usually provide an adequate seal (see Figure 20.11). This test gives valuable guidance during surgery but is only appropriate when the operation itself has the correct indications, that is, gravitational downflow in the superficial veins indicating simple incompetence. Demonstration of valve incompetence in a vein that is acting as a collateral past deep veins damaged by previous thrombosis does not indicate that this vein should be stripped since its collateral function may be far more important than the component of incompetence (see Chapter 8). This should have been detected and fully evaluated before any decision for surgery*

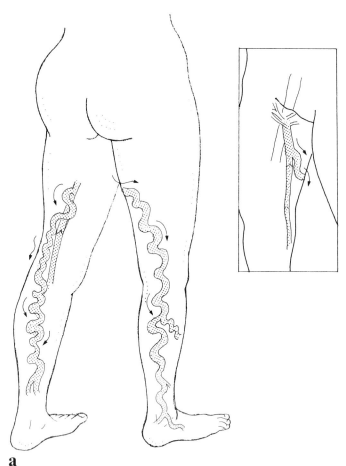

**a**

**Figure 5.8** *Varicose veins seen on the back of the thigh.*
*(a)* Right limb (and inset). *Varicose veins arising from postero-medial branch of long saphenous vein; these usually run down to disperse in the calf and commonly continue down to the ankle and foot.*
Left limb. *Varicose veins arising from a short saphenous vein that extends to a high level in the thigh. There are many variations of this (see Figure 5.9). The short saphenous vein may terminate at high level in the upper popliteal or superficial femoral vein, or it may continue up to join the profunda femoris vein, or it may sweep across to the inner aspect of the thigh to join the long saphenous vein or its posteromedial branch. Some of these variants are indicated in the subsequent figures.*

**Figure 5.8** *(continued)*

*(b)* Right limb (and inset). *Varicosity extending down the limb and arising from the superficial external pudendal branch of the long saphenous vein. This may continue down across the ankle to the foot.*

Left limb. *The short saphenous vein has a high termination which is competently valved but interconnection from an incompetent long saphenous vein joins it below the valve(s) so that if the remainder of the short saphenous is incompetent varicosities may arise from it in the calf, and at the ankle.*

*(c)* *Deceptive origin of varicosities arising in mid-posterior thigh of a lady, aged 45. The varicosities had been confined to the thigh for some years but recently had rapidly extended below the knee. These varicose veins could not be controlled by long saphenous occlusion but strong Doppler downflow shown in them after exercise was prevented by finger pressure over the upper popliteal fossa; the same manoeuvre was found to give complete control of the varicosities. Doppler flowmetry detected upflow in a concealed vein running from the fossa up to join the varicose vein, down which the same pattern of flow continued. Origin from an upward extension of the short saphenous vein was suspected and functional phlebography carried out.*

> *1. Photograph to show the varicose veins on the back of the thigh, calf and outer ankle; other varicosities were present over the front of the ankle.*
>
> *2, 3. Composite phlebogram and outline diagram showing a large coiled vein running upwards from the vicinity of the short saphenous termination (not seen). The long saphenous vein is also shown and is well valved and normal in appearance; it does however show a branch communicating with the varicose vein, suggesting that the*

*latter has developed from an upward extension of the short saphenous vein, which commonly connects the saphenous systems in the thigh (see page 92).*

*4. Diagram showing overall arrangement of flow pattern from popliteal vein, through the coiled vein and upwards to emerge superficially and then flow downwards to join a valveless portion of short saphenous vein in the lower leg; a branch varicosity runs round to the front to join the long saphenous vein. Both saphenous veins give off further varicosities at the ankle; the upper parts of the saphenous veins are valved and competent (see page 92).*

*5. Appearance 4 months postoperatively (see page 92)*

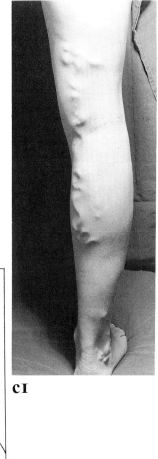

**c1**

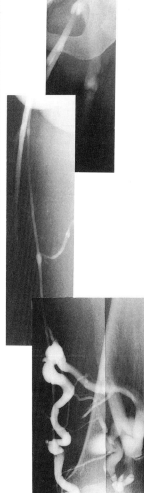

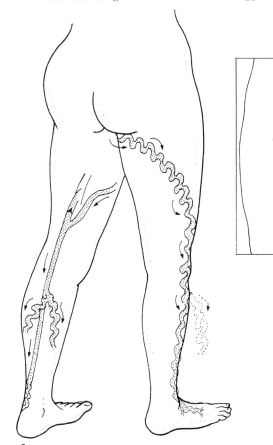

**b**

**c2**

**Figure 5.8** *(continued)*

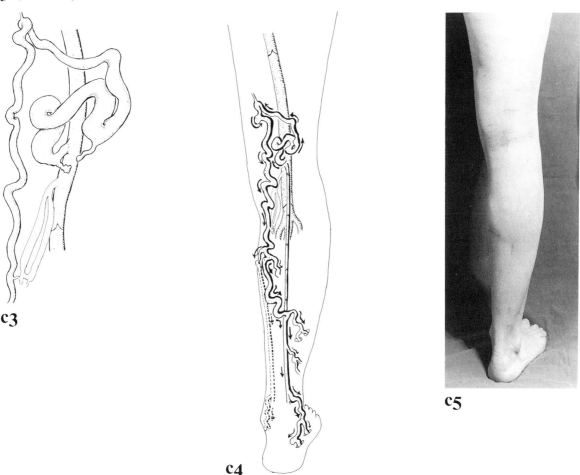

c3

c4

c5

Similar varicosities may arise from a short saphenous vein with an unusually high termination or having an upward extension (Figures 5.8(b) (left limb), (c), 5.9) or from an interconnecting branch between the long and short saphenous veins (Figures 5.8(b) (left limb), 5.9(b) (right limb), (c); see also Figures 1.5(c), 4.22–4.24, 5.11(d)).

Thigh varicosities arising from pelvic veins are seen on the uppermost, inner aspect of the thigh, usually accompanied by a history of vulval varicosities persisting from pregnancy, and this is yet another source seen in women. Varicose veins with this origin are considered further presently. Incompetent perforating veins from the profunda femoris vein may occasionally cause a set of varicose veins meandering down the posterior thigh and the outer aspect of the calf; these may arise at quite a high level and usually respond well to sclerotherapy. Care must be taken not to diagnose them too readily because the other causes for posterior thigh varicosities discussed above are more likely, although often obscured by obesity.

## Interconnection between long and short saphenous systems

It is commonplace for a branch from the upper part of the long saphenous system to run superficially round the back of the thigh to join the short saphenous vein behind the thigh or knee according to the level of its termination (Figure 5.8(b) (left), or run into an upward extension of it (Figure 5.9(b) (right), (c)). In the calf region a major branch from the long saphenous may run across to join the short saphenous vein (Figure 5.10 (left)), or from short saphenous to long saphenous system (Figure 5.10 (right)), with much variation in the details of positioning. The importance of these interconnections at any level is that they commonly share in the process of incompetence either due to valvular failure or, in many cases, due to apparent absence of any valves. This means that a long saphenous incompetence may be switched across to a short saphenous vein and is then, perhaps, the main source of incompetence in the short saphenous system. Similarly behind the knee or at calf level a short saphenous incompetence may be channelled across to join the lower part of the long saphenous system and the cause of varicosities there (Figure 5.10 (right)). Less commonly, an upward extension of the short saphenous

**Figure 5.9** *Some anatomical variants in termination of the short saphenous vein. The site at which this vein passes through the deep fascia on its way to the popliteal fossa is very variable and may be anywhere between mid-calf and the popliteal fossa itself. The commonest position is between upper and middle thirds.*

(a) Right limb. *Termination in the upper part of the popliteal vein.*
Left limb. *Termination in the superficial femoral vein.*

(b) Right limb. *The short saphenous vein joins the popliteal vein but a large component continues upwards in continuity with the posteromedial branch of the long saphenous. Incompetence in this upward extension is a common cause for varicosities arising from the short saphenous vein, as illustrated here. These may be controlled by a Trendelenburg test in the upper part of the thigh and so misdirect the surgeon. Careful use of the tapwave technique in mapping out can usually detect this arrangement of the veins.*
Left limb. *The short saphenous vein extends up to join the profunda femoris vein and, if this is incompetent, ligation of the short saphenous at knee level may be inadequate and further varicosities are likely to develop from the portion of vein remaining above this. The same is true with any form of high termination of the short saphenous. See Figure 5.11 for possible interconnection with pudendal varicose veins of pelvic origin.*

(c) *An unusual source of incompetence from an upward extension of the short saphenous vein connecting with the long saphenous vein in the upper inner thigh and causing varicosities running down from here. The patient, a female aged 31 years, complained of discomfort in varicose veins on the posterior thigh and outer aspect of the knee. Her veins are illustrated by phlebograms; these were obtained because Doppler downflow was not found at any level in the long saphenous vein itself although present in the varicosities; a separate pelvic origin was suspected. Functional phlebography was carried out in various head-up tilts, with opaque medium injected into varicosities in the upper inner thigh; several phases of filling are shown; rotation of the limb was varied several times and for this reason the composite pictures are not exact matches (see page 94).*

*1. Initial stage of injection into upper thigh varicosity; downflow has been prevented by a mid-thigh bandage in order to direct medium to the groin but no likely source was found here. Note the oblique vein in the lower part of the picture; this is the upper end of a connection with the short saphenous vein.*

*2, 3. Bandage removed to allow downward display and to follow the 'oblique' vein. Well-valved long and short saphenous veins are seen and are most unlikely to be at fault; the paired perforating veins between profunda femoris and long saphenous vein in upper thigh are normal and not incompetent. A valveless vein runs obliquely up from the short saphenous vein towards the uppermost varicosities and injection needle. On the image intensifier screen, and faintly on X-ray films, complete continuity was demonstrated but is not fully seen here. The commencement of this connecting vein shows sacculation and tortuosity indicating a leaking valve and reversed flow. The tortuous varicosities evident across the lower thigh are on its posterior aspect.*

*4. After exercise, the lower part of the connecting vein from the short saphenous has partially cleared due to upflow in it.*

*5. Diagram of the arrangement of the veins shown in the phlebograms. The interconnecting vein from the short saphenous vein is shown running upwards and across the back of the thigh to join long saphenous branches in its upper part. Two sets of varicose veins descend from here; one set winds posteriorly (shown in interrupted outline) down the thigh and round its outer aspect to the front of the leg where it joins the other set which has descended medially (not appearing in phlebograms), so that together they encircle the limb. Arrows indicate direction of flow on exercise, up the interconnecting vein and down the varicosities.*

*At surgery the connecting vein was syringe tested and found to allow only upward flow due to a single valve in its upper part; this vein was removed together with the larger varicosities but the long saphenous vein was left intact; some outlying varicosities required subsequent injection but overall the result was good.*

Conclusion: *The presence of the interconnecting channel (commonly present), and a particular pattern of valve failure, has allowed upflow from the short saphenous vein to the upper thigh from where it spills down the varicose veins*

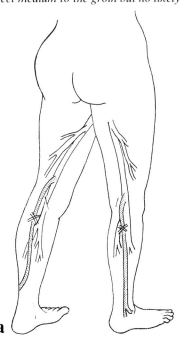

**a**

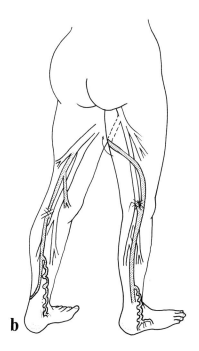

**b**

**Figure 5.9** *(continued)*

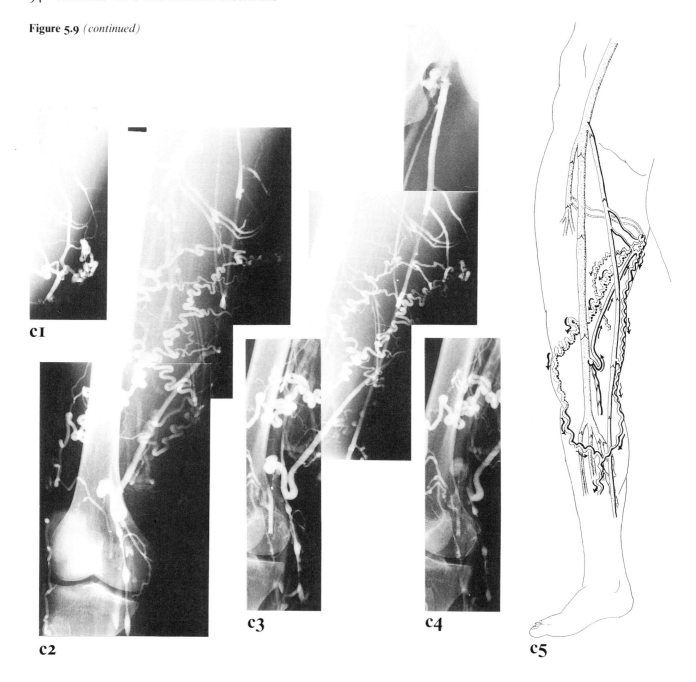

cI

c2

c3

c4

c5

vein, connecting with a posteromedial long saphenous branch in the upper thigh, is the source of varicose veins running down from here (Figure 5.9(c)).

Interconnections of this sort are common diagnostic traps (Hubner and Schultz-Ehrenburg, 1986) which may lead to misdirected surgery failing to remove the real source of incompetence. Putting this differently, the pathway of incompetence not infrequently starts in one saphenous system and transfers across to the other saphenous system by an interconnecting channel and the surgeon must be fully prepared to meet this.

*Manometric filling of long saphenous vein*

A common variety of incompetence is found in the first few inches of the short saphenous vein with a major branch conducting this to the long saphenous vein in the mid-leg with varicosities arising from this. Although the long saphenous vein is fully competent in its upper part, the rapid inflow from the short saphenous system causes filling and slight distension of the long saphenous vein at the knee and in the lower thigh so that it is mistaken for an enlarged and incompetent vein. In fact it is filling like a fluid manometer (manometric filling) rapidly registering the deep vein pressure at popliteal level. A Trendelenburg test selectively applied to the long saphenous vein in the lower thigh, will fail to control the varicose veins and the

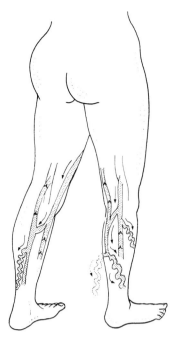

**Figure 5.10** *Interconnection between the saphenous veins in the lower thigh and calf.*

Right limb. *The short saphenous vein may send a large branch across to join the long saphenous vein or one of its major tributaries. In this way short saphenous incompetence may be transferred to the lower part of the long saphenous system which has good valves above this level.*

Left limb. *The reverse can occur; the long saphenous vein commonly sends a large branch across to communicate with the short saphenous vein and in this way long saphenous incompetence can be transferred to the short saphenous system. The lower long saphenous vein is, perhaps, well valved and does not show varicosities but these will arise from the short saphenous vein even though it is adequately valved in its upper part*

characteristic Doppler downflow after exercise will not be present in the thigh portion of the long saphenous vein. When the Doppler fails to show this, in spite of the presence of varicosities arising from this vein lower down, then there should be immediate suspicion that the real origin of the varicosities is the short saphenous vein. Interconnection between the varicosities and the short saphenous vein may be readily demonstrated by the tap-wave technique and, of course, a selective Trendelenburg test applied by thumb pressure to the uppermost short saphenous will control the varicosities; this is confirmed by a Doppler flowmeter showing strong downflow in the short saphenous vein after exercise.

Even more deceptive is a simultaneous incompetence in both long and short saphenous veins with interconnection between them (for example see Figure 22.11 (e)). The diagnostician is alerted to this because a Trendelenburg test applied with localized fingertip pressure may fail to control the varicosities and the tapwave technique shows interconnection between the two systems; Tren-

delenburg's test repeated with careful positioning of finger pressure over both long and short saphenous veins may give firm proof of the double source of filling. This topic is referred to again later in this chapter under the section 'Patterns of failure in the treatment of varicose veins'.

Varicosities may of course be given off at any level from the incompetent portions of the saphenous veins and the interconnecting channels between them. As a rather separate aspect of this, it must be pointed out that large varicosities from one saphenous vein may run across to lie over the other saphenous vein but not necessarily communicating with it. It is insufficient to rely on the position of varicose veins as a guide to their origin, which can only be reliably indentified by systematic mapping out of veins and demonstrating full control with a Trendelenburg test by localized digital pressure over the correct pathway of incompetence.

## Pelvic veins as a source of incompetence – pudendal varicose veins

During pregnancy it is common for massive enlargement and incompetence to occur in the veins throughout the lower limbs and the pelvis. This includes veins communicating between superficial and deep veins within the pelvis so that outflow to the upper thigh and vulval regions occurs, setting up pathways of incompetence and causing vulval and perineal varicosities. The veins usually involved are the internal pudendal and the obturator veins (Lea Thomas *et al.*, 1967; Lea Thomas, 1976). After childbirth the veins rapidly recede and often disappear, but some, although reduced, will persist as obvious varicosities. These may dissipate harmlessly by running down the thigh for a short distance and into perforators here but may connect up with long saphenous incompetence or, on their own, establish a pathway of incompetence running right down the limb to form popliteal, calf or even foot varicosities (Figure 5.11(a)–(c)). The varicose veins derived from the pelvis in the uppermost part of the limb cause little in the way of local symptoms and the patients are usually much more concerned with any varicose veins that may be obvious in the lower part of the leg. Because the patient is not complaining of the varicosities in perineum or upper thigh their contribution to the general pattern of incompetence in the limb may be underrated. They should never be ignored but always assessed as far possible and if surgery is to be carried out upon, say, the long saphenous system then it is only a small extension to remove these 'pelvic' varicosities from the perineum and uppermost inner thigh. It is true that similar veins in the perineal region may arise from the long saphenous vein via its superficial external pudendal branch, but unless clinical tests prove this beyond doubt it is best to assume a pelvic origin and at surgery trace the vein as far as possible towards the pelvic sources. A

**Figure 5.11** *Varicosities on the thigh arising from pelvic veins. In the first patient ((a)–(c)), high ligation and stripping of the long saphenous vein had failed to cure varicosities running down the thigh and calf, and these were subject to recurring thrombophlebitis.*

*(a) In this photograph, varicosities in the pudendal region can be seen leading to a varicose vein running down the length of the thigh. Finger pressure at high level completely controlled all these veins; Doppler flowmetry confirmed strong downflow after exercise.*

*(b) Phlebogram obtained during operation in the same patient. The thigh varicosity has been divided in its uppermost part and contrast medium sent upwards into the pudendal varicosities from here. These varicosities dominate the picture but they can be seen to be in easy communication with at least five sets of veins and these are clarified in (c).*

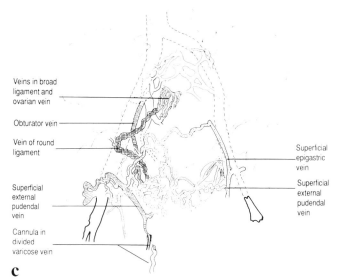

Veins in broad ligament and ovarian vein

Obturator vein

Vein of round ligament

Superficial external pudendal vein

Cannula in divided varicose vein

Superficial epigastric vein

Superficial external pudendal vein

**c**

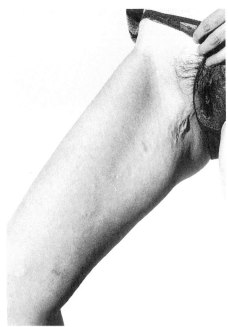

**a**

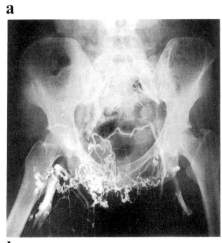

**b**

*(c) Diagram indicating the principle connections shown in the preceding phlebogram (b). The pudendal varicosities form a convoluted mass but study of the original X-ray films showed the following connections, some only appearing faintly in (b): with the superficial external pudendal vein, disconnected at the time of previous saphenous ligation, which has established a tortuous*

*communication with the profunda femoris vein; with the vein accompanying the round ligament of the uterus which passes through the inguinal canal and arches back to join the venous plexus in the broad ligament; with the obturator vein which enters the pelvis to join the internal iliac vein; by interconnection with pudendal veins on the opposite side and via the left superficial external pudendal vein to join the saphenous termination on that side – from here the superficial epigastric vein runs upwards to anastomose across the pubic region to connect again with the pudendal varicosities on the right side; a vein believed to be the internal pudendal vein has filled from the obturator vein but it has not shown any direct filling from the pudendal varicosities.*

*Varicography, such as this, always tends to fill the veins capriciously and when the direction of flow is 'upwards' will be travelling in the direction allowed by valves. Thus, the veins outlined are not necessarily at fault and may be fully competent. Moreover, this phlebogram was taken at operation with the patient lying horizontally and gives no indication of function within the veins when the patient is upright and moving, that is to say, when the retrograde circuit is active. If ovarian veins were enlarged and incompetent it is unlikely that a phlebogram of this sort would outline them. The vein accompanying the round ligament and the obturator vein were believed to be the sources filling the pudendal and thigh varicose veins. The role of other veins is uncertain but the pudendal varicosities are the focal 'point' through which downflow must pass; there may have been a component of cross-over incompetence from the left side.*

*(d)–(f) Phlebograms of another patient who presented, soon after the birth of her third child, with severe discomfort and engorgement of small varicosities behind the right knee at menstruation. Pudendal varicosities were present but short saphenous incompetence was suspected (see pages 97 and 98).*

*(d) 1, 2. Phlebograms by needle into a calf varicosity showing (postero-anterior views) a short saphenous vein joined near its termination by a large vein coming down the back of the thigh and in its upper part in direct communication with the pudendal varicosities; a gastrocnemius vein has also filled but is not abnormal.*
*3. Competent valves are seen in common and superficial femoral veins, with a well-valved and competent long saphenous vein.*

*Insufficient importance was given to the vein connecting pudendal varicosities with the short saphenous and an operation carried out removing the upper part of the short saphenous vein together with the lowermost 3 cm of the*

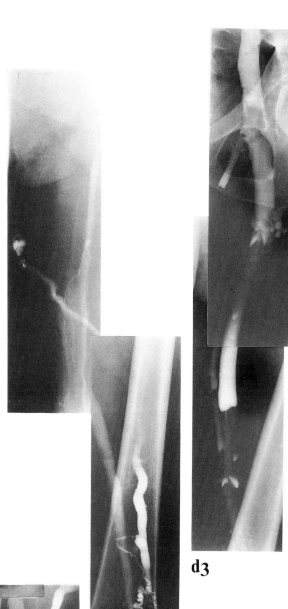

**Figure 5.11** *(continued)*
*upwardly extending connecting vein. The patient returned a few months later with her symptoms unchanged and showing severe venous congestion in the popliteal fossa and upper calf at period times. The importance of the pudendal varicosities was now apparent and further phlebography was carried out. See (e).*

*(e)   Second phlebogram in the patient illustrated in (d). This has been obtained by injection into the pudendal varicosities with the patient in a near-upright position. These views are antero-posterior (unlike the preceding ones) and slightly oblique.*

*1. A composite view extending from pudendal region down to knee level. Opacified blood has outlined the pudendal varicosities and from these the varicose vein identified at previous phlebography runs posteriorly down the thigh to the popliteal fossa where it connected with the popliteal vein and with branches distributed over the upper calf (see (f)3) including numerous subdermal varicosities and a gastrocnemius perforator.*

*2. Diagram illustrating the arrangement of the veins shown in 1 and (f). In the upright patient pudendal varicosities fill from an incompetent internal pudendal vein; the veins accompanying the round ligament and the obturator vein are not involved (see page 99).*

Subsequent examination with a Doppler flowmeter located the varicose vein in the upper popliteal fossa and here it showed strong downflow after exercise which ceased when finger pressure was applied to the pudendal varicosities. Thus, Doppler flowmetry and phlebography both confirmed the connection between pudendal veins and the popliteal region. Phlebography of the ovarian veins by transfemoral catheterization was considered but it was decided to try sclerotherapy to the pudendal varicose veins first. This proved easy and closed these veins with a firm cord. The patient's symptoms were completely relieved so

**d3**

**d2**

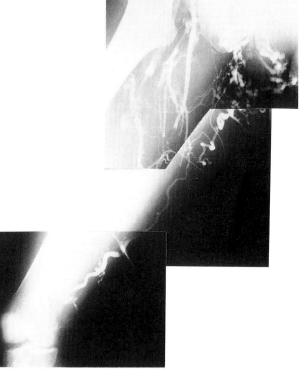

**e1**

**d1**

**Figure 5.11** *(continued)*

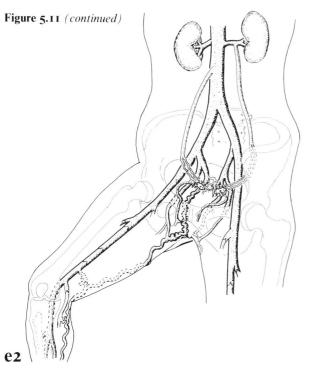

e2

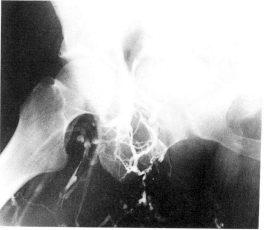

f2

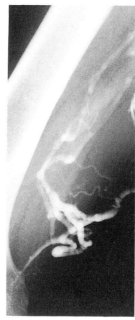

f3

*that investigations were not pursued further and it is not known whether ovarian vein incompetence played a part here. Further details of phlebography in this patient are given in (f).*

*(f)   Additional details of phlebograms in (e).*
*1. The obturator vein is clearly shown.*
*2. Further examination shows it has a competent valve so that this vein is unlikely to be acting as a source to the pudendal varicosities. However, an enlarged, faintly outlined internal pudendal vein was shown to be in communication posteriorly and this vein was believed to be*

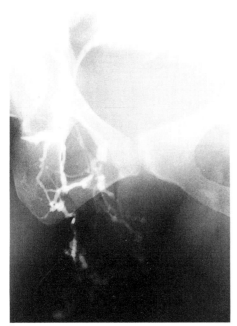

f1

*the main source of the varicosities. Filling it from below, with the patient nearly upright, against the incompetent stream was inevitably unsuccessful and attempts at clearer visualization with the patient near-horizontal were unsatisfactory.*
*3. The thigh varicose vein in the upper popliteal fossa showing a tortuous communication with the underlying deep vein. Valves in the superficial femoral vein, shown at previous phlebography, would cause the pressure difference after exercise required to create flow from pelvic veins, down the varicose veins and into the popliteal vein. This part of the pathway of incompetence survived because surgery was too limited; another vein has substituted for the portion of vein that was removed and extends downwards to the upper calf where a branch flowed into a gastrocnemius vein by a perforator.*

*(g)   Gross ovarian vein incompetence running to varices in the broad ligament is the female equivalent of the male varicocele and is sometimes referred to as 'varicocele of the broad ligament'. This is distinct from iliac vein occlusion with enlarged pelvic veins acting as collaterals. It occurs in multiparous women and*

usually involves both ovarian veins, and may affect both lower limbs. This diagram illustrates the extensive pathway of incompetence which may be found in these patients. Thus, when the patient is upright and moving, flow passes down ovarian vein(s), enters the venous network of the broad ligament which has free communication with the veins accompanying the round ligament(s) and, through the internal iliac branches, with obturator and internal pudendal veins. One or more of these veins allows flow to the pudendal varicosities from which varicose veins may run the full length of the limb, even to the venous plexus on the underside of the foot. Perforators communicate with the deep veins at various levels to form a series of retrograde circuits. There may also be interconnection with either of the saphenous systems at and below knee level but in the thigh the pudendal pathway of incompetence is often quite separate from the long saphenous vein and will therefore survive its surgical removal.

(h) Phlebograms of bilateral ovarian vein incompetence. The patient, aged 39 and the mother of three children, had suffered increasingly from severe premenstrual pelvic pain, accompanied by visible enlargement and considerable discomfort of varicosities in the lower limbs. Several attempts to treat the varicosities, including pudendal veins, proved unsuccessful and the patient was referred to Mr Hobbs who diagnosed pelvic

congestion syndrome. Descending bilateral ovarian phlebograms, shown here, were obtained by transfemoral catheterization. (1) Right side on Valsalva manoeuvre; (2) Additional detail of initial filling of right ovarian vein to show its large size; (3) Left side on Valsalva manoeuvre. On both sides, in head up tilt, medium passes easily down the ovarian veins to outline the parametrial and internal iliac pelvic veins, and onwards to perivulval and upper thigh veins. On the left side opacified blood flows down incompetent superficial veins in the thigh and is seen at knee level. Bilateral ligation of the ovarian veins, with removal of as much as possible of the plexus at their lower ends was carried out, together with extensive removal of dilated superficial veins in the limbs. Subsequently the patient reported a remarkable relief in her premenstrual pain and an associated frequency of micturition, present for many years. (Mr J. Hobbs' patient; phlebograms reproduced here with his kind permission)

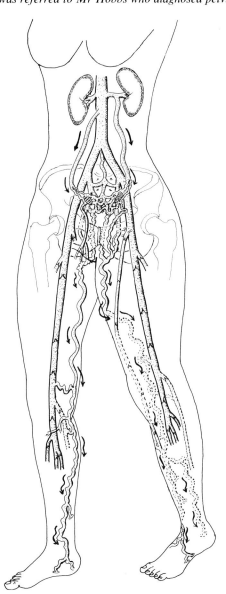

g

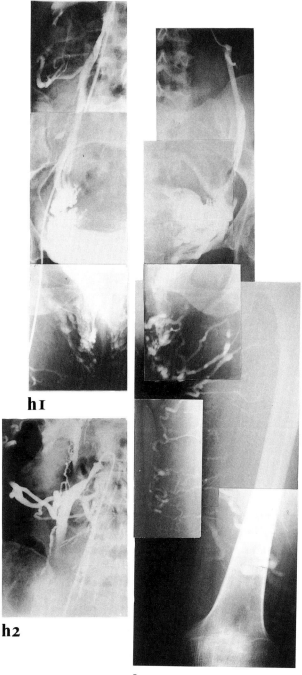

h1

h2

h3

preoperative venogram into these veins should give a good indication of their connections and the extent of removal required (Figure 5.11(b)). However, functional phlebography carried out as an outpatient with the opaque medium injected into a pudendal varicosity is easy to carry out and much more informative than the limited outlining possible on the operating table; the patient history illustrated by phlebograms and diagram in Figure 5.11(d)–(f) is a good example of how deceptive these veins may be.

Pudendal varicosities of pelvic origin, of the sort just described, are quite common and treatment by injection or by surgical excision of the veins and their downward extension is usually successful. However, similar veins may be associated with an extensive form of varicosis within the pelvis caused by ovarian vein incompetence, described below, or by veins acting as collaterals to post-thrombotic occlusion of an iliac vein. In this case a history of previous deep vein thrombosis and the presence of pubic varicosities will suggest this diagnosis, easily confirmed by phlebography. Treatment here is not usually advisable because not only will it prove ineffective but it may damage a valuable collateral mechanism. It might be permissible in a complex pattern of disorder (see later) where the pudendal varicose veins arise from simple incompetence, proved by Doppler flowmeter downflow, descending from collateral veins; even here treatment is limited by the need to preserve collateral flow.

*Note on treatment*

If varicosities derived from the pelvis are an isolated problem then treatment by sclerotherapy is usually effective and should be first choice. Alternatively surgery under local anaesthetic can be employed but these veins are very thin walled and troublesome to handle because they collapse to thread-like proportions and break easily. If surgery is required for other varicose veins in the limb then the best answer is to include the pudendal veins with this operation. Sclerotherapy or surgery outside the pelvis should always be tried first before considering tackling the source from within the pelvis. Such a procedure would require most careful prior evaluation by phlebography, clearly identifying the source of incompetence. A venogram demonstrating inward flow from limb to pelvis (the normal direction) is not sufficient evidence; there must be unequivocal evidence of gravitational outflow in a well-defined path before surgery within the pelvis is contemplated. Indentification of an obturator vein at surgery within the pelvis is feasible but the internal pudendal may prove inaccessible. Care in selection is necessary because enlarged perineal veins caused by iliac vein or inferior vena caval occlusion may be mistaken for the incompetent pudendal veins referred to above. In this case the history and the pattern of varicosities acting as collaterals at the level of the pelvis and lower abdomen, together with swelling in the limb(s), should make this diagnosis clear. Examination of pudendal varicose veins should certainly include an enquiry for possible previous deep vein thrombosis, and careful inspection made for collaterals, before concluding the veins are due to no more than a localized pelvic vein incompetence as an aftermath to pregnancy. In cases of real doubt phlebography should be employed.

## Ovarian vein incompetence causing pudendal varicose veins

In multiparous women the presence of pudendal varicosities may be associated with an extended form of pelvic vein incompetence. This is not caused by previous thrombosis but is due to massive incompetence in one or both ovarian veins which creates a state corresponding to varicocele in the male. In fact, the ovarian vein is forming the first part of an extensive retrograde circuit, with a pathway of incompetence running from the inferior vena cava or left renal vein down one or both ovarian veins to a plexus of pelvic veins and out by pudendal or obturator veins to varicosities extending down the limb, and finally into deep veins there; the return pathway is up the deep veins, the iliac veins and inferior vena cava. Retrograde flow only occurs when the patient is upright and moving (Figure 5.11(g)) but its activity is greatly increased by pelvic vascularity just before and during menstruation. The patient has often suffered large vulval varicosities during pregnancy and now complains of lower abdominal discomfort which becomes much more severe around menstruation, together with pain and engorgement of varicosities in the affected limb. The latter features may be quite striking to the clinical observer when compared with the non-active stage between periods.

Phlebography by transfemoral ovarian vein catheterization, with the patient tilted feet down, will show one or both of these veins to be greatly enlarged and without any competent valves (Figure 5.11(h)). The opaque medium runs rapidly down to join the pelvic veins and out via obturator or pudendal veins to varicosities in the lower limb where, for example, a vein lying posteriorly in the thigh runs down to a cluster of varicosities behind the knee and similar to that shown in Figure 5.11(e). This explains the symptoms of popliteal engorgement and discomfort at period time so often described by the patient. This clinical state has been described by Hobbs (1976, 1990) and Lechter, Alvarez and Lopez (1987) who have published a well-documented account of 50 cases. It is now an accepted cause for premenstrual discomfort but it is important to distinguish this from symptoms of gynaecological origin.

The treatment advocated by Lechter, Alvarez and Lopez is to interrupt the ovarian veins by abdominal surgery and, no doubt, in the more severe forms this is justifiable when the evidence, including phlebography, is unequivocal. However, understanding of this condition is still evolving and the author counsels caution. The phlebography involved is not to be taken lightly and the implication of an abdominal operation by way of treatment is somewhat daunting when the patient's main concern is with varicose veins in the lower limbs! A patient with severe premenstrual discomfort associated with engorgement of varicosities, particularly in the popliteal region, may well have ovarian vein incompetence, but a gynaecological opinion (Beard *et al.* 1984, 1986) should always be obtained before considering venous catheterization and phlebography of these veins. If no pelvic pathology or hormonal disorder is found then sclerotherapy (or surgery) to the pudendal and other varicosities should be the next step. This may relieve the symptoms that have brought the patient to a venous specialist. If these measures fail then phlebography and the possibility of subsequent treatment by ovarian vein interruption should be discussed with the patient. The fully developed syndrome is comparatively uncommon but pudendal varicose veins as a localized aftermath of pregnancy are quite common and, as stated above, usually require no more than the simple measure of sclerotherapy.

## Varicosities below the knee and on the foot

Varicose veins may be seen on any aspect of the leg below the knee and, as usual, if the cause is simple incompetence, are based on a retrograde circuit of high-level outflow from deep veins falling to the low pressure areas beneath the pumping mechanisms provided by the leg muscles and the foot. The possible sources are listed below:

- The long saphenous vein and its branches giving varicosities mainly on the inner and front aspects of the legs but not exclusively so.
- The short saphenous veins and its branches, giving varicosities predominately on the back of the calf and ankle but not infrequently winding round to either side and to the front.
- Both long and short saphenous systems may be providing downflow into the same varicosities but usually one will predominate and may fill the varicose veins so fast that the contribution from the other saphenous system is concealed and does not have the opportunity to develop fully until surgery has removed the dominant pathway of inflow. This 'blocking phenomenon' is discussed further under recurrent varicose veins later in this chapter.
- Perforating veins from the pelvis and from various thigh perforators may be the source for a pathway of incompetence running to varicosities anywhere on the leg or foot.
- Perforating veins in the upper calf may be the source for a retrograde circuit falling down to the foot.

- The venous sinuses of gastrocnemius and soleus muscles may have incompetent veins communicating with the surface to give a powerful surge of blood in and out, with varicosities radiating from them (see Chapter 11).
- Other perforators, particularly in the lower leg following localized thrombosis or in the inborn valveless state, may give strong surge with each muscle contraction, again creating varicosities and retrograde circuits running to the underside of the foot (see Chapter 11).
- Varicosities may arise from the enlarged superficial veins of long or short systems that are acting as collaterals past post-thrombotic deformity and occlusion of deep veins (see Chapter 8). These varicose veins are not necessarily part of the collateral system but may be caused by retrograde circuits with gravitational downflow (just as in simple varicosities) to below any surviving pumping mechanisms, especially the foot. This is discussed further, later in this chapter, under complex patterns.

Numerically, by far the largest group of leg varicosities is derived from long or short saphenous incompetence and easily distinguished by a Trendelenburg test with localized finger pressure applied to the suspected pathway of incompetence.

### *Foot varicosities*

Varicosities running from the lower leg across the ankle and onto the foot are often seen. The great majority are derived from incompetence in the long or short saphenous systems and therefore represent the final part of a pathway of incompetence running to the underside of the foot-pumping mechanism (Figures 5.12, 5.13). They are one expression of simple incompetence in the lower limb and should, at least, be interrupted at the time of surgical treatment since otherwise they are likely to acquire some other source of filling and give persisting unsightly varicose veins, capable of aggravating any tendency to venous stasis (see Chapter 4). Their undesirable state is greatly compounded by heavy surge upwards every time the foot is put to the ground when walking.

Any of the sources given in the previous section on leg varicosities may provide gravitational flow to the underside of the foot and hence cause foot varicosities. Although varicose veins on the foot are often a true downward extension of the venous disorder above this level, this is not necessarily so. For example, foot varicosities in a post-thrombotic limb will seldom be acting as collateral vessels past deep vein occlusion but are usually due to gravitational leak back from whatever source may be available above this level and aggravated by surge with each footstep; the foot varicosities are an additional but different state taking advantage of the

**Figure 5.12** *Varicose veins running to the foot.*

*(a) Varicosities arising from the long saphenous vein and running to the underside of the foot pump.*

*(b) Varicose vein running to the underside of the foot from perforating vein(s) on the inner side of the lower leg. This may be a continuation of simple incompetence in the saphenous system, or, from localized incompetence in deep veins and a perforating vein, or, from a perforator which is part of an outward pumping collateral mechanism from deep to superficial veins past impaired deep veins at a higher level*

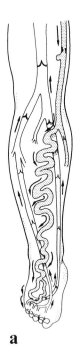

**a**

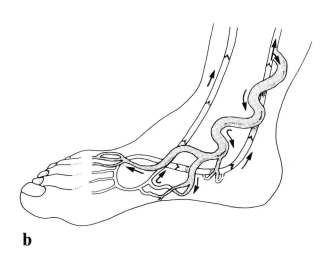

**b**

abnormalities higher up but nevertheless an added disadvantage to the limb.

*Foot varicosities as a hindrance to upward venous pumping*

Foot varicosities will usually be associated with considerable movement of blood to the underside of the foot as it is raised. Thus, at the very moment that blood should be entering the deep vein pumping mechanisms it is sequestered in the foot (Figure 5.13(d),(e)). As soon as the foot is placed down again the blood surges back into the lower leg and in this way must be a substantial hindrance to venous return and an important factor in venous stasis (Figure 5.13(d)).

**Note on treatment** The footpiece of an elastic stocking may have an important role to play in controlling surge to the foot (see Chapter 21). At surgery, when venous stasis and ulceration is caused by massive but simple incompetence in the superficial veins, it would seem particularly important to eliminate the most obvious varicosities running to the foot so that the rapidity of pooling in the foot is limited as far as possible.

### Lateral varicose veins of congenital origin

Persistence of the lateral embryonic vein to the limb will occasionally give rise to a vast channel often associated with other vascular abnormalities, such as haemangiomas and overgrowth in the limb (Klippel–Trenaunay's syndrome) and these are discussed in Chapter 12. The gross examples of this, with a huge vein running up the length of the limb (Figure 5.14) and disappearing in the upper thigh or gluteal region, leave no doubt as to its identity especially if there are associated abnormalities also present. However, the large meandering varicosity quite often seen on the outer side of the limb and illustrated in (Figure 5.3) is sometimes said to be based upon the lateral embryonic vein. This is possible but it seems more likely to be derived from linking of the numerous networks of small superficial veins normally present. A large tortuous varicosity does not necessarily develop from a pre-existing defined single channel and it seems probable that

**Figure 5.13** *Varicose veins running to the foot (see page 103).*

*(a),(b) Foot varicosities of long saphenous origin.*

*(c) Long saphenous incompetence causing venous stasis and ulceration with a large varicosity extending down to the foot. This patient refused surgery and was successfully treated by sclerotherapy to the enlarged vein (see also Figure 4.8).*

*(d) Phlebogram of foot varicosities arising from saphenous incompetence.*

*(e) Composite functional phlebogram of massive varicosities arising from the long saphenous vein and extending down to the foot*

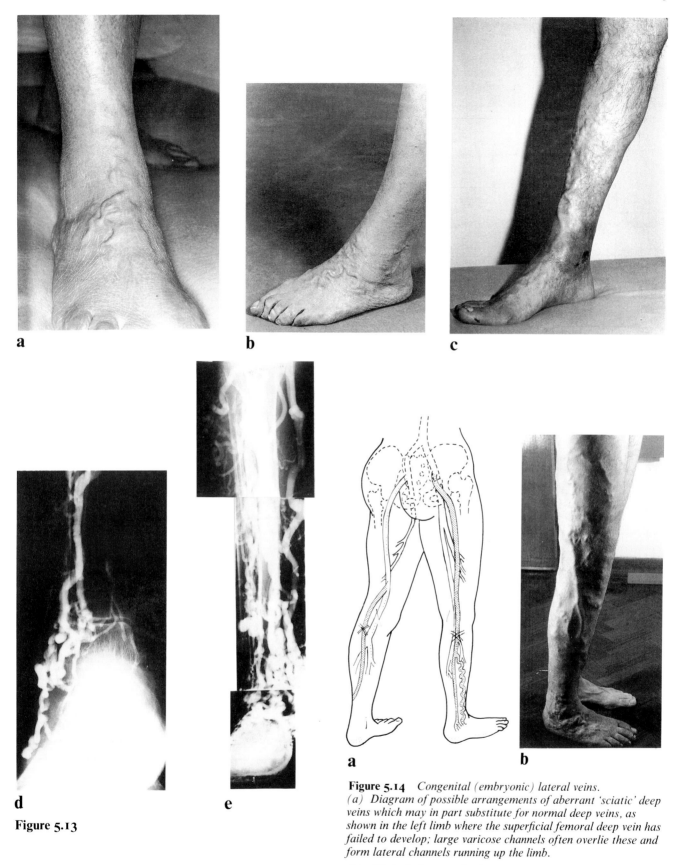

**Figure 5.13**

**Figure 5.14**  *Congenital (embryonic) lateral veins.*
*(a)  Diagram of possible arrangements of aberrant 'sciatic' deep veins which may in part substitute for normal deep veins, as shown in the left limb where the superficial femoral deep vein has failed to develop; large varicose channels often overlie these and form lateral channels running up the limb.*

*(b)  Clinical photograph of congenital lateral vein in a patient with Klippel–Trenaunay syndrome (see Chapter 12). This patient had 3 cm of lengthening in the tibia*

that when very small veins have established a pathway of incompetence, they may develop into massive varicosities with very thin walls over a number of years. The author has reviewed many cases, recorded as accurate diagrams, followed over the last 25 years and where treatment has been postponed by the patient. These give a clear indication that insignificant veins are capable of becoming very large varicosities over, say, a 10-year period. There is considerable variation between patients in the capacity of their veins to do this and those most prone we have termed, for convenience, the 'weak vein syndrome' (see Chapter 7). Other factors, such as high consumption of alcohol, may contribute to this.

## Complex patterns of superficial vein incompetence

Complex patterns of incompetent superficial veins arise when they are derived from simple incompetence in the opposite limb (cross-over incompetence), or are combined with post-thrombotic damage to deep veins and take origin from the collateral veins resulting from this, either in the same limb, or from veins crossing over from the opposite side (Tibbs, 1986).

### Cross-over incompetence

This term is given to superficial vein incompetence which has its source in the opposite limb. Probably, this will never occur unless the normal superficial or deep vein anatomy has been disturbed by surgical interference or by previous thrombosis. Two groups may be recognized:

*I. Incompetence derived from remnants of the long saphenous termination left by inadequate surgery on the opposite limb*

Here the deep veins of both lower limbs are normal throughout, including the iliac veins. A Trendelenburg operation to one side has left the superficial epigastric vein intact and this has been able to establish a pathway of incompetence across the pubic region and into the uppermost long saphenous vein of the opposite side (Figure 5.15), usually via the superficial epigastric vein or the superficial external pudendal vein, or both. This probably will not occur unless there is a pre-existing incompetence in the long saphenous system of that side, allowing downflow and creating the low pressure necessary to set up this pattern of flow. Once established, flow from, say, a left saphenous stump across the pubic region and down the right long saphenous vein will follow every movement of the limb. This causes progressive enlargement of the veins involved, so that, after a year or two, large varicosities may be seen running across the pubic region and into a typically incompetent long saphenous

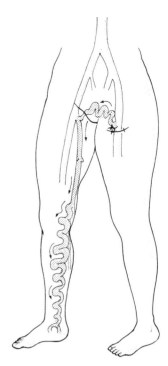

**Figure 5.15** *Diagram of cross-over incompetence arising from a long saphenous stump left by inadequate surgery on the opposite side*

vein with varicosities arising from it, and, in some cases, even causing venous stasis at the right ankle (Figure 5.16). In this example, proof that cross-over incompetence is occurring is given by the following features:

- Continuity of pubic varicosities with right long saphenous vein is evident by inspection, by touch and by use of the tapwave technique.
- The varicosities on the right side may be controlled by digital compression of the pubic veins. This will depend on whether the pubic contribution is entering via an external pudendal vein below a competent saphenous valve. In other cases, there is a dual source of incompetence from pubic veins and, in usual fashion, from the termination of the saphenous vein itself so that this test is less clear cut.
- A Doppler flowmeter placed over the pubic varicosities shows strong downflow across to the side of long saphenous incompetence immediately after each movement of the limb in the upright position. Similarly, this Doppler flow can be interrupted by digital compression of the long saphenous vein. Variations of this can be obtained by putting the Doppler probe over the saphenous vein in mid-thigh and demonstrating intermittent cessation of downflow with repeated pressure to the pubic veins.
- Functional phlebography, with the patient upright and the medium introduced into the veins of the left side, will demonstrate flow, stimulated by exercise, from a saphenous remnant, crossing over the pubic region and down the long saphenous vein of the opposite side.

It will also show that the iliac and other deep veins are normal (Figure 5.16(b)), confirming that the pubic veins do not have any collateral function but are acting solely as a pathway of incompetence.

**Note on treatment** This condition is fully amenable to surgery removing the source, the saphenous stump, together with the superficial epigastric vein arising from it and the pubic varicosities as far as possible; the operation is completed by flush ligation of the long saphenous termination on the opposite side, together with stripping of the saphenous vein and appropriate dissection of varicosities. However correct identification of the condition is important because it is easily confused with incompetence arising from pubic collaterals caused by iliac vein occlusion, described in the next section, and injudicious surgery here could prove harmful. Clinical diagnosis must be backed by the additional evidence of functional phlebography, outlined above, and it would be unwise to proceed to operation without this corroboration.

*II. Cross-over incompetence derived from pubic collateral veins in iliac vein occlusion*

This has many similarities with the condition just described but the essential difference is that a significant deep vein occlusion is present in the iliac veins, causing pubic collateral veins. These cross over the pubes via the terminal branches of the long saphenous veins to drain into the deep veins of the opposite side where it is not uncommon to find saphenous incompetence being fed by the collateral veins which are providing a significant source for downflow (Figure 5.17).

**Note on treatment** Surgery to the incompetent long saphenous vein receiving cross-over flow via pubic collaterals is permissible, but only after confirming that the deep veins on that side are normal and that the operation can be carried out without damage to the collateral circulation. Selective occlusion (Trendelenburg) test should give satisfactory control of the varicose veins in the limb and Doppler flowmeter tracings from the long saphenous vein should show downflow after exercise, both tests indicating that these veins show simple incompetence only and are not part of a collateral mechanism. In addition functional phlebography should be used to clarify the state of the deep vein throughout both lower limbs and the iliac veins; it should also give details of the collateral circulation and give reassurance that surgery is possible without interrupting this.

At operation, in order to ensure that the collateral circulation is left undisturbed, it may be necessary to leave the uppermost branches of the long saphenous vein intact by carrying out ligation at a lower level than usual. In this case it will be essential to strip the incompetent saphenous vein since otherwise communication with it would soon be re-established. Even so, the benefits of

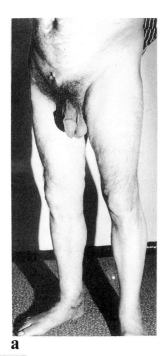

**a**

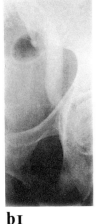

**b1**

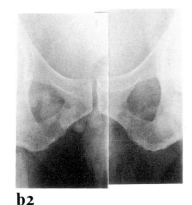

**b2**

**Figure 5.16** *(a) Clinical photograph of cross-over incompetence arising from a saphenous stump in the left groin and crossing over to the right side where there is saphenous incompetence down the length of the limb, causing marked venostatic changes with threatened ulceration at the right ankle.*

*(b) Functional phlebograms in:*
*1. The patient shown in (a).*
*2. Another patient with an identical pattern of cross-over incompetence. In both, opaque medium injected into the superficial veins on the left side outlines normal deep veins, including the iliac veins, and after exercise can be seen crossing pubic varicosities to descend down an incompetent right long saphenous vein. Note: the opaque medium is very diluted by the time it crosses over and gives only a weak outline so that it is only just visible in these photographs. The original X-rays show it beyond doubt and it was clearly seen on the image-intensifier screen. Surgery confirmed the presence of a left saphenous stump with its uppermost branches intact and connecting with the enlarged pubic veins*

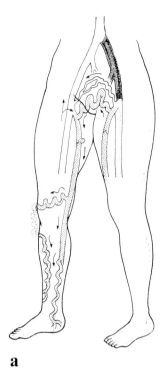

**a**

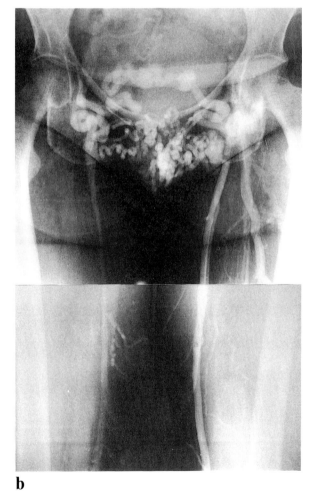

**b**

**Figure 5.17** *(a) Diagram of cross-over incompetence arising from a pubic varicosity which is acting as a collateral to the occluded iliac vein on the left side. Blood reaching the right side passes into the deep veins and upwards, but also spills down an incompetent right long saphenous vein and varicosites arising from it.*

*(b) Functional phlebogram illustrating this form of cross-over incompetence. The patient was known to have suffered left iliac vein thrombosis at the time of pregnancy 30 years previously with residual oedema and venostatic changes on that side; more recently varicose veins, with early skin changes at the ankle, had appeared on the right side. Opaque medium injected into calf veins of the left side travels across to the opposite side and with exercise descends down the right saphenous vein. Surgery was avoided and the patient responded well to knee-length elastic support*

such an operation may be short lived because low ligation, preserving the terminal branches, is known to be an inadequate safeguard against recurrence. This is further explained later in this chapter (see section on 'Measures to ensure adequacy of surgical operation. 2. Ligature flush with deep vein') but, in essence, the network of collateral veins running into the upper part of the limb will constantly seek to find any incompetent superficial veins that can establish a pathway of incompetence down to the low pressure areas beneath the pumping mechanisms of the limb. In each case an individual decision must be made but, unless the surgeon can see a clear opportunity for long-term improvement, it may be wiser to recommend elastic support rather than an operation that will be prone to early recurrence.

## Superficial incompetence combined with deformity and occlusion of the deep veins in the same limb

Superficial incompetence may be seen in association with two categories of post-thrombotic damage to deep veins on the same side.

### Superficial incompetence beneath iliac vein occlusion

It is not uncommon to find typical long saphenous incompetence with varicosities in the limb below a common iliac post-thrombotic occlusion (Figure 5.18(a)). This is seen in its clearest form when the iliac vein occlusion has occurred without any real damage to the common femoral vein or other deep veins below this level and good collateral veins across the pelvis have compensated well for the venous obstruction. This means that the limb has an undamaged pumping system capable of creating low pressure beneath it; the long saphenous vein will not be serving any collateral function and if its valves are incompetent there is no reason why the manifestations of incompetence should not develop. A typical example is shown in Figure 5.18(b)–(d). The patient gave a history

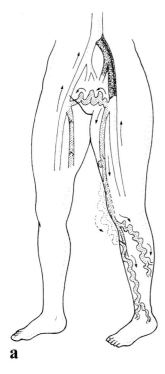

**a**

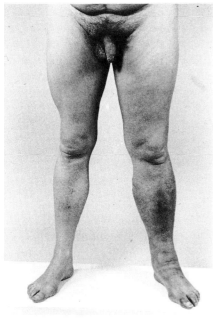

**b**

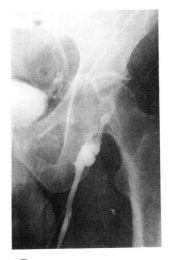

**c1**

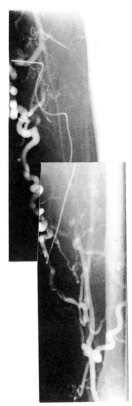

**c2**

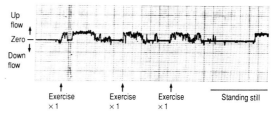

**d**

**Figure 5.18** *(a) Diagram of varicose veins arising from typical long saphenous incompetence in the left lower limb but below post-thrombotic iliac vein occlusion. The deep veins below the inguinal ligament are undamaged and provide the effective pumping mechanism necessary for gravitational downflow in the long saphenous vein and its varicosities.*

*(b) Photograph of patient with typical long saphenous varicosities, but with limb swollen up to the groin and a history suggesting deep vein thrombosis. (c) 1, 2 and (d) are all from the same patient.*

*(c) 1. Upward trace phlebogram in the same patient and showing post-thrombotic occlusion in the external iliac vein with the superficial circumflex iliac vein acting as a collateral.*

*2. Functional phlebogram outlining varicosities arising from the long saphenous vein in the calf. In the upright position, with exercise, opacified blood travelled down these veins and into the deep veins of the leg; there was no upward movement in the long saphenous vein itself but deep veins filled steadily as far as the inguinal ligament and were seen to be normal.*

*(and see page 108)*

**Figure 5.18** *(continued)*
*(d) Tracings of directional Doppler flowmeter applied to long saphenous vein in left thigh showing downflow with exercise and varicosity crossing the groin showing continuous upflow, accentuated by exercise (see page 107).*

Note. *In this patient, the left long saphenous vein could have been divided in the lower thigh, mobilized and swung across to be anastomosed with the right common femoral vein to provide a substantial additional venous return from the left limb. This was not done, however, because the patient's symptoms were minimal and well controlled by elastic support. Moreover, in a saphenous vein used in this direction, flow is counter to the valve cusps which, although incompetent, will distend and may fill with clot. Measures may be used to overcome this but success is doubtful*

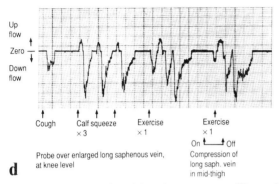

Up flow
Zero
Down flow

Cough  Calf squeeze ×3  Exercise ×1  Exercise ×1
On ⌐ Off
Compression of long saph. vein in mid-thigh

**d** Probe over enlarged long saphenous vein, at knee level

of deep vein thrombosis with subsequent swelling of the limb but not following too severe a course and with only mild residual effects in the limb. The patient noticed varicosities in the limb but these had been previously regarded as collateral veins (so-called secondary varicose veins) because of the history of thrombosis. Examination of the patient showed moderate swelling of the limb and venotensive change; pubic varicosities were visible. An enlarged long saphenous with varicosities arising from it was present and was well controlled by a selective Trendelenburg test; a Doppler flowmeter showed downflow after exercise characteristic of a simple superficial incompetence. Functional phlebography confirmed the presence of an iliac vein occlusion with pelvic collateral vessels but the deep veins below the inguinal ligament showed little abnormality. Exercising the upright patient during phlebography confirmed the diagnosis by showing opacified blood from the common femoral vein spilling over and down the long saphenous system.

Valve failure in the long saphenous system in a case of this sort may be the result of overenlargement whilst acting as a collateral at the time of deep vein thrombosis or by having suffered thrombosis itself at that time. These explanations presume that a very complete recovery from any thrombosis in deep veins below the inguinal ligament has occurred. Whatever its origin, this condition is not infrequently seen in association with occlusion in the iliac vein above it. It is most often seen on the left side in keeping with the preponderance of thrombosis to the left iliac veins.

**Note on treatment** Surgery to an incompetent long

saphenous system such as this is perhaps permissible provided it does not interfere with the collateral veins arising from the terminal branches of the long saphenous and running across the pubes. Thus, ligation will have to be below these branches and, as explained in the section above, such a procedure will have an increased likelihood of recurrence because of the incomplete nature of the operation. This will be minimized by stripping the long saphenous vein but, nevertheless, the benefits are likely to be short lived so that the operation may not be justifiable. Each case requires careful individual assessment and this should include functional phlebography to show flow patterns in the veins concerned. If the surgeon does not see a clear opportunity for removing the incompetent saphenous without significant damage to collaterals in the groin he should not embark on the operation but settle for appropriate elastic support. Caution is advised in such cases.

In some circumstances it may be possible to put the incompetent saphenous vein of the affected limb to good use to provide an additional cross-over channel to the normal side (a 'reversed' Palma operation). It must be remembered that the valves in this vein, although incompetent, will tend to oppose flow and may require division. This procedure is outside the author's experience but conceivably might be of value. However, it is only likely to bring advantage when the long saphenous vein is typically incompetent and it should not be contemplated if the saphenous vein is acting as an important collateral, as in the state described in the next section, but will be best left serving that function.

*Superficial incompetence accompanying post-thrombotic occlusion and deformity in common femoral, superficial femoral and popliteal veins*

Where the deep veins of the thigh are extensively occluded or deformed the long saphenous system (or remnants of it after inappropriate surgery) will act as a valuable collateral set of veins allowing escape of blood upwards. However, the deep veins below the knee may be undamaged and capable of effective pumping action via collateral veins and succeed in creating low pressure at the ankle and underside of the foot. These are the circumstances in which superficial incompetence can allow gravitational downflow (Figure 5.19(a)). Such patients are unlikely to have severe venous stasis but quite often large varicosities are seen running down the leg, across the ankle and to the foot (Figure 5.19(b)). These are branches of the long saphenous vein that are allowing spillage of blood down to the foot every time it is raised. Thus, the long saphenous vein and its major branches are acting as collateral veins with upward flow at each step whilst other branches are allowing spillage from the saphenous system to the low pressure area below the foot. A Doppler flowmeter will demonstrate this and also show

**Figure 5.19**  *(a) Diagram of occlusion in popliteal and/or superficial femoral deep veins, with the long saphenous vein acting as a collateral: varicosities arise from it and run down to below the foot pumping mechanism.*

*(b) Clinical photograph of varicosities running to the foot below occlusion of the popliteal vein. The patient, aged 47, gave a history of deep vein thrombosis following hysterectomy 8 years previously (possible stirrup injury). There was moderate swelling but little tendency to venous stasis at the ankle.*

*(c) Directional Doppler tracings in the same patient showing upward movement in the long saphenous vein, accentuated by exercise, because this is acting as collateral. Varicosities running to the foot show downflow on foot raising but no evidence of collateral function.*

*(d) Functional phlebogram of the same patient showing severe post-thrombotic deformity and occlusion in the popliteal vein with both saphenous veins acting as collaterals; the short saphenous has a wide upward extension in continuity with profunda femoris vein. The long saphenous gives off a large varicose vein running down to the foot and opacified blood could be seen running down this when the foot was raised (see page 110).*

Note.  *The enlarged saphenous veins are providing excellent collateral channels; any surgical interference with them is most unlikely to improve on this (see Chapter 21)*

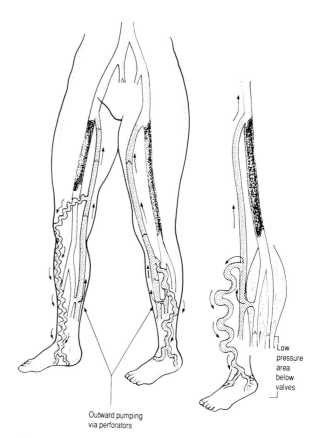

Outward pumping via perforators

Low pressure area below valves

**a**

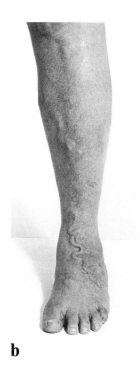

**b**

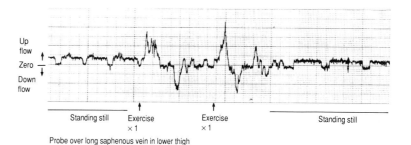

Up flow
Zero
Down flow

Standing still | Exercise × 1 | Exercise × 1 | Standing still

Probe over long saphenous vein in lower thigh

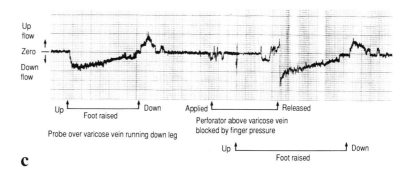

Up flow
Zero
Down flow

Up | Foot raised | Down | Applied | Released

Perforator above varicose vein blocked by finger pressure

Probe over varicose vein running down leg

Up | Foot raised | Down

**c**

a heavy surge back again when the foot is placed to the ground (Figure 5.19(c)). Functional phlebography can confirm this phenomenon (Figure 5.19(d)).

**Note on treatment** Treatment by surgery or by sclerotherapy to varicose veins running to the foot is theoretically possible but if stasis is mild then the veins are presumably comparatively harmless and controlled most appropriately by a below-knee elastic support. Sclerotherapy is not always easy to limit in its effect and if it is to be employed should be only used in very small doses for fear of thrombosis spreading into collateral channels. Treatment by surgery or sclerotherapy should only be carried out after careful evaluation by Doppler flowmeter and plethysmography to demonstrate that no ill-effects are caused by occluding the vessels which are to be removed or sclerosed. This should be backed by the findings at functional phlebography which should not show any significant post-thrombotic damage in the deep veins below the knee although it is not always easy to obtain an effective demonstration when the deep veins above this level are blocked; the varicosities being considered for removal should not show any collateral upflow but only downflow when the foot is raised, and surge up again when it is placed on the ground again.

The sections above are only considering superficial incompetence seen in combination with various patterns of deep vein occlusion. The other aspects of post-thrombotic occlusive deep vein states are considered in Chapters 8 and 9.

## Persistent and recurrent varicose veins

By far the largest part of treatment in venous disorders is concerned with the elimination of retrograde circuits of incompetence and it is perhaps best to start this section by restating (see Chapter 4), in simple terms, the basic thought behind this. The cause for most varicose veins in the lower limb, and in many cases of venous stasis, is gravitational downflow in incompetent veins (the pathway of incompetence); this runs from a higher level, somewhere above a pumping mechanism, to a lower level, somewhere below a pumping mechanism. Turbulent flow down these veins enlarges them to become varicose and, in some cases, the downflow may be sufficient to overwhelm the musculovenous pump so that venous hypertension, and its clinical changes, ensue. In a much smaller group of patients the condition being treated is caused by, or accentuated by, surge through perforators (see Chapter 11) and this aspect is considered separately.

The basis of treatment is the elimination, as completely as possible, of the pathway of incompetence by surgical removal or obliteration by sclerotherapy. Success will therefore depend upon the accurate recognition of the pathway of incompetence and the source of flow down this. The various patterns of failed treatment, the reasons

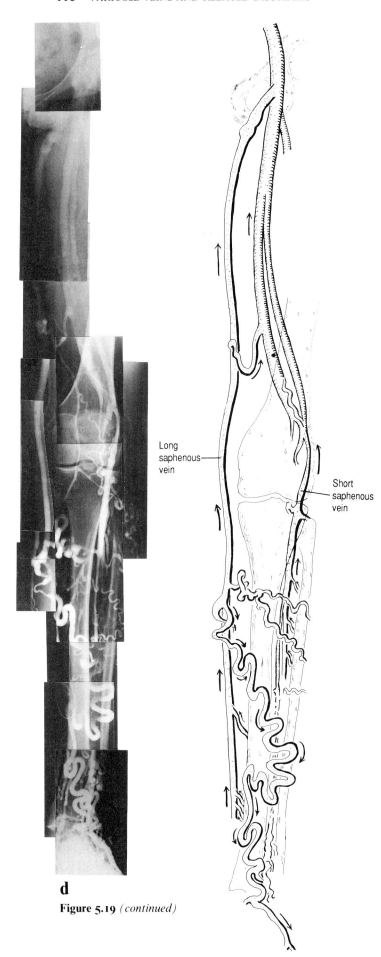

Long saphenous vein

Short saphenous vein

**d**

**Figure 5.19** (*continued*)

for these and the methodical approach required to minimize failures will now be considered.

## Patterns of failure in the treatment of varicose veins

Following surgical treatment for varicose veins, various forms of failure may become evident; similar considerations may also apply after sclerotherapy.

### Persisting or residual varicosities

The original varicosities may persist so that failure of treatment is apparent from an early stage after surgery. Here it is evident that there are two factors:

1. The varicosities are still substantially intact and the operation has disconnected rather than removed them (Figure 5.20) and they may represent a large part of the original pathway of incompetence.
2. The true origin of the veins has not been accurately

located, or the varicosities have a second source of filling which has not been previously recognized. In the former case, an example might be where inadequate assessment before operation has attributed the incompetence to the short, instead of the long, saphenous vein, or vice versa, a mistake that can occur all too easily in calf varicosities (Figure 4.22(e)). Alternatively, the varicosities may have filled from both long and short incompetent saphenous veins and only one of these veins has been dealt with (Figure 5.21). It is quite common for incompetence in, say, the long saphenous vein to fill the varicosities so quickly that another contributary incompetence, for example, from the short saphenous vein, only has a brief opportunity to provide downflow to the varicosities before these are filled to capacity awaiting the next muscle contraction. This 'blocking' phenomenon will limit the development and enlargement of the lesser origin until it is uncovered by removal of the principle source of incompetence. The lesser source then has opportunity for unlimited downflow and may rapidly enlarge up to declare its presence. Thus the fast filling from one source has obscured slow filling from another source which will take over if given the opportunity. This may be apparent at an early stage after operation or appear after an interval of many months, perhaps years, during which time the surviving source has

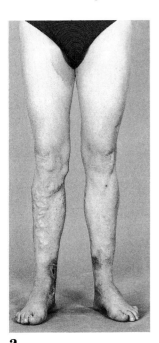 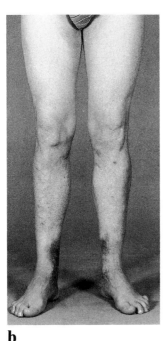

**a**        **b**

**Figure 5.20** *A patient before and after surgery, illustrating persisting veins.*

*(a) Substantial long saphenous varicosities right side with venous stasis at the ankle before operation.*

*(b) Surgery to the long saphenous vein has removed the main pathway of incompetence and the skin at the ankle is much healthier. However, a large varicosity on the outer side of the right leg was not removed and has remained open. Not only is this cosmetically disappointing for a patient but a large incompetent channel such as this is likely to find a new source for flow down it, to cause progressive enlargement and eventually renewed venous stasis. It is best to remove these varicosities at the time of surgery but, failing this, such an obvious persisting varicosity, especially if it shows strong Doppler downflow on exercise or foot raising, should be obliterated by sclerotherapy to complete treatment*

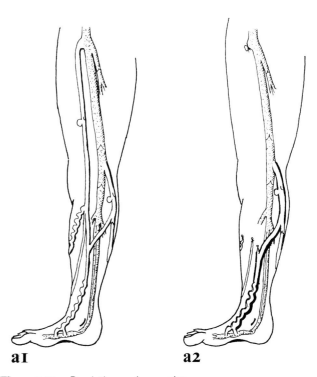

**a1**        **a2**

**Figure 5.21** *Persisting varicose veins.*

*(a) 1. Diagram to show varicose veins with a double source of filling.*
*2. Removing only one source will not bring any lasting benefit to the patient.*

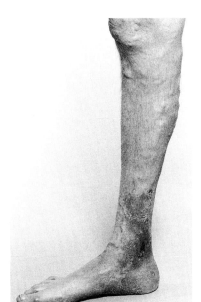

**b1**

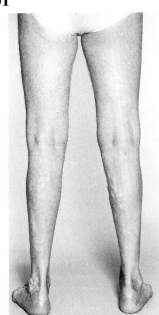

**b2**

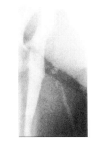

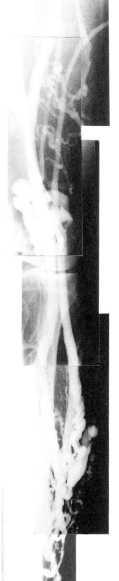

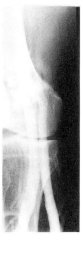

**Figure 5.21** *(continued)*
*(b) 1, 2. Clinical photographs of varicose veins persisting after*
*high ligation and stripping of long saphenous vein.*
*Pigmentation and ulceration at the ankle remains indolent.*
*Clinical tests showed that the varicosities were now filling*
*from the short saphenous vein.*

*3. Phlebogram of the same patient; composite picture with*
*limb in external rotation to show calf varicosities filling*
*from the short saphenous vein which terminates at normal*
*level but has an upward extension winding round the back*
*and inner thigh to join remnants of the long saphenous*
*system; some lesser varicosities on the front of the thigh are*
*faintly seen arising from this. A large convoluted varicose*
*vein arises from the short saphenous vein behind the knee*
*and runs down to join long saphenous varicosities on the*
*inner leg. High ligation and stripping of the short saphenous*
*vein, together with removing its upward extension and the*
*varicosities on thigh and inner leg, gave a good result.*

*(see page 113 for explanatory drawing)*

**b3**

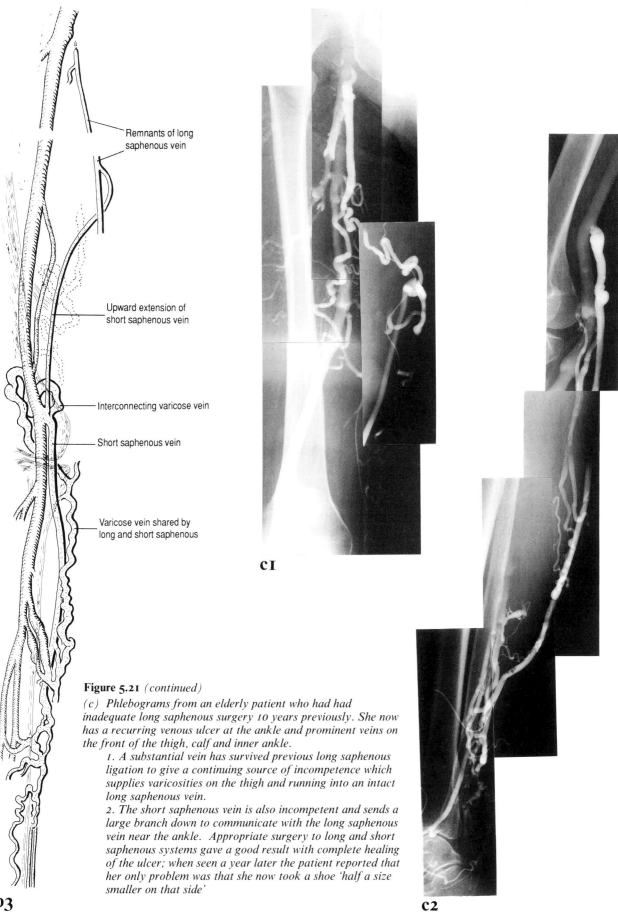

Remnants of long
saphenous vein

Upward extension of
short saphenous vein

Interconnecting varicose vein

Short saphenous vein

Varicose vein shared by
long and short saphenous

**Figure 5.21** *(continued)*

*(c) Phlebograms from an elderly patient who had had
inadequate long saphenous surgery 10 years previously. She now
has a recurring venous ulcer at the ankle and prominent veins on
the front of the thigh, calf and inner ankle.*

*1. A substantial vein has survived previous long saphenous
ligation to give a continuing source of incompetence which
supplies varicosities on the thigh and running into an intact
long saphenous vein.*

*2. The short saphenous vein is also incompetent and sends a
large branch down to communicate with the long saphenous
vein near the ankle. Appropriate surgery to long and short
saphenous systems gave a good result with complete healing
of the ulcer; when seen a year later the patient reported that
her only problem was that she now took a shoe 'half a size
smaller on that side'*

**b3**

**c1**

**c2**

steadily enlarged so that the varicose veins become clinically evident again and are regarded as recurrent rather than persisting varicosities.

Another possibility is the existence of a complex state in which the varicose veins are filled from two different types of source, one due to simple superficial vein incompetence and the other to incompetent communication with deep veins. Veins communicating with the gastrocnemius venous sinuses, for example, may sometimes provide a concealed second source of varicose veins. Initially this may have been overshadowed by saphenous incompetence and only develops fully after removal of this dominant source (Figures 5.32, 5.33).

*Substitute varicosities*

Again these are noticed at an early stage after surgery but, although the original varicosities have gone, a new and different set of veins have now appeared (Figure 5.22). This usually means that surgery has not adequately removed the origin of the previous incompetence, although perhaps much of the original pathway has been removed by stripping of a saphenous vein and dissection of the varicosities. The survival of a ready source of outflow at a high level has soon found a new pathway of incompetence which catches the eye of the patient. This is often seen on the anterolateral thigh as a slender tortuous vein not seen before, and can respond well to a single injection given soon after it is recognized; if left untreated it is likely to enlarge progressively over the years.

*Recurrent varicose veins by anatomical routes or by re(neo)vascularization of saphenous stump*

Recurrence is the return of varicosities at the original site and may be noticed some years after a good initial result. They are often based on the original pathway of incompetence which has not been completely removed and has found a new source of outflow from the deep veins at high level to give renewed and ever-increasing flow down it. There are a variety of causes for this, including the following:

1.  Incomplete surgery to the origin leaving behind a branch which enlarges steadily over the next year or two, utilizing the pathway provided by previous varicosities (Figures 5.23–5.26).
2.  Communication between the original source, for example, the termination of the saphenous vein, and its pathway of incompetence has been established by a completely new and non-anatomical channel that has developed, possibly by canalization of haematoma following surgery (Figures 5.23(a) (left), 5.27, 5.28). This possibility is increasingly recognized and is discussed further below.

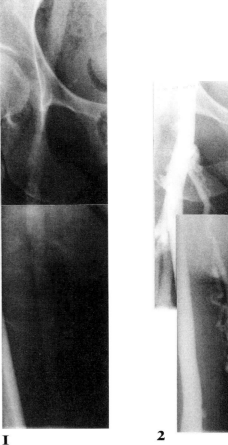

**1**          **2**

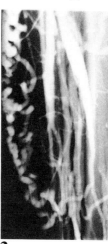

**3**

**Figure 5.22** *Substitute varicose veins following surgery for incompetence of the right long saphenous system. This functional phlebogram shows that one of the branches at the termination of the long saphenous vein has been left intact and has established a new pathway of incompetence to form varicosities on the front of the thigh and winding down the outer aspect to the lower leg. These varicosities had enlarged progressively over the 2 years following operation.*
*1. Before exercise.*
*2. After exercise, with opacified blood spilling down varicosity.*
*3. The same varicosity in lower leg, with flow from it into the deep veins*

**Figure 5.23** *Diagrams of incomplete surgery to upper long saphenous vein leading to early recurrence.*

*(a)* Right limb. *Ligation of long saphenous vein has not been flush with common femoral vein and the saphenous vein has not been stripped. An uppermost branch has survived and connects with the saphenous vein which provides a new and active pathway of incompetence.*
Left limb. *Flush ligation has been carried out but the saphenous vein has not been stripped. Varicosities have established communication with the saphenous vein, renewing the pathway of incompetence down this. This is not necessarily caused by uppermost saphenous branches being left intact but may be due to revascularization of haematoma at the saphenous stump to form a complex of veins communicating between the common femoral vein and long saphenous vein (non-anatomical reconnection). This will be encouraged by low venous pressure in the divided but still incompetent saphenous vein; in the upright and exercising patient, the pressure difference between this and the common femoral vein will be considerable.*

*(b)* Right limb. *Recurrence from a secondary source, the pelvic veins, emerging via internal pudendal or obturator veins. This flows into an unstripped long saphenous vein, or a new pathway of incompetence based on remnants of the saphenous system, and fills original varicosities down to the foot.*
Left limb. *Anterolateral branch from the saphenous stump has re-established connection with an unstripped long saphenous vein.*

*(c)* Right limb. *Mid-thigh perforator has established outward flow to remaining long saphenous vein after partial stripping of its upper part.*
Left limb. *Short saphenous vein takes over varicose veins left intact after stripping of the long saphenous vein from which they arose*

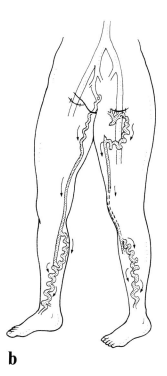

**b**

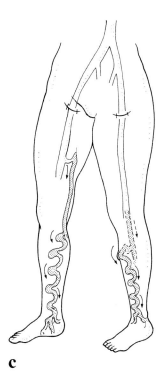

**c**

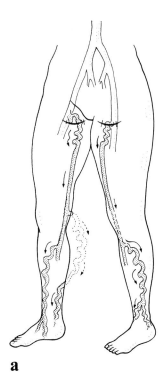

**a**

3. The original varicosities may find a completely new source or one that has been previously obscured by a much larger source (see above) and is now uncoverd by its removal, for example, a mid-thigh perforator that connects with the original varicosities and thereafter progressively expands (Figures 5.23(b) (right), (c) (both sides), 5.29, 5.30).

4. A short saphenous vein, previously obscured, has taken over as described above under 'persisting veins'.

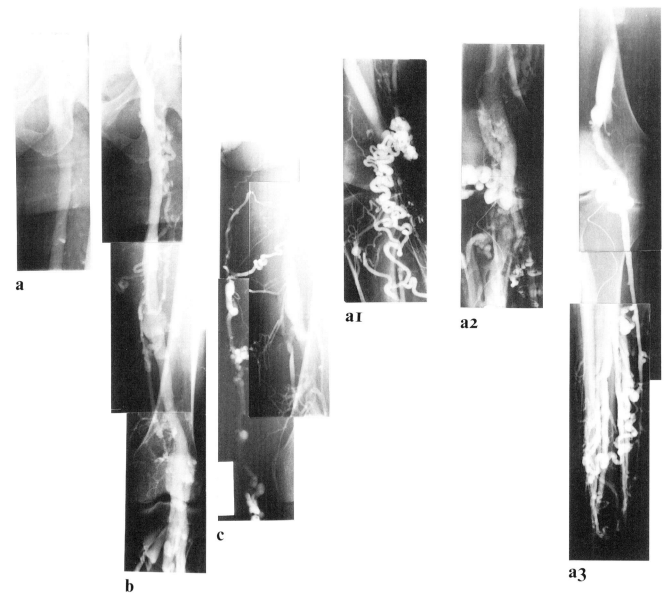

**Figure 5.24** *Example of a persisting tributary in a long saphenous stump on the left side connecting with thigh varicosities not removed at previous operation. Functional phlebography in near-upright patient shows:*

*(a) Femoral vein passively filling with patient standing still.*

*(b) After exercise downflow is seen in recurrent varicosities.*

*(c) A slightly later phase. Connection with original thigh varicosities on inner aspect of thigh is seen. This sort of recurrence may be misdiagnosed as an incompetent perforator with disappointing results at further surgery*

**Figure 5.25** *Some examples of incomplete surgery to the short saphenous vein; all are posterior views.*

*(a) Bilateral short saphenous recurrence.*
*1. Right side. Upward trace with patient near horizontal to show convoluted varicosity taking off from short saphenous stump.*
*2, 3. Left side:*
*2. Functional phlebogram with patient upright showing rather high termination of short saphenous vein which appears intact with a large varicosity taking off in mid-popliteal fossa.*
*3. Composite view, including upward trace and shown in partially rotated limb. The short saphenous vein is clearly seen joining the upper popliteal deep vein; varicosities arise in the popliteal fossa and in mid-calf where blood can be seen recycling into the deep veins of the leg; this portion of the composite picture was obtained with the patient upright.*

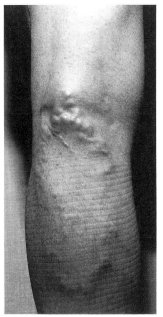

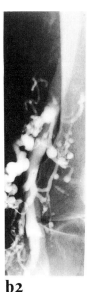

**b1**          **b2**

**Figure 5.25** *(continued)*
*(b) 1. Clinical photograph of varicose veins appearing behind the knee in a 60-year-old man, 2 years after ligation and stripping of the short saphenous vein for calf varicosities.*
*2. Phlebography outlining origin of the varicose veins arising from a substantial stump of short saphenous vein. Further surgery, with flush ligation, gave a good result without recurrence when reviewed 2 years later*

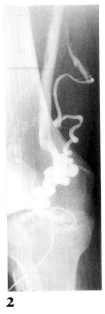

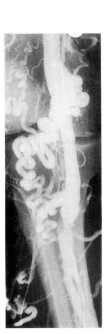

**2**

**1**

**Figure 5.26**    *A further example of incomplete surgery to the short saphenous vein.*
*1. A functional phlebogram with the patient upright shows a large varicosity arising from a remnant of short saphenous vein.*
*2. Upward trace to show saphenous remnant more clearly; the upper 3 cm is intact and includes a branch penetrating the deep fascia; this has become a new pathway of incompetence from which a large new varicosity has formed over the popliteal fossa and descending down the calf*

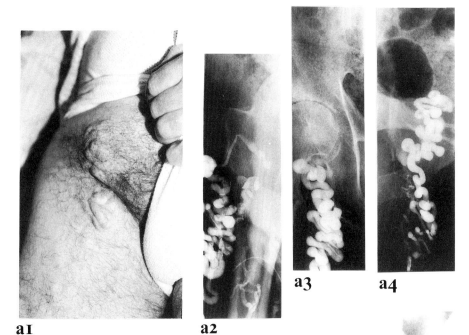

**a1**   **a2**   **a3**   **a4**

**Figure 5.27** *Non-anatomical new connections as a cause for recurrence.*

*(a)* 1. *Clinical photograph of massive recurrent varicose veins in the groin of a patient who had had two previous attempts to remove these.*

  2–4. *Upward trace phlebograms in the same patient, at various stages, and in three different rotations to show connection with underlying common femoral vein. There was no clear demonstration of a saphenous stump and at surgery it was confirmed that flush ligation had been previously carried out but a large venous 'spongework' of varicosities, without any anatomical basis, had been established from the site of ligation and connected with remnants of the saphenous system. This appears to be an example of non-anatomical revascularization, perhaps encouraged by haematoma left at operation. Further surgery completely removing the groin varicosity, together with the thigh varicose veins descending from it, proved successful.*

*(b)* *Phlebograms of long saphenous vein recurrence seen 10 years after operation. The 51-year-old male patient, a keen tennis player, disliked the large varicosities on his inner thigh and calf.*

  1. *A spongework of small veins in the area of saphenous ligation joins an anterior saphenous branch which runs down to remnants of the saphenous system; normal perforating veins to the profunda femoris are seen.*

  2. *A slightly later view with flow entering varicosities and an unstripped long saphenous vein.*

*The appearances at the saphenous stump do not suggest an origin from a surviving branch but one of revascularization; the findings at surgery were in keeping with this. Appropriate clearing of the spongework from the front of the common femoral vein and removing the superficial veins involved gave a good result when reviewed a year later*

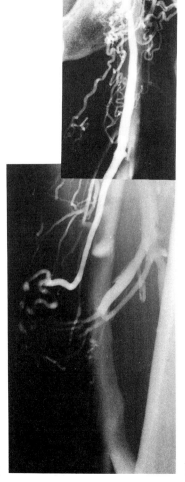

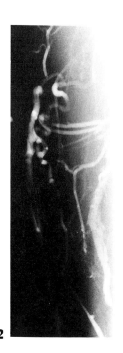

**b1**   **b2**

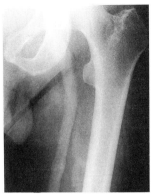 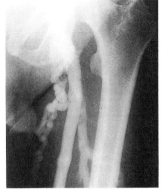

**a1**　　　　**a2**

**Figure 5.28**　*Non-anatomical recurrence after high ligation for saphenous incompetence.*

*(a) Phlebograms 3 years after long saphenous ligation without stripping it, in a male patient, aged 48, with massive incompetence in the long saphenous vein, recurrent varicosities and venotensive changes. Functional phlebograms in the upright patient show:*

> *1. Passive filling of the deep veins before exercise.*
> *2. Immediately after exercise, opacified blood spills down a coiled mass of varicosities running from the site of saphenous ligation to connect with the unstripped long saphenous vein. The phlebogram does not show any evident saphenous stump and, at surgical exploration, previous flush ligation appeared to have been complete without evidence of any persisting anatomical connection but communication was through a mass of small veins. This seems likely to be an example of revascularization with development of a venous spongework connecting with the incompetent long saphenous vein still* in situ. *Connection of this sort probably requires the pressure difference that would exist between the femoral vein and the detached long saphenous vein when the patient is upright and exercising.*

*(b) Revascularization at site of ligated perforator arising from an upward extension of short saphenous vein. Phlebogram from man, aged 42, ten years after unsuccessful operation ligating the short saphenous vein, and subsequent ligation of 'recurrent perforator' in posterior thigh.*

> *1. The deep vein is faintly shown with a 1 cm stump of short saphenous vein; running from this is a large upward extension in continuity with profunda femoris vein; at the site of perforator ligation is a convoluted mass of veins, connecting with a superficial varicose vein.*
> *2. This was found to join the long saphenous vein and flowed down it to enter the deep veins by a large perforator in mid-leg*

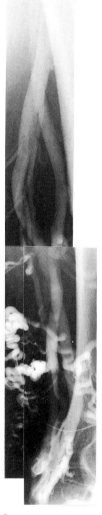 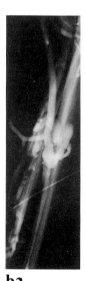

**b2**

**b1**

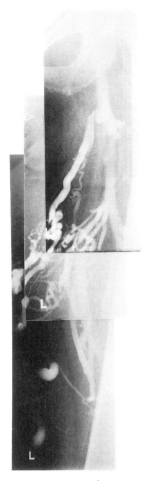

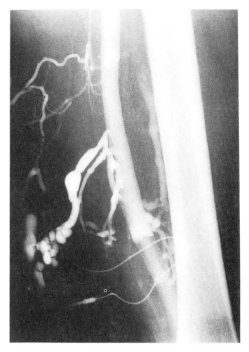

**Figure 5.30**  *Recurrence due to acquisition of a new source. High ligation and stripping of the long saphenous vein had been carried out some years before recurrent varicosities developed. These appeared to fill from a source in the mid-thigh and phlebography confirmed this by showing a large perforating vein running from the superficial femoral deep vein to varicosities based on remnants of the saphenous system. Note the effective deep vein valve a short distance below the origin of this perforator; this, and any other valves below it, provide the pressure difference following exercise necessary to cause flow down the incompetent perforator and superficial veins to the low pressure areas beneath the valves*

**Figure 5.29**  *Recurrent varicosities by acquisition of a new source. Flush ligation and stripping of the long saphenous vein had been carried out some years before but without removing thigh varicosities. This composite phlebogram shows a large vessel running from the lowermost common femoral vein to the thigh varicosities. This arises from the deep vein about 3 cm below the usual site of the long saphenous termination and appears to be a high-level perforating vein which is now the new source of the pathway of incompetence. The rounded bulge is probably due to a neighbouring valve in the deep vein; from this single view the possibility of an unusually low termination to the long saphenous vein, with a residual stump, would have to be considered; other views showed this to be most unlikely*

*New varicosities*

These appear within a year or two but do not correspond with those originally present. Here a new system of varicose veins has been established. This may be based on:

1. An old source that has not been properly eliminated and has set up a new and different pathway of incompetence which eventually enlarges to become visible as the new varicosities (Figure 5.31 (right)). These are equivalent to the substitute varicosities described above that are not immediately apparent after operation but have enlarged since then.

*or*

2. A short or long saphenous vein, or one of the less usual sources such as a pelvic vein, not previously at fault (Figure 5.31 (left)). This is not strictly a failure in treatment but the development of a new and separate set of varicosities. Nevertheless, if one saphenous system has been at fault there is an increased possibility of an incipient incompetence in the other system that will reveal itself sooner or later. However, this is not sufficiently likely to justify a precautionary removal of the second saphenous system until such time as it has clearly declared itself.

*Varicosities not due to simple incompetence*

Varicosities may persist, or became worse, after surgery, because the basic diagnosis is incomplete or at fault and the veins are not just simple (primary) varicosities caused by retrograde flow from above a pumping mechanism to below it; surgery based on that assumption has been inappropriate and indeed the condition may not be amenable to surgery. Examples of this include: a communicating gastrocnemius vein sending high pressure surge back and forth (Figures 5.32, 5.33 and see Chapter

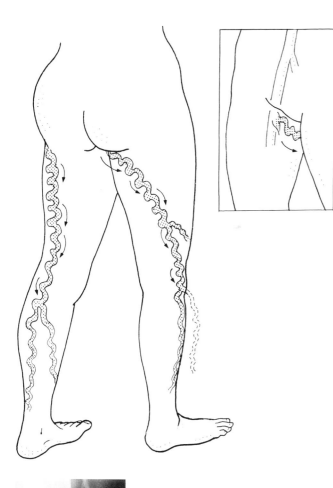

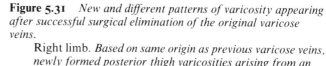

**Figure 5.31** *New and different patterns of varicosity appearing after successful surgical elimination of the original varicose veins.*

*Right limb. Based on same origin as previous varicose veins, newly formed posterior thigh varicosities arising from an external pudendal vein surviving inadequate surgery to the saphenous termination. Inset shows origin of this from saphenous stump.*

*Left limb. New set of varicosities, unrelated to previous varicose veins, due to filling from an unusual pelvic source, the inferior gluteal vein. A more common pelvic origin would be an enlarged internal pudendal vein persisting after pregnancy (not illustrated here but see Figure 5.11)*

**Figure 5.32** *Recurrence of short saphenous varicosities due to a double origin from short saphenous vein and from incompetent communication with a gastrocnemius vein.*

*(a) Original phlebograms (upright, posterior views).*
*1. In internal rotation, showing incompetent short saphenous vein running down the back of the calf.*
*2. A view in mid-rotation showing free communication with a gastrocnemius venous sinus; the possible significance of this was overlooked because it was assumed to be superficial to deep perforator inward flow, commonly seen during phlebography.*
*3. A lateral view from the inner side to show detail of a large varicose vein arising from the short saphenous vein in the upper calf.*

*(b) Further phlebogram taken 1 year after high ligation and stripping of short saphenous vein (upright, anterior view). The varicosities at this stage had reappeared and enlarged progressively. A small bulge due to the residual stump of the short saphenous vein is seen in mid-popliteal but this is not at fault. A large incompetent gastrocnemius vein is seen communicating with superficial varicosities and is the cause of their recurrence. This is the same communication, now much enlarged, as that shown in the original phlebogram. Further views of this patient are shown in Figure 11.22*

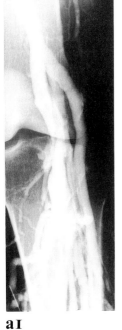

**a1**

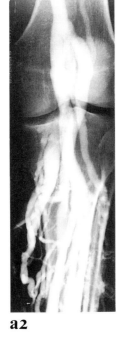

**a2**

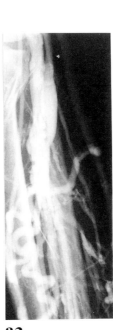

**a3**

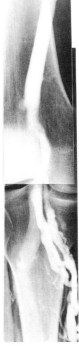

**b**

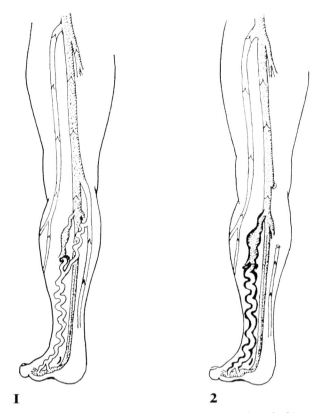

**I**                                    **2**

**Figure 5.33**   *Diagrams to explain the changes described in Figure 5.32.*
> *1. The original state, with substantial short saphenous incompetence filling the varicose veins but these also communicate with a gastrocnemius venous sinus. Short saphenous incompetence dominates and by the rapidity of its filling tends to oppose development of the alternative gastrocnemius source.*
> *2. After high ligation and stripping of the upper short saphenous vein the gastrocnemius source rapidly enlarges because it is no longer 'blocked' by the dominant source.*

*An incompetent gastrocnemius vein is likely to cause more than gravitational downflow and may pump blood outwards at each contraction of the muscle. Phlebography or ultrasonography is usually required to elucidate the origin of this pattern of veins (see Chapter 11 on the role perforating veins)*

11), post-thrombotic syndrome (see Chapter 8), valveless syndrome (see Chapter 7), congenital venous abnormality (see Chapter 12), or the presence of acquired or congenital arteriovenous fistula(s) (see Chapter 17).

## Measures to minimize failure in treatment: the importance of preoperative assessment

Some forms of failure, for example, due to two sources of incompetence, are difficult to avoid altogether so that a second operation will be necessary from time to time. However, a proper assessment of the patient initially should give a clear confirmation of the suitability for surgical treatment and predict reliably the outcome of such surgery. This is also true if sclerotherapy is being considered, but here the effectiveness in closing off veins is less precise than with surgery and this, together with other considerations (see Chapter 18), gives less certainty to the outcome. Precision in the good selection of patients for treatment depends on:

1. Accurate mapping of enlarged veins and interconnections between them. Thoroughness in this is essential so that a clear picture is built up without any doubt upon the likely pathway of incompetence leading down to the varicose veins. Such mapping will entail:
   (a) Tracing the veins visually, but, although this is assisted by oblique illumination, it is the least effective method.
   (b) Locating and following veins by light touch.
   (c) *Use of the tapwave technique* (see Chapter 2). This is by far the most valuable method for mapping out veins which cannot otherwise be detected clinically.
   (d) Doppler flowmeter, but this is a somewhat tedious way of mapping veins if it is used extensively.

   In some cases phlebography is necessary to understand the pattern and interconnection of the veins, especially when the normal anatomy of the superficial veins has been disturbed by previous operations and recurrent varicosities are present.

2. Demonstration that the pathway of incompetence mapped out, and including the varicosities themselves, shows the typical features of a simple incompetence. This is proved by:
   (a) A selective Trendelenburg test, using fingertip compression over the pathway of incompetence, controls the varicosities; exercise during this test, without appreciable filling of the veins, gives it added conviction.
   (b) Perthes' test, again with fingertip control to the pathway of incompetence, gives undoubted softening of the varicosities.
   (c) A directional Doppler flowmeter over the pathway of incompetence, including the varicosities, shows characteristic downflow after exercise.
   (d) A photophlethysmograph, or similar test, shows that an abnormally shortened recovery period after exercise is improved to near normal by temporary occlusion of the pathway of incompetence. This is especially valuable when venotensive change is present but in varicose veins without stasis there may be insufficient departure from normal for the test to be valid.

Usually a selective Trendelenburg test alone is sufficient evidence of simple incompetence but when supported by one or more of the tests given above is conclusive proof of this and, moreover, gives absolute confirmation that the pathway of incompetence has been accurately localized by the fingertips; its removal can only bring benefit to the patient and the surgeon can proceed with confidence.

If the above tests are not convincing the surgeon must think again before deciding upon surgery; perhaps the wrong vein is under suspicion or during the tests the fingertips have not been accurately positioned over it. Examine the other saphenous system in the limb carefully, or perhaps both systems may be at fault and simultaneous control will give the answer. Perhaps the problem is not one of simple incompetence and the various possibilities given above in 'Varicosities not due to simple incompetence' have to be considered. If further examination does not give a clear answer, and the patient's clinical condition justifies it, then functional phlebography will be needed.

## When venotensive changes are present

Special care is required when the clinical manifestations of venous hypertension (venous stasis) are present (venous flares around the ankle, pigmentation, induration, oedema, eczema, threatened or actual ulceration). Over half of new patients showing ulceration will be due to post-thrombotic or valveless syndrome, and those due to simple, but often concealed, incompetence of a saphenous vein, suitable for surgery, must be distinguished with great care. To fail to recognize a concealed incompetence is a great disservice because leaving this curable state will unnecessarily condemn the patient to prolonged disability. If the cause is simple incompetence of the superficial veins the following features will be found:

### Simple incompetence

1. Usually there is no history of deep vein thrombosis or of a fracture in the limb. However, if there is, it must not be assumed that residual damage to the deep veins is the cause. Some of these cases do recover completely from deep vein thrombosis and go on to develop massive incompetence in a saphenous vein, possibly because at one stage it was used as a collateral or because thrombosis and recanalization has occurred in it too. Moreover history can be misleading over the occurrence of deep vein thrombosis.
2. Venotensive changes tend to be localized and heavily grooved.
3. An enlarged long or short saphenous vein can be mapped out by using the tapwave technique. One or more saccules may be recognized along it, particularly in the thigh.
4. Trendelenburg's test gives good control with fingertips accurately over the saphenous vein (often made easy by a deep groove in the thigh in elevation). Exercise during this test does not cause appreciable filling of

varicosities; release of control leads to rapid and complete filling.
5. Directional Doppler flowmetry shows downflow after exercise or on lifting the foot off the ground.
6. *Photoplethysmography shows a shortened recovery period after exercise but this reverts to near normal with localized fingertip control to the saphenous vein under suspicion.* Use of plethysmography in this fashion to confirm a concealed superficial incompetence is its most valuable role.

By contrast, when venous hypertension is not due to superficial incompetence, the following features will be recognized:

### Post-thrombotic or inborn valveless states

1. The history will prove important and usually there is a clear history of deep vein thrombosis or of a major fracture in the limb. A congenital abnormality may be suggested by the first manifestations appearing in childhood.
2. The saphenous vein may be enlarged but a selective Trendelenburg test fails to control this or any associated veins.
3. Doppler flowmetry over enlarged principal superficial veins in post-thrombotic states shows continuous upflow, accentuated by exercise.
4. *Photoplethysmography shows a shortened recovery period after exercise and this is not improved by any manipulation blocking superficial veins.*
5. Functional phlebography confirms deformed and obstructed deep veins with collateral, preferential upflow in superficial veins alongside; similarly other deep vein abnormalities may be shown in keeping with the valveless syndrome or congenital disorders.

Surgery to the veins here is likely to be inappropriate and should be avoided unless there is special evidence of the benefit it may bring.

## Measures to ensure adequacy of surgical operation

### 1. Good preoperative assessment

The operation may be misdirected because of poor initial assessment and this has been considered in some detail above.

### 2. Ligature flush with deep vein

A common error in high ligation of the long or short saphenous vein is a lack of thoroughness so that the uppermost branches are left intact and capable of continuing or re-establishing incompetence. This is particularly prone to produce recurrent varicosities when the pathway of incompetence, for example, a long saphenous vein, is not removed and remains as a massive conduit ready to receive any outflow that may find its way from the incompetent surviving branches at the saphenous stump. A quick operation ligating the long saphenous vein an inch below its termination, without stripping of the vein, is particularly prone to heavy recurrence and the same applies to short saphenous ligation carried out low in the popliteal fossa without the guidance of venography to display its termination and connections. In the long saphenous vein high ligation should be flush with the common femoral vein, disconnecting all the branches at the termination and combined with an effective removal of the pathway of incompetence by stripping of the saphenous vein and dissection of the main varicosities. This alone will accomplish the principles of treatment, namely, effective shutting off of the outflow from the deep vein, together with as complete as possible removal of the pathway of incompetence, including major varicosities. Unfortunately this is a time-consuming procedure but the long-term results are so superior to those given by an inadequate operation, with the complex recurrences it may produce within a few years, that this has to be accepted.

A combination of flush ligation of the long saphenous vein without stripping it and subsequent sclerotherapy to the vein and its varicosities saves time and may be permissible but, in the author's experience, does produce an undue number of recurrences which eventually take far longer, and require a far greater degree of skill to put right, than an effective operation in the first place (see Chapter 20). In the case of the short saphenous vein, with its very variable termination, there is much to be said for a phlebogram being obtained with views in various rotations (see Chapter 22) a few days beforehand or, as advocated by Hobbs (1985), on the operating table as a preliminary. Ligation to this vein must be carried out above its uppermost branches and flush with the popliteal vein, if possible. An upward extension of the short saphenous vein, winding round the back of the thigh to join the long saphenous vein, is often present and may require removing since it is otherwise a potent source of recurrence.

*3. Prevention of neovascularization at saphenous stump*

All authorities are agreed that the commonest form of recurrence is due to inadequate operation as just described, that is, the leaving of one or more branches at the termination which are able to re-establish communication with an unstripped saphenous vein. Many examples of this are seen. However, not all recurrences, for example, from a long saphenous stump, give the appearance of this being due to an anatomically recognized terminal branch vein being left intact. An incompetent channel between the ligated saphenous stump and

a residual long saphenous vein, or one of its branches, may not conform to any recognized anatomy but is composed of a very thin-walled, immensely convoluted channel; moreover in these cases the long saphenous stump may be so small that the terminal branches have been almost certainly removed. Davy and Ouvry (1986) describe the findings in 21 out of 107 recurrences here as 'reconstitution of a parasaphenous venous network, or presence of cavernous angioma, that is, an irregular varicose knot replacing the terminal section of the saphenous vein'; in these patients re-operation confirmed that flush ligation had been carried out. A possible explanation here is that a haematoma around the stump after the original operation has eventually recanalized into the communication just described. Certainly the author has a strong impression that this may happen (Figures 1.8(a), 5.27, 5.28) and is not alone in this view (J. L. Villavicencio, 1985, personal communication; Sheppard 1986). Recently Glass (1987a,b) has described restoration of continuity by neovascularization in saphenous veins known to have been effectively ligated; he puts forward a good case for the pressure difference between the saphenous stump (higher pressure) and a retained long saphenous vein (lower pressure), during the healing phase, being a critical factor in the development of vessels aligned to encourage flow from stump to saphenous vein. Experiments on blood clot enclosed in permeable membrane have shown the formation of primitive blood channels (Ghani and Tibbs, 1962). One does see cases with an angioma-like lesion on hand, forearm or leg, with a clear history of this developing after a crush injury as a child, in a previously normal limb. Canalization of haematoma seems sufficiently real as a mechanism in recurrence of varicose veins for the following precautions to be advised:

(a) Haemostasis at the long saphenous termination or in the popliteal fossa must be meticulous so that haematoma is minimized. There must be no avulsion of branches here, all must be ligated.

(b) At the end of operation all haematoma in the track of the long saphenous vein must be expelled.

(c) Ligation of the saphenous vein itself must be with a non-absorbable material preferably with two separate ligatures.

(d) Where there is a strong overlying fascial covering, as in the popliteal fossa, this should always be carefully sutured since haematoma filling the space from deep vein to superficial tissues, without interruption, could form a ready means for communication between superficial and deep veins. Recurrent varicosities from the short saphenous vein in the popliteal fossa invariably emerge through a deficiency in the fascial layers.

*4. Verification of veins at fault during operation*

During the course of a varicose vein operation the

pathway of incompetence should be consciously identified and inspected for evidence of its incompetence. It should show the following features:

(a) It will be unnaturally large when first exposed, possibly with one or more saccules visible; it will, of course, contract down within a few seconds so that its true size is masked.

(b) Evidence of its incompetence can readily be obtained by cannulating it and syringing peripherally with normal saline (Figure 5.7; see Figure 20.11). Incompetence is confirmed if there is no resistance to 20 ml or more of saline put in swiftly and, often, the varicosities lower in the limb respond with an obvious bulge. The latter feature may not be present, however, with a saphenous vein so capacious that the syringeful of saline is lost within it. Confirming the correct identification of an incompetent vein in this way should be a routine and is particularly valuable when the main incompetence is in one of the uppermost branches of the long saphenous, rather than the saphenous vein itself. The greatly enlarged branch vein, together with the lack of resistance and bulging of the varicosities on retrograde syringing, gives good evidence that it is the vein at fault; the saphenous vein itself may be of normal size and show complete resistance to the syringe and in this case need not be stripped, at least in its upper part. An accessory long saphenous running centrally down the front of the thigh, may give off massive varicosities which rejoin the long saphenous vein in the lower thigh (see Figure 4.21) so that it requires stripping from this level downwards.

## Policy in treating persisting or recurrent varicose veins

The principles in management of varicose veins appearing after treatment are no different to those used in veins not previously treated. However, detailed diagnosis and actual surgery are undeniably more difficult once the normal superficial vein anatomy has been broken up by surgical interference and the scar tissue it creates. The following approach is recommended.

When recurrent veins are detected there should always be a critical reappraisal of the basic diagnosis. Is the condition one of simple incompetence; is it possible that there is an underlying post-thrombotic state, perhaps with iliac vein occlusion; is a congenital venous abnormality or an arteriovenous fistula present; is a valveless state present where any improvement by surgery may not be feasible? The veins must be specifically examined to make sure that they do show the typical features of simple incompetence.

The usual clinical methods are used, that is mapping out by the tapwave technique, employment of a Trendelenburg test by selective digital pressure, and by use of the Doppler flowmeter. These tests should confirm the characteristic downflow of simple incompetence, identify the pathway of incompetence, and often will locate the source at its uppermost part. However, the source may not be evident from this examination, or the diagnosis remains in doubt, and here phlebography is indispensable.

Successful surgical treatment will depend on accurate recognition of the source so there should be no hesitation in using phlebography for this. It is best carried out by the functional method described in Chapter 22 and if this does not reveal the source of downflow to the varicosities an 'upward trace', with the patient near-horizontal, will usually do so (varicography). It must be emphasized, however, that the 'upward trace' technique can be treacherous because of the unpredictable route the opaque medium will follow by travelling 'upwards' in a horizontal patient and although it will show various physical connections, it does not necessarily outline the pathway of incompetence and its source; moreover the veins are partially collapsed so that it is difficult to decide upon their importance.

Clinical examination will usually have given good indication of the approximate location of the source so that particular attention can be given to this area during phlebography. Without this guidance from the clinician it is unreasonable to expect the radiologist to give useful information.

### Methods of treatment

Sclerotherapy can be especially useful in treating recurrent varicosities when they are not unduly large and take the form of tortuous veins, meandering down the thigh or leg. The initial success rate here can be high but, not infrequently, sclerotherapy fails to obliterate the source so that the veins will eventually reappear.

For larger veins surgery may be the only effective way of eliminating them. Unless the source is clinically evident beyond doubt, phlebography must be used to identify it. This is probably best done a few days before operation in the X-ray department so that a full examination, in various positions and assisted by the image intensifier, can be carried out; a single shot method on the operation table has severe limitations and may fail to show the functional pathway of incompetence. Surgery will often involve crossing the scar tissue of a previous operation area and dealing with fragile recurrent veins overlying the source; this is considered in more detail in Chapter 20. A determined effort must be made to carry out ligation of the source at its origin, flush with the deep vein. The pathway of incompetence, usually remnants of long or short saphenous systems, must be removed as completely as possible down the length of the limb by stripping, multiple dissections or avulsions, whichever is appropriate. To be successful, such a procedure will usually take far longer than a corresponding one carried out on previously untreated veins.

In some of the more intricate longstanding patterns, even extensive surgery may fail to eliminate lesser outlying varicosities and here sclerotherapy can be used to complete treatment.

## References

Beard, R. W., Highman, J. W., Pearce, S. and Reginald, P. W. (1984) Diagnosis of pelvic varicosities in women with chronic pelvic pain. *Lancet*, **ii**, 946–949

Beard, R. W., Reginald, P. W. and Pearce, S. (1986) Pelvic pain in women. *British Medical Journal*, **293**, 1160–1162

Davy, A. and Ouvry, P. (1986) Possible explanations for recurrence of varicose veins. *Phlebology*, **1**, 15–21

Ghani, A. R. and Tibbs, D. J. (1962) Role of blood-borne cells in organisation of mural thrombi. *British Medical Journal*, **1**, 1244–1247

Glass, G. M. (1987a) Neovascularization in restoration of continuity of the rat femoral vein following surgical interruption. *Phlebology*, **2**, 1–5

Glass, G. M. (1987b) Neovascularization in recurrence of the varicose great saphenous vein following transection. *Phlebology*, **2**, 81–91

Goren, G. and Yellin, A. E. (1990) Primary varicose veins: topographic and hemodynamic correlations. *Journal of Cardiovascular Surgery*, **31**, 672–677

Hobbs, J. T. (1976) The pelvic congestion syndrome. *Practitioner*, **216**, 529–540

Hobbs, J. T. (1985) A new approach to short saphenous vein varicosities. In *Surgery of the Veins* (eds J. J. Bergan and J. S. T. Yao), Grune and Stratton, New York, pp. 301–321

Hobbs, J. T. (1990) The pelvic congestion syndrome. *British Journal of Hospital Medicine*, **43**, 200–205

Hubner, H. J. and Schultz-Ehrenburg, U. (1986) Simple and hidden atypical refluxes of the leg veins. In *Phlebology* (eds D. Negus and G. Janket), John Libbey, London, pp. 58–60

Lea Thomas, M. (1976) *Phlebology of the Lower Limb*, Churchill Livingstone, Edinburgh

Lea Thomas, M., Fletcher, E. W. L., Andress, M. R. and Cockett, F. B. (1967) The venous connections of vulval varices. *Clinical Radiology*, **XVIII**, 313–317

Lechter, A., Alvarez, A. and Lopez, G. (1987) Pelvic varices and gonadal veins. *Phlebology*, **2**, 181–188

Sheppard, M. (1986) The incidence, diagnosis and management of sapheno-popliteal incompetence. *Phlebology*, **1**, 23–32

Tibbs, D. J. (1986) The intriguing problem of varicose veins. *International Angiology*, **4**, 289–295

# 6

# Complications of superficial vein incompetence and varicose veins

Superficial vein incompetence is usually, but not always, accompanied by varicose (tortuous) veins. It is not uncommon for substantial incompetence to be present without obvious varicose veins and here the pathway of incompetence is the straight-through variety (see Figure 4.18) running down to perforating veins without intervening varicosities. Typical of this variety is massive concealed incompetence of the long saphenous vein and in Chapter 4 it was pointed out how easily this state is overlooked and its effects misdiagnosed as a deep vein disorder or perforator incompetence.

Both patterns of incompetence, with and without varicose veins, may develop pigmented skin, degenerative fibrotic tissue changes (liposclerosis) and eventually ulceration. This process is a response to a sustained venous hypertension resulting from loss of effective valves in superficial veins and occurs where pressure is highest in the lower part of the limb. There are, however, other causes for venous hypertension, all capable of giving rise to similar tissue changes but requiring very different policies of management and treatment; the various causes are reviewed briefly after a comment upon terminology.

## Terminology

The terms used to describe changes in skin and subcutaneous tissue in response to venous hypertension have varied over the years in accordance with the current beliefs. 'Venous stasis', implying inadequate venous flow, is time honoured but is no longer considered very appropriate because flow may actually be increased and the term does not express the most significant abnormality. Likewise, 'varicose' fails to include cases where venous hypertension is present without varicose veins. 'Venous induration' and 'venous ulceration' are permissible, making it clear that the condition referred to is venous in origin, but still not sufficiently expressive. 'Gravitational ulcer' is a term proposed by Dickson Wright in 1931 (a paper well worth reading even today), stressing the relationship of the ulcer to the upright position; it is still

acceptable, indicating the influence of gravity in causation and, when reversed by elevation, in healing.

Terms describing the condition (dermatitis, induration, pigmented, etc.), rather than indicating the abnormal physiology causing it, are safer but often not specific enough for the circumstances and require qualifying to indicate the causative venous disorder. A descriptive term, 'lipodermatosclerosis', often shortened to 'liposclerosis', was suggested by Browse and Burnand (1978) and associated specifically with the tissue changes seen in venous hypertension. It has become a widely used and valuable code-name for the tissue changes caused by venous hypertension. However, there are a number of different venous disorders all with venous hypertension as the common denominator but the term 'liposclerosis' gives no hint of this. Although 'liposclerosis' has established a tacit association with 'venous hypertension' it is still frequently necessary to add this term in order to be specific but, equally important, the cause for the hypertension must be clarified beyond doubt, for example, 'venous hypertension due to superficial vein incompetence (or post-thrombotic syndrome, or arteriovenous fistula, etc.)'.

In this book 'venous hypertension' is often abbreviated to 'venotension'. When 'lipodermatosclerosis' or 'liposclerosis' are used it must be taken that the changes of pigmentation, oedema, induration and, often, ulceration (not merely sclerotic skin and fat) are present in varying degree. It must also be appreciated that these changes are steadily progressive and may be seen at any stage of increasing severity, varying from a mere hint of things to come, through the stage of a well-established, discoloured and thickened area giving clear warning of impending ulceration, and finally to extensive pigmentation, swelling, sclerosis and severe ulceration.

The first part of this chapter considers the relationship of superficial incompetence to venous hypertension and the skin and subcutaneous tissue changes that may result. Varicose veins are themselves a consequence of superficial incompetence rather than a cause but they produce particular problems of their own, notably superficial thrombophlebitis and haemorrhage, discussed later in this chapter.

## Summary of the various causes of venous hypertension and consequent tissue changes (liposclerosis)

Venous hypertension will arise when the musculovenous pump proves inadequate in returning venous blood against gravity when the patient is upright. This may occur in the following states:

1. When the best efforts of the musculovenous pump are overwhelmed by downflow in incompetent superficial veins (see this chapter).
2. When there is an inborn weakness or deficiency in the valves of the pumping mechanism or in major deep veins (see 'Valveless syndrome' – Chapter 7).
3. In post-thrombotic damage to deep veins and their valves (see 'Impaired deep veins' – Chapters 8 and 9).
4. In any combination of the above conditions (see 'Mixed and complex states' – Chapters 5 and 10).
5. In congenital venous abnormalities reproducing any of the conditions given above (see Chapter 12).
6. In arteriovenous fistula, which may be congenital and multiple, traumatic or iatrogenic in origin (see Chapter 17).

Any of these may show, in varying severity, the features of brown pigmentation of the skin, oedema, induration and, eventually, ulceration and the common denominator is venous hypertension.

## Histopathological effects of venous hypertension from any cause

The mechanism by which venous hypertension causes tissue damage is still not completely understood but in a series of clinical and experimental studies Browse, Burnand et al. (Browse and Burnand, 1978; Burnand et al., 1981, 1982; Browse, 1985) found four significant changes:

1. The intracapillary pressure is raised.
2. The permeability of the capillary wall is increased.
3. There is an increase in the number of capillaries.
4. Fibrinolytic activity in the tissues, which normally prevents formation of fibrin, is reduced.

The probable sequence of events is that venous hypertension stimulates proliferation of capillaries, raises capillary pressure, and increases the permeability of the capillary wall through which an excess of exudate passes. This contains electrolytes and the smaller protein molecules, including fibrinogen. The reduced fibrinolytic activity in tissues allows fibrinogen to coagulate (poly-

merize) to form fibrin, a large molecule, which accumulates as dense cuffs around the capillaries. These perivascular cuffs act as barriers to nutrition and the passage of oxygen. This leads to tissue damage in the form of diffuse fibrosis and increasing induration, devitalization of the skin and subdermal tissues and eventually ulceration. The tissues involved are easily injured and show poor healing; indeed, a small injury may fail to heal and be the start of an ulcer. The characteristic pigmentation of the skin is probably related to the increased capillary permeability and leakage of iron products to be deposited as haemosiderin.

## Venotensive skin and subcutaneous tissue changes (liposclerosis) and ulceration

### Incidence

One in five patients presenting with varicosities, and hence superficial incompetence, will show at least some evidence of venotensive tissue change, such as an area of slight subcutaneous thickening and brown discolouration of the overlying skin. In all new patients presenting with active liposclerosis from any cause, often with ulceration, one-half are due to superficial incompetence, with or without varicosities (Tibbs and Fletcher, 1983). This is a common, potentially disabling complication of superficial incompetence and the underlying cause is venous hypertension due to heavy downflow in superficial veins overwhelming a comparatively weak pumping mechanism.

### Clinical features

The clinical features of venotensive tissue change (liposclerosis) are brown pigmentation of the skin, with oedema and fibrosis of the underlying subcutaneous tissue and, eventually, devitalization of the skin leading to ulceration (Figure 6.1). Eczema is a frequent but separate accompanying condition (Figure 6.2). These changes are not necessarily all present together and there is a considerable variation in the appearances from case to case, with little relationship to the size of accompanying varicose veins. Indeed varicose veins may be virtually absent in concealed saphenous incompetence with substantial skin changes and, conversely, massive varicosities may develop no venotensive change. In its least extensive form there is a thickened, indurated area, no more than, say, 4 cm across and with brown overlying skin (Figure 6.3); in its most extensive form it may encircle the entire ankle and extend well up the leg (Figure 6.4). The most common site is on the inner aspect of the leg just above the ankle but, depending on the origin and distribution of the veins causing it, may be seen on the posterior or outer aspect (Figure 6.5) of the leg at varying levels and even on the dorsum of the foot and toes. Position alone is not the key

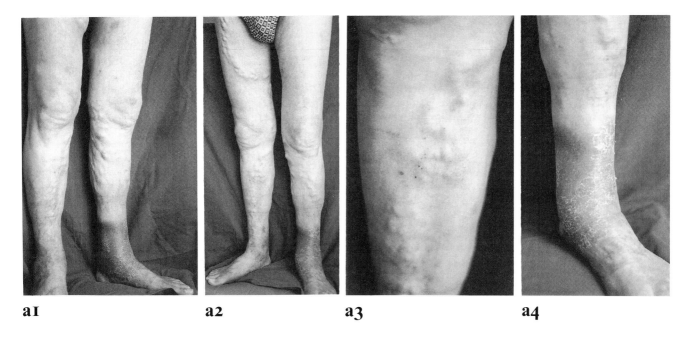

**a1**          **a2**          **a3**          **a4**

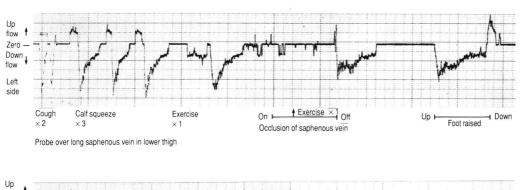

Probe over long saphenous vein in lower thigh

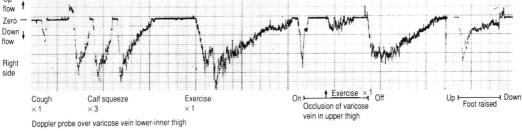

Doppler probe over varicose vein lower-inner thigh

**a5**

**Figure 6.1** *Superficial vein incompetence causing venous hypertension and the severe changes it may cause, including painful ulceration.*

*(a) 1,2. A man, aged 62, with a long history of bilateral varicose veins, a gradual development of pruritus, great discomfort, and swelling. Clinical examination identified gross incompetence in superficial veins on both sides; selective Trendelenburg tests gave complete control of all varicosities. The illustrations show in two views:*
Right side*(1). A large anterolateral varicose branch of the long saphenous vein at the commencement of a pathway of incompetence running down to the foot.*
Left side*(2). Massive varicosities arising from an incompetent long saphenous vein and running down to the lower leg where they are lost in oedema. The skin here is pigmented and eczematous, and was frequently exuding fluid; scattered areas of eczema are seen on the left thigh.*
*3. Scratch marks due to pruritus, overlying varicosities on the right leg.*
*4. On admission to hospital, after a week of elevation and elastic support at home. There has been a marked improvement in response to this.*
*5. Doppler tracings from a varicose vein in the right thigh and the left long saphenous vein in the lower thigh. The characteristic downflow after squeezing the calf or exercising is seen (and see page 130).*

**Figure 6.1***(a) (continued)*

*6. Photoplethysmograms from both sides. When the pathways of incompetence are occluded by compression with fingertips, the recovery times revert to normal, confirming the severe incompetence in these veins.*

*7, 8. Four months after surgery removing the incompetent veins. The varicosities have been eliminated, swelling and skin pigmentation is much less, the eczema has subsided and the patient expressed great relief that all discomfort and pruritus had gone. Postoperative photoplethysmograms are also shown and both sides are normal at over 20 seconds recovery time. A very satisfying result but nevertheless the patient was advised to stand less (he is a publican and will delegate more), elevate whenever he can and to use medium-weight elastic support up to the knees, when he is at work. Undoubtedly the patient's way of life had contributed to the severity of the reaction to venous hypertension.*

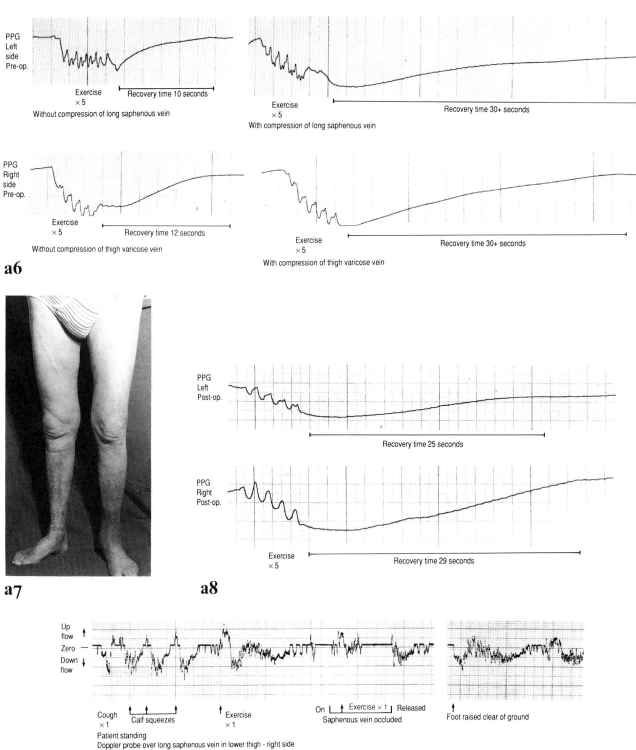

PPG Left side Pre-op.

Exercise ×5 — Recovery time 10 seconds
Without compression of long saphenous vein

Exercise ×5 — Recovery time 30+ seconds
With compression of long saphenous vein

PPG Right side Pre-op.

Exercise ×5 — Recovery time 12 seconds
Without compression of thigh varicose vein

Exercise ×5 — Recovery time 30+ seconds
With compression of thigh varicose vein

**a6**

**a7**

PPG Left Post-op.

Recovery time 25 seconds

PPG Right Post-op.

Exercise ×5 — Recovery time 29 seconds

**a8**

Up flow
Zero
Down flow

Cough ×1     Calf squeezes     ↑ Exercise ×1      On ⌐ Exercise ×1 ¬ Released      ↑ Foot raised clear of ground
                                                  Saphenous vein occluded

Patient standing
Doppler probe over long saphenous vein in lower thigh - right side

**b2** *(and see page 131 opposite)*

**Figure 6.1** (*continued*)

(*b*) *1. Typical venotensive tissue changes caused by massive incompetence of the long saphenous vein and its branches. An area of skin has become heavily pigmented with thickening and induration of the underlying tissue. At its centre, devitalization of the skin has led to an ulcer 3 cm across. The diagnosis was confirmed by: complete control of all enlarged veins by selective occlusion of the long saphenous vein; characteristic downflow in the saphenous vein following exercise; photoplethysmography showing very reduced recovery time after exercise but reverting to normal with selective occlusion of the long saphenous vein; rapid healing of the ulcer following appropriate surgery to the saphenous system.*

*2. Page 130: directional Doppler flowmeter over the long saphenous vein in the lower thigh, on squeezing the calf and with exercise. Page 131: simultaneous recordings from a Doppler flowmeter over the long saphenous vein in the upper calf and from a photoplethysmograph with sensor on the lower leg, patient sitting with the feet clear of the ground. With five exercise movements substantial downflow is*

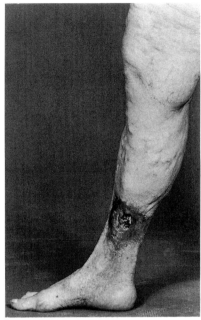

**b1**

*recorded and the phlethysmogram falls, indicating venous emptying and reduced venous pressure. On cessation of exercise the Doppler downflow dwindles away over 10 seconds as venous filling occurs and this is paralleled by a rise in the photoplethysmogram over the same time. When the long saphenous vein is occluded by finger compression in the lower thigh, the same exercise sequence causes no Doppler movement but the photoplethysmogram shows increased venous emptying (steeper slope) and a recovery time increased to over 30 seconds. After this time, on release of the saphenous vein, venous filling is rapidly completed. The results were easily repeatable and indicate with certainty that the long saphenous vein is at fault.*

*3. Surgical removal of this vein was followed by immediate mobilization of the patient and this photograph was taken 6 weeks later. The ulcer has now healed, the surrounding discolouration has lessened and no varicose veins are evident. When seen 2 years later the ulcer remained healed without further problems. This example shows the severity of ulceration that may be caused by simple incompetence in either long or short saphenous systems*

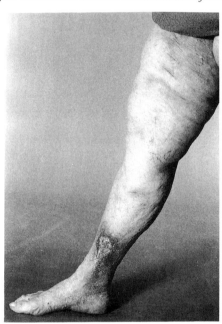

**b3**

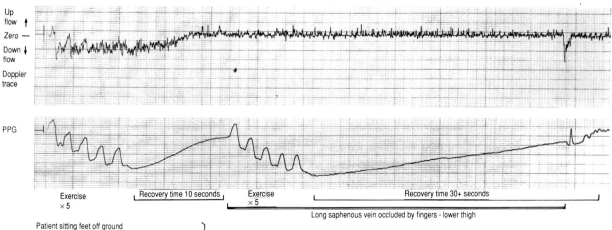

Up flow ↑
Zero —
Down ↓ flow

Doppler trace

PPG

| Exercise ×5 | Recovery time 10 seconds | Exercise ×5 | Recovery time 30+ seconds |

Long saphenous vein occluded by fingers - lower thigh

Patient sitting feet off ground
Doppler probe over long saphenous vein in upper calf ⎫ Carried out simultaneously
PPG sensor on lower leg ⎭

**b2** *(and see page 130 opposite)*

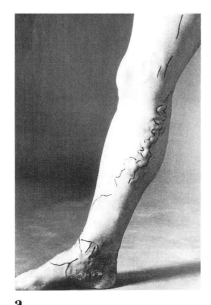
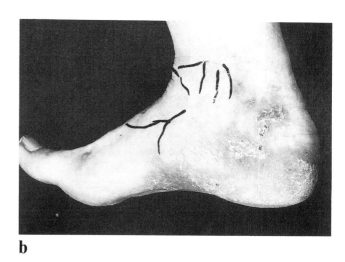

**a**                    **b**

**Figure 6.2**   *Eczema overlying varicosities.*

*(a)  Massive long saphenous varicosities running down to the foot which showed active eczema just below the ankle spreading onto the sole of the foot.*

*(b)  Closer view of the foot to show the eczematous areas with pigmentation. Ankle and foot varicosities were easily palpable underlying the eczema*

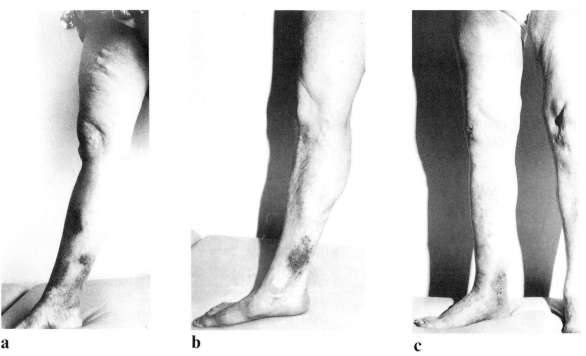

**a**                    **b**                    **c**

**Figure 6.3**   *Examples of venotensive changes (pigmented liposclerosis) with poor relationship to size of visible varicose veins.*

*(a)  Diffuse pigmentation with slight thickening and induration of tissues in the lower leg, due to long saphenous incompetence with few visible varicosities. All tests gave positive confirmation and appropriate surgery gave a good result.*

*(b), (c)  Two patients with localized areas of venotensive change causing discomfort and pruritis. Both show pigmented skin with eczematous change but varicose veins are not conspicuous. However, all tests gave positive confirmation that the long saphenous vein was grossly incompetent. The skin changes subsided after surgery removing this vein*

**Figure 6.4**   *Pigmented liposclerosis and threatened ulceration encircling the leg.*

*(a)  Venotensive changes (pigmented liposclerosis) encircling the lower leg. The pigmented skin showed active eczema with continuous exudate and several small areas of shallow skin ulceration. Massive incompetence in the long saphenous vein was present and the bulge of a sacculation in it can be seen in the lower third of the thigh. Selective occlusion of this vein gave excellent control of all enlarged veins; Doppler and photoplethysmogram gave positive confirmation that the saphenous vein was at fault and this vein was surgically removed.*

*(b)  Postoperative result 6 weeks later, the eczema has subsided and the skin is now healthy although still heavily pigmented. This patient was advised to use elastic support up to the knee as a long-term policy and was trouble free on this side when he returned 3 years later with problems on the left side*

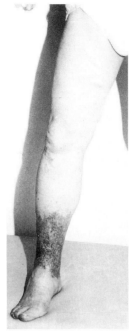
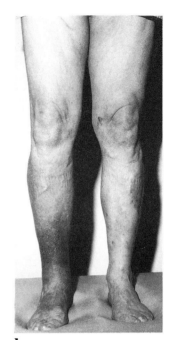

**a**          **b**

**Figure 6.5**   *Example of pigmented liposclerosis with a 2 cm ulcer on the outer side of the leg. This was caused by venotension at the lower end of the large varicose vein that can be seen meandering down the entire limb, from long saphenous termination to the ankle where its tributaries surround the ulcer. (By kind permission of S. Rose)*

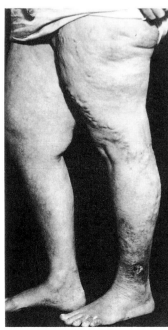
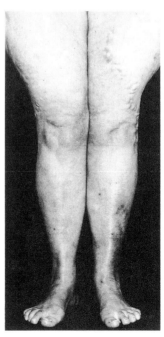

**I**                            **2**

to diagnosis and the combination of features already given, pigmentation of skin, thickening and induration of the underlying tissues, is the most evocative. There should never be undue complacency about the diagnosis as even the most typical of cases may produce a surprise as Figure 6.6 shows. Additional evidence is given by the presence of a large varicose vein running to the venotensive area (Figure 6.7) and, if the limb is elevated to collapse the veins, it is often possible to feel a hollow or groove marking the site of the varicosity underlying the area itself. A lesion of this sort is likely to be progressive and the forerunner to eventual ulceration.

Pruritis, which may be severe if eczema is present, is often the first warning of the venotensive changes described above and there is usually also some discomfort when these are fully established. Ulceration is not

**Figure 6.6** *Tales of the unexpected! This was to have been presented as a small venous ulcer from massive varicose veins.*

*1. A 1 cm ulcer with a small area of pigmentation and induration surrounding it, in a patient with massive varicosities arising from simple long saphenous incompetence; the ulcer is covered with a firm scab. The varicosities were easily controlled by fingertip compression of the saphenous vein in the lower thigh.*
*2. Doppler flowmeter tracings, typical of simple incompetence, and a photoplethysmogram recorded with simultaneous saphenous Doppler flowmeter tracing to show the effect of temporary occlusion of the long saphenous vein. Note the striking improvement in the plethysmogram after retrograde flow in the saphenous vein has been prevented.*
*3. Seen 1 year later all varicose veins had gone, the pigmentation and induration under the ulcer were no longer present; the photoplethysmogram was normal at 15 seconds recovery time.*
*4. However the ulcer remained unhealed with a thick scab over it and had a slightly beaded edge. It was excised surgically and histology confirmed that it was a rodent ulcer (basal cell carcinoma). It is not known whether this was a rodent ulcer from the outset or a subsequent change in a small venous ulcer, but very few cases of this are recorded (see also Figure 13.7(c))*

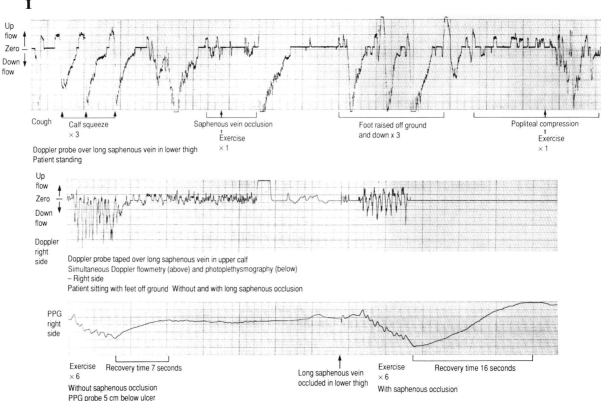

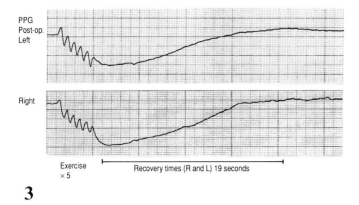

PPG
Post-op.
Left

Right

Exercise
×5

Recovery times (R and L) 19 seconds

**3**

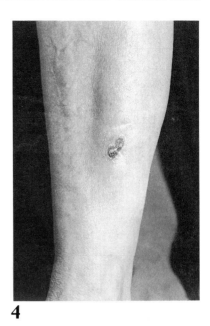

**4**

**Figure 6.6** *(continued)*

necessarily painful but can cause real pain if it is infected with a pathogen, such as *Staphylococcus aureus*.

Differential diagnosis of an ulcer must always be given careful thought and there must not be an automatic assumption that it is venous in origin. In this respect

perhaps the most likely pitfalls are ulcers of ischaemic origin or an ulcer due to a diabetic neuropathy but it may be the result of a combination of possible causes. Chronicity caused by anaemia or a persisting infection with a damaging pathogen, such as staphylococcus, must

**Figure 6.7** *The evidence that superficial vein incompetence is the cause of venotensive change.*

*(a) 1. Massive incompetence and enlargement of the long saphenous vein. This has caused slight swelling in the ankle region with diffuse pigmentation and some thickening of the tissues. On elevation, collapsing the enlarged veins, hollows caused by underlying varicosities were easily palpable and particularly marked in the pigmented areas. All enlarged veins were easily controlled by selective occlusion of the long saphenous vein in the thigh.*

*2. Doppler and plethysmograph tracings in the same patient. The right Doppler flowmeter shows characteristic downflow after squeezing the calf or exercise. Photoplethysmograms, on the right side, following five exercise movements, show the recovery time is very brief at 6 seconds. When this is repeated with the long saphenous vein occluded by fingertip compression in the thigh, the plethysmogram indicates increased venous emptying in response to exercise and the recovery time improves to 30 seconds, in keeping with the left side which had no evident venous problems (and see page 136).*

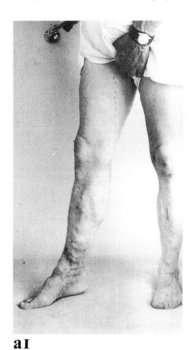

**a1**

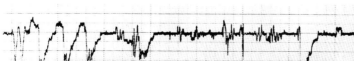

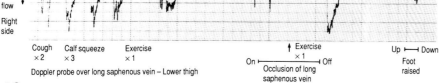

Up
flow
Zero
Down
flow

Right
side

Cough ×2   Calf squeeze ×3   Exercise ×1    Exercise ×1   On ⊢ Off   Up ⊢ Down

Doppler probe over long saphenous vein – Lower thigh    Occlusion of long saphenous vein    Foot raised

**a2**

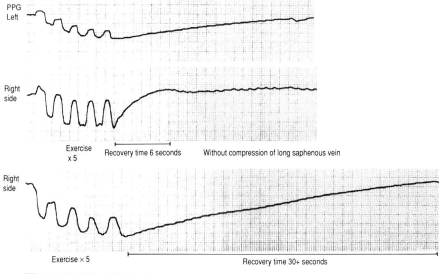

PPG
Left

Right
side

Exercise
× 5    Recovery time 6 seconds    Without compression of long saphenous vein

Right
side

Exercise × 5    Recovery time 30+ seconds

With compression of long saphenous vein

**a2**

**Figure 6.7** *(continued)*

*(b)* 1. *Further example of pigmented liposclerosis with a 1 cm ulcer, under which a massive long saphenous varicosity can be seen to run. With the limb in elevation, the groove marking the track of this vein could be traced under the ulcer. The clinical tests gave strong evidence that the long saphenous vein was at fault.*

*2. Doppler flowmeter tracing from the long saphenous vein in the right thigh shows downflow after squeezing the calf or exercise; there is also a large flow down to the foot when it is raised. Photoplethysmography is normal on the left side which had only moderate superficial incompetence; on the right side recovery time is reduced to 12 seconds; the arterial pulsation evident on this tracing is often seen when venous filling is complete and appears within 9 seconds. The recovery time improves to 28 seconds when the long saphenous vein is selectively occluded. Surgery was carried out removing the saphenous vein and varicosities.*

*3. The patient was mobilized immediately after operation and this photograph shows the result 6 weeks later. The ulcer has healed and all discomfort has gone, swelling is less and the pigmentation less intense. When seen 2 years later the patient had remained at work without further problems (see page 137)*

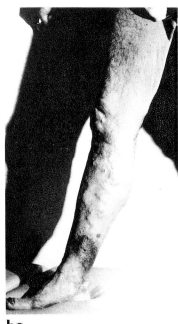

**b1**

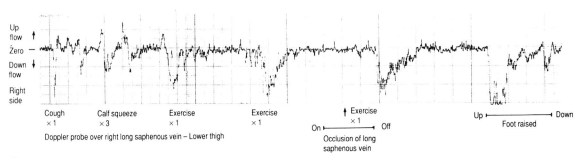

Up
flow
Zero
Down
flow

Right
side

Cough
× 1    Calf squeeze
× 3    Exercise
× 1    Exercise
× 1    ↑ Exercise
× 1
On ⊢————⊣ Off    Up ⊢————⊣ Down
Foot raised

Doppler probe over right long saphenous vein – Lower thigh    Occlusion of long
saphenous vein

**b2** *(and see page 137)*

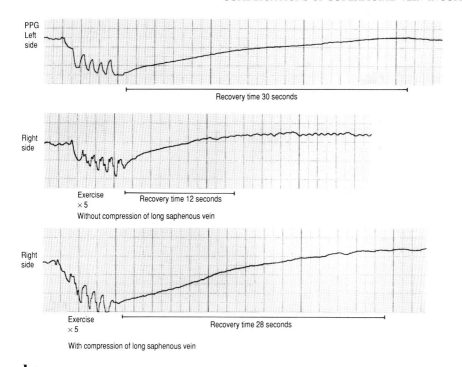

PPG
Left
side

Recovery time 30 seconds

Right
side

Exercise
×5
Recovery time 12 seconds

Without compression of long saphenous vein

Right
side

Exercise
×5
Recovery time 28 seconds

With compression of long saphenous vein

**b2**

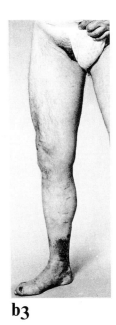

**b3**

**Figure 6.7** *(continued)*

not be underrated. Differential diagnosis and special factors in ulceration are discussed in Chapter 13.

Eczema shows much variability in its site and distribution but is most commonly seen when venous hypertension and liposclerosis are present (Figure 6.3). However, it may occur without obvious liposclerosis but

then usually overlying a large varicosity (Figures 6.2, 6.8). Its causation shares something in common with venotensive change so that both appear in similar circumstances. Eczematous skin shows increased sensitivity and is easily aggravated by materials containing allergens (see Chapter 13) applied as treatment (Figures 6.9, 6.10).

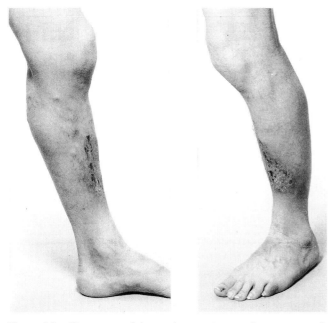

**Figure 6.8** *Eczema overlying varicose veins may be encountered almost anywhere below the knee or even on the thigh. In this illustration a large area of eczema overlies varicose veins running obliquely across the shin and forming a communication between long and short saphenous systems*

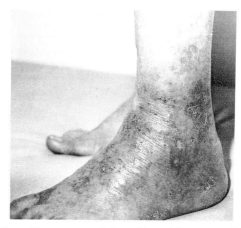

**Figure 6.9** *Eczema around the ankle and foot, severely aggravated by sensitivity to an antibiotic (neomycin) cream. A number of very small ulcers can be seen and these exuded fluid when the patient was up and about. Venous hypertension caused by short saphenous incompetence was present but the patient had eczema on other parts of the body and it is possible that venotension was a precipitating factor rather than truly causative. This skin reaction subsided with withdrawal of the antibiotic preparation and elevation of the limb; treatment was completed by mobilization in a support bandage and surgery to the veins soon afterwards*

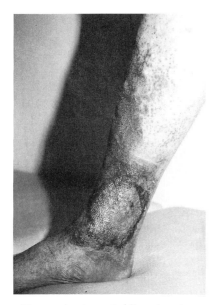

**Figure 6.10** *Eczema in pigmented liposclerosis, greatly exacerbated by sensitivity to tulle gras impregnated with antibiotic (sodium fusidate). This patient is also illustrated in Figure 13.16. The area involved, still bearing the imprint of the gauze, has an extreme reaction with loss of the surface layers. This subsided with a short spell of elevation and withdrawal of all medicated applications. As soon as the eczematous reaction had receded, surgery to the incompetent saphenous system was carried out and the patient mobilized, with a successful result*

### Ethnic skin colouring and venous pigmentation

The brown pigmentation (haemosiderin) characteristic of venous hypertension from any cause is a most valuable sign easily seen in a white skin. However, an obvious question is, how useful is this when obscured by the natural pigmentation (melanin) of tropical and subtropical races? The two pigments are entirely different materials but of similar colour not easily distinguished visually one from the other. In venous ulceration occurring in a black patient the surrounding skin will often show an increased darkening by a combination of the two pigments. However, on its own this cannot be regarded as a reliable indicator of venous origin because the black skin may react to any prolonged disease process by increased melanin production to give pronounced darkening around a non-venous ulcer (see Colour Plate 23). Nor can the absence of such darkening be regarded as reliable in excluding a venous origin because the venous pigmentation may be insufficient to darken a strong concentration melanin, or, the combined colour may be reduced by a melanin depigmentation that can occur in the vicinity of any longstanding skin disease. For these reasons, the skin colour around an ulcer is not a reliable indicator of venous disease in dark skinned races (T. Ryan, 1991, personal communication). The other tissue changes of oedema and induration are not specific to venous disease but fortunately the diagnosis is easily confirmed by the presence of abnormal veins, by Doppler flowmetry and plethysmography identifying an accompanying venous disorder.

African and other dark skinned races are said to have a low incidence of both simple varicose veins and post-thrombotic syndrome (Burkitt, 1972), and in tropical countries where venous ulcer is rare in comparison with other causes there seems a real possibility that its true nature may be overlooked but, again, the evidence of accompanying venous disorder is likely to be immediately apparent. In the United Kingdom, where there is a mixed community of races, venous disease and its complications are not uncommon in black patients, and localized darkening of the skin around an ulcer is usually present, but any uncertainty is quickly dispelled by finding the typical features of an accompanying venous insufficiency.

### Superficial incompetence as a cause for venous hypertension and its consequences

Amongst surgeons there is still much debate upon the role of superficial incompetence in the cause of venotensive change and ulceration (Sethia and Darke, 1984), and it is correctly pointed out that often the most massive of varicose veins are not accompanied by any sign of this, let alone ulceration (Cockett, 1955). There is however general agreement that the basic cause of ulceration is unrelieved venous hypertension due to some form of inadequacy of the pumping mechanism. A really strong mechanism will not be overwhelmed even by a massive downflow in a retrograde circuit of superficial incompetence but if the pumping mechanism is weak then a substantial superficial downflow will overload the pump and the resulting venous hypertension will cause liposclerosis and ulceration. Our own studies, backed by phlebography in over one hundred cases, have shown that, in patients with large varicose veins *without* any liposclerosis the deep vein valves are invariably good and plethysmography gives every indication of a strong pumping system. By contrast when superficial incompetence, with or without varicosities, is accompanied by liposclerosis, the deep veins often appear deficient in valves; plethysmography shows a poor pumping performance with a rapid refilling after exercise but this is improved, at least in part, by temporary occlusion of the pathway of incompetence. Thus, the determining factor whether venous hypertension and liposclerosis develop in superficial incompetence is the ability of the deep vein pumping mechanism to withstand the extra burden. This explains the apparent paradox of massive varicose veins without ulceration in contrast to less striking veins with severe ulceration. To this must be added the quite sizeable number of patients with straight-through (concealed) incompetence, without varicose veins, in whom the important component of superficial incompetence is not recognized. Experience has shown abundantly that removal of superficial downflow will bring a dramatic improvement by reducing the unnecessary load upon the musculovenous pump so that a reasonable balance is restored (Figures 6.1, 6.3, 6.4, 6.6, 6.7). Thus, when venotensive tissue changes are present, the ability to diagnose superficial incompetence overwhelming a weak pumping mechanism is of considerable importance. This will depend upon careful mapping by tapwave of the likely pathway of incompetence and demonstration that a selective Trendelenburg test by fingers applied to this gives prolonged control to prominent veins and varicosities; evidence is completed by a Doppler flowmeter showing characteristic downflow after exercise. Without such positive confirmation, surgery is insecurely based and it will be necessary to clarify further by plethysmography and, if need be, by functional phlebography.

*Importance of distinction between the various causes of venotensive tissue changes (liposclerosis)*

Pigmented liposclerosis is the response to venous hypertension whether this is caused by overwhelming of the musculovenous pump in superficial vein incompetence or some other venous disorder. It is important to understand that venous hypertension can be produced by any of the following:

- Superficial vein incompetence (with or without varicose veins).
- Valveless syndrome.
- Impaired deep veins, as in the post-thrombotic syndrome.
- Mixed and complex venous states.
- Many congenital venous disorders.
- Arteriovenous fistulas.

Surgical treatment or sclerotherapy may be entirely inappropriate or harmful for some of the conditions given above so that it is certainly not sufficient to diagnose just 'liposclerosis due to venous hypertension'. The cause for the hypertension must be fully understood and diagnosed with certainty before any decision on treatment is made. However, undue caution may loose the opportunity to treat a potentially disabling condition and positive identification of the state most likely to respond well to surgery, that is, superficial vein incompetence, is summarized below.

*Summary: positive recognition of venous hypertension due to superficial downflow overwhelming the musculovenous pump*

Various features which will confirm the diagnosis when superficial vein incompetence is a major (and removable) factor in the development of venotensive tissue changes (liposclerosis) are summarized below.

1. An obvious pattern of varicosities which can be traced, by tapwave, to one of the saphenous systems and can be controlled by a selective Trendelenburg test applied by finger compression to the pathway of incompetence; a Doppler flowmeter will confirm downflow after exercise or foot raising. (In post-thrombotic syndrome, with impaired deep veins, scattered varicosities may be present but a satisfactory Trendelenburg test will not be obtained and a Doppler flowmeter over enlarged superficial veins will not show characteristic downflow but is likely to find upflow accentuated by exercise.)

2. Absence of varicosities does not exclude superficial vein incompetence (see 'straight through' or concealed pattern of incompetence in Chapter 4), but here an enlarged saphenous vein can usually be detected by tapwave and controlled by a selective Trendelenburg test applied to it; a Doppler flowmeter shows downflow in it after exercise or foot raising and confirms its incompetence. Photoplethysmography is particularly valuable in finally resolving any doubts (see below).

3. A large varicosity, or an enlarged saphenous vein or major branch, can usually be traced to the centre of the skin changes. This is most easily done by palpation with the limb in high elevation so that the veins become represented by hollows or grooves in the subcutaneous fat. However, it must be remembered that a venous hollow merely marks the position of the vein and does not tell you whether this vein is part of a pathway of superficial incompetence or performing a collateral role in deep vein obstruction; it is only of value in detecting or confirming the presence of a large vein or varicosity and not in making deductions from this.

4. A Doppler flowmeter to a suspected pathway of incompetence or to any varicose vein should confirm downflow after exercise or foot raising. If further evidence is needed photoplethysmography can be of great value when marked venotensive change is present, by giving positive identification of superficial incompetence and its pathway. Here a photoplethysmogram will show reduced recovery time which reverts to near normal when the incompetent veins are occluded, and this is clear confirmation of the diagnosis. If there is still uncertainty then functional phlebography can be employed but this is not usually necessary in the case of superficial incompetence. These special investigations are described further in Chapters 22 and 24.

*Additional factors with ulceration*

When ulceration is present, thought should always be given to the possibility of any background states that might be aggravating factors and, indeed, whether the cause is unrelated to the enlarged veins that are visible. All ulcers should be cultured for the presence of pathogens and other investigations should include haemoglobin level, full blood picture, blood sugar and urea estimations. The arterial supply to the foot should always be checked. Ulceration is considered further in Chapter 13. The incidence and disability caused by this is well discussed by Callam *et al.* (1985) and Cornwall, Dore and Lewis (1986).

*Treatment of venotensive tissue changes and ulceration caused by superficial incompetence*

When liposclerosis, with threatened or actual ulceration, is present and it is clear from the tests outlined above that superficial vein incompetence is the cause, and the pathway of incompetence has been clearly established, then surgery removing the veins concerned is undoubtedly the best form of treatment. This is detailed in Chapter 20 and does not differ from the case without ulceration, except for possible difficulties caused by the skin changes and underlying fibrotic tissue when incisions are required in this area. If heavily infected ulceration is present, as shown by purulent discharge and sloughing base, then it is best to obtain a healthier background for the operation by a preliminary few days in high elevation (with a programme of active exercise), frequent dressings (see Chapters 13 and 18) and an appropriate antibiotic. Surgery should not be delayed by waiting for an ulcer to heal as this may lead to a long and demoralizing wait. As soon as the ulcer presents a surface of clean healthy granulation tissue, without slough or pus, pathogen free on culture, and, best of all, visible ingrowth of epithelium at the edges, then surgery is permissible. Antibiotic cover can be given as an extra precaution; incisions may be made within the area of venostatic skin changes, or nearby, without harm but should not be made through the ulcer itself. If the ulcer is very large and it is in a healing phase (epithelial ingrowth at the edges) then a split skin graft can be applied to the ulcer at the same time as the operation to the veins and this should not interfere with the patient's postoperative mobility.

If for any reason, such as old age or infirmity, surgery is not possible then conservative treatment will be necessary by a policy of high elevation (but see warning on ischaemia given below), with short spells of active walking and other exercise, local dressings to the ulcer and, if eczema is present, sparing use of steroid cream to the affected skin, but not to the ulcer. The proportion of the day that is given to elevation should vary according to the severity of the condition but, for example, with an active ulcer, elevation for 55 minutes in the hour with 5 minutes walk-about for exercise and for essential tasks should be strictly adhered to. As soon as the ulcer is clean and enters a healing phase a non-elastic external support of paste bandage, lightly applied with the limb in elevation (see 'Inelastic containment' in Chapters 13 and 18), may be used and full mobility encouraged, but returning to elevation when not purposefully active. The time given to elevation is reduced as the condition improves but, without surgical removal of the cause or use of external support (non-elastic is always best), it may be necessary to follow a policy of dividing the day into spells of alternating elevation and mobility as a long-term measure to keep the ulcer from recurring. Raising the foot of the bed is a valuable measure in gaining maximal benefit overnight.

**Warning on ischaemia** If high elevation is to be advised, especially in the elderly patient, the arterial supply to the foot must be carefully assessed and, as a minimum, maintenance of good colour in the elevated position must be checked upon. Photoplethysmography, in arterial mode, is very helpful in confirming that pulsatile flow is maintained in elevation. Ischaemic ulcers may well be mistaken for venous and in this case elevation can only cause increased pain and do harm. A combination of ischaemia and venous problems is not rare in the elderly, adding to possible confusion. This sort of error, overlooking arterial insufficiency, can be greatly compounded by additional use of compression bandaging and the combination of this with elevation can cause loss of the limb. Compression bandaging brings no advantage in the elevated position and is best avoided in this category of patient. If there is any suspicion of diminished arterial supply, positioning at horizontal level will have to suffice and no compression used. The matter of combined states of ischaemia and venous disorder is given further thought in Chapter 17 and the hazards well documented by Callam *et al.* (1987a,b).

**Elastic support** In any patient with superficial incompetence awaiting operation, or who is at the ambulatory stage of conservative treatment, elastic support is of especial value. Here it will limit downflow in the superficial veins and allow the pump to reassert itself. For reasons of comfort it should be limited to knee level if possible but if large thigh varicosities indicate a higher level then an excessively strong stocking must be avoided as this is likely to be too uncomfortable for the patient who may cease to wear it. Elastic support is reviewed in Chapter 18. The arterial supply must be checked before prescribing an elastic stocking, particularly if it is to give strong compression.

## Comment upon oedema caused by superficial vein incompetence

The many causes for oedema in the lower limbs are considered in detail in Chapter 14 and here only a brief reminder is given that oedema must not be automatically ascribed to any varicose veins that are present. If superficial incompetence is sufficient to cause significant venous hypertension, as described above, then oedema may well accompany the venotensive changes. In this case it will be localized to the affected area and will seldom encircle the limb in the way in which deep vein impairment can. In less severe circumstances, substantial superficial incompetence may cause mild to moderate oedema at the ankle, or show as slight puffiness on the foot. Anything more may be because some additional factor is present, for example, the deep veins are involved. Such cases must be considered carefully before acting on the assumption that superficial varicosities are the cause. This is especially true if the oedema is bilateral because here a systemic cause, such as renal or cardiac disease, must be excluded.

## Complications of varicosities: thrombophlebitis (phlebothrombosis) and haemorrhage

Varicosities are liable to two very different but specific complications, thrombosis and haemorrhage.

### Superficial thrombophlebitis in varicose veins

Thrombosis in a superficial vein is usually accompanied by an obvious inflammatory response and for many years it was referred to as phlebitis because it was thought that bacterial infection was the prime cause. When it was shown that this was not so, the terms 'thrombophlebitis' or 'phlebothrombosis' were introduced to emphasize that the perivenous inflammatory changes that accompany it were the result of thrombosis without bacterial invasion (Hobbs, 1977). This distinguishes it from the much feared suppurative thrombosis of old, which occurred as a result of a cellulitic or purulent infection surrounding a vein, causing it to thrombose and shed infected clot into the circulation, giving rise to pyaemia, usually fatal.

#### Thrombosis in a previously normal vein

Thrombosis may occur in a previously normal superficial vein for a variety of reasons, such as injury by trauma or the injection of an irritant, or it may be provoked by some generalized change in blood disease or malignancy (Bergqvist and Jaroszewski, 1986; Efem, 1987; Chiedozi and Aghahowa, 1988). A recurring superficial thrombosis at variable sites, described by Buerger as 'phlebitis migrans', may be caused by the arterial disease he described or some other systemic disease; it is always ominous and usually signifies a serious underlying condition. A superficial thrombophlebitis may remain localized to a small area or spread progressively over days or weeks to an extensive run of veins. However, varicose veins are a special case, peculiarly prone to thrombosis, and require separate consideration.

#### Thrombosis in varicose veins

Here we are concerned with phlebitis in a disordered superficial vein, a varicose vein. Experience shows that varicosities are peculiarly prone to undergo an apparently spontaneous thrombosis and their vulnerability must lie

in the features unique to them. The typical varicosity is greatly oversize for normal (upward) flow requirements, the walls are unnaturally thin and flow within it varies from turbulent, reversed flow when the patient is up and about, to almost complete stagnation over prolonged periods in a fully distended state when the patient is standing or sitting without movement. Production of fibrinolysins in the wall, the natural local defence against thrombosis, may be reduced in these circumstances (Wu and Mansfield, 1979; Wolfe, Morland and Browse, 1979).

A thrombus forming in a varicose vein does not prevent flow through it, even if it is packed and grossly distended with clot. This is easily demonstrated with a Doppler flowmeter which will show the usual downflow after exercise characteristic of varicose veins in the upright patient; similarly phlebography will show opacified blood streaming past by the thrombus to give the 'tramline' effect (Figure 6.11). In this way the condition tends to be self-feeding and once the process has started, further thrombus will tend to accumulate every time the vein distends

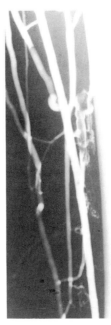

**Figure 6.11** *A phlebogram in a case of recurrent superficial thrombophlebitis. A varicosity is seen largely filled with thrombus but opacified blood is flowing freely past it, thus allowing further build up of thrombus. Firm bandaging prevents this*

with blood on standing so that eventually it becomes packed with successive layers of clot and the walls tightly stretched, causing pain (Figure 6.12). This gives the clue to one aspect of treatment and that is the use of firm bandaging to limit the cycle of further filling and renewed thrombosis; the efficacy of this treatment confirms the importance of this mechanical aspect. This principle of firm support bandaging is used to control the thrombosis induced by sclerotherapy which otherwise would give a prolonged, active thrombophlebitic reaction.

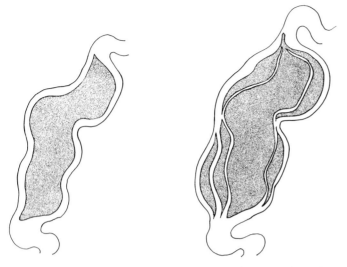

**Figure 6.12** *Diagram illustrating the cumulative build up of thrombus in varicose veins with superficial thrombophlebitis. When the patient is upright and moving, blood flows down past thrombus already there (easily detected by Doppler flowmeter) and more thrombus is deposited. In this way successive layers of thrombus are laid down and painfully distend the varicosity. An essential in treatment is the use of firm bandaging to prevent blood from entering the vein and continually adding to the thrombus in this way*

Superficial thrombosis in varicosities gives rise to a painful swelling, often with reddened overlying skin so that understandably it may be attributed to bacterial infection, but in most cases there is no other evidence of this and cultures prove negative; antibiotics, although often given, do not appear to influence its progress. It is best viewed as thrombosis occurring in abnormal veins which stagnate in an overfilled state for long periods, and once started it has a strong tendency to propagate along the vein. In some cases it will involve the long saphenous vein and spread right up to the groin. In its later phase of recovery, the inflammatory appearance goes and only a firm discoloured cord remains to mark the occurrence. At this stage the vein is likely to be occluded but eventual recanalization often occurs. At first sight the process, if sufficiently extensive, may appear to have cured a set of varicose veins but often they reappear eventually and the process may repeat itself. Any previous valve function will be lost by thrombotic damage of the cusps and the recurrent state may be more severe than the original one, as is often the case in recurrences following sclerotherapy.
**Differential diagnosis** Because it resembles an inflammatory process it may be mistaken for an area of cellulitis or, because of its alignment, a lymphangitis. In both these conditions the skin is likely to show some break through which the infection has entered and there will not be the underlying firm knotty cord of vein which is usually so distinctive in phlebitis. Lymphangitis usually has enlarged lymph glands in the groin but care must be taken not to misinterpret the upper end of a thrombosed long saphenous vein. All these conditions may cause some

malaise and fever but this is seldom severe in the case of superficial thrombophlebitis.

The presence of varicosities is, of course, important support for the diagnosis of superficial thrombosis but at the same time may lead to unjustified suspicion of a deep vein thrombosis. An extensive superficial phlebitis may give such widespread changes that the differentiation is not easy, particularly in pregnancy which is liable to develop either of these conditions. Even if extensive, a superficial phlebitis can usually be seen to involve a broad line running up the limb in the distribution of former varicose veins with a firm, tender cord following this subcutaneously; deep vein thrombosis causes a more general swelling circumferentially without being confined to a broad strip of redness and tenderness. Figure 6.13 summarizes the features distinguishing the main causes for widespread swelling and apparent inflammation of the lower limb, namely, lymphangitis, superficial vein and deep vein thrombosis. Usually the distinction can be

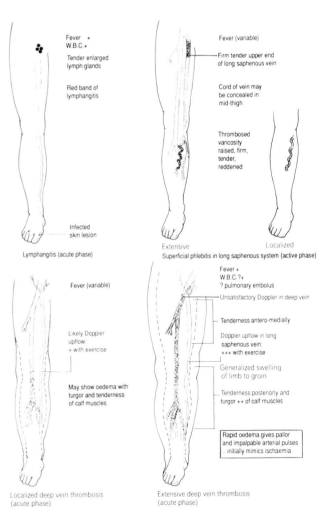

**Figure 6.13** *Diagram summarizing the differences between three major causes for painful swelling along the length of the lower limb: superficial thrombophlebitis, deep vein thrombosis and lymphangitis*

reliably made on clinical grounds and phlebography avoided, especially in pregnancy, but if necessary this can be used to give reassurance upon the deep vein state.

**Course** The condition tends to be self-limiting but may continue for a considerable time if effective treatment by firm bandaging is not given.

**Pulmonary embolism** Embolism arising from thrombosis in varicose veins is rare, partly because the thrombus is firmly adherent but also it is not subject to the same forces of compression and upflow of blood as in the deep veins; in fact when upright the flow in these veins will be peripherally, downwards. However, embolism can occur occasionally when the long saphenous vein is extensively involved and it is important to be aware of this possibility if the clinical state suggests it. The author can recall three cases, one of whom was a well-known political figure whose embolus was diagnosed as a virus pneumonia until it was realized that he had thrombosis filling a massive long saphenous vein; none of these cases was fatal but all were unpleasant enough. Incautious, tight bandaging in the treatment of thrombosis involving a long saphenous vein could conceivably dislodge clot to cause pulmonary embolus and is worth bearing in mind.

*Treatment of superficial thrombophlebitis*

**Conservative** A small area of superficial phlebitis may well require no more than 2 weeks' firm bandaging for it to settle but a severe and widespread attack may be sufficient to justify a few days of elevation and use of an anti-inflammatory agent, such as indomethacin, to relieve the discomfort. In this case the patient should be instructed to exercise frequently whilst elevated; when mobility is permitted then a firm supporting bandage must be kept applied so that the phlebitic vein is not allowed to refill, even briefly, when the patient is upright. As soon as the more obvious inflammatory changes recede then an ambulatory policy should be followed; here the emphasis must be upon firm supporting bandage, put on whilst the limb is in elevation (a non-elastic paste bandage is very suitable and can remain in place for many days) and abundant exercise both by walking and limb movements when 'at rest'. The limb must not be allowed to stagnate in a vertical position, so that standing still or sitting with the legs down is not permitted and, when upright, the patient should either be walking or intermittently marking time; on sitting the legs should be raised to high elevation, again with frequent movements or, if this is not feasible, with repeated foot movements in the down position. This programme may be required for as long as 3 weeks until the condition has settled sufficiently for resumption of normal life with simple elastic (medium weight) compression to the leg for perhaps a further 2 months.

Anticoagulants and antibiotics are not usually beneficial but may be prescribed in cases of real uncertainty as an insurance. In some cases the phlebitis may run such a protracted or recurring course that anticoagulants are employed. However in such circumstances the diagnosis must be carefully reviewed to make sure that some other background state is not present and, when reassured upon this, thought given to surgical treatment of the underlying cause, superficial vein incompetence.

**Evacuation of haematoma within thrombosed varicosities** The discomfort in superficial thrombosis is caused by the tight distension of the vein with clot. If this is removed and the vein firmly supported to prevent its refilling, then the patient has immediate relief and the condition does not recur. If the vein is filled with fluctuant clot, strong aspiration through a 15 gauge needle can be very effective (just as in decompressing haematomas in veins following sclerotherapy). However, if the clot is too firm to be sucked out, a small stab incision, using local anaesthesia by spray or injection, allows the clot to be squeezed out. This can be used fairly extensively by multiple incisions if necessary and followed by firm bandaging (Hobbs, 1977; Zelikovski *et al.*, 1986) (again a method widely used for postsclerotherapy haematomas).

Evacuation in this fashion is suitable for the moderately extensive superficial thrombosis when it is clear that the patient has much discomfort, likely to last for many days and to be followed by a long period of slow absorption of the thrombus.

**The role of surgery in superficial thrombophlebitis** Surgery to remove the causative varicose veins is often left until the phlebitis has completely subsided but this need not be so. Once the diagnosis is secure and has been additionally confirmed by subsidence of the more acute manifestations, then there is no contraindication to surgical cure at an early stage. The usual operation for the pattern of incompetence is carried out, including high ligation and stripping of a saphenous vein even if this has thrombosed as well; any thrombosed varicosity can be readily dissected away, thus sparing the patient the slow process of natural resolution.

Return to full normality is usually hastened by using surgery in this fashion but against this must be balanced the possibility that the attack of phlebitis might prove curative. In practice this is seldom so as the original state of superficial incompetence usually emerges again eventually. When considering surgery it must be born in mind that the phlebitis may confuse accurate recognition of the origin of the varicosities and it is essential that there is no uncertainty about the appropriateness of the operation to be carried out. In cases of doubt surgery should be delayed until the condition has settled and full evaluation carried out then.

**Note on pulmonary embolus** If the thromboplebitis extends in massive fashion to the uppermost long saphenous vein then early surgery to remove this vein is strongly indicated as this is the category that may release a pulmonary embolus. Care is needed not to dislodge clot at surgery; clamps should not be applied to the saphenous termination for fear of breaking the clot, which should be gently extracted as the vein is divided and the clamp then applied. If embolus has already occurred surgery may still be advisable to prevent recurrence but the alternative is treatment by heparin, with surgery at a later stage.

## Haemorrhage from varicosities

The slow expansion of a varicose vein in the subcutaneous tissues not only creates a substantial hollow in the fat, which is very evident when the vein is emptied by elevation, but if directly under the skin will cause its progressive stretching and thinning. In addition the vein becomes very adherent to the skin and inseparable from it so that the blood within is contained by a fragile membrane of paper-thin skin backed by little more than vein intima. When the patient is upright, and the vein tense with blood, any small injury may rupture this precarious covering giving rise to copious haemorrhage. If the patient remains upright a considerable quantity of blood may be lost and only cease when he/she collapses in a faint. This condition is most commonly seen in the elderly where the tissues tend to be more fragile but may be seen at a much younger age if the veins started early and have been present for some years. The areas most usually affected are the foot and ankle, presumably because here the venous pressure and vulnerability to injury are greatest but any level can be affected, although progressively less likely up the limb.

The appearance of a vein at risk from haemorrhage is characteristic; the dark blue blood shows with striking clarity through its tense thin covering when the patient is standing; on elevation the colour goes and the bulge subsides into a hollow which is both visible and palpable. There may have been small warning haemorrhages or the possibilty of bleeding has been realized and advice sought because of this, but the patient is often oblivious to the danger and will have to be warned of the need to have treatment. Usually the surrounding skin is heavily pigmented with clear evidence of venotension and sometimes is actually ulcerated so that haemorrhage may occur from an ulcer, large or small. Bleeding, once it has occurred, is likely to be repeated as the vein does not show any great tendency to close off spontaneously. Any of the circumstances outlined above is a clear indication for treatment to obliterate the vein at risk either by injection or by surgical excision.

**Treatment** The immediate treatment to stop haemorrhage is to lie the patient down, elevate the limb and apply a pad firmly bandaged into position. This is always effective and the ruptured vein soon seals with clot; the patient can resume activity within the next day or two with the safeguard of a secure bandage over the affected area. However the devitalized tissue that has given way

has no recuperative power so that effective closure is unlikely to take place. Meanwhile the underlying vein remains open with the aperture precariously sealed by recent clot and sooner or later it will bleed again. Prolonged elevation may produce a degree of fragile healing but more positive treatment is necessary to restore lasting stability. If the vein at fault arises from typical superficial vein incompetence, surgery to this, including excision of the varicosity, is by far the best answer. Surgical cure is a relatively minor procedure but if the patient is elderly and too infirm for operation then sclerosing the vein by injection followed by a firm bandage for 3 weeks is usually effective (Figure 6.14) in dealing with the local problem

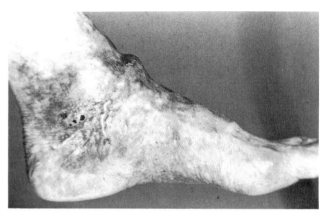

**Figure 6.14** *This patient had suffered four episodes of alarming haemorrhage from a superficial varicosity overlying the medial malleolus. The typical changes of pigmentation from venous hypertension were evident and massive varicosities were present on the leg. In this photograph, a small scab can be seen marking the site of recent haemorrhage; a large varicose vein immediately under this showed ink-blue through paper-thin skin. Note the massive varicosity on the front of the ankle, again covered with only the thinnest of skin. This patient was elderly and infirm but a good arterial supply was present and treatment by sclerotherapy was decided upon. This successfully solved the problem by sealing the veins most likely to bleed. Sclerotherapy in this vicinity is usually avoided because of the proximity of the anterior and posterior tibial arteries and should be used with great care only on special indication*

(but check upon the arterial supply to the limb first); other varicosities may be relatively harmless if supported with suitable elastic support and the patient urged to elevate the limb when nothing purposeful is being done.

Regarding injection to sclerose the vein, this in no way conflicts with surgery a few weeks later and can certainly be used as a stopgap measure to ensure no more episodes of bleeding whilst the patient is awaiting operation. The needle is best introduced 1–2 cm away from the actual point of bleeding where the skin is less fragile.

# References

Bergqvist, D. and Jaroszewski, H. (1986) Deep vein thrombosis in patients with superficial thrombophlebitis of the leg. *British Medical Journal*, **292**, 658–9

Browse, N. (1985) The pathogenesis of venous ulceration. In *Surgery of the Veins* (eds J. J. Bergan and J. S. T. Yao), Grune and Stratton, New York, pp. 25–31

Browse, N. and Burnand, K. (1978) The postphlebitic syndrome: a new look. In *Venous Problems*, (eds J. J. Bergan and J. S. T. Yao), Year Book Medical, Chicago, pp. 395–405

Burkitt, D. P. (1972) Varicose veins, deep vein thrombosis, and haemorrhoids: epidemiology and suggested aetiology. *British Medical Journal*, **2**, 556–561

Burnand, K. G., Whimster, I. W., Clemenson, G. *et al.* (1981) The relationship between the number of capillaries in the skin of the venous ulcer bearing area of the lower leg and the fall in foot vein pressure during exercise. *British Journal of Surgery*, **68**, 297–300

Burnand, K. G., Whimster, I., Naidoo, A. *et al.* (1982) Pericapillary fibrin in the ulcer bearing skin of the lower leg. The cause of lipodermatosclerosis and venous ulceration. *British Medical Journal*, **285**, 1071–1072

Callam, M. J., Ruckley, C. V., Harper, D. R. and Dale, J. J. (1985) Chronic ulceration of the leg: extent of the problem and provision of care. *British Medical Journal*, **290**, 1855–1856

Callam, M. J., Harper, D. R., Dale, J. J. and Ruckley, C. V. (1987a) Arterial disease in chronic leg ulceration: an underestimated hazard. *British Medical Journal*, **294**, 929–931

Callam, M. J., Ruckley, C. V., Dale, J. J. and Harper, D. R. (1987b) Hazards of compression treatment of the leg from Scottish surgeons. *British Medical Journal*, **295**, 1382

Chiedozi, L. C. and Aghahowa, J. A. (1988) Mondor's disease associated with breast cancer. *Surgery*, **103**, 438–439

Cockett, F. B. (1955) The pathology and treatment of venous ulcers of the leg. *British Journal of Surgery*, **43**, 260–278

Cornwall, J. V., Dore, C. J., Lewis, J. D. (1986) Leg ulcers: epidemiology and aetiology. *British Journal of Surgery*, **73**, 693–696

Dickson Wright, A. (1931) The treatment of indolent ulcer of the leg. *Lancet*, **i**, 457–460

Efem, S. E. E. (1987) Mondor's disease in the groin. *British Journal of Surgery*, **74**, 468

Hobbs, J. T. (1977) Superficial thrombophlebitis. In *The Treatment of Venous Disorders*, (ed. J. T. Hobbs), MTP, Lancaster, pp. 414–427

Sethia, K. K. and Darke, S. G. (1984) Long saphenous incompetence as a cause of venous ulceration. *British Journal of Surgery*, **71**, 754–755

Tibbs, D. J. and Fletcher, E. W. L. (1983) Direction of flow in superficial veins as a guide to venous disorders in lower limbs. *Surgery*, **93**, 758–767

Wolfe, J. H. N., Morland, M. and Browse, N. L. (1979) The fibrinolytic activity of varicose veins. *British Journal of Surgery*, **66**, 185–187

Wu, A. V. O. and Mansfield, A. (1979) The fibrinolytic activity of the vein following venous stasis. *British Journal of Surgery*, **66**, 637–639

Zelikovski, A., Haddad, M., Sahar, G. and Reiss, R. (1986) The role of ambulatory surgery of thrombosed varicose veins. *Phlebology*, **1**, 135–137


# Bibliography

Mani, R., White, J. C., Barrett, D. F. and Weaver, P. W. (1989) Tissue oxygenation, venous ulcers and fibrin cuffs. *Journal of the Royal Society of Medicine*, **82**, 345–346

Michel, C. C. (1990) Oxygen diffusion in oedematous tissue and through pericapillary cuffs. *Phlebology*, **5**, 223–230

Stacey, M. C., Burnand, K. G., Layer, G. T. and Pattison, M. (1988) Calf pump function in patients with healed venous ulcers is not improved by surgery to the communicating veins or by elastic stockings. *British Journal of Surgery*, **75**, 436–439

Stibe, E., Cheatle, T. R., Coleridge Smith, P. D. and Scurr, J. H. (1990) Liposclerotic skin: a diffusion block or a perfusion problem. *Phlebology*, **5**, 231–236

Travers, J. P., Berridge, D. C. and Makin, G. S. (1990) Surgical enhancement of skin oxygenation in patients with venous lipodermatosclerosis. *Phlebology*, **5**, 129–133

# 7

# Widespread valve failure in superficial and deep veins: valveless syndrome and weak vein syndrome

In Chapter 3 reference was made to a deficiency in the number of valves in the deep veins of many patients with superficial vein incompetence and in whom there is no history or phlebographic evidence of previous deep vein thrombosis. In this way a spectrum of valve deficiency (Figure 7.1) exists; at one end the deep vein valves are normal but, on moving along the spectrum, there is an increasing lack of effective deep valves with a corresponding weakening of the pumping mechanism which is, therefore, more easily overwhelmed by downflow from the incompetent superficial veins (see also Chapter 6). At the extreme end of the spectrum there is a severe deficiency of valves and we have called this state the 'valveless syndrome' but the term 'primary valve failure' is being increasingly used by others recognizing this condition.

There is no sharp boundary to the 'valveless syndrome' in the spectrum and the distinction is made arbitarily to include only the most severe overall valve deficiencies. At the borderline, the pumping mechanism is barely adequate and is easily overwhelmed to produce venotensive tissue changes (liposclerosis), but if superficial incompetence is eliminated by treatment these changes will recede (Figure 7.2). In the valveless syndrome, beyond the borderline, the deficiency of valves in the deep veins is so complete that no manipulation of the surface veins, either during special tests or by surgical removal, will restore effective pumping action sufficiently to prevent venous hypertension. The resulting state of venotensive changes and ulceration, without any preceding history of deep vein thrombosis and, on phlebography, showing severe widespread deficiency of superficial and deep valves, is characteristic of the valveless syndrome.

## The valveless syndrome

This condition is likely to be due to an inborn overall deficiency of valves both in numbers and in quality and

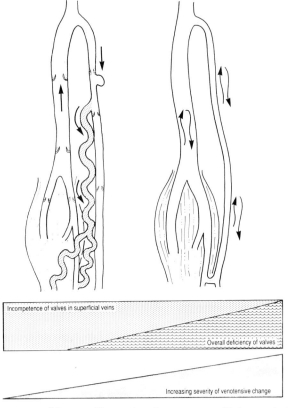

**Figure 7.1** *Diagram illustrating the spectrum of inborn valvular insufficiency in the lower limb. At one end there is no more than simple incompetence in superficial veins. Here, there is an adequate number of valves but some have become incompetent, setting up a retrograde circuit and causing varicose veins; there is a normal distribution of competent valves in the deep vein and these provide an effective pumping mechanism so that venotensive changes do not occur. Moving along the spectrum, an increasing proportion of patients have deficiency both in the number and the quality of the valves in superficial and deep veins; the more marked this deficiency the greater the tendency for venous hypertension with liposclerosis and ulceration. At the far end of the spectrum, the deficiency in valves of the superficial and deep veins is so widespread that the pumping mechanism is severely impaired giving severe venotensive changes and intractable ulceration*

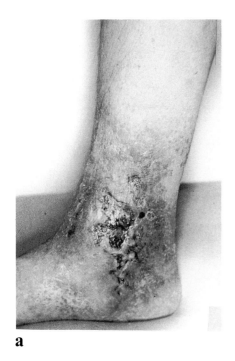

a

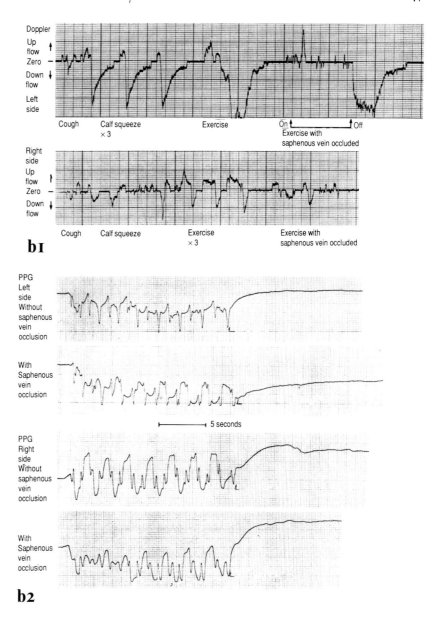

**Figure 7.2** *Borderline valveless syndrome.*

*(a) An actively deteriorating ulcer on the right leg of a patient with massive incompetence of the long saphenous vein and poorly valved deep veins. There was no history of possible deep vein thrombosis. Selective saphenous occlusion gave delayed filling of enlarged leg veins. On the left side there was a large incompetent saphenous vein but no ulcer.*

*(b) 1. Doppler flowmeter tracing from the right saphenous vein with exercise shows considerable surge suggesting deficient deep vein valves; the left side does not show surge.*
*2. Photoplethysmograms: right side, showing abnormally short (under 10 seconds) recovery time after exercise but this was not improved by saphenous occlusion; the left side shows similar shortening of recovery time but with some improvement on saphenous occlusion.*

*This unpleasant ulcer was in need of urgent treatment if further deterioration and increasing disability were to be prevented. The precarious musculovenous pump had been overwhelmed by massive downflow in the saphenous vein. Surgery removing this vein was carried out to restore a better balance, so that, with care, the patient could avoid recurrence once the ulcer had healed. This was achieved by a spell of elevation, followed by mobilization in an inelastic (paste) bandage and subsequent surgery to the saphenous vein. Long-term use of below-knee elastic support was advised*

it may correspond to the 'postphlebitic leg' without evidence of a previous thrombosis, described by Browse, Clemenson and Lea Thomas (1980). It may first become evident in the young adult but clinical changes may not appear until later in life; this suggests that a precarious pumping mechanism, at first adequate, undergoes some form of deterioration over the years, perhaps by breakdown of the few valves originally present (Figure 7.3). Incomplete valves, with a single cusp, may be seen on phlebography supporting the possibility of valves both

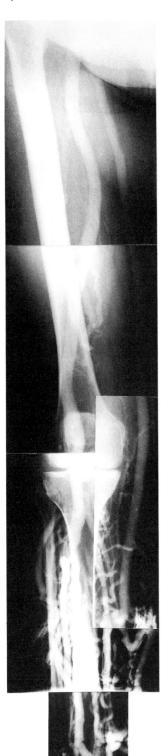

**Figure 7.3** *Composite phlebogram of a patient with longstanding venous hypertension with pigmented liposclerosis and ulceration. There was no history of deep vein thrombosis. Attempts to display valves during phlebography by using the swill technique (rapid change in position from upright to horizontal and back again) have failed to reveal any valves. The deep veins have wide lumens without any suggestion of post-thrombotic deformity, a massive long saphenous vein is present which communicates in mid-leg with the deep veins and here blood could be seen to surge back and forth during exercise. In the femoral vein, exercise by rising on the toes caused upward movement at the moment of contraction but on relaxation blood rapidly receded down again. Similarly, with a change of posture from vertical to horizontal and back again, blood in the principal deep vein could be seen moving upwards and then down again without any evidence of control by valves. The pumping mechanism is unable to give purposeful progressive upward movement of blood against gravity*

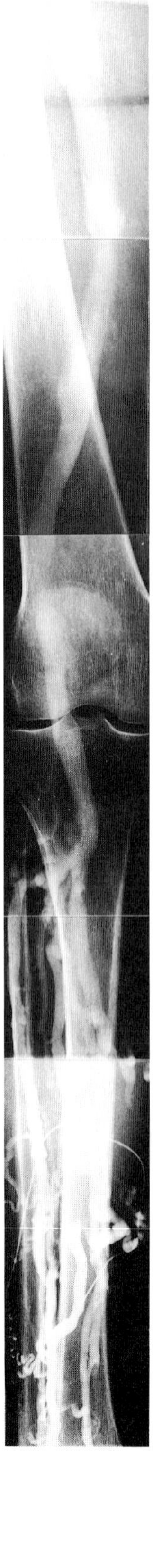

**Figure 7.4** *The deficiency of valves in the valveless syndrome is not only in their number but their quality may also be defective. This patient had longstanding venous hypertension with pigmented liposclerosis and ulceration at the ankle. There was no history of previous deep vein thrombosis. Doppler flowmeter confirmed heavy surge back and forth in the superficial veins with exercise. Photoplethysmography showed a poor response to exercise and a very reduced venous refilling (recovery) time; this could not be changed by any manipulation of the superficial veins. Phlebography, illustrated here, showed large deep veins without any evidence of post-thrombotic deformity. Attempts to display valves in the deep veins showed one valve with well-formed cusps in the upper part of the femoral vein but opacified blood could be seen streaming downwards through these cusps after exercising or repositioning (Figure 1.11(c)). Two expansions lower down in the femoral vein suggest the presence of valves but one of these contained only a single cusp and the other no cusps, and there was no suggestion of resistance to venous reflux with repositioning of the patient from horizontal to vertical positions. Beneath this level repositioning techniques, normally revealing an abundance of valves, showed few, if any, valves. A perforator in mid-leg showed heavy surge back and forth with exercise and this corresponded with Doppler flowmeter findings*

poor in numbers and quality (Figure 7.4). In a study of 527 patients attending a vein clinic, Tibbs and Fletcher (1983) found 42 (8%) with marked or severe venostatic (venotensive) changes, many with ulceration, were in this category. Often, these patients have unusually wide veins suggesting that the deficiency is not confined to the valves but is a more generalized change. Our understanding upon this is incomplete and this is further emphasized by the observation that some patients are found who have a remarkable deficiency of deep vein valves (using techniques of phlebography designed to show valves – see Chapter 22) but yet appear to have an adequate pumping action; present methods of investigation are not sufficiently sophisticated to show why these patients are able to maintain a precarious balance whilst the others cannot.

The belief that this is an inborn condition is based upon the absence of any history of previous deep vein thrombosis and, on phlebography, the lack of any deformity in the deep veins that might suggest a thrombosis in the past (Turner Warwick, 1930; Lockhart-Mummery and Hillyer-Smitham, 1951; Ludbrook, 1966). Moreover, congenital aplasia of the valves in the veins of the lower limbs running within families is well documented (Plate et al., 1986; Friedman, Taylor and Porter, 1988). Of course, in a normal limb a limited deep vein thrombosis may pass unnoticed but yet cause valve damage, or, conversely, thrombosis may arise as an additional complication in a 'valveless syndrome' so that it becomes post-thrombotic. However, when all the evidence is weighed up, the two groups, thrombotic and non-thrombotic, stand apart with few cases of uncertainty. In clinical practice, if surgery is not being considered, the distinction is not too critical since treatment by conservative management is likely to be the same for both conditions. The distinction does, however, become important if surgery is contemplated because of the real possibility of doing harm in post-thrombotic syndrome by removing valuable collateral veins.

The valveless sydrome we recognize certainly comes within the term 'venous insufficiency syndrome' recommended by Taheri et al. (1985) to acknowledge that many cases previously termed 'postphlebitic' are, in fact, unlikely to have origin in previous thrombosis. It seems probable that it also includes the condition referred to by Kistner (1980, 1985) as primary valve incompetence and due to prolapse of a valve cusp; this would scarcely have great significance unless there were a deficiency of other valves in femoral or popliteal veins; certainly we have seen the occasional case with a solitary femoropopliteal valve, leaking heavily (see Figures 1.11(c), 7.4) and apparently suitable for the repair operation described by Kistner. Both these authors make clear distinction between primary valve incompetence in deep veins and the thickened damaged cusps in post-thrombotic conditions.

## Clinical features

The condition becomes apparent in men or women over a wide age group, from young adults through to old age. The presenting feature is severe, pigmented venotensive change, usually with ulceration, which may be extensive, but without any history of deep vein thrombosis (Figure 7.5). In connection with this, an episode during pregnancy 30 years before, or following a fractured limb, may not be regarded by the patient as relevant and carefully framed questions will be needed to ensure this is not overlooked.

On examination, the superficial veins are not necessarily unnaturally enlarged or tortuous. A selective Trendelenburg test applied to the superficial veins does not give control, nor does a Perthes' test show any response.

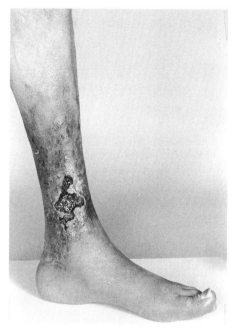

**Figure 7.5** *Severe venotensive changes with pigmented liposclerosis and ulceration in a male patient of 65 years. This had gradually developed over the last 15 years and proved resistant to all forms of treatment. Although the patient was thin there was no undue enlargement of superficial veins and varicosities were not present. There was no history of any deep vein thrombosis or circumstances, such as fracture, that might have led to this. Doppler flowmeter to superficial veins showed strong surge back and forth with exercise. Photoplethysmography showed a poor response to exercise with an abnormally short recovery time; temporary selective occlusion of superficial veins did not cause any improvement. Phlebography showed the deep veins to be patent throughout with good, undeformed lumens but no satisfactory valves were demonstrated. This case suggests that the patient may have been born with too few valves and these of poor quality, so that they failed progressively in adult life. The opposite limb had similar but less severe changes*

## Special investigations

Directional Doppler flowmetry to superficial veins shows that at the moment of muscle contraction blood surges out through leg perforators, up superficial veins and then subsides back again when the muscles relax. Purposeful onward movement, as determined by valves, is not present, only a displacement first in one direction and back again (Figure 7.6). This Doppler flow pattern is strongly suggestive of widespread absence of functioning valves in both superficical and deep veins. It does not show the continuous upflow, accentuated by exercise, seen in post-thrombotic deep vein impairment.

Photoplethysmography shows a poor response to exercise and a very short recovery period confirming an ineffective pump, unguarded by valves. Temporary occlusion of a suspected pathway of superficial incompetence does not bring any improvement because the main fault lies within the valveless deep veins.

Phlebography should usually be carried out in these patients who have a potentially disabling condition and in whom the important decision, for or against surgery, must be based upon reliable evidence. This examination (see Chapter 22 for more technical details) is carried out in the upright position with a needle into a superficial leg vein. A small initial injection of medium, followed by the patient exercising by rising on the toes several times, confirms that on muscle contraction a substantial surge of blood occurs outwards through leg perforators with immediate return of the displaced blood on relaxation (Figures 7.3, 7.4). With the patient standing still, deep and superficial veins opacify in parallel as further medium is put in, to show veins with wide undeformed lumens, but no valves. A rapid repositioning of the patient from upright to horizontal and back again (the swill test) fails to display any satisfactory valves in femoral, popliteal or the leg deep veins although the occasional vestigeal or single cusp may be seen (Figure 7.4); major branches,

such as the profunda femoris, do not necessarily share in the defect and well-formed valves may be demonstrated here. The saphenous veins and their major tributaries are usually valveless, completing the picture of overall valvular deficiency. The deep veins do not show any deformity that might suggest old thrombosis.

With exercise, a considerable volume of blood in the deep veins can be seen to be displaced upwards as muscle contracts but with relaxation there is a rapid clearing of medium from the upper levels as the blood falls down again. A similar effect is seen when the patient is put to a near-horizontal position and then to vertical again, with apparent disappearance of opacified blood as it drops down the valveless deep veins. Return of venous blood is largely passive, driven by arterial inflow, but surge back and forth gives a considerable mixing effect so that opacified blood rapidly spreads through the limb giving the illusion of purposeful upward movement. The opposite limb usually shows a similar but possibly less extreme state of valve deficiency.

**Treatment**

The significant defect is a scarcity of effective valves in the deep veins and there is no reliable means for remedying this although various operations designed for this are described (see Chapter 21). As predicted by the clinical and special tests, surgery removing the superficial veins will not bring any benefit. However, in this state with widely open, undeformed deep veins, the superficial veins are not acting as collaterals so that their removal does not involve the same risk of damage as in deep vein impairment (see Chapter 8) and operation is permissible in borderline cases. Nevertheless, in view of the clinical

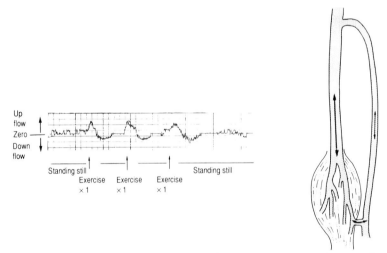

**Figure 7.6** *Doppler flowmeter recording from a patient with deficiency of superficial and deep vein valves. The Doppler probe is over the long saphenous vein in the lower thigh. With each exercise movement there is a substantial upflow of blood which on relaxation is followed by a corresponding downflow. The impression is one of surge back and forth without any purposeful flow and this is in keeping with the findings at phlebography where, with exercise, blood could be seen to surge between deep and superficial veins*

similarities between the valveless syndrome and deep vein impairment, great care is needed and a wise rule is that superficial veins, such as long or short saphenous veins, should not be removed without convincing control by a selective Trendelenburg test and a phlebogram showing widely open deep veins without hint of deformity. Photoplethysmography can give valuable guidance by the response to exercise with and without temporary occlusion of the superficial vein under suspicion; an adverse response to occlusion indicates that removal of this vein is likely to prove harmful, for example, in the post-thrombotic syndrome.

Often the decision will be against surgery and in the first place conservative treatment will be employed to heal the ulcer. Depending on the severity of the ulcer, this may be either a week or two with the leg in high elevation and actively exercised, or, an ambulatory policy with the affected leg encased in a non-elastic support, a paste bandage. When the ulcer has healed, reasonable mobility can be allowed, with elastic or inelastic support, but still giving a good proportion of the day to elevation. This will usually prevent recurrence, but the price for this is perpetual vigilance. The principles of care in venotensive change and ulceration are considered in detail in Chapters 13 and 18.

## Weak vein syndrome

The term 'weak vein syndrome' is used in this book to describe a rather different state from that just described above. It may be an inborn condition but in many patients there are features suggesting an acquired component is present.

The surgeon seeing venous conditions recognizes that a significant number of patients develop massive varicose veins. This is not just a measure of the severity of venous incompetence or of its duration because the saphenous vein involved may have several well-formed, but incompetent, valves and the patient is not necessarily old. Men and women are equally affected and phlebography shows that the deep veins share the same tendency to be oversize (Figure 7.7, see also Figure 4.17). Surgery to these patients may give a good result at first but eventually the same type of massive varicose vein will reappear. These veins do not seem especially prone to cause venotensive tissue changes although this occurs in many. It seems that this category of patients has some form of inborn or acquired weakness in the vein walls which readily yield to pressure and become oversized. The valve rings, supporting the cusps, share in the process so that incompetence is increased and the reversed flow in the veins encourages further enlargement and tortuosity to give massive varicose veins to an extent not seen in the usual patient. After treatment, new pathways of incompetence are easily re-established so that recurrence of massive

veins is quite common. An unduly high proportion of these patients seems to be obese and in professions involving prolonged standing, combining conviviality with high consumption of alcohol, for example, wine merchants, innkeepers or hoteliers. This indicates an acquired component but the youth of some patients points to an inborn tendency.

This is an important category of patient to recognize as the long-term results do not flatter the surgeon! It is often recognized by the response to previous surgery and, in this case, as the condition is usually bilateral and the patient often still quite young, it is best to advise that the benefits gained by further surgery should be protected by wearing an elastic support up to the knee as a long-term measure. This is easy enough in the case of a man (see Chapter 18) but less easily accepted by a woman. Elastic support hose as tights may prove a reasonable compromise, or if events have proved this to be inadequate, a below-knee stocking up to the knee is comfortable to wear and neat in appearance. If there is any uncertainty about the diagnosis of 'weak veins' it may be better to warn of possible recurrence but not condemn the patient, perhaps unnecessarily, to an elastic stocking at this stage, but to let events decide the matter. The obese patient should be advised to lose weight and, when appropriate, to reduce intake of alcohol but this advice is seldom followed.

There is substantial evidence based on studies with the electron microscope showing that fragmentation of the circular muscle layers occurs in the veins of many varicose vein patients (Rose, 1986a,b, and see below). Structural weakness appears to be an important factor in the development of superficial vein incompetence and varicose veins in many patients and the 'weak vein' syndrome, described above, may be an extreme form of this.

## Inborn deficiency of valves and weakness of the vein walls as non-thrombotic causes for venous disorder

It must be pointed out that the valveless and weak vein syndromes, referred to above, are not generally recognized categories, although all experienced venous specialists will be familiar with the type of case described, especially as these patients tend to be amongst the least satisfying to treat. In this chapter attention has been drawn to the probability that states with valves deficient in number or durability exist, and may be inborn. Many authorities believe that such cases are in fact the end product of subclinical attacks of deep vein thrombosis. This may be the case but the author has been impressed by the absence of any history of possible thrombosis and the lack of any tell-tale evidence on phlebography.

The other category, described above, of weakness in the walls of the veins has much in common with the

**Figure 7.7** *An example of weak vein syndrome illustrated by phlebography. The patient was a male aged 40 years who had massive bilateral varicose veins with severe venotensive changes and threatened ulceration. There was no history suggestive of past deep vein thrombosis and a previous surgical attempt, by high saphenous ligation without stripping, had soon been followed by massive recurrence. The patient was a large man, 6 feet in height, and very obese, with marked ankle oedema; he worked in the wine trade and admitted to a high consumption of alcohol. Clinical examination showed massive varicosities largely concealed in ample subcutaneous fat. These could not be controlled by any form of Trendelenburg test; Doppler flowmetry showed no distinctive movement on exercise and the vast size of the varicosities made meaningful examination difficult. Photoplethysmography showed poor venous emptying with exercise and abnormally brief venous refilling time. The illustration shows a composite phlebogram of the right side. The femoral and iliac veins have been outlined by passive filling with the patient standing still and are seen here after three exercise movements. The long saphenous vein is visualized along its length and the deep veins are unusually large but no valves could be demonstrated. The long saphenous vein is massive and in the lower thigh gives off a large varicosity running to mid-calf where it communicates with gastrocnemius and tibial veins. The large saccule in the popliteal fossa is probably in the uppermost short saphenous vein.*

*Both sides were similarly affected. Because the deep veins were widely open it was considered safe to remove the long saphenous vein and some of the varicosities. This brought little improvement to the venous hypertension and the patient has to rely upon strong elastic support to prevent deterioration. The impression is of veins with weak walls and capable of massive enlargement. It is not certain whether there is a widespead failure of valves due to separation of the valve cusps by distension of the valve rings, or there is a widespread deficiency in the number of valves as in the valveless syndrome*

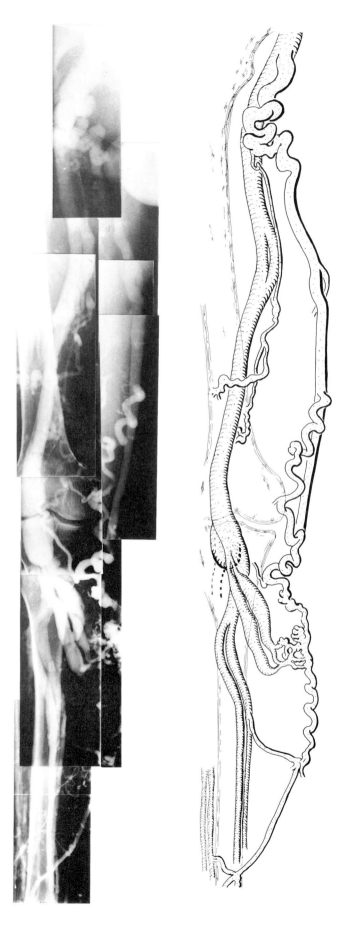

valveless state but its identity seems sufficiently real to describe it separately, especially in view of its association with obesity and alcoholism. If weak vein walls wreak such havoc as to cause widespread failure of valves in deep and superficial veins, the question arises whether this may occur in more localized fashion to account for the everyday phenomena of simple, uncomplicated varicose veins. S. Rose (1986a,b, and by personal communication) has made a special study of the structure of the vein wall in varicose conditions using conventional light microscopy and transmission electron microscopy. He found that varicose veins invariably have degenerative changes breaking the regular pattern of the muscle layer by invasion with fibrous tissue. On electron microscopy, these changes are clearly seen with separation of the muscle cells by increased fibrous tissue laid down as irregular collagen fibres and by isolated groups of elastic fibres. The appearances are as though the muscle cells have formed a pericellular layer of amorphous fibrous tissue. The cytoplasm shows increased vacuole formation possibly related to collagenase and elastase production. Hemidesmosomes on the basement membrane are more widely separated than usual and this may interfere with their function of communicating contraction from one muscle cell to another. As a result of these changes, support provided by the muscle layers becomes less effective, with the vein wall loosing its tone and stretching to form a varicosity. With further development, the intermuscular space becomes filled with collagen and scattered elastic tissue, so that the ability of the vein to contract is reduced. The valve rings are involved in the overall distension of the vein wall, leading to incompetence by separation of the cusps. Rose believes that this process is the initiating pathology in simple superficial vein incompetence. Many share this belief and the following arguments may be produced to support this:

1. The rapid development of florid varicosities in pregnancy, and their remarkable disappearance within a few weeks of childbirth, is best explained by temporary relaxation of the vein walls and valve rings, caused by circulating hormones, particularly oestrogens. This provides a common example of recoverable valve failure in circumstances where the vein wall is known to undergo gross overdistension.

2. Many cases of varicose veins are found to have a full complement of well-formed valves in the saphenous vein, but yet, the clinical tests, Doppler flowmetry, photoplethysmography, phlebography and testing the valves by syringe at operation, all give unequivocal evidence of their incompetence. Often the cusps appear indistinguishable from normal and it is hard to explain this except by overdistension of the valve rings with separation of the valve cusps.

3. The competence of valves is variable from one time to another. In Chapter 2 it was noted that many patients find that the severity of their varicose veins increases just before menstruation or after a hot bath, both circumstances leading to maximal relaxation of muscular tone in the vein walls. During syringe testing of a saphenous vein that has contracted down at operation, a valve can sometimes be felt to yield and become incompetent as pressure by the syringe expands the vein.

4. The ability of veins to withstand high pressure shows individual variation. A normal saphenous vein used as an arterial bypass withstands the sustained arterial pressure without any tendency to become varicose. This is true whether it is a reversed graft or an 'in situ' bypass. (It should be noted, though, that in the former flow is in the natural direction allowed by valves and, in the latter, the important factor of reversed flow, counter to the valves, has been 'neutralized' by deliberate destruction of the valves.) In contrast to this, an incompetent long saphenous vein giving rise to varicosities may not be suitable for use as an arterial graft and may soon show gross overdistension or even rupture of any pre-existing saccules in its wall, whether it is used as a reversed graft or 'in situ'. This suggests inherent weakness in the wall.

There are many questions unanswered in this matter but it does seem that weakening in the vein wall is likely to be a major factor in the typical incompetent saphenous vein. The key question is whether this change in structure is secondary to stress in the walls of any portion of vein exposed to excess pressure (as in the theory of sequential failure of valves), or is a primary process, for reasons unknown, which causes veins to dilate and the valves to give way. This question remains unanswered but it is probable that both factors can operate, each encouraging the other.

## References

Browse, N. L., Clemenson, G. and Lea Thomas, M. (1980) Is the postphlebitic leg always postphlebitic? Relation between phlebographic appearances of deep vein thrombosis and late sequelae. *British Medical Journal*, **281**, 1167–1170

Friedman, W. I., Taylor, L. M. and Porter, J. M. (1988) Congenital venous valvular aplasia of the lower extremities. *Surgery*, **103**, 24–27

Kistner, R. L. (1980) Primary venous valve incompetence of the leg. *American Journal of Surgery*, **140**, 218–224

Kistner, R. L. (1989) Venous valve surgery. In *Surgery of the Veins* (eds J. J. Bergan and J. S. T. Yao), Grune and Stratton, New York, pp. 205–217

Lockhart-Mummery, H. E. and Hillyer-Smitham, J. (1951) Varicose ulcer. *British Journal of Surgery*, **38**, 284–295

Ludbrook, J. (1966) *Aspects of Venous Function in the Lower Limbs*, Charles C. Thomas, Springfield, IL

Plate, G., Brudin, L., Eklof, G. *et al.* (1986) Physiological and therapeutic aspects of congenital vein valve aplasia of the lower limb. In *Phlebology '85* (eds D. Negus and G. Jantet), John Libbey, London, pp. 780–782

Rose, S. (1986a) The aetiology of varicose veins. In *Phlebology '85* (eds D. Negus and G. Jantet), John Libbey, London, pp. 6–9

Rose, S. (1986b) The aetiology of varicose veins. In *Progress in Flebologia* (eds M. Tesi *et al.*), Edizioni Minerva Medica, Torino, pp. 47–48

Taheri, S. A., Heffner, R., Meenaghan, M. A. *et al.* (1985) Technique and results of venous valve transplantation. In *Surgery of the Veins* (eds J. T. Bergan and J. S. T. Yao), Grune and Stratton, New York, pp. 219–231

Tibbs, D. J. and Fletcher, E. W. L. (1983) Direction of flow in superficial veins as a guide to venous disorders in lower limbs. *Surgery*, **93**, 758–767

Turner Warwick, W. (1930) Valvular defect in relation to varicosis. *Lancet*, **ii**, 1278–1286

## Bibliography

Almgren, B. (1990) Non-thrombotic deep venous incompetence with special reference to anatomic, haemodynamic and therapeutic aspects. *Phlebology*, **5**, 255–270

El-Gohary, M. A. (1984) Boyhood varicocele: an overlooked disorder. *Annals of the Royal College of Surgeons of England*, **66**, 36–38

Lodin, A., Lindvall, N. and Gentele, H. (1958/59) Congenital absence of venous valves as a cause of leg ulcers. *Acta Chirurgica Scandinavica*, **116**, 256–261

Lodin, A. and Lindvall, N. (1961) Congenital absence of valves in the deep veins of the leg. A factor in venous insufficiency. *Dermato-Venereologica (Stockholm)*, **41**, Suppl. 45, 7–91

# 8

# Impaired deep veins and venous pump failure: the post-thrombotic (postphlebitic) syndrome

In this state the deep veins have suffered widespread damage to both lumen and valves from a previous deep vein thrombosis or by direct injury. The consequences of this, such as ulceration, may be apparent within 2 or 3 years but often the time interval from thrombosis to the full clinical manifestations of unresolved damage in the deep veins may be very much longer, with a latent period of 10 or even 20 years before real problems arise. The original thrombosis may have arisen in various circumstances, for example: during pregnancy or after childbirth, as a complication accompanying any serious illness, or following injury and fractures in lower limbs or pelvis. Sometimes the condition arises without any immediately obvious cause and investigation may show enhanced thrombogenesis due an inherited coagulation disorder (see Chapter 16) or an acquired state, such as use of the contraceptive pill; it may be the response to systemic changes accompanying malignancy (Rickles and Edwards, 1983) but here the patient may not survive long enough to develop the long-term consequences of a deep vein thrombosis. However, it is not our purpose to review the active phase of thrombosis but rather the type of long-term damage that it may cause and the manifestations arising from this, a state often referred to as the post-thrombotic or postphlebitic syndrome.

## Venous hypertension: the key factor and its causes

Unfortunately the term 'post-thrombotic (or postphlebitic) syndrome' has often been loosely applied to any condition which shows similar manifestations but is not necessarily the result of previous deep vein thrombosis. In this case, 'post-thrombotic' is being used as a convenient label to designate a particular syndrome of physical signs which has several very different causes but, nevertheless, all sharing in common the feature of *venous hypertension*. This is the common denominator which determines whether the patient suffers the worst features of venous disorder. Encountering the set of symptoms and signs arising from it does not on its own justify the term 'post-thrombotic' and far better would be, perhaps, 'venotensive syndrome', or even 'post-thrombotic type of syndrome', in order to signify the typical appearances caused by venous hypertension have been recognized but without indicating what form of venous failure has lead to this. The main causes of venous hypertension have been considered in Chapter 6 but are summarized below:

1. Overwhelming of the musculovenous pumping mechanism by incompetence in the superficial veins (see Chapter 6).
2. Inborn weakness or deficiency of valves in the pumping mechanism and major deep veins; this may be combined with superficial vein incompetence (see Chapter 7).
3. Post-thrombotic damage to deep veins and their valves with corresponding failure in the venous pump mechanism (considered in this chapter).
4. Combination of any of the above conditions (see Chapters 5 and 10).
5. Congenital venous abnormalities reproducing any of the conditions given above (see Chapter 12).
6. In arteriovenous fistula, which may be congenital and multiple, traumatic or iatrogenic in origin (see Chapters 12 and 17).

It must be admitted that in practice there is a sizeable group of patients showing all the manifestations of venous hypertension but in whom it is not possible to be certain about the nature of the process that has lead to failure of the deep vein pumping mechanism. This aspect will be returned to later in this chapter and our starting point will be the well-defined *true* post-thrombotic (postphlebitic) state.

# Post-thrombotic deep vein impairment

## Incidence of true post-thrombotic deep vein impairment

It has been established beyond doubt that deep vein thrombosis can cause lasting damage leading to venous hypertension and progressive deterioration in the limb. Homans (1917) recognized this association and used the term 'post-thrombotic'. A notable contribution was made by Bauer (1942), supported by phlebographic evidence, which traced the fate over 10 years of limbs sustaining thrombosis and demonstrating an increasing proportion with swelling, induration, pigmentation and ulceration as the years passed. Many workers have subsequently confirmed this and Dodd and Cockett (1976) in reviewing the experience of a number of authorities, together with their own findings, quote figures suggesting that over 50% of recognized deep vein thromboses develop these changes in due course and state that the evidence is 'indisputable'. More recently Widmer et al. (1986) have presented further strong confirmation of the relationship in a study of 341 patients. Certainly this is in keeping with our own experience and various patients in this category are illustrated throughout this chapter.

Since deep vein thrombosis itself occurs over a wide age group, including the young (most commonly caused by intravenous drip in infancy or childhood (Rabe, 1987, see Figure 8.7)), it is not surprising to find patients with the post-thrombotic state from the late teens onwards and increasing with age. Women have a somewhat higher incidence, particularly in those with iliofemoral thrombosis; in this latter group, the left side is affected about twice as commonly as the right side and the reasons for this are considered presently. All authorities are agreed upon the chronicity of the condition. Once it is established there is strong tendency for increasing deterioration over the years, eventually giving rise to ulceration which may be healed by appropriate measures (see Chapters 13 and 18) but may recur repeatedly over the patient's lifetime.

Most authorities agree that the incidence of venous ulcer from all causes is about 1% (Hobbs, 1977) of the population at some stage in their lives. The proportion of those directly caused by a recognizable deep vein thrombosis and having evidence of deep vein deformity on phlebography is not accurately known but probably accounts for about one-half of all venous ulcers, that is, about one person in two hundred will suffer from recurring ulcer related to identifiable deep vein thrombosis.

## Medical and social importance: relationship to venous ulceration

Hobbs (1977) quotes various authorities including Boyd, Dodd and Cockett, Gjores, and Widmer, indicating that between 0.5% and 3% of people in European countries suffer from one or more episodes of venous ulceration at some time in their lives. Callam et al. (1987), based on a study of 600 patients with chronic leg ulcers, arrive at a similar approximation of 1% of the population are affected at some point in their lives. However, it must be noted that many venous ulcers are not strictly the result of a previous deep vein thrombosis so that the figures just given are not precise, and our own experience suggests that approaching half are caused by superficial vein incompetence or are due to a deep vein incompetence without any evidence, by history or phlebography, of a preceding deep vein thrombosis. With such differing criteria in selection of cases, an exact figure is not possible but it seems that something in the order of one person in 200 suffers appreciable disability as a long-term consequence of deep vein thrombosis and a sizeable additional group have similar disability from a different set of venous causes.

## The importance of medical history

In any venous disorder it is important to know if there is any possible history of deep vein thrombosis and it must be explained to the patient that one is asking about an event occurring many years ago, even 20 years or more, and possibly long since forgotten. Some of the most useful questions in this respect are upon 'white leg of pregnancy', prolonged swelling of one limb following surgery, serious illness or injury, especially a fracture in the lower limbs (Wolfe, 1987), and upon the use of long-term anti-coagulants or the occurrence of pulmonary embolus. Although a significant history of this sort points strongly to old thrombotic damage being the cause of a patient's present state, in fact, a number of cases of deep vein thrombosis do resolve without any evident persisting deep vein impairment. The present condition may be a separate development, or, quite simply, superficial phlebitis has been confused with a deep vein thrombosis, not an uncommon error. Moreover, it is possible that a thrombosis, which has resolved completely, may have encouraged superficial vein incompetence in two ways:

1. Superficial valve rings, overexpanded by the veins acting as collaterals at the time of thrombotic occlusion, may not recover.
2. The valve cusps have been damaged by thrombosis extending into the superficial veins.

Thus, a positive history indicates a probability, but not a certainty, of deep vein impairment being the dominant defect. Because such a history can be misleading, it is important to carry out the usual clinical and special tests with care to ensure that a simple treatable condition is not mistaken for an intractable deep vein impairment.

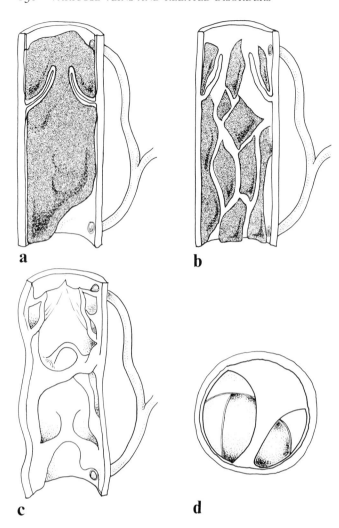

a   b

c   d

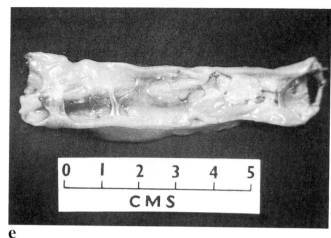

e

**Figure 8.1** *Changes within a deep vein following thrombosis.*

*(a) Recent thrombus filling a deep vein and surrounding valve cusps. A thin flow of blood around the clot is possible and will give a characteristic 'tramline' appearance on phlebography.*

*(b) Over many weeks, resolution of the thrombus takes place. This is a combination of fibrosis and recanalization with endothelial-lined channels.*

*(c) The final outcome is a deformed and often multiple lumen. The interior is irregular, perhaps crossed by fibrous webs, and with valves that are thickened and immobilized by adhesions. At this stage, the interior, with all its irregularities, is covered by intima and capable of conducting blood without thrombosis.*

*(d) End-on view of the irregular interior of a vein impaired by previous thrombosis. A vein such as this will offer appreciable resistance to flow and will not have any effective valves.*

*(e) Photograph of a vein thrombosed 2 years previously and showing a deformed lumen following recanalization. A shining intimal surface is evident throughout.*

## The nature of the damage

The original deep vein thrombosis will have filled the veins with adherent thrombus over an extensive area and inevitably involved the delicate valves as well. The level and extent of this can vary from massive involvement of deep veins throughout the limb to a localized area of thrombosis confined to, say, veins and muscle sinuses of the calf or a localized segment of a major deep vein. The iliac and pelvic veins may well be involved at the same time (see Chapter 9). The ultimate long-term picture will be related to the severity and positioning of the original thrombosis (Figure 8.8(a)) but, unless original phlebograms are available, the information on this is so incomplete, and the degree of resolution following thrombosis is so variable, that it is of little value in understanding the present state. When the initial active phase of thrombosis has settled then repair processes commence attempting to restore normality. The thrombus is absorbed and by endothelial proliferation new channels are formed (Figure 8.1). However intimal regeneration is accompanied by fibrosis and often the new channels are multiple, narrow and deformed (Scott, 1970). If recognizable valves emerge they are likely to be distorted and

ineffective. The final picture is one of irregular deep veins without functioning valves. This has two consequences: first, there is resistance to return of blood up the deep veins so that alternative collateral routes, established at the time of the thrombosis, are likely to persist; secondly, the normal pumping function within the deep veins, dependent upon a good lumen and sound valves, is permanently lost in the affected veins. According to the extent of the original thrombosis, the musculovenous pump, essential for proper venous return in the upright position, may suffer irreparable damage which may be severe. The valves that normally prevent venous reflux after muscle contraction, or after rising to an upright position, will have lost this protective function so that full venous pressure is only inadequately and briefly reduced by exercise, that is to say, the state of venous hypertension (venous stasis) occurs.

## Reflux in collateral veins

Veins acting as collaterals, in both superficial and deep layers, often become greatly expanded and loose all valve function, so that they will allow heavy reflux to occur which increases the rapid build up of full venous pressure (a continuous column of venous blood from foot and heart) in the upright position. Although their collateral contribution is very desirable, possibly essential, they may be an important cause for the rapid return of venous pressure after exercise, the very feature that is so damaging in venous hypertension. This adverse affect is usually outweighed by their collateral benefits and great care has to be used in assessing this if removal of a superficial vein is being considered. A large saphenous vein serving as a collateral *and* which is shown on venogram to have a good set of valves is to be greatly prized and should never be removed because it is bringing only the benefits without the serious disadvantage of reflux. Even if this is not so, blind removal of enlarged veins (or perforators) is not justifiable when the means of proper assessment is so easily available by Doppler flowmetry, photoplethysmography and functional phlebography. For example, the effect of selective occlusion (by pressure with fingertips) of a vein suspected of being harmful should always be ascertained; the photoplethysmogram may register an immediate congestive effect giving warning that its collateral role is significant and should be preserved (see example in Figure 8.8(d)).

## The haemodynamic effects

If the deep veins are fully or partially obstructed by severe deformity, blood can only return by collateral channels which will include the superficial veins. These veins will become unnaturally prominent, but not necessarily tortuous because flow is in their natural direction. Outflow from patent deep veins below the obstruction will be through multiple perforating veins but often one perforator takes on a major role and acts as the principal outlet to the superficial collateral circulation (Figure 8.2(a)). In the upright exercising patient each muscular contraction will pump blood out through the perforators and up the superficial veins and this is easily detected by the directional Doppler flowmeter (Figure 8.2(b)). This outward and upward pumping (Figure 8.2(c),(d)) is very different from the gravitational downflow occurring in simple incompetence in the superficial veins from a source above a pumping mechanism to the low pressure below it. The two states (Figure 8.3(a),(b)) are in direct contrast because in the collateral state blood is being pumped outwards and upwards from deep veins at low level, whilst in superficial incompetence it is spilling over at high level and falling down to enter deep veins at low level. The implications and methods of treatment of these two conditions differ correspondingly. Both may be associated with one or more enlarged perforating veins and the term 'incompetent perforator' is often misleading since it can be applied with some justification to both these states. It is best avoided in favour of more specific

terms such as 'deep vein impairment' or 'superficial vein incompetence'. In either condition the perforator is usually playing an incidental part, secondary to the more fundamental failure in deep or superficial veins, and it should not be accorded a leading role too readily. This is further considered in Chapter 11.

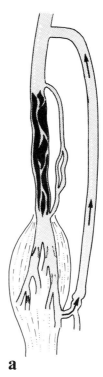

**a**

**Figure 8.2** *The changed haemodynamics with impaired deep veins.*

*(a) Diagram of the effect of extensive occlusion or deformity in popliteal and femoral deep veins. Venous blood under pressure from muscular contraction finds the easiest route is via perforator veins to superficial veins so that it is returned against gravity by preferential flow up them and the saphenous veins are usually involved in this. One perforator conducting blood out to them may predominate so that its useful role as a collateral vein may be misinterpreted.*

*(b) Upward flow in the superficial veins when the patient is standing is easily detected by a Doppler flowmeter and this is a valuable diagnostic indicator in many patients. A typical tracing from saphenous vein in lower thigh in a postphlebitic limb is shown, with upward flow when standing still and accentuated by squeezing of the calf or exercise by rising on the toes. There is no component of downflow following exercise (unlike simple incompetence of the long saphenous vein) but there may be a compensatory pause in upflow after exercise (see page 158).*

*(c) The late consequences of thrombosis in tibial, popliteal and femoral veins in a man aged 61 years. This composite phlebogram during functional phlebography shows failure of upper tibial and popliteal vessels to fill and marked deformity in the lower femoral vein. The deep veins in the lower leg can be seen but outlet from them is by multiple, tortuous perforating veins to the superficial veins so that venous return from below the knee is two main routes, preferential flow up the long saphenous vein, and by the short saphenous vein, now enormously enlarged and substituting for the popliteal vein (see page 158).*

**Figure 8.2** *(continued)*

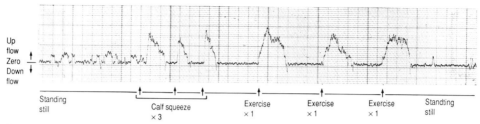

**b**

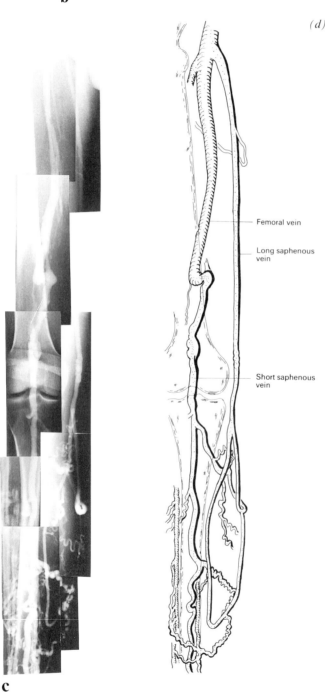

Femoral vein

Long saphenous vein

Short saphenous vein

**c**

*(d)* *1, 2. Post-thrombotic occlusion of the popliteal vein in a patient aged 78 years, following hip joint replacement. Two phases of filling during phlebography are shown. The deep veins below the knee are grossly disorganized and occluded in many places; multiple tortuous veins communicate with the superficial veins but one large perforating vein in the inner, lower leg is particularly evident sending preferential flow up the long saphenous vein. This dominant perforator is performing a valuable collateral role in the presence of extensive deep vein impairment and its destruction by surgery or sclerotherapy would be unwise in most circumstances (see Chapter 11)*

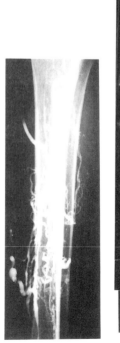

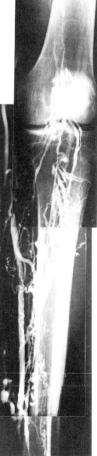

**d**

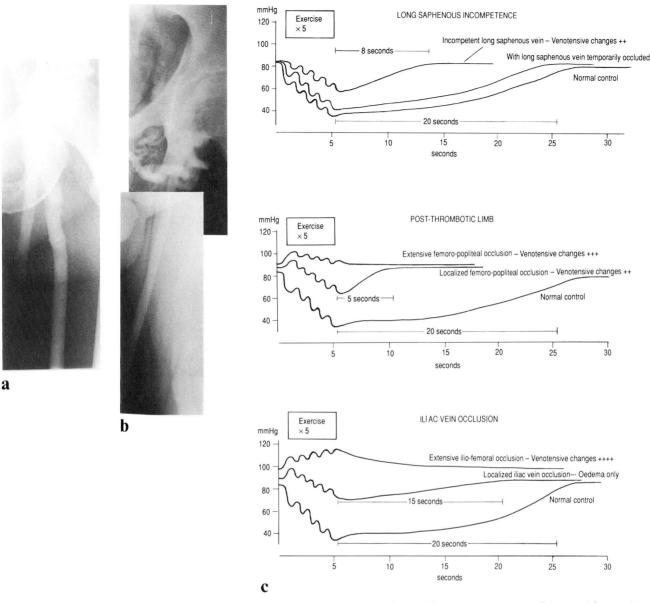

**Figure 8.3** *Functional phlebograms comparing the flow patterns in the upper long saphenous vein; pressure changes with exercise in several venous disorders compared with the normal.*

*(a)  Saphenous valvular incompetence, with normal deep veins. The deep veins have been outlined passively with the patient upright and are seen here immediately after two exercise movements. Opacified blood can be seen spilling down the long saphenous vein.*

*(b)  Extensive deep vein impairment of femoral and iliac veins due to thrombosis following a fractured pelvis 2 years previously. The iliac veins are obstructed and the common and superficial femoral deep veins are severely deformed. With the patient near upright, opacified blood is seen travelling preferentially up the long saphenous vein which is an important collateral. Flow continues from here into pubic varicosities across to the normal right side.*

*In the first case, the saphenous vein is allowing gravitational flow downwards and is creating an extra load for the musculovenous pump; it can be removed with benefit to the patient. In the second case, the saphenous vein is acting as a valuable collateral and compensating for the inability of the deep veins to allow easy flow up their length; it should be preserved.*

*(c)  Venous pressure changes at the ankle in response to five exercise movements in the upright position. Three venous disorders, each sufficiently severe to cause venous hypertension are portrayed, together with the response in a normal limb. With long saphenous incompetence, the fall in pressure is small and brief but temporary occlusion restores normality. Two degrees of severity of post-thrombotic syndrome are shown; with extensive deep vein impairment, the reduction in pressure achieved is very small; in the less severe state a modest fall occurs but this is soon lost by downward reflux in deep veins and collateral channels. In localized iliac occlusion, the resting venous pressure is slightly above normal but shows a moderately good fall and refilling time; the raised resting level will cause oedema in the limb. With extensive iliofemoral occlusion, the resting level is markedly raised and on exercise there is an actual rise in venous pressure that is slow to subside. All gradations in severity and degree of response are found in practice*

## The key consequence: inadequately relieved venous pressure and venous hypertension

The combination of reduced output by the pumping mechanism, and the rapid reflux of blood downwards in valveless deep veins and collateral channels, causes the return of blood to the heart against gravity to be severely impaired. When upright, the response to exercise, a fall in pressure, is inadequate and brief so that the venous pressure remains at high levels for prolonged periods. Venous hypertension is the most significant and harmful feature of venous disorder and its manifestations are often seen at their most severe in the post-thrombotic (postphlebitic) syndrome. The pressure changes with exercise in this syndrome and in superficial vein incompetence are compared with the normal by diagrams in Figure 8.3(c).

## The symptoms and clinical manifestations of the true post-thrombotic syndrome

The symptoms and clinical manifestations of the changes described above are essentially those of venous hypertension and will vary greatly in severity according to the extent and distribution of the venous damage. When fully developed the symptoms will include a heavy, uncomfortable limb with swelling becoming more marked as the day progresses. Added to this may be the discomforts of venotensive skin changes with pruritus and those due to any accompanying eczema, and possibly pain, if an ulcer is present.

An early physical sign of unrelieved venous pressure will be increasing development of numerous venules in the skin, often arranged in a radiating fashion as venous flares. This will be followed by increasing pigmentation and oedema which in severe cases with iliofemoral occlusion may extend up to the groin. This is followed by increasing induration of the subcutaneous tissues which may eventually so encase the limb that oedema becomes less evident. These indurative changes are often referred to as lipodermatosclerosis or liposclerosis, and are prone to develop slightly cyanotic, tender areas of low grade inflammatory change (panniculitis). This state will persist and slowly deteriorate if effective treatment is not carried out and eventually prove to be the forerunner to active ulceration. At times more active cellulitis due to bacterial invasion may be present especially alongside an open ulcer and then fluid exudate or purulent discharge will add to the patient's discomforts. The induration may be accompanied by extensive fibrosis which will tend to restrict ankle movement and, if progressive, eventually prevents any movement at the ankle, which further reduces any remaining venous pump action. Thus, the patient may finally have such pain and stiffness that walking is limited to a painful hobble, with the added misery of an open ulcer. It is unlikely that the patient can continue in employment or household duties in this state.

## Venous claudication

In certain patterns of venous obstruction a disabling symptom will be venous claudication, that is to say, pain on walking for a short distance. This is often described as an unbearable feeling of tightness in the calf, as if it were going to burst, so that the patient is forced to stop. This is most likely to occur in the weeks following acute venous thrombosis and may diminish as the thrombus resolves and collaterals expand. The exact incidence of venous claudication in longstanding post-thrombotic states is not known, perhaps because it is often overshadowed by other manifestations which limit walking in any case, but it does not appear to be particularly common. It is a distinctive phenomenon of venous obstruction restricting the outflow of blood from the exercising limb and its occurrence is accompanied by a rise in venous pressure and increasing girth of the calf as the patient walks (Bollinger and Jager, 1986; Woodyer, Walker and Dormandy, 1986). Most authorities agree that it does not occur in venotensive states without venous obstruction, considered later in this chapter. Venous claudication is discussed further under obstructed venous outlet syndrome in Chapter 9 and is mainly found in iliofemoral obstruction. There is no specific treatment, except in the occasional case that proves suitable for venous reconstruction, considered further in Chapters 9 and 21. However, it is worth bearing in mind that it may improve spontaneously by development of collateral channels in the months following first onset.

## The patterns of deep vein impairment

The term 'impairment' is used here to describe any deep vein that has either remained permanently obstructed after thrombosis or has recanalized to leave a damaged vein offering resistance to flow and with ineffective valves. So great is the variation in the degree of impairment, and its extent, that it is impracticable to cover all the possibilities but certain broad patterns can be distinguished both in the localizaton of the damaged veins and the effects of this upon the venous function of the limb.

Venous function may be disturbed in three ways:

1. Resistance to blood flow by obstructed or deformed deep veins will lead to the venous pressure rising above the normal range (hydrostatic pressure between foot and heart) with exercise and this will cause a tendency to generalized swelling below this level.
2. The widespread loss of effective valves will not only reduce the stroke volume of the musculovenous pump but will allow rapid reflux of blood that has been pumped upwards so that the usual lowering of venous pressure in response to exercise is inadequate and brief (Negus, 1970; Dodd and Cockett, 1976; Bjordal, 1977; Hobbs, 1977; Strandness, 1978; Wright et al., 1978;

May, 1979; Lawrence and Kakkar, 1980; Nicolaides, Zukowski and Kyprianov, 1985; Sumner, 1985). Depending on the severity of the defect a sustained, unrelieved state of venous hypertension arises when the patient is standing or moving about, and as a result the clinical manifestations of venotension (venous stasis) will develop progressively. As explained above, absence of valve function in collateral veins will contribute significantly to this.

3. Repeated peaks of excessive venous pressure, well above the usual maximal, may occur in the lower leg:
    (a) By blood forced up from enlarged veins on the underside of the foot as it is placed to the ground at each step.
    (b) Locally, over points of perforator collateral outflow, as blood is pumped outwards and upwards during exercise.

This is a complex process with a slow build up of undesirable effects and at first the limb may show little more than a persistent swelling but gradually a diffuse fibrosis develops in the subcutaneous fat (lipodermatosclerosis or liposclerosis). Raised capillary pressure causes exudation of fluid containing small molecule proteins, particularly fibrinogen, leading to the development of a cuff of fibrin around the capillaries. This cuff increasingly interferes with tissue nutrition and appears to be a key factor in the ultimate development of skin ulceration (Burnand *et al.*, 1982; Browse, 1985). Increased capillary permeability

**Figure 8.4** *Diagram indicating the main patterns of post-thrombotic deep vein impairment by occlusion or severe deformity. The collaterals that may develop in saphenous veins and lesser deep veins are indicated (superficial veins in dotted lines).*

Below the knee. *The multiplicity of veins, with several parallel principal veins, allows easy re-routing of blood past damaged areas and on phlebography it is difficult to define localized damage. Substantial damage to the pumping mechanism and incompetence of valves may be present but not easy to demonstrate. This probably accounts for many ill-defined venous problems including 'incompetent perforating veins' (see Chapter 11). If the damage below knee also involves the popliteal vein then there is a considerable obstructive component and the venotensive changes (post-thrombotic syndrome) will be severe (see Figure 8.5); collateral flow through both saphenous systems will be important together with collateral veins developed around the original deep veins but the latter are greatly expanded and lacking effective valves.*

Upper popliteal, superficial and common femoral veins. *Thrombotic occlusion and deformity will produce a variable degree of obstruction and generate correspondingly large collaterals from small veins around the deep veins and, of course, in the saphenous veins, including an extension upwards from the short saphenous vein (Giacomini vein).*

*Overexpansion of these veins, particularly the deep collateral channels, causes their valves to fail so that they are virtually valveless and provide a massive source of incompetence; this may be more important than valve damage in recanalized deep*

veins. *However, a saphenous vein that is enlarged may still have good valves and is to be greatly prized and preserved. Collateral outflow through enlarged perforators to superficial veins is part of a compensatory mechanism that should not be destroyed without good reason and evidence that it will bring benefit and not harm.*

Common iliac vein. *Permanent occlusion here may be so well compensated by collaterals, crossing the pelvis internally or superficially by pubic veins, that its effects are minimal but usually there is at least some resistance to venous outflow and consequent oedema throughout the limb (lymphatic involvement may add to this); the pump mechanisms in the limb may be intact. However, when this is combined with femoropopliteal vein damage, as is often the case, then the obstructive effect can be severe and combined with the worst features of pump failure, so that the limb is oedematous to the groin with pigmented, indurative change (liposclerosis) and ulceration at the ankle (see Figure 8.8(d))*

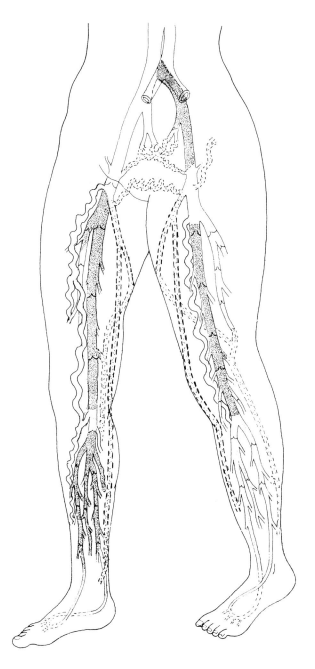

also allows extravasation of haemosiderin, with consequent brown pigmentation of the skin. These are the characteristic changes caused by venous hypertension but, as emphasized above, identical changes may also arise from other causes and are not specific to deep vein impairment, although the most severe examples are found here. Venotensive tissue changes have been considered from the viewpoint of superficial incompetence in Chapter 6.

A more recent hypothesis, based on observations by microscopy to capillary loops in the skin in the legs of patients with chronic venous insufficiency, has been advanced by Coleridge Smith, *et al.* (1988) and Thomas, Nash and Dormandy (1988), and adds a further factor to the role of capillary perfusion and the diffusion of nutrients in the causation of liposclerosis and ulceration. These authors found evidence of substantial accumulation of white cells in the capillaries when the legs are dependent, but reversible when elevated. They suggest that a prolonged aggregation of white cells has the effect of:

1. Plugging capillaries to cause ischaemia.
2. The release of enzymes from the white cells, which damage the endothelium and cause increased capillary permeability; this leads to pericapillary deposition of fibrin cuffs described by Browse and Burnand (1978).

The patterns of deep vein impairment and the collateral flow patterns that may develop are summarized in Figure 8.4 and in the various phlebograms illustrating this chapter. The main patterns are detailed below.

### I. Persisting damage to the deep veins at and below the knee, including the veins of the calf muscles

The importance of this is that the main pumping mechanism of the lower limb is impaired, possibly severely. As a result, venous pressure may not be satisfactorily reduced, and perhaps even more damaging, there may be peaks of excessive venous pressure by blood forced up from the foot at each step. In this way, the lower part of the limb is particularly prone to liposclerosis and ulceration (Figure 8.5).

### II. Deformity of the lumen and destruction of the valves in popliteal, superficial femoral and common femoral deep veins

The predominant effect is obstructive so that oedema is likely to occur, particularly in the early stages before collaterals have expanded to meet requirements of venous return; the efficiency of the musculovenous pump will also be reduced so that venotensive changes and eventually ulceration will accompany this. The below-knee portion of the limb will show chronic enlargement (sometimes referred to as hypertrophy). The superficial veins will

**Figure 8.5** *A typical consequence of severe deep vein obstruction at popliteal level. The patient, a man aged 40 years, gave a history of osteomyelitis in the right lower limb as a child. At the age of 20 years he had an operation for varicose veins in the left lower limb. This entailed high ligation of the long and short saphenous veins. Immediately after this operation the left lower limb became very oedematous and steadily deteriorated with increasing pigmentation and ulceration. It is not clear whether the surgical operation removed important collateral vessels resulting from thrombotic occlusion at the time of hospitalization for osteomyelitis, or whether the popliteal vein had been mistaken for the short saphenous vein and ligated, an error compounded by ligating the best potential collateral, the long saphenous vein, at the same time.*

*(a) Clinical photograph showing an intractable ulcer near the ankle with widespread pigmentation in the lower leg; 2 cm of swelling was present at this level with dense induration (lipodermatosclerosis). In the upper calf a prominent superficial vein can be seen but there are no evident varicosities. Doppler flowmetry to this vein showed upflow, accentuated by exercise (see Colour Plate 6).*

*(b) Doppler tracing from long saphenous remnant in the lower thigh, when standing. There is no component of downflow, and upflow is accentuated by squeezing the calf or exercise. Compression over the popliteal fossa increases the upflow and exercise accentuates this still further (phlebography showed extensive collateral formation in the fossa).*
*Photoplethysmograms comparing the two limbs. On the left side the recovery time following exercise is brief at 8 seconds, indicating a severely reduced effectiveness of the musculovenous pump and this could not be improved by any manipulation of the superficial veins. On the normal right side the recovery time following exercise is above 20 seconds, within the normal range (see page 163).*

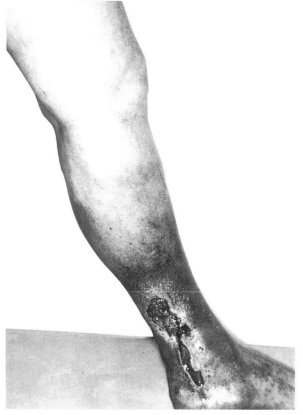

**a**

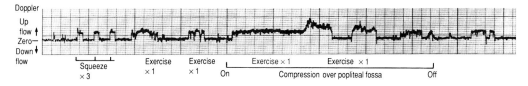

Doppler

Up flow ↑
Zero—
Down flow ↓

Squeeze ×3 | Exercise ×1 | Exercise ×1 | On | Exercise ×1 | Exercise ×1 | Off
Compression over popliteal fossa

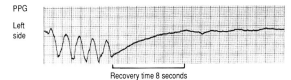

PPG

Left side

Recovery time 8 seconds

Right side

Exercise ×5 | Recovery time 20+ seconds

Patient sitting
Sensors on lower legs

**b**

**Figure 8.5** *(continued)*

*(c) 1–3. Functional phlebography in the same patient. Opaque medium introduced into the foot in the upright position outlined few deep veins but travelled preferentially up the superficial veins. The popliteal vein is completely obstructed in its middle part where gastrocnemius veins and the short saphenous vein are acting as collaterals. An upward extension of the short saphenous joins the femoral vein which appears undamaged. The findings are of extensive damage to the musculovenous pump in the calf region and obstruction to outflow. It is inevitable that such a patient will not be able to tolerate prolonged standing at work and will develop ulceration. Conservative treatment by elevation and subsequent mobilization with external support bandage was successful in healing the ulcer (see Chapter 13) and in training the patient in a way of life that would prevent recurrence*

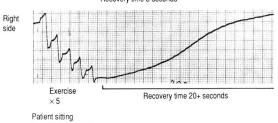

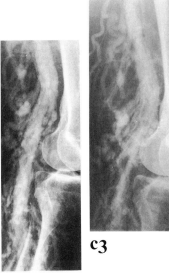

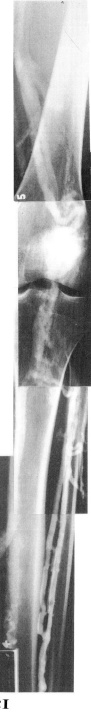

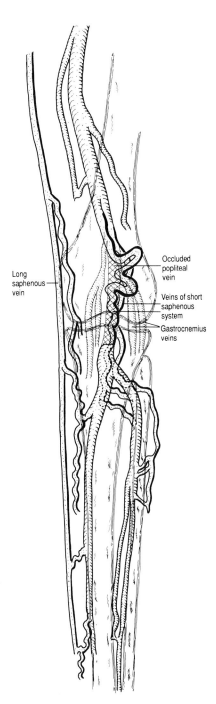

Long saphenous vein

Occluded popliteal vein

Veins of short saphenous system

Gastrocnemius veins

**c2**

**c3**

**c1**

usually be enlarged and a Doppler flowmeter shows upflow in them, accentuated by exercise; a Trendelenburg test, however performed, does not control these veins which instead fill quickly from below and cannot be controlled by any manipulation (Figures 8.6, 8.7). They are acting as collaterals, providing the line of least resistance to venous return and, although enlarged, usually do not show tortuosity because the flow is in their natural

**Figure 8.6** *Patients with popliteal and femoral vein post-thrombotic occlusion and deformity of varying severity.*

*(a) A patient aged 27 years and the mother of one child, who requested treatment for unsightly enlarged veins on the inner left thigh and calf. Examination confirmed unusual prominence of the long saphenous vein and some of its branches but these could not be controlled by a saphenous occlusion test and a Doppler flowmeter showed continuous upflow accentuated by exercise when standing. Further enquiry revealed that 4 years previously she had sustained a severe fracture of the left ankle whilst skiing and this had been treated by some months in plaster but had not been followed by any undue swelling. Deep vein impairment was suspected and functional phlebography carried out. A composite phlebogram from this is shown and it can be seen that the short saphenous vein has filled preferentially and this communicates with the profunda femoris by a tortuous upward extension; the upper half of the popliteal vein is totally obstructed and the femoral vein is deformed over much of its length. Additional views at knee level, in different rotations, are also shown. The tibial and lower popliteal veins filled with difficulty and it was clear that they emptied by perforators into superficial collateral channels provided by long and short saphenous veins. There is little doubt that an unsuspected thrombosis in popliteal and adjoining femoral vein had occurred during treatment of her fracture. There was no significant disability in this limb and the patient was advised that it would be most unwise to remove the enlarged collateral superficial veins but protective measures should be employed by the use of elastic support hose and elevation of the limb whenever possible.*

*(b) A female patient aged 65 years, with bilateral varicose veins. On the right side massive varicosities due to simple incompetence in the long saphenous vein were present, well controlled by saphenous occlusion and showing downflow after exercise with Doppler flowmeter. On the left side the varicose veins could not be controlled by saphenous occlusion and a Doppler flowmeter showed upward flow with strong surge on exercise. A composite functional phlebogram on the left side is illustrated and shows that the upper popliteal vein is occluded; above this a slender, valved vein runs in place of the superficial femoral vein; an upward branch of the short saphenous connects with the profunda femoris vein and another large varicosed branch connects with the long saphenous system; the long saphenous vein is also acting as a collateral. The iliac veins on both sides were normal. There was no history of a deep vein thrombosis and it is assumed that a silent thrombosis occurred during one of her pregnancies 30 years before. The varicosities on the right lower limb were treated surgically together with removal of one varicosity running down onto the foot on the left side, which showed all the features of simple incompetence; other enlarged veins on the left side from knee level upwards were retained undisturbed because of their collateral function (see page 165).*

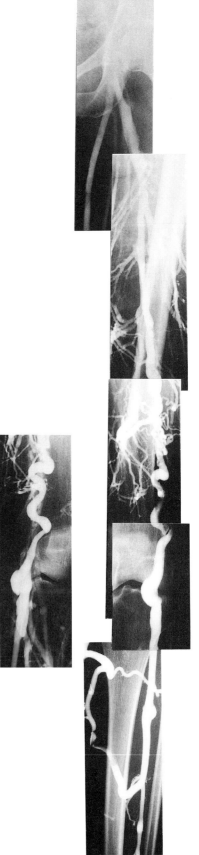

**a**

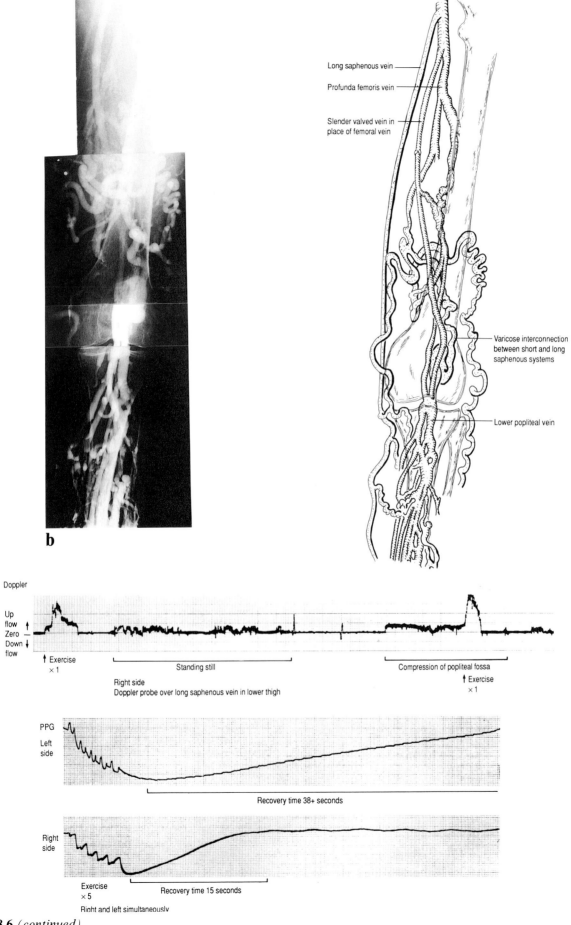

Long saphenous vein

Profunda femoris vein

Slender valved vein in
place of femoral vein

Varicose interconnection
between short and long
saphenous systems

Lower popliteal vein

b

Doppler

Up
flow
Zero
Down
flow

↑ Exercise
× 1

Standing still

Compression of popliteal fossa

↑ Exercise
× 1

Right side
Doppler probe over long saphenous vein in lower thigh

PPG
Left
side

Recovery time 38+ seconds

Right
side

Exercise
× 5

Recovery time 15 seconds

Right and left simultaneously

cI

**Figure 8.6** *(continued)*
*(see caption on page 166)*

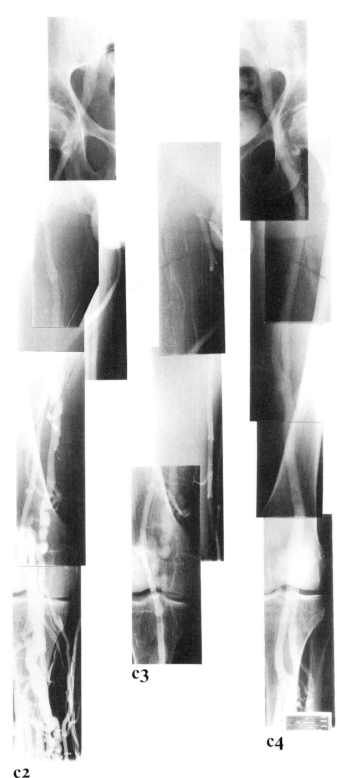

**c3**

**c4**

**c2**

**Figure 8.6** *(continued)*

*(c) Investigations in a man aged 36 years who had sustained a fracture of the right tibia and fibula 3 years previously. Subsequently the limb had developed slight swelling, pigmentation induration and early ulceration.*

*1. Doppler flowmeter tracing taken from the right long saphenous vein with the patient standing shows upflow, accentuated by exercise; compression of the popliteal fossa increases the upflow and this is further accentuated by exercise (phlebography confirmed important collaterals in popliteal fossa) but is not followed by any component of downflow (unlike simple incompetence) (see page 165). Photoplethysmograms comparing the two sides are also illustrated. On the uninjured left side recovery time following exercise is normal at 38 seconds but on the right side this is reduced to 15 seconds, indicating a significant reduction in effective venous return against gravity (see page 165). Composite phlebograms from this patient are also illustrated.*

*2. The right side, showing an obstructed popliteal vein and very abnormal looking upper tibial vessels. Upward flow is occurring through an enlarged short saphenous vein and an upward extension from it; this runs to the upper thigh where it winds round to the medial aspect (this collateral pathway is commonly present) to join the long saphenous vein which is also acting as a collateral with preferential upflow. An abnormal vein takes off from the remnant of the lower popliteal vein and follows the course of the deep veins to join the femoral vein.*

*3. Showing the right long saphenous vein after a swill test. It is seen to be well valved, and a collateral vein such as this with good valves preventing reflux is particularly effective in assisting venous return against gravity and should be carefully preserved.*

*4. Phlebogram of the normal left side in the same patient; no preferential upflow in the superficial veins is shown and opacified medium injected at low level has travelled easily up the deep veins by passive flow, giving a normal outline (the deep vein in mid-thigh shows a double channel for a short distance but this is a common variant); this X-ray has been included to emphasize by comparison the abnormal changes on the right side.*

Conservative treatment was advised.

*(d) A female patient aged 38 years with a history of left deep vein thrombosis whilst on the contraceptive pill 3 years previously. At that time a venous thrombectomy had been carried out through the left common femoral vein, with subsequent use of anticoagulants. The patient now had moderate swelling of the leg, induration, pigmentation and early ulceration. The long saphenous vein was prominent and a Doppler flowmeter showed upflow accentuated by exercise. A composite functional phlebogram from this patient is shown in various phases (see page 167).*

*1. The popliteal vein has not filled and upward flow is carried by a tortuous extension of the short saphenous vein and by a leash of gastrocnemius veins which join a valveless double channel in the position of the superficial vein; only the upper long saphenous vein shows valves.*

*2. Two rotated views of the popliteal region are also given to show further the connections of the gastrocnemius veins. An extension of the short saphenous vein also carries flow upwards to join collateral flow in the long saphenous vein.*

*3. The common femoral vein, at the site of thrombectomy, is occluded and varicosities in the vicinity are acting as collaterals across to the opposite side and upwards to the external iliac vein of the same side which was seen to lead into a normal common iliac vein. Conservative treatment was advised, using a graduated elastic stocking and elevating the limb whenever possible*

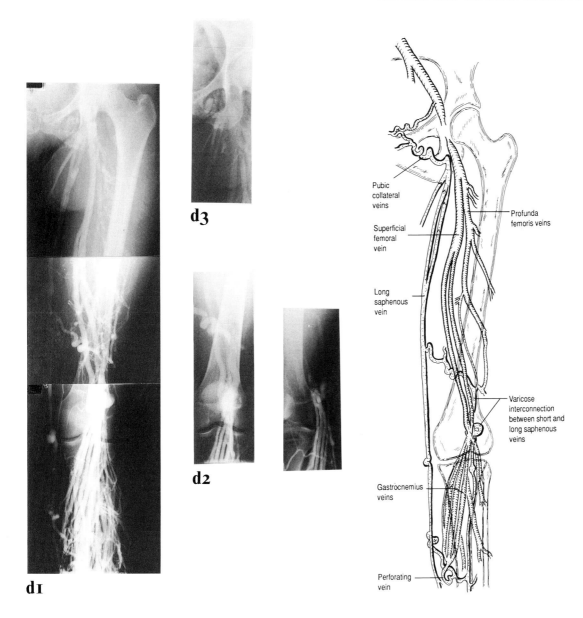

direction. Nevertheless, tortuous superficial veins may be present for any of the following reasons:

1. Superficial branch veins, acting as collaterals in their apparent natural direction of flow, sometimes do develop tortuosity.
2. Simple varicose veins which were present before deep vein thrombosis have changed their role to a collateral one.
3. A complex pattern is present, with an incompetent branch of a principal superficial collateral vein, such as a saphenous vein, allowing retrograde flow down to the lower leg or foot. In such a vein, blood may surge back and forth with each footstep and so cause it to so become enlarged and tortuous (and see below).

### III. Persisting obstruction of the iliac veins (venous outflow obstruction syndrome) (and see Chapter 9)

Thrombosis in the iliac veins seldom resolves satisfactorily and recannulation is uncommon. The iliac veins are not usually valved, that is to say, they are not part of the pumping mechanism, so that the efficiency of this aspect is not reduced provided the limb below this has not also been involved in the thrombosis. If the damage is confined to the iliac veins, the main effect is resistance to venous outflow from the limb and oedema up the groin is likely to occur. However, in some patients the collateral network of veins, both superficial and deep, across the pelvis is so good that oedema may be insignificant (Figure 8.8). If the pumping mechanism and deep veins below are unaffected then it is possible for simple incompetence in the superficial veins of the limb to coexist

**Figure 8.7**  *Persisting occlusion of the common femoral vein in a young woman aged 20 years, who complained of moderate swelling in the limb and varicose veins in the right lower limb. The varicosities were mainly concentrated in the upper thigh and running onto the lower abdomen. Further enquiry revealed that the patient had sustained severe burns as an infant which required prolonged treatment in hospital. This included intravenous drip by 'cut-down' into the long saphenous vein at the ankle; the scar of this was clearly visible. A high-level deep vein obstruction was suspected and functional phlebography carried out.*

*(a)  Composite phlebogram showing that the common femoral vein is obstructed, with side branches of the superficial femoral vein acting as collaterals; the upper long saphenous vein could not be filled and appears occluded. It seems likely that common femoral and saphenous vein thrombosis occurred as a result of the intravenous therapy 20 years before.*

*(b)  Photoplethysmograms in the same patient comparing the two limbs. The left side is a good normal with recovery time of 40 seconds; on the right side the recovery time following exercise is just within normal limits at 21 seconds, in keeping with a relatively undamaged pumping mechanism but some resistance to outflow at the groin. The patient had no real disability and was not unduly worried by the collateral veins in the groin which had compensated so well for the femoral vein obstruction. Conservative management was advised*

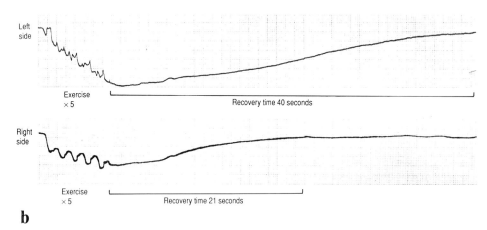

**Figure 8.8**  *Extensive deep vein thrombosis including iliac vein and giving rise to iliofemoral combined patterns of deep vein impairment (see pages 169–173).*

*(a)  Iliofemoral vein deformity and occlusion in a man aged 23 years, following acute deep vein thrombosis in the left lower limb 3 years previously. The history prior to thrombosis included an operation for pilonidal sinus 5 months before and a story of recurring bouts of alcoholism, so that the cause of thrombosis was uncertain. Phlebograms at that time, and subsequently, suggested that left common iliac vein compression by the overlying right common iliac artery may have been an important factor.*

*1. A composite phlebogram, taken at the time of the acute thrombosis, shows clot outlined by opacified blood (tramline sign) in calf veins; the common femoral and iliac veins could not be made to fill and were thought to be obstructed by thrombus.*
*2. The second phlebogram shows a composite picture 3 years later. Severe deformity in superficial and common femoral veins and external iliac veins is present; only the lower part of the common iliac vein has filled and blood can be seen passing up an ascending lumbar vein acting as a collateral*

*past the uppermost common iliac vein, which appears to be totally obstructed. The clinical picture at this stage was one of oedema up to the groin in the left lower limb, with induration, pigmentation and ulceration in the lower leg. The saphenous vein could be identified in the lower thigh and showed strong upward Doppler flow, accentuated by exercise; large collateral veins could be seen running across the pubes subcutaneously and upwards in the iliac fossa.*
*3. On photoplethysmography, recovery time was abnormally brief at 9 seconds and was not improved by saphenous compression. Conservative management was advised (see page 169).*

*(b)  A patient with a typical post-thrombotic limb of moderate severity with oedema to the knee, liposclerosis and threatened ulceration in the lower leg. Sixteen years previously, at the age of 32 years, she had sustained a deep vein thrombosis on the left side during the late stage of pregnancy. Oedema had persisted and the limb slowly deteriorated to its present state. The composite fuctional phlebogram shows strong preferential flow up a well-valved long saphenous vein; the upper popliteal and the superficial femoral veins cannot be identified but appear to have been replaced by abnormal, tortuous channels. The common*

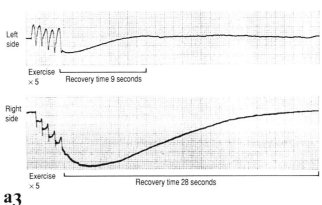

a3

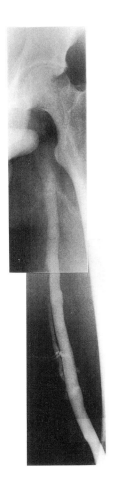

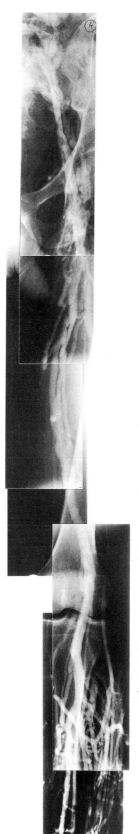

*femoral vein is grossly irregular and a superficial external pudendal vein is acting as a collateral across the pubes. The external iliac is open and some collateral veins crossing the pelvis can be seen faintly. The common iliac vein could not be visualized and was believed to be occluded. Surgery by Palma's operation (swinging over the opposite saphenous vein to act as a collateral) was considered but a maximal venous outflow test showed little reduction from normal, suggesting collateral veins at pelvic level provided an adequate outlet and conservative management was advised (see page 170).*

*(c)  Post-thrombotic syndrome on the left side, in a patient aged 29 years, who sustained thrombosis in pregnancy 3 years previously. Clinical changes were comparatively mild with some oedema and slight pigmentation in the lower leg. The long saphenous vein was slightly enlarged and Doppler flowmetry showed upward flow accentuated by exercise. Pubic varicosities were present. A functional phlebogram is shown. There is preferential upflow in the long saphenous vein and the deep veins below the knee look normal, but above this level there is gross irregularity in the mid-popliteal and the superficial femoral veins; a large channel is seen communicating between the upper popliteal and the profunda femoris veins; the upper superficial femoral and common femoral veins show gross deformity. Two varicosities formed from the external pudendal veins can be seen taking flow to the opposite side. The iliac veins could not be demonstrated but large irregular channels, presumably pelvic veins acting as collaterals, were seen in their vicinity. Palma's cross-over operation was considered but the patient's disability was not great and the special investigations were reassuring. A maximal venous outflow test indicated that collateral veins had compensated well for obstructed and deformed veins; plethysmography was near normal, implying that sufficient valve function remained to give a reasonably effective pumping mechanism; conservative management was advised (see page 171).*

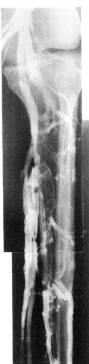

a1                              a2

**Figure 8.8** *(continued)*

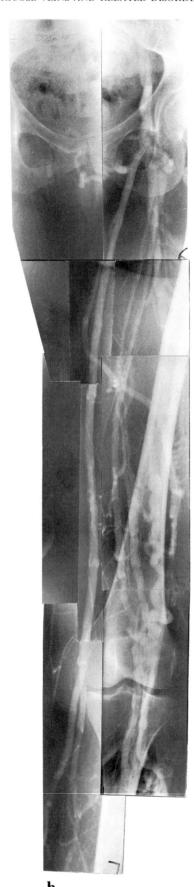

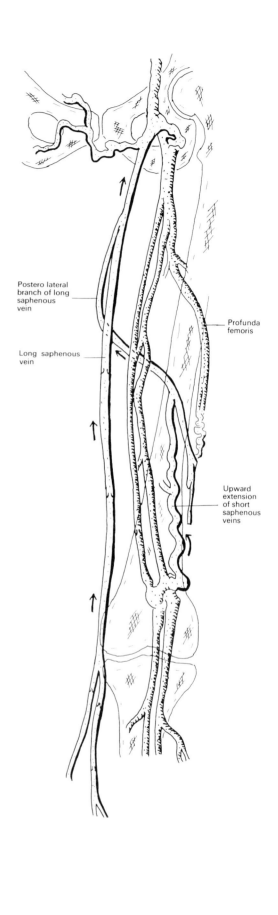

Postero lateral
branch of long
saphenous
vein

Profunda
femoris

Long saphenous
vein

Upward
extension
of short
saphenous
veins

b

**Figure 8.8** *(continued – caption on pages 168 and 169)*

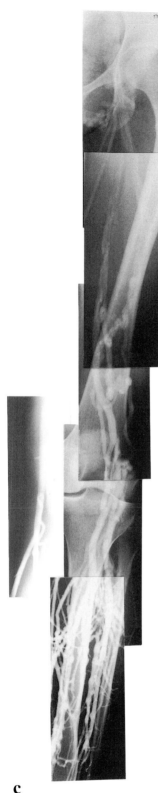

c

*(caption on page 169)*

**Figure 8.8** *(continued)*

*(d) Bilateral post-thrombotic syndrome in a man aged 61 years, due to bilateral fractures of tibia and fibula in a road traffic accident 5 years previously. He was admitted with severe oedema extending up to the groin in the left lower limb and with extensive pigmentation, induration and early ulceration in the lower leg. On the right side similar but less severe changes were present. The oedema rapidly receded with a short spell of high elevation and active movement. This patient had not previously been instructed in the importance of elevating the limbs whenever possible and the use of external support. Following suitable rehabilitation and instruction he was able to maintain his lower limbs in reasonably good condition and increase his range of active participation in life.*

*1, 2. Clinical photographs showing the state of the legs after maximal improvement has been obtained. Considerable*

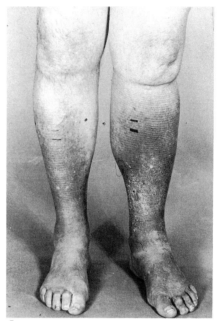

d1

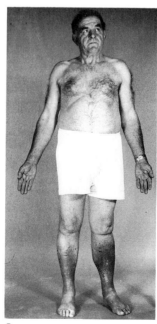

d2

*enlargement of the left side is still evident, in keeping with obstruction to venous outflow from this limb at pelvic level. Venotensive skin changes are extensive in the lower leg but changes on the right side are less severe (see Colour Plate 1).*

*3–5. Composite phlebograms, referred with the patient from another department, show various orthopaedic screws originally used to stabilize the fractures. On the more severely affected left side the iliac veins have failed to fill and appear to be occluded, with various collateral vessels running across to the right iliac veins, which are normal.*

*6. Doppler flowmeter tracings from the saphenous veins show upflow, accentuated by exercise.*

*Photoplethysmograms show, on the left side, little response to exercise and a very brief recovery time at 4 seconds, giving the impression of a severely defective pumping mechanism. On the right side, the response to exercise is more definite but the recovery time is still very short at 5 seconds; compression of the long saphenous vein appears to cause some venous congestion, presumably by impeding an important collateral vein (see page 173)*

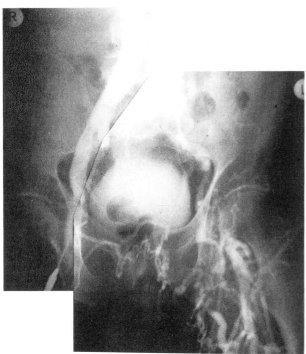

d3

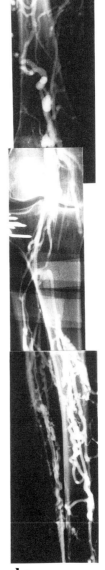

d4

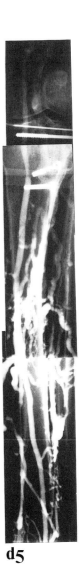

d5

**Figure 8.8** *(continued)*

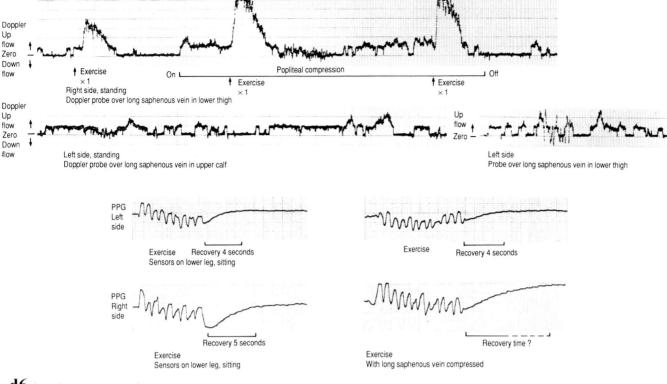

**d6** *(caption on page 172)*
**Figure 8.8** *(continued)*

and, in fact, this is quite often seen (and see below). The presence of simple varicosities in the limb, controlled by saphenous occlusion, does not necessarily exclude a possible iliac vein occlusion above. The main clinical evidence of obstructed iliac veins is the presence of varicosities (collaterals) across the pubic region or lower abdomen, together with enlargement of the limb up to the thigh and groin (Lea Thomas *et al.*, 1967). These features should always be looked for if there is any history suggesting previous deep vein thrombosis.

*IV. Combined patterns of deep vein impairment*

The individual patterns of damage given above seldom occur on their own but arise in various combinations with each other so that the effects may be much more severe. The worst examples of venous hypertension with ulceration and oedema are nearly always the result of widespread involvement of the deep veins. The extent is best revealed by appropriate phlebography and it is important to demonstrate this at some stage to understand the magnitude of the problem. Duplex and Triplex ultrasonography can also give clear visualization at various levels below the inguinal ligament but not quite so comprehensively as fuctional phlebography (see Chapter 22). Imaging with radioactive isotopes and gamma camera can be helpful but lacks detail (see Chapter 23).

*V. Complex patterns of deep vein impairment combined with superficial vein incompetence*

These may arise, as indicated above and illustrated in Chapters 5 and 10 and Figure 8.9. The importance of this is the possibility that a deep vein impairment may be underrated because of the evidence of superficial vein incompetence, perhaps leading to surgical interference which could prove harmful, for example, by taking away important collateral veins when removing varicose veins arising from them. The main warnings of deep vein problems will come from routinely enquiring for any history of possible thrombosis in the past and, if so, checking for enlargement of the limb and the presence of lower abdominal or pubic varicosities. There should always be reluctance to accept that even massive varicosities are the cause for extensive oedema or apparent 'hypertrophy' of the limb, because these changes are seldom caused by superficial incompetence alone. If there is underlying deep vein impairment the key examinations of selective saphenous occlusion and Doppler flowmetry to the superficial veins are unlikely to give satisfactory evidence of straightforward superficial incompetence suitable for surgery, and further clarification by functional phlebography will be needed. Other causes for oedema, such as lymphoedema or oedema of renal or cardiac origin, will also have to be considered (see Chapter 14).

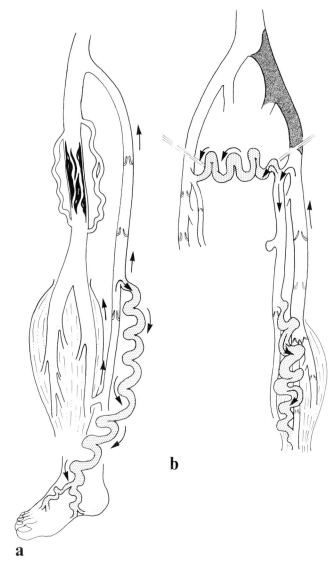

a

**Figure 8.9** *Diagrams of superficial vein incompetence coexisting with deep vein impairment to give complex patterns of venous disorder.*

*(a) The long saphenous vein is acting as a collateral past post-thrombotic occlusion and deformity in the femoral vein. The deep veins below the knee and in the foot provide sufficient pumping action to reduce venous pressure so that it is possible for a varicosity arising from the saphenous vein to allow counterflow down to the underside of the foot. Thus, with each footstep, some of the collateral flow pumped up the saphenous vein spills down to the foot when it is raised and then surges back again as it is replaced on the ground.*

*(b) An incompetent long saphenous system giving rise to varicosities in the limb beneath obstructed iliac veins is not uncommon. In this diagram the iliac veins on the left side are obstructed but the deep veins below the inguinal ligament have not been damaged and form an effective pumping mechanism sending blood via pubic collaterals to the opposite side. This is succeeding in reducing pressure in the lower leg and foot, and in this way gives opportunity for retrograde flow down an incompetent long saphenous vein and the varicose veins arising from it. This and further examples of paradoxical flow in complex venous disorders of this sort, including cross-over incompetence, are illustrated in Chapters 5 and 10*

## Policy on management of impaired deep veins (post-thrombotic syndrome)

When the history suggests the possibility of previous deep vein thrombosis it must not be assumed that lasting deep vein impairment has occurred. Some patients with a suggestive history nevertheless have good deep veins and the explanation for their present trouble lies with the superficial veins. Careful mapping out of superficial veins and performance of a selective saphenous occlusion (Trendelenburg) test upon them is a minimal requirement. Good control of the veins by this test immediately indicates the probability of superficial vein incompetence but, with absence of control, care is needed as this may be caused by failure to recognize concealed long saphenous incompetence (see Chapter 4); it would indeed be unfortunate to label this curable condition as a deep vein problem when it is not so. For this reason, when a saphenous occlusion test does not give control, further evidence must be sought, for example, a Doppler flow-meter may provide this by showing strong upflow in a long saphenous vein, indicating collateral function past impaired deep veins. However, before pronouncing that deep vein impairment is present, with all that this implies, it is usually best to carry out functional phlebography to demonstrate beyond doubt the state of the deep veins. If these are shown to be in good order, and particularly if high-level spillover down an enlarged long saphenous vein is seen (as opposed to preferential flow up it), then it is clear that no significant deep vein damage has occurred in the past and a curable state in the superficial veins is present. Conversely demonstration of deformed or occluded deep veins gives clear evidence that surgery may be unwise or, at best, will be unhelpful.

Assuming that superficial vein incompetence has been excluded with absolute certainty, then the decision has to be reached whether surgery has any part to play in the treatment of the patient. Probably it will not unless some form of deep vein reconstruction (Gruss 1988) is being considered (see Chapter 21); at the time of writing, this has not become a regularly practised form of surgery and should only be attempted by surgeons specializing in this field. The small number of successful cases published so far (1991) probably signifies the limitations of surgical reconstruction. The advice will therefore be upon conservative management and this will usually be to follow a policy of high elevation whenever the opportunity presents and the use of graduated elastic support whenever the patient is up and about. This is more fully discussed in Chapters 13 and 18 upon the care of venotensive changes (venous stasis) and ulceration but the principles are summarized below.

## Summary of the principles in the long-term care of the post-thrombotic limb

The harmful factor is the unrelieved high venous pressure in the lower part of the limb when the patient is upright. This must be counteracted as far as possible by:

1. Giving a considerable proportion of the day to high elevation of the limb because then venous return is good and the pressure minimal.
2. Improving the effectiveness of the pumping mechanism when the patient is upright and moving about. This is usually possible by use of external support. This will limit the size of the venous 'pool' in the lower limb and foot which otherwise creates a large volume of blood surging back and forth with each footstep giving high peaks of pressure as the foot is put down. It is beyond the capacity of the pump to reduce this unaided. Moreover, the support will resist venous reflux down the limb and to some extent diminish this burden on the pump.

*Important medical note.* Always check that there is a good arterial supply to the limb. This is essential if there is pain or the patient is elderly. If the arterial supply is in doubt the limb must not be elevated above the horizontal, nor should any form of compression be applied.

The patient has to understand that successful care can only come through his or her own efforts; all the time the limb is elevated it is improving, but when down it is deteriorating. Every opportunity must be taken to put it into high elevation, the foot of the bed should be elevated at least 50 cm, and a sedentary job should be obtained. This must become a way of life but, nevertheless, the patient must not be physically inactive and should move the feet often.

External support, by bandage or stocking, is usually beneficial. Inelastic containment is the most effective, for example, encasement in a paste bandage, but this is somewhat troublesome to use and best kept for times of crisis, such as development of an ulcer. Elastic support, as a stocking, is more convenient and this should be of the graduated variety to avoid undue tightness in the upper part that might cause constriction of venous return in collateral vessels. Increasing strength of compression does not bring increasing benefit but may do harm and a maximum of 40 mmHg should not be exceeded. A stocking is probably achieving little if the patient finds it excessively uncomfortable; if it causes pain it is inappropriate and should not be used further until its suitability had been checked upon and the arterial supply to the limb verified. The fitting of a venous stocking in the post-thrombotic limb is a skilled task best carried out by a specialist orthotist.

Treatment of active ulceration in the post-thrombotic syndrome is described in Chapter 13. The use of pharmacological agents given orally to enhance fibrinolysis of the pericapillary fibrin cuff (Burnand *et al.*, 1980), to decrease capillary permeability or to alter blood viscosity are also discussed in Chapter 13 but the evidence in their favour is weak and they have not gained universal acceptance.

## The unidentified group: venous hypertensive syndrome without evidence of preceding deep vein thrombosis

(In the discussion that follows it must be assumed that superficial vein incompetence (see Chapter 4) and arteriovenous fistula (see Chapter 17) have been excluded as a cause.)

So far in this chapter a substantial group of patients have been described who have clear evidence of mild to severe venotensive changes caused as a direct result of one or more known episodes of deep vein thrombosis in the limb and iliac veins. Here the relationship between thrombotic damage, leaving clearly recognizable phlebographic changes in the deep veins and their valves, and causing varying degrees of failure in the proper return of venous blood against gravity, seem beyond doubt. However, at the beginning of the chapter, and in Chapter 7, it was pointed out that there was also a group of patients in whom the nature of the process leading to venous pump inadequacy was not clearly identified and it is this group which is now to be considered further.

The author's findings may be of some interest in connection with this (Tibbs and Fletcher, 1983; Tibbs, 1986). In a study by image intensifier-assisted phlebography in over 150 patients with typical venotensive changes it was found that a significant number did not have any suggestion of deformity in the deep veins in keeping with an old deep vein thrombosis, nor could their condition be explained by superficial incompetence; instead, the deep veins were widely patent without deformity but apparently deficient in valves. The term 'valveless syndrome' or 'primary valve failure' has been used in this book (see Chapter 7) to describe this group. One limitation in studying this is the difficulty in displaying satisfactorily the complex arrangement of deep veins below the knee. Nevertheless, we had no doubt that this 'valveless' group could not be regarded as 'post-thrombotic' from the evidence available to us. Other authors, for rather different reasons, have also concluded that there may a sizeable group of patients in whom a clear-cut relationship between a deep vein thrombosis and subsequent development of venotensive changes cannot be substantiated.

Browse, Clemenson and Lea Thomas (1980) examined 130 legs in 67 patients 5–10 years after phlebography for suspected deep vein thrombosis and showed 47 of these limbs to be normal and 83 limbs to have thrombus present. Their findings do much to throw doubt upon the inevitability of venotensive syndrome following an episode of thrombosis. For example, out of 12 limbs originally with iliofemoral thrombosis, five had no symptoms at all and only two had severe symptoms; 33% of legs which originally had severe thrombosis had no residual symptoms. By contrast, of the 47 limbs originally found to be normal at phlebography, 32% had symptoms. It was clear that not every limb with a thrombosis will develop venous problems and many limbs without thrombosis will subsequently develop venous symptoms. These authors were able to show that the extent of the original thrombosis made little difference to the eventual severity of symptoms. Of legs found to be normal by a fibrinogen uptake test soon after an operation, up to 11% had venous symptoms 3 years later and even those with minimal lesions were capable of developing moderate to serious symptoms; moreover, many patients had evidence of venous changes well before the thrombotic episode that brought them into the study. Was thrombosis, therefore, an incidental event superimposed on a separate, progressive, degenerative process in the deep veins? These authors admit, however, the weakness of not being able to obtain phlebograms at the late follow-up which could have indentified the true nature of the final venous state.

Mudge, Leinster and Hughes (1988) published a paper, extending earlier similar work, studying 564 patients over 5–10 years after laparotomy, to see whether 'post-thrombotic (type of) syndrome' may occur after an operation not complicated by deep vein thombosis and to assess the importance of preceding and subsequent thrombotic episodes apart from the qualifying laparotomy. Like Browse, Clemenson and Lea Thomas (1980) they challenge the concept established by Bauer (1942) that the post-thrombotic *type of* syndrome is always the result of deep vein thrombosis and the two studies have much in common. Both suffer from a lack of precise evidence by phlebography in the final 'post-thrombotic' state and Mudge *et al.* have no phlebographic evidence to confirm or exclude various episodes diagnosed as thrombotic at the outset; nevertheless, these and other papers produce strong evidence of the following:

1. Many patients with proven deep vein thrombosis do not develop the 'post-thrombotic' (venotensive) syndrome. This suggests that complete resolution is possible but phlebographic evidence of this is lacking in the studies quoted above. Our own experience shows that many patients who have no symptoms in their good limb some years after a major thrombosis in the opposite limb, nevertheless, have evidence of deep vein damage on the good side, but well compensated by collateral veins. Absence of symptoms quoted in many papers is not reliable evidence of an undamaged deep venous system but this is not to deny that thrombosis shown on phlebography can disappear without discernible trace on subsequent phlebography, possibly because the changes are too subtle or inaccessible to be demonstrated.

2. Many patients without known episodes of deep vein thrombosis, including those with normal venograms at the time of suspected thrombosis, do eventually develop the venotensive syndrome. Again phlebograms of the venous state associated with this are lacking in the studies referred to, but our own series of phlebograms suggests that about half of these limbs have undeformed widely patent deep veins, with an apparent deficiency of valves, that is to say, with no convincing evidence of thrombotic damage. Some degenerative process is at work but not producing the deformed veins known to follow many cases of thrombosis.

3. Patients developing the venotensive syndrome often have a long history of venous symptoms and signs well before any episode of possible deep vein 'thrombosis', perhaps indicating that an overt thrombosis was merely one additional incident and not a unique provoking episode.

4. Commonly both lower limbs are involved in the eventual venotensive state whether or not there is a history of thrombosis, or even when thrombosis has been shown to be on one side only (Stacey *et al.*, 1987), suggesting that something more than a single, localized event has occurred. Certainly our own experience supports this and, if thrombosis due to local trauma or compression are excluded, the explanation must include a recurring or widespread process (see below).

5. There is little relationship between the severity or extent of an original thrombosis, proved phlebographically, and the eventual state. Even severe thrombosis may eventually have only mild or no symptoms a few years later, but, as already expressed, symptoms prove to be a poor guide to the extent of persisting damage in the veins when this is assessed by phlebogram.

6. A number of factors confuse our evaluation of these cases and have altered circumstances since Bauer's original concept nearly 50 years ago:
   (a) Treatment of deep vein thrombosis by anticoagulation may have reduced the severity of damage and likelihood of true post-thrombotic syndrome.
   (b) Phlebograms, particularly using high dosage of old style opaque medium, may themselves have provoked damage to the veins, either by direct chemical action or by precipitating thrombosis.
   (c) There is evidence that, in some patients, procedures intended to treat venous disorders, either by surgery or by sclerotherapy, have actually been a damaging influence. This possibility has long been recognized and is an important reason behind the present-day drive to improve understanding and, by accurate diagnosis, to ensure that only surgery entirely appropriate

to the patient's state is carried out; for similar reasons sclerotherapy should be scrupulously regulated to minimize any hidden damage to the deep veins. Nevertheless, unsuitable or excessive treatment may have been a factor obscuring the natural history of the condition in the past and possibly still is.

It is clear from the foregoing section that there is a considerable area of uncertainty, with a number of issues yet to be resolved. If superficial vein incompetence and arteriovenous fistula are excluded, possible explanations, compatible with the observations given above, for the development of venotensive states without evident preceding thrombosis are as follows:

1. Recurring small episodes of thrombosis, often subclinical, in subjects prone to this; major episodes may be superimposed on this in some patients. The small episodes may immobilize valve cusps without causing deformity of the veins, thus giving an apparently valveless state. In our own group the phlebograms looked so clean that it is hard to accept this possibility in many of the cases we have seen.

2. An inborn deficiency in the number and integral strength of deep vein valves and/or the vein walls. This could lead to the progressive deterioration seen in these patients. Such states may be more vulnerable to thrombosis, perhaps due to reduced fibrinolytic activity and confusing the scene still further.

3. The progressive destruction of valves, possibly because they are weak or deficient, by wear and tear as the years pass. This may be part of an ageing process to which some are more susceptible than others, comparable to the loss of skin elasticity and many other changes in older people.

## Conclusions

It seems reasonable to conclude that Bauer's (1942) belief that deep vein thrombosis is followed eventually by a true post-thrombotic syndrome in many patients (rising to 72%) is still correct, although it is to be hoped that early diagnosis and treatment of the thrombosis can greatly improve the outcome he forecast. However, the development of the 'post-thrombotic' type of syndrome (due to venous hypertension) is not always the consequence of a deep vein thrombosis. Some will be, but a significant number of patients with this type of syndrome have a long story of its progressive development without known episodes of deep vein thrombosis, and phlebology at the late stage does not show recognizable evidence of previous thrombosis. An inborn state of valve deficiency and/or weak vein walls may explain this, but silent, repeated, small episodes of thrombosis, destroying valves, is still a possibility to be considered.

*Comment*

Speculation without more precise understanding of the nature of venous failure in these patients can only serve the purpose of suggesting possible avenues to be explored. More information is required by accurate visualization with phlebogram or ultrasonography. Fortunately phlebography by modern non-irritant opaque media, and using the image intensifier, makes it possible to perform this in a trouble-free fashion so that its use by experts in problem cases is justifiable. A real difficulty is that the deep veins below the knee are notoriously difficult to display satisfactorily by the techniques available. Radiological computerized scanning techniques, combined with digital subtraction of unwanted background, or further development of ultrasonic scanning, should certainly be capable of giving a considerable improvement upon this. The main barrier to this is the great expense of developing such equipment suitable for veins in the lower limbs and pelvis, but with continued effort this can surely be achieved and here lies the best prospect of improved understanding. For the present an open mind should be kept upon this group. It is best to acknowledge that this is an area of uncertainty and that it is not justifiable to label all these patients as 'post-thrombotic' on the present evidence. The term 'post-thrombotic' should not be used indiscriminately because this can only prolong confusion in this area.

## Nomenclature: the post-thrombotic (post-phlebitic) syndrome

These terms are widely used to sum up the clinical consequences of impaired deep veins described above. Although this may vary in localization of the deep veins involved and in severity, the characteristic features are of swelling, induration, pigmentation and, often, ulceration in the lower part of the limb; these changes are immediately brought to mind by use of the term. When the cause is known to be a previous deep vein thrombosis, however caused, then it is wholly appropriate and makes it clear that the underlying fault is due to thrombotic damage to the deep veins and their valves (true post-thrombotic syndrome). However, as is repeatedly emphasized in this book, other conditions (see Chapter 6) may also create venous hypertension giving similar clinical changes, and here the term 'post-thrombotic' or 'postphlebitic' would not be appropriate but misleading. When the clinical state is first encountered, before the precise cause is known, informative but less specific terms, such as 'venous hypertensive changes', or less satisfactory, 'venostatic changes', should be used, or even 'post-thrombotic type of syndrome'; 'chronic venous insufficiency' or 'venous insufficiency syndrome' are also widely accepted terms; in this book 'venotensive changes' or 'venotensive syndrome' have been frequently used. If phlebography has displayed the features described in Chapter 7, then 'valveless syndrome' or 'weak vein syndrome' is descriptive without defining the causation of this.

The proof in diagnosing true post-thrombotic (post-phlebitic) syndrome should include the following:

*History* of a known previous thrombosis or an injury leading to it.

*Clinical examination* finding swelling, induration, pigmentation and often ulceration (liposclerosis), *plus* evidence by Doppler flowmetry of upflow, accentuated by exercise, in principal superficial veins. Photophlethysmography showing a very shortened recovery time (below 10 seconds) that cannot be improved by selective saphenous occlusion is in keeping with the post-thrombotic syndrome but not specifically so because the valveless syndrome gives a similar response.

*Functional phlebography* demonstrating: preferential upflow in superficial veins; deformed or obstructed deep veins; collateral flow in tortuous veins crossing the pelvis or running upwards in the limb itself.

*Ultrasonography* gives a particularly effective display of the major conduit veins, such as popliteal or superficial femoral veins. It may detect loss of continuity or deformity, or show that they have been replaced with collateral channels. Preferential upflow in superficial veins can be a valuable pointer to disturbed function.

# References

Bauer, G. A. (1942) Roentgenological and clinical study of the sequelae of thrombosis. *Acta Chirurgica Scandinavica*, **74**, 1

Bjordal, R. I. (1977) Haemodynamic studies of varicose veins and the post-thrombotic syndrome. In *The Treatment of Venous Disorders* (ed. J. T. Hobbs), MTP, Lancaster, pp. 37–55

Bollinger, A. and Jager, K. (1986) Intermittent venous claudication evaluated by strain-gauge plethysmography during treadmill exercise. In *Phlebology 85* (eds. D. Negus and G. Jantet), John Libbey, London, pp. 571–573

Browse, N. (1985) The pathogenesis of venous ulceration. In *Surgery of the Veins* (eds. J. J. Bergan and J. S. T. Yao), Grune and Stratton, New York, pp. 25–31

Browse, N. and Burnand, K. (1978) The postphlebitic syndrome: a new look. In *Venous Problems* (eds J. J. Bergan and J. S. T. Yao), Year Book Medical, Chicago, pp. 395–405

Browse, N. L., Clemenson, G. and Lea Thomas, M. (1980) Is the post-phlebitic leg always post-phlebitic? *British Medical Journal*, **281**, 1167–1170

Burnand, K., Clemenson, G., Morland, M. *et al.* (1980) Venous lipodermatosclerosis: treatment by fibrinolytic enhancement and elastic compression. *British Medical Journal*, **280**, 7–11

Burnand, K. G., Whimster, I., Naidoo, A. and Browse, N. L. (1982) Pericapillary fibrin in the ulcer bearing skin of the lower leg. The cause of lipodermatosclerosis and venous ulceration. *British Medical Journal*, **285**, 1071–1072

Callam, M. J., Harper, D. R., Dale, J. J. and Ruckley, C. V. (1987) Chronic ulcer of the leg: clinical history. *British Medical Journal*, **294**, 1389–1391

Coleridge Smith, P. D., Thomas, R., Scurr, J. H. and

Dormandy, J. A. (1988) Causes of venous ulceration: a new hypothesis. *British Medical Journal*, **296**, 1726–1727

Dodd, H. and Cockett, F. B. (1976) *The Pathology and Surgery of the Veins of the Lower Limb*, Churchill Livingstone, Edinburgh

Gruss, J. D. (1988) Venous reconstruction, Part 1 and 2. *Phlebology*, **3**, 7–18, 75–87

Hobbs, J. T. (1977) The post-thrombotic syndrome. In *The Treatment of Venous Disorders* (ed. J. Hobbs), MTP, Lancaster, pp. 253–271

Homans, J. (1917) The aetiology and treatment of varicose ulcer of the leg. *Surgery Gynecology and Obstetrics*, **24**, 300

Kakker, V. V., Howe, G. T., Flanc, C. J. and Clarke, M. B. (1969) Natural history of postoperative deep vein thrombosis. *Lancet*, **ii**, 230

Lawrence, D. and Kakkar, V. V. (1980) Post-phlebitic syndrome – a functional assessment. *British Journal of Surgery*, **67**, 686–689

Lea Thomas, M. (1982) *Phlebography of the Lower Limbs*, Churchill Livingstone, Edinburgh

Lea Thomas, M., Fletcher, E. W. L., Cockett, F. B. and Negus, D. (1967) Venous collaterals in external and common iliac vein occlusion. *Clinical Radiology*, **18**, 403–411

May, R. (1979) *Surgery of the Veins of the Leg and Pelvis*, Georg Thieme, Philadelphia

Mudge, M., Leinster, S. J. and Hughes, L. E. (1988) A prospective 10-year study of post-thrombotic syndrome in a surgical population. *Annals of the Royal College of Surgeons of England*, **70**, 250–252

Negus, D. (1970) The post-thrombotic syndrome. *Annals of the Royal College of Surgeons of England*, **47**, 92–105

Nicolaides, A. N., Zukowski, A. and Kyprianou, P. (1985) Venous pressure measurements in venous problems. In *Surgery of the Veins* (eds J. J. Bergan and J. S. T. Yao), Grune and Stratton, New York, pp. 111–119

Rabe, E. (1987) Acute and chronic venous insufficiency. *Phlebology*, **2**, 249–255

Rickles, F. R. and Edwards, R. L. (1983) Activation of blood coagulation in cancer: Trousseau's syndrome revisited. *Blood*, **62**, 14–32

Scott, G. B. D. (1970) Concerning the organization of thrombi. *Annals of the Royal College of Surgeons of England*, **47**, 335–343

Stacey, M. C., Burnand, K. G., Pattison, M. *et al.* (1987) Changes in the apparently normal limb in unilateral venous ulceration. *British Journal of Surgery*, **74**, 936–938

Strandness, D. E. (1978) Applied venous physiology in normal subjects and venous insufficiency. In *Venous Problems* (eds J. J. Bergan and J. S. T. Yao), Year Book Medical, New York, pp. 25–45

Sumner, D. S. (1985) Applied physiology in venous problems. In *Surgery of the Veins* (eds J. J. Bergan and J. S. T. Yao), Grune and Stratton, New York, pp. 3–23

Thomas, P. R. S., Nash, G. B. and Dormandy, J. A. (1988) White cell accumulation in dependent legs of patients with venous hypertension: a possible mechanism for trophic changes in the skin. *British Medical Journal*, **296**, 1693–1695

Tibbs, D. J. (1986) The intriguing problem of varicose veins. *International Angiology*, **5**, 289–295

Tibbs, D. J. and Fletcher, E. W. L. (1983) Direction of flow in superficial veins as a guide to venous disorders in lower limbs. *Surgery*, **93**, 758–767

Tibbs, D. J. and Fletcher, E. W. L. (1986) Further experience with directional Doppler flowmeter applied to superficial veins in the diagnosis of venous disorders of the lower limbs. In *Progressi in Flebologia* (ed. M. Tesi), Edizioni Minerva Medica, Torino, pp. 90–96

Widmer, L. K., Zemp, E., Widmer, M. Th. and Voelin, R. (1986) Thromboembolic recurrence and post-thrombotic syndrome after deep vein thrombosis. In *Phlebology 85* (eds D. Negus and G. Jantet), John Libbey, London, pp. 556–559

Wolfe, J. H. N. (1987) Postphlebitic syndrome after fractures of the leg. *British Medical Journal*, **295**, 1364–1365

Woodyer, A. B., Walker, R. T. and Dormandy, J. A. (1986) Venous claudication. In *Phlebology 85* (eds D. Negus and G. Jantet), John Libbey, London, pp. 524–527

Wright, C. B., Hobson, R. W., Swan, K. G. and Rich, N. M. (1978) The pathophysiology of extremity venous occlusion. In *Venous Problems* (eds J. J. Bergan and J. S. T. Yao), Year Book Medical, Chicago, pp. 451–467

## Bibliography

Cockett, F. B. (1991) Venous valves: history up to the present day. *Phlebology*, **6**, 63–73

Gajraj, H. and Browse, N. L. (1991) Fibrinolytic activity and calf pump failure. *British Journal of Surgery*, **78,** 1009–1012

Shull, K. C., Nicolaides, A. N., Fernandes, F. *et al.*, (1979) Significance of popliteal reflux in relation to ambulatory venous pressure and ulceration. *Archives of Surgery*, **114,** 1304–1306

Stacey, M. C., Burnand, K. G., Lea Thomas, M. and Pattison, M. (1991) Influence of phlebographic abnormalities on the natural history of venous ulceration. *British Journal of Surgery*, **78,** 868–871

# 9

# Obstructed venous outlet syndrome: iliac vein occlusion

Obstruction of a major venous outlet has already been given some consideration in Chapter 8 but is worth special thought because its presence is easily overlooked and this may lead to inadvertent surgical damage to important collateral veins. The basic feature of the condition is the occlusion of a deep vein positioned at a 'bottleneck' in venous return, that is to say, where the main venous return from the limb is channelled through a single deep vein with the only alternative of side-branches and superficial veins. Notable examples of this are the popliteal, common femoral, iliac and axillary veins. Obstruction to any of these veins will of necessity cause side-channels to take over venous return from the limb below this level, in other words, to develop as collateral veins. These may be clearly visible or palpable but not always so, and special means such as the Doppler flow-meter or functional phlebography may be needed to detect them.

If the deep veins and pumping mechanisms below the obstruction are undamaged, the resting and exercising venous pressures below the block will be raised by the resistance to venous return. This causes an increase in the mean pressure without necessarily affecting the overall pattern in response to exercise. This general setting of pressure at a higher level encourages capillary trans-udation and collection of fluid in the tissue spaces. In this way, an obstructed venous outlet can cause oedema without other venotensive changes. The severity of oedema will depend upon the adequacy of the collateral return, which can be so good that clinical consequences are negligible. However, the original thrombosis has often also involved the deep veins at a lower level so that the manifestations of a defective pumping mechanism will obscure those solely attributable to an obstructed venous outlet. This is particularly true of the main topic of this chapter, occlusion of the common iliac vein, which on its own may cause only mild symptoms but, when combined with extensive impairment of the deep veins and pumping mechanisms following iliofemoral thrombosis, the manifestations may be severe and cause real disability (Negus

and Cockett 1967; Negus 1970; Lawrence and Kakkar, 1980).

## Obstructed common iliac vein

The left common iliac vein is decidedly more prone to thrombosis than the right side in a ratio of around 2:1 (Negus, 1970; Dodd and Cockett, 1976). This is likely to be related to its passage under the right common iliac artery (Cockett and Lea Thomas, 1965; Cockett, Lea Thomas and Negus, 1967; Lea Thomas, 1982). Many studies have shown that, when viewed by phlebography, it is not unusual for the vein to appear flattened at this point due to compression by the artery (Figure 9.1). This may never cause any problem but in the more severe examples it makes it more vulnerable to thrombosis, especially during pregnancy or after childbirth, prolonged illness, following fractures of the lower limbs or pelvis, or in any state of heightened thrombosis. Another aeti-ological factor in left common iliac vein thrombosis is the occurrence of one or more spurs or bands within the lumen at its termination, directly underlying the point at which it is compressed by the artery, and present in around 20% of people (May and Thurner, 1957; Negus, 1970; Dodd and Cockett, 1976; May, 1979). These seldom cause obstruction unless accompanied by thrombosis. They may be the result of compression by the artery but yet are to be found in over 4% of infants, suggesting a developmental origin (Jones, Taylor and Stoddard, 1976), at least for some.

The left common iliac vein shows little tendency to recanalize following thrombosis, and continuing compression by the overlying common iliac artery may play a part in this, so that the vein remains permanently closed. The thrombosis may extend down to the external iliac vein to close the entire run of iliac veins on that side but parts may recanalize to give a narrowed remnant of external iliac vein, or fragments forming a collateral pathway, for example, an internal iliac vein emptying via

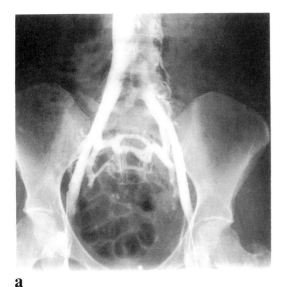

a

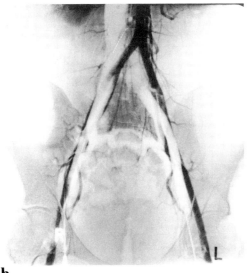

b

**Figure 9.1** *Combined views by phlebogram and aortogram showing compression of the left common iliac vein by the right common iliac artery in a woman aged 26 years.*

*(a) Phlebogram showing occlusion in the left common iliac vein with probable thrombus protruding into the inferior vena cava. Presacral collateral veins are shown taking venous return across to the right internal iliac vein.*
*(b) An aortogram in the same patient and taken immediately after the phlebogram; subtraction films have been superimposed on the phlebogram, so that the exact relationships of artery to vein can be seen. The right common iliac artery coincides precisely with the occluded portion of the common iliac vein*

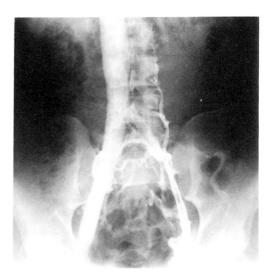

**Figure 9.2** *Phlebograms from a male patient, aged 20, who had sustained a major fracture in the lower limbs 2 years previously. Two phases of filling are shown; the termination of the common iliac vein shows post-thrombotic occlusion but the open remnant forms part of a collateral chain between the internal iliac and the ascending lumbar vein. The external iliac vein is deformed and narrowed by its involvement in the original thrombosis. An enlarged and tortuous circumflex iliac vein carrying collateral flow can be seen faintly*

a remnant of common iliac into an enlarged ascending lumbar vein (Figure 9.2).

Collateral circulation will be provided in variable degree by superficial veins and deep veins within the pelvis (Lea Thomas *et al.*, 1967). Of the superficial veins the external pudendal and superficial epigastric veins anastomosing with those of the opposite side will form varicose pubic and lower abdominal veins (Figure 9.3), whilst the superficial circumflex iliac veins may similarly estab-

lish tortuous communication with the lateral abdominal and thoracic veins of the same side. These varicose superficial veins are often clearly visible (Figures 9.4, 9.5) and palpable, and are a distinctive feature. The pelvic veins that take over collateral function include branches of the inferior epigastric, pubic and obturator veins, perivesical branches of the internal iliac vein and the parametrial veins anastomosing variously with those of the other side, the sacral plexus and upward to ascending lumbar veins and the vertebral plexus; the ovarian veins may enlarge to form important collaterals but this is most usually seen in occlusion of the inferior vena cava. These veins will not, of course, be visible on clinical examination but are characteristic on phlebography (Figures 9.2, 9.6).

It is necessary to distinguish clearly between the collateral veins just referred to and states of incompetence in ovarian veins, causing pelvic congestion and, via obturator and internal pudendal veins, communicating with the upper thigh to cause superficial vein incompetence there (see Chapter 5). In the former, the collateral veins crossing the floor of the pelvis must be preserved with care during gynaecological operations such as hysterectomy, because their destruction may cause deterioration in a post-thrombotic limb relying upon them for venous return. In the latter, removal of the enlarged and tortuous veins in the pelvis may bring benefit by eliminating pelvic congestion and a source of superficial incompetence in the lower limb. Great care must be taken in the interpretation of 'varicose veins' demonstrated in the pelvis by phlebography and they should not be surgically interfered

**Figure 9.3**  *Superficial collateral veins in left common iliac vein occlusion.*

*(a) Diagram showing pubic varicosities acting as collaterals between superficial external pudendal (or superficial epigastric) vein on the left side crossing over to join corresponding veins on the right side. The superficial circumflex iliac vein is also shown acting as a collateral taking blood to join the lateral abdominal and thoracic veins.*

*(b) Doppler flowmeter tracing with the probe placed over pubic varicosities in a patient with left post-thrombotic iliac occlusion. With the patient standing still there is steady movement from the left side across to the right side. This is accentuated by five exercise movements and is then followed by a compensatory pause before the cross-over flow recommences.*

*(c) Phlebograms from a patient giving a story of 'white leg of pregnancy' 30 years previously with only mild swelling in the left limb since then. Her present complaint was of recurring phlebitis in varicosities on the right calf; all tests, including Doppler flowmetry, confirmed typical simple, right long saphenous incompetence but pubic varicosities were found on inspection. These phlebograms were taken with the patient in a near upright position with opaque medium injected into a calf vein on the left side.*

*1. With the patient standing still and 100 ml of medium injected. Passive filling has occurred and preferential flow can be seen passing up the long saphenous vein and the profunda femoris vein to join the common femoral vein. From here flow is directed by extensive varicose collateral veins across the pubic and vulval region to the right side; the iliac veins do not fill.*

*2. After the patient has given two exercise movements; it can be seen that this has increased filling in the pubic varicosities and begun to fill the right external iliac vein. The right long saphenous vein has outlined with downflow because it is incompetent (cross-over incompetence – see Chapters 5 (Figure 5.17) and 10). The vulval set of varicosities are derived from the superficial external pudendal vein and the suprapubic one from the superficial epigastric vein; both link with the corresponding veins on the other side*

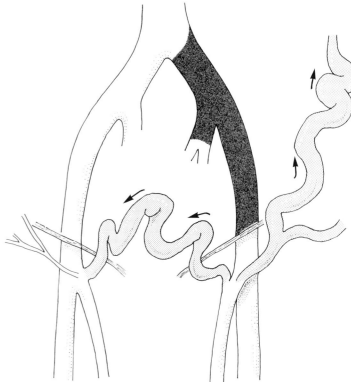

**a**

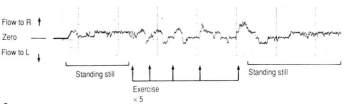

Flow to R

Zero

Flow to L

Standing still          Standing still

Exercise
× 5

**b**

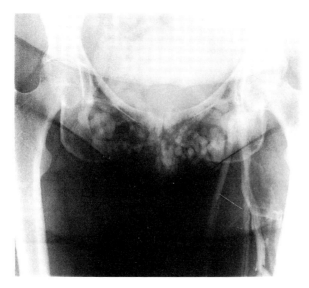

**c1**

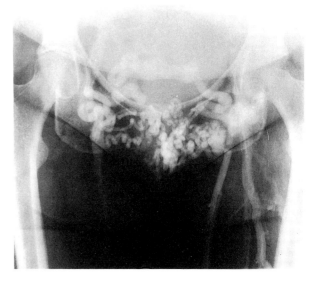

**c2**

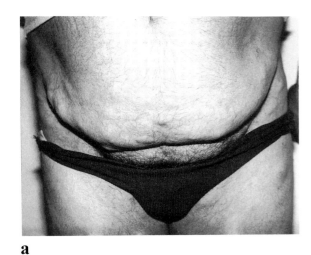

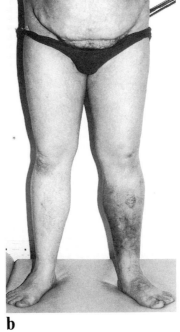

**Figure 9.4** *Pubic and lower abdominal varicosities following injury. Photographs and phlebograms in a young man, aged 20 years, who had sustained a fractured pelvis 2 years previously in a motorcycle accident, followed by many weeks in hospital. His left lower limb showed at least 4 cm of swelling up to the groin and marked venotensive (liposclerotic) changes were evident in the leg.*

*(a) The clinical photographs show extensive suprapubic varicosities partly concealed by obesity but readily recognized by touch.*

*(b) General appearance with moderately severe post-thrombotic changes on the left side.*

*(c) 1. Doppler flowmeter tracings from pubic varicosity, showing crossflow from left to right, and strong upflow in the left long saphenous vein, both accentuated by exercise.*
*2. Photoplethysmography: left side has a shortened recovery period of 9 seconds but the right side is normal at over 25 seconds.*

*3. The phlebogram shows strong preferential upflow in the left long saphenous vein and, at its termination, tortuous collateral veins derived from the superficial external pudendal vein can be seen crossing the pubes and entering the common femoral vein on the right side. The left external iliac vein has outlined faintly, there was no filling of the common iliac vein. There was also extensive deep vein impairment down the left lower limb accounting for the venotensive changes on that side and this is shown in a more complete composite phlebogram of this patient in Figure 11.27*

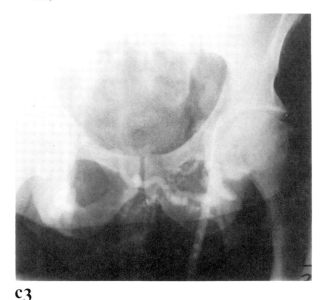

**c3**

**Figure 9.4** *(continued)*

**Figure 9.5** *Further examples of pubic and lower abdominal varicosities.*

*(a) An elderly patient with common iliac occlusion and extensive post-thrombotic changes in the left lower limb. This was probably*

*the result of thrombosis in pregnancy. The pubic varicosities are unusually large but even these could be missed if this area is not properly inspected in all cases of the post-thrombotic syndrome. The lower limb is not unduly swollen, presumably because the enormous pubic varicosities provide an excellent venous outlet. Post-thrombotic damage to the venous pump below the knee has caused extensive ulceration. Much improvement was obtained by careful training in the care of her limb.*

*(b) 1, 2. Another example of left iliac occlusion in a patient aged 60 years and arising from pregnancy some 40 years previously; two views are shown. Her history also included a lower abdominal operation at the age of 45 years. In this patient the pubic varicosities are more typical in size than the preceding patient but could easily be seen and felt. Both limbs show moderate venotensive changes with little swelling, partly because of good collateral veins but also because the patient was very conscientious with elevation and wearing of elastic support. It is likely that at the time of her several pregnancies, and possibly following the abdominal operation, successive thrombotic damage occurred in both lower limbs in addition to the left iliac occlusion. Doppler flowmetry showed surge back and forth in the prominent superficial veins on 'marking time'; on photoplethysmography there was a very shortened recovery time, under 6 seconds, on both sides. Scarring at the left ankle can be seen due to an ulcer healed by a split skin graft taken from the thigh. Only conservative measures were practicable here but the patient had already stabilized her condition by good self-management and was given all encouragement to continue.*

*(c) Varicosities above and below a horizontal suprapubic scar in a patient of 58 years following hysterectomy 5 years previously. There is moderate swelling in the limb with venotensive changes and a small ulcer at the ankle. The clinical picture is one of iliac vein occlusion with some accompanying post-thrombotic impairment in the deep veins of the leg (see page 185).*

*(d) A 40-year-old male patient who sustained fractures in both lower limbs some years previously and reported with bilateral*

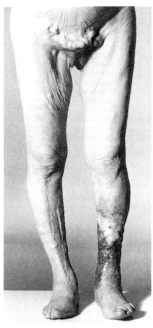

**a**

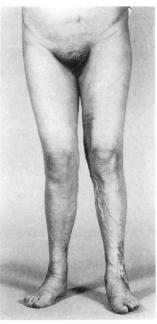

**b1**

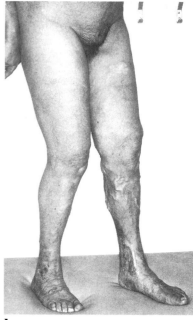

**b2**

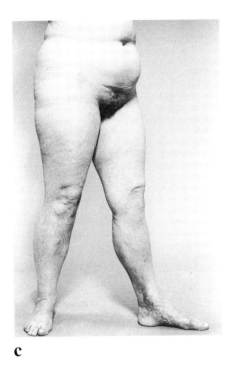

**c**

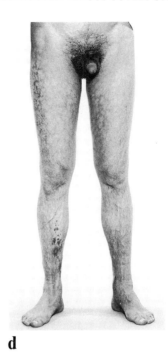

**d**

*post-thrombotic changes. A pubic varicosity is visible and readily confirmed by palpation. It showed typical cross-over flow with a Doppler flowmeter, confirming occlusion in the left common iliac vein; the prominent superficial veins just below the right knee showed upward flow indicating impairment in the underlying deep veins and similar changes were found on the left side.*

*(e) Tortuousity and enlargement in the right superficial circumflex iliac vein, indicative of right common iliac vein occlusion and caused by a fractured femur and subsequent treatment in hospital some years previously. (By courtesy of Mr S. Rose)*

**Figure 9.5** *(continued)*

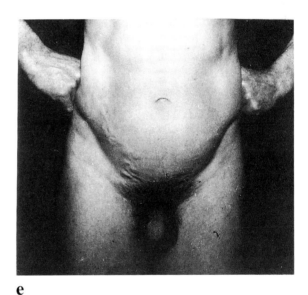

**e**

with without a clear understanding of these two very different categories.

## Clinical manifestations

In its least complicated form oedema of the corresponding limb is the presenting manifestation (Figure 9.6) and this leads to discovery of pubic and lower abdominal collateral varicosities. It may be a relatively harmless state but often the damage has extended to the veins in the lower limb so that the full picture of venous hypertension, with pigmentation, induration and ulceration, is present. In these circumstances, where venotensive changes predominate, it is all too easy to overlook the possibility of an accompanying iliac vein obstruction and the rule must be that all patients with evidence of venous hypertension should be carefully examined for tell-tale pubic varicosities and, likewise, if phlebography is carried out it must include examination of the iliac

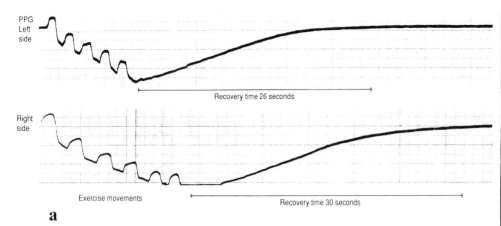

PPG Left side

Recovery time 26 seconds

Right side

Exercise movements

Recovery time 30 seconds

**a**

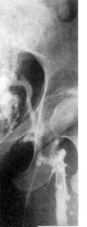
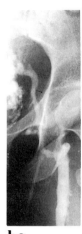

**b2**

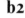

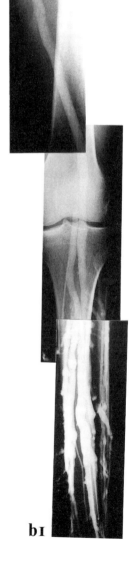

**Figure 9.6** *Photoplethysmogram and phlebograms in a patient who reported with swelling in her left lower limb. This had commenced 2 weeks after the birth of twins, 4 months previously. Initial treatment by heparin, and subsequently by warfarin, had been given for deep vein thrombosis. Examination showed 2 cm of swelling in the left lower limb up to the groin but no prominent or varicose veins were visible in the limb or pubic region. Doppler flowmeter to the long saphenous vein showed no abnormal flow.*

*(a) Photoplethysmogram showing that on the left side the recovery period following exercise is within normal range. The story and the physical findings of oedema in the limb without any evidence of deep vein impairment suggested that a deep vein thrombosis had caused occlusion of the left common iliac vein but without any significant damage to the deep veins in the limb below.*

*(b) Phlebograms confirming the diagnosis:*
   *1, 2. Composite picture showing full limb and left pelvis; a normal deep system has been easily outlined up to the groin but, here, normal upflow is interrupted and replaced by a large collateral vessel, probably an obturator vein filling from the deep external pudendal vein.*
   *3. Slightly later picture showing extensive collateral flow across the pelvis, principally in parametrial veins of the broad ligament, and filled by the obturator vein*

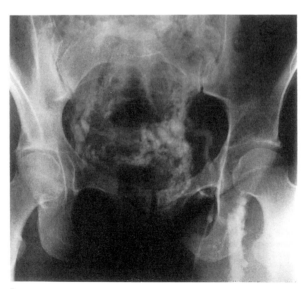

**b3**

**b1**

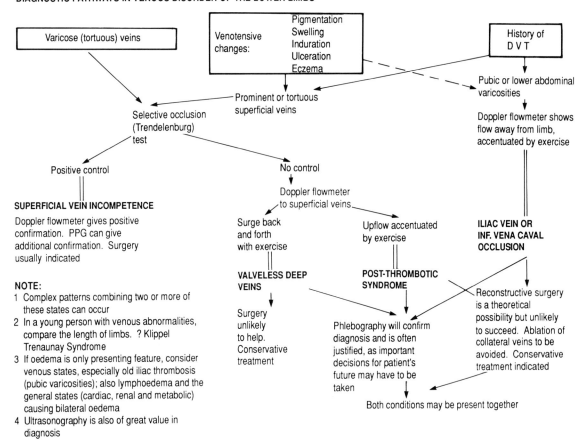

**DIAGNOSTIC PATHWAYS IN VENOUS DISORDER OF THE LOWER LIMBS**

**Figure 9.7** *Diagram of the diagnostic pathways in venous disorder of the lower limbs. With iliac vein occlusion, the starting point might well be in the right-hand top corner because there is a significant history of previous deep vein thrombosis, or pubic varicosities have been found during the routine inspection that should be carried out in any patient with venotensive (liposclerotic) changes*

veins. The diagnostic flow-chart in Figure 9.7 may help in unravelling the interrelationship between the main venous disorders.

As stated in Chapter 8, an extensive combination of femoral and iliac vein occlusion, caused by iliofemoral thrombosis, will eventually give considerable disability with liposclerosis and ulceration. It may take many years for the full severity of the condition to develop, as some of the case histories in the accompanying figures illustrate. Many authorities have emphasized the inevitability of these changes sooner or later (Kakkar *et al.*, 1969; Negus, 1970; Dodd and Cockett 1976; Hobbs, 1977; May, 1979; Widmer *et al.*, 1986) after iliofemoral occlusion; this may be determined by the loss of functioning valves in key veins, such as the popliteal (Shull *et al.*, 1979). It is in this group, where there is severe venous outlet obstruction, not adequately compensated for by collaterals, that venous claudication may be found, with the patient's ability to walk limited by pain within a few minutes.

*Venous claudication*

Claudication (a limping, so named after the Roman Emperor Claudius) is the term given to a painful limitation in walking. Intermittent claudication describes the state in which pain, brought on by walking a short distance, causes limping and may force the patient to stop. This may arise from restriction of arterial supply, obstruction to venous return, or from a neurological disorder due to compression of the lumbar spinal cord or cauda equina. All these three specialties tend to use the term with the tacit assumption that it only applies to their area of interest and confusion is best avoided by adding the qualification, arterial, venous or neurological to clarify its origin. In the case of venous claudication the concept of its causation is quite simple. Exercise by walking increases the blood flow through the muscles and this is forcibly ejected into the veins with each contraction. If the venous outlet is inadequate then the veins below the obstruction become painfully distended at an unnaturally high pressure.

Many patients with longstanding induration and active ulceration at the ankle have pain in that area on standing and walking but this must not be confused with venous claudication. In the literature it is not always clear how effectively this type of pain has been separated from that of venous claudication which gives a bursting pain in the calf or behind the knee, increasing with walking and halting the patient after a minute or two. A severely restricted arterial supply or a stenosis in the spinal canal can both cause a rather similar pattern of pain related to muscular effort and developing all the more quickly on hurrying or climbing a gradient. In the case of venous claudication a number of studies have described this condition and shown that the onset of pain is accompanied by increasing girth of the calf and a rise in the venous pressure to well above the maximum resting level in the upright position (Negus 1970; Hobbs, 1977; Villavicencio *et al.*, 1985; Woodyer, Walker and Dormandy, 1986; Bollinger and Jager, 1986). This is certainly in keeping with venous blood being pushed out from the muscles faster than a restricted venous outlet can allow it to escape. Various authors who have also carried out phlebography conclude that the combination of claudication with increased calf volume and raised venous pressure is only found in obstructed states of the major deep veins, particularly when the main outlet from the lower limb, the iliofemoral veins, is involved. It probably requires a relatively undamaged set of veins in the main venous pumps provided by the muscles of the calf. It does not occur in the majority of venotensive states because of the following circumstances:

1. In venous hypertension caused only by superficial vein incompetence and where the deep veins have a good lumen throughout, without any component of deep vein obstruction; excess (greater than foot to heart level) pressures cannot be generated by the musculo-venous pump.

2. When deep vein valvular failure rather than obstruction is the principal cause of venous hypertension, as in those cases we have called the valveless syndrome (see Chapter 7). In these cases the deep veins are widely open throughout and offer no resistance to venous return; pressures above foot to heart level cannot be generated.

3. When the extent and positioning of a venous block is not critical and alternative channels of venous return are easily available.

4. In extensive iliofemoral block where a good collateral venous circulation has developed to compensate for the obstructed veins. This may be demonstrated by a near normal maximal venous outflow test and confirmed by phlebography displaying liberal collateral vessels circumventing the obstructed veins. Most outlet syndromes fall in this category and do not experience claudication.

In the weeks following major acute iliofemoral thrombosis the symptom of venous claudication may be at its most severe but gradually becomes less with time, presumably due to recanalization of thrombosed veins and expansion of collateral vessels.

## Treatment

In any limb disabled by venous hypertension the patient must be taught the principles behind treatment to ameliorate the condition. The extensive iliofemoral post-thrombotic syndrome, if neglected, can produce the full range of venotensive changes and much discomfort is added by gross oedema up to the groin giving a tightly distended limb. The patient may have pain on walking but the limb can improve greatly with a suitable programme of elevation to reduce the oedema. The author has seen limbs where amputation was being seriously considered until it was pointed out that the patient at no time raised the limb(s) above the horizontal and often spent all day and all night in a chair with the legs down! In such limbs a period of high elevation and active movement may transform the limb. The improvement can be maintained once the patient understands the great benefit of elevating the limb whenever possible and giving a good proportion of the day to this (see Figure 8.8(d)). In some, the limb may be improved by such measures but venous claudication may remain as a disabling symptom.

*Warning: swelling accompanying ischaemic rest pain.* The patient with severe ischaemia due to arterial insufficiency may find that ischaemic rest pain is relieved by putting the leg in a dependent postion, for example, by hanging it out of bed or sleeping in a chair with the legs down. In these circumstances the limb becomes swollen because of the prolonged dependency and lack of movement. There is a real danger that this may be mistaken for a venous condition. It must always be remembered that a patient with a painful, swollen lower limb may have severe ischaemia and high elevation of the limb would be a grave error which could lead to its loss. The positioning desirable for a critically ischaemic limb and that for one swollen from venous outlet obstruction are in direct contrast. The ischaemic limb should never be elevated above the horizontal because this may totally deprive it of its precarious arterial supply, but the oedematous venotensive limb will benefit greatly by high elevation. Every case of painful swollen limb must have its arterial supply assessed with great care to ensure that a critical ischaemia is not overlooked (see Chapter 17).

As regards other aspects of treatment, a well-fitted graduated stocking, up to the knee (not higher in case it should impede venous return through superficial veins acting as collaterals), should be given trial but the patient may find that this actually increases his discomfort on walking and may abandon it. If venous claudication continues to be disabling a year after the causative thrombosis and it appears that maximal improvement has occurred then venous reconstruction can be considered. This type of operation should not be lightly embarked upon nor should it be performed by the inexperienced, and detailed phlebography identifying the veins to be used is an essential preliminary. The various surgical possibilities are:

1. Rearranging superficial veins, such as the long saphenous vein, in order to bypass the obstructed venous outlet. In Palma's operation the long saphenous vein from the opposite limb is swung over for anastomosis with the deep vein below the obstruction in the affected limb (Halliday, Harris and May, 1985). In patients with extensive occlusion in both superficial and profunda femoral veins, May–Husni operation, re-routing the long saphenous vein within its own limb, to act more effectively as a collateral past the block, may prove helpful and a small number of successful cases are reported in the literature (Gruss, 1985, 1988).

2. The use of venous prostheses made from Teflon or Dacron (Dale, 1985).

3. Free grafts of the patient's own vein may succeed in expert hands. Taheri et al. (1985) report success using portions of valved brachial vein, but only short lengths can be obtained and only of rather small calibre. This type of operation has its real application in attempts to reconstruct valveless deep veins rather than obstructed deep veins and will seldom apply in iliofemoral outlet syndrome.

4. The use of the patient's own tissues, especially peritoneum, to fashion a living endothelial-lined tube. Experimental evidence here is encouraging but at the time of writing there are few reports upon its use in accepted surgical practice, however it may find a role in future developments.

5. Heterografts using animal tissue are most unlikely to succeed. Any degree of immune response will soon precipitate thrombosis. The possibility of various biological preparations of living tissue, matched to the patient's, from which vein substitutes can be prepared, is looking increasingly promising for the future.

6. 'Cleaning out' operations, akin to endarterectomy in arteries, are not successful even if supported by an arteriovenous fistula below them in order to encourage full distension and rapid flow. However, if carried out sufficiently early as a thrombectomy within a few days from onset there is some prospect of success in a limited length of vein and when backed by temporary arteriovenous fistula (Eklof, Einarsson and Plate, 1985).

7. Operations designed to repair incompetent valves (Kistner, 1985), or grafting valves from elsewhere, are not likely to improve the symptom of venous claudication but may improve certain other categories of venous hypertension where the cause is predominantly incompetence in deep vein valves.

## Discussion

Surgical reconstruction in some form (Gruss, 1988) is naturally tempting for obstructed veins and, for example, Palma's cross-over procedure, bringing over the saphenous vein from the other side as a substantial additional collateral channel, is capable of giving the occasional good result. These and other operations are described in Chapter 21. However good long-term results are not easily obtained by these means and it may be wiser to settle for conservative treatment.

The problems of venous reconstructive surgery are twofold: such procedures are prone to undergo thrombosis postoperatively and although various methods of preventing this are described, such as construction of a temporary arteriovenous shunt, the overall success rate remains limited; the other factor is that open deep veins in the vicinity, upon which the reconstruction depends, are likely to be deformed and thickened by some involvement in the original thrombosis. This is not a favourable background for such procedures and the greater the patient's need for help the more probable it is that no satisfactory vein will be found to which the new venous outlet may be anastomosed. The procedure should not be embarked upon unless a suitable vein has been identified by phlebography beforehand. There is a real need for reliable techniques of venous reconstruction to be developed (see end section of Chapter 21), but until that time it is wisest for this form of surgery to be left to those who take a specialized interest in it.

### Surgery to coexistent superficial vein incompetence

As explained in Chapters 5, 8 and 10, simple incompetence may coexist in the limb below a common iliac vein obstruction and for this reason surgical removal of veins, as opposed to reconstruction, may have an occasional role to play. Theoretically, a reconstruction is possible by utilizing an incompetent long saphenous vein to swing it over to the opposite side for anastomosis there, thereby 'removing' a troublesome vein and providing an additional collateral channel. However, few successful cases are reported perhaps because the valve cusps, although incompetent, may hinder flow and predispose to thrombosis, even if valvulotomy is performed. If the saphenous vein is not to be used in this fashion, care is needed in selection and carrying out surgery to incompetent veins because it is important that enlarged superficial veins acting as collaterals should be preserved; for example, a high ligation of the long saphenous will deprive the limb of the superficial epigastric vein which is usually a principal collateral vein; on the other hand, not taking it may give inadequate control of the incompetence so that recurrent varicosities soon appear with this vein as the source. Any surgical effort along these lines must be based upon unequivocal control of the suspected incompetence by a selective saphenous occlusion Trendelenburg test, clear Doppler downflow in the suspect veins after exercise and a good phlebogram which has shown that the superficial veins being considered for removal are not part of a collateral mechanism; this in its turn implies that the deep veins at that level are healthy and undeformed with no need for collateral function in the overlying superficial veins and the phlebogram should confirm this. However, with so many cautions and reservations it may be advisable to avoid any thought of ablative surgery and settle for appropriate elastic support, which, although tedious, will be effective in controlling the superficial incompetence and limiting the oedema arising from outflow obstruction.

Conservative treatment depends upon the patient understanding the nature of the problem and the means of mitigating it. The basis of this is in giving a sufficient proportion of the day to high elevation of the limb, raising the foot of the bed, the use of external support bandage or stocking if this is found to bring improved comfort to the limb, and possibly the judicious use of diuretics.

## Venous disorders in the limb opposite to iliac vein occlusion

Venous disorder in the limb opposite to common iliac vein occlusion is usually due to post-thrombotic changes caused by deep vein thrombosis having occurred in that limb at the time of the original iliac thrombosis. Another possibility is a coincidental incompetence in the superficial veins of the limb and taking its source from collateral veins crossing the pubes (cross-over incompetence; Tibbs 1986) as described and illustrated in Chapters 5 and 10. This is not particularly rare and confusion between these two conditions may arise so that care is needed in interpreting such cases, and especially in deciding upon any form of surgery. Another complex pattern, superficial vein incompetence below common iliac occlusion of the same side, has been already referred to above and also in Chapters 5, 8 and 10. Thus, in any limb with a history suggesting deep vein thrombosis, the groins and lower abdomen must be carefully examined for collateral veins indicating iliac occlusion and the venous state of both limbs assessed for evidence of previous bilateral thrombosis having occurred or whether a superficial incompetence exists below an iliac occlusion or even takes it origin from the collaterals of one on the opposite side. In that case, it may be possible to improve the component of superficial incompetence by carefully selected surgery.

## Occlusion of the inferior vena cava

Thrombosis of the inferior vena cava leading to permanent occlusion in its infrarenal portion is uncommon and may occur without apparent cause but more usually as a complication of serious illness, injury or malignancy. The commonest cause for inferior vena caval obstruction of recent years has been iatrogenic, due to surgical ligation, or following the insertion of a vena caval filter, in the prevention of pulmonary embolus. Occasionally, it may arise in young people and should not be forgotten at any age when unusual superficial veins and swelling are encountered bilaterally in the lower limbs, especially if there is any preceding history of prolonged illness. The clinical picture is usually unmistakable if the abdomen and upper thighs are included in the inspection with the patient standing. Really it is an extension of the features already described for common iliac vein occlusion. The lower limbs are swollen in variable degree up to the groins but this may not be easily apparent when both limbs are involved and one limb cannot be compared against the other. Suspicion should be aroused by a number of tortuous veins on the thighs which do not conform to any usual pattern and cross the groins onto the lower abdomen; from here further tortuous veins may be seen running upwards in the course of the superficial epigastric and circumflex iliac veins (Figure 9.8). These veins may be traced to the epigastrium, the lower thorax and the axilla in a thin patient. This characteristic network of veins may be evident even when the patient is lying, and testing for the direction of flow in traditional Harvean fashion confirms the 'upward' flow in them. The directional Doppler flowmeter gives striking confirmation of this and if further evidence is required phlebography can remove all doubts (Figure 9.9).

Occlusion of the inferior vena cava does not necessarily cause great disability to the patient because this is determined by the extent of the occlusion, the degree of involvement of the deep veins in the lower limbs and the quality of the collateral veins that have developed. Regarding treatment, as with iliac occlusion, reconstructive surgery is a specialized task not to be lightly considered and the conservative management already described is usually the wisest course.

## Concurrent venous disorder in the limbs below inferior vena caval occlusion

Deep vein thrombosis in either, or both, of the lower limbs may have occurred at the time of thrombosis in the inferior vena cava and leave its legacy of mild to severe post-thrombotic changes. Superficial vein incompetence in the limbs below an occluded inferior vena cava is theoretically possible if the deep veins of the limb concerned have not shared in the thrombosis. In both cases conservative management is advised.

## External compression of veins

Compression of major veins by neighbouring structures, or pathological processes surrounding them, is an occasional cause for venous congestion and swelling, and

**Figure 9.8** *Collateral veins on the abdomen in occlusion of the inferior vena cava.*

*(a) Obstruction due to malignancy showing an enlarged tortuous superficial circumflex iliac vein running up the flank to join the lateral thoracic vein (calcarine vein – so called after the vein in horses endangered by the rider's spur).*

*(b) Similar vein and similar cause in a different patient, photographed by infrared light.*

*(c) 1, 2. In this patient the cause of inferior vena caval occlusion is unknown. Anterior view of the abdomen shows extreme enlargement and tortuousity of the superficial circumflex iliac veins of both sides and the right superficial epigastric vein. Photograph 2 is by infrared light. (By courtesey of Mr S. Rose)*

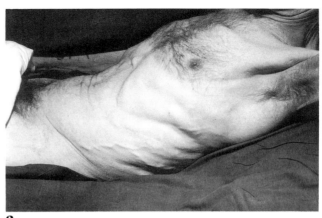

a

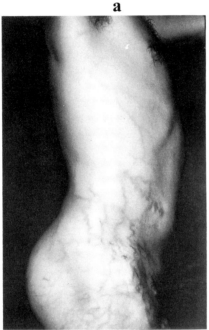

b

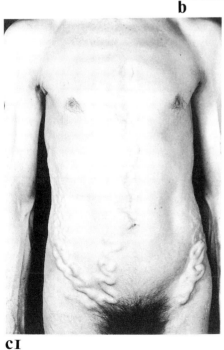

c1

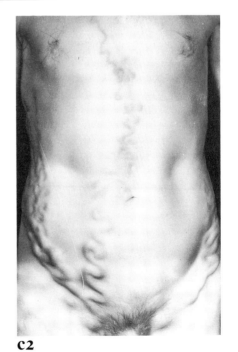

c2

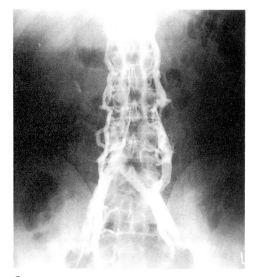

a

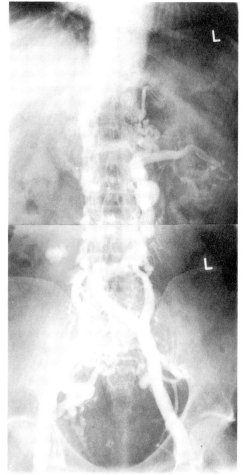

b

**Figure 9.9** *Examples by phlebogram of collateral veins developed within the abdomen in response to occlusion of the inferior vena cava.*

*(a) Collateral veins formed from the ascending lumbar vein on both sides.*

*(b) Collaterals formed from presacral, vertebral and ascending lumbar veins. On the left side the ascending lumbar is particularly large and crosses the second lumbar vertebra to join an enlarged azygos vein. The ovarian vein on the left side has shown faintly in its upper part*

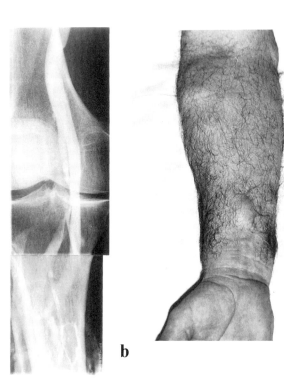

b

a

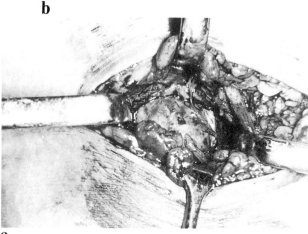

c

**Figure 9.10** *Partial obstruction of veins in the popliteal fossa by a lipoma. The patient, a man aged 42 years, had numerous lipomas over the trunk and limbs but complained of intermittent swelling in the right ankle and lower leg, usually brought on by kneeling.*

*(a) Phlebogram showing displacement and narrowing of the uppermost tibial veins as they join to form the popliteal vein which commences at a higher level than usual.*

*(b) The right forearm showing multiple lipomas which were present subcutaneously in all parts of the body.*

*(c) View at operation after incision of popliteal deep fascia. The rounded mass of a firm lipoma, 5 cm across, has been revealed. Removing this relieved the patient's symptoms*

some aspects of this are considered in Chapter 14 on the oedematous limb. The main causes for external compression are summarized below.

## Causes common to most sites

- Tumours; innocent tumours, such as lipoma (Figure 9.10) or neurofibroma; a wide variety of malignant neoplasms and secondary lymph nodes from them, especially in the abdomen; lymphadenoma (Figure 9.11) and other reticuloses; secondary lymph glands from melanoma in a limb.
- Aneurysm.
- Haematoma within an enclosed anatomical compartment.
- Cysts, including Morrant Baker (synovial) cyst from nearby joint.
- Infective processes giving rise to a large abscess.
- Following injury with displacement of fractured bones.
- Fibrosis following injury by a variety of agents, including radiotherapy and surgery.

*Note.* Lymphoedema from lymphatic obstruction is likely to be an important consequence of many of the processes given above and is often present together with venous thrombosis.

## Entrapment of veins by anatomical structures

In the popliteal fossa the deep vein may take an aberrant course through or around a head of the gastrocnemius muscle or between divisions of the major nerves so that intermittent obstruction or thrombosis arises (Connell, 1978; Iwai *et al.*, 1987); similarly, entrapment of the femoral vein by an abnormal arrangement of the inguinal ligament may occur (May, 1979). Compression of the left common iliac vein by the right iliac artery is a form that may lead to thrombosis. In the upper limb, entrapment at the thoracic outlet by costoclavicular compression is not rare and a probable cause for axillary vein thrombosis; this has also been attributed to other anatomical structures in the vicinity (Boontje, 1979). A cervical rib seldom causes venous problems because the vein lies beyond the scalenus anterior muscle, unlike the subclavian artery which passes between it and the extra rib or a ligamentous extension, and is subject to aneurysm and thrombosis as a result of pressure from this (see Chapter 15).

## Encirclement of a limb or digit by a band

A tight band around a limb or digit will of course threaten both artery and vein if it is not soon removed. The deliberate application of a tourniquet puts a heavy responsibility upon the medical attendant and should never be employed without good cause; its use in venous

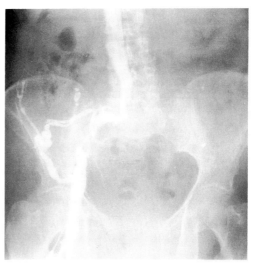

**Figure 9.11** *Phlebogram of external compression of right iliac veins by malignant lymphoma in a man aged 44 years. This patient, known to suffer from lymphadenoma, developed extreme swelling of the right lower limb and a mass could be felt in the right iliac fossa. The phlebogram confirms narrowing and displacement of the external and common iliac veins, probably compounded by thrombosis. The deep circumflex iliac vein is acting as a collateral. A mass of malignant glands, whether from a primary reticulosis, as in this case, or secondary involvement from other forms of malignancy, such as bronchial carcinoma, may compress the iliac veins and obstruct the lymphatics to cause severe oedema in the lower limb. It may be the presenting evidence of malignancy and this possibility should always be considered when there is rapid development of unexplained oedema up to the groin on one or both sides*

surgery is seldom justifiable. Constriction by a band may occur by accident in infants ensnared in strands of knitted woollen gloves or clothing. Self-adminstered application of a band to an upper or lower limb, in order to produce an alarming venous congestion and oedema, may be secretly practised as a form of hysteria when a patient wishes to capture attention (see Chapter 14). It is an occasional diagnostic problem the venous specialist should be aware of.

## References

Bollinger, A. and Jager, K. (1986) Intermittent venous claudication evaluated by strain-gauge plethysmography during treadmill exercise. In *Phlebology 85* (eds D. Negus and K. Jager), John Libbey, London, pp. 571–573

Boontje, A. H. (1979) Axillary vein entrapment. *British Journal of Surgery*, **66**, 331–332

Cockett, F. B. and Lea Thomas, M. (1965) The iliac compression syndrome. *British Journal of Surgery*, **52**, 816

Cockett, B., Lea Thomas, M. and Negus, D. (1967) Iliac vein compression – its relation to iliofemoral thrombosis and the post-thrombotic syndrome. *British Medical Journal*, **2**, 14

Connell, J. (1978) Popliteal vein entrapment. *British Journal of Surgery*, **65**, 351

Dale, W. A. (1985) Synthetic grafts for venous reconstruction.

In *Surgery of the Veins* (eds J. J. Bergan and J. S. T. Yao), Grune and Stratton, London, pp. 233–239

Dodd, H. and Cockett, F. B. (1976) *The Pathology and Surgery of the Veins of the Lower Limb*, Churchill Livingstone, Edinburgh

Eklof, B., Einarsson, E. and Plate, G. (1985) Role of thrombectomy and temporary arteriovenous fistula in acute iliofemoral venous thrombosis. In *Surgery of the Veins* (eds J. J. Bergan and J. S. T. Yao), Grune and Stratton, New York, pp. 131–144

Gruss, J. D. (1985) The saphenopopliteal bypass for chronic venous insufficiency (May–Husni operation). In *Surgery of the Veins* (eds J. J. Bergan and J. S. T. Yao), Grune and Stratton, New York, pp. 255–265

Gruss, J. D. (1988) Venous reconstruction. Parts 1 and 2. *Phlebology*, **3**, 7–18, 75–87

Halliday, P., Harris, J. and May, J. (1985) Femoro-femoral crossover grafts (Palma operation): a long term follow-up study. In *Surgery of the Veins* (eds J. J. Bergan and J. S. T. Yao), Grune and Stratton, New York, pp. 241–254

Hobbs, J. (ed.) (1977) The post-thrombotic syndrome. In *The Treatment of Venous Disorder*, MTP, Lancaster, pp. 253–271

Iawi, T., Sato, S., Yamada, T. *et al.* (1987) Popliteal vein entrapment caused by the third head of the gastrocnemius muscle. *British Journal of Surgery*, **74**, 1006–1008

Jones, W. M., Taylor, I. and Stoddard, C. J. (1976) Common iliac vein compression syndrome occurring in siblings. *British Journal of Surgery*, **60**, 663–664

Kakkar, V. V., Howe, G. T., Flanc, C. J. and Clarke, M. B. (1969) Natural history of postoperative deep vein thrombosis. *Lancet*, **ii**, 230

Kistner, R. J. (1985) Venous valve surgery. In *Surgery of the Veins* (eds J. J. Bergan and J. S. T. Yao), Grune and Stratton, New York, pp. 205–217

Lawrence, D. and Kakkar, V. V. (1980) Post-phlebitic syndrome – a functional assessment. *British Journal of Surgery*, **67**, 686–689

Lea Thomas, M. (1982) *Phlebography of the Lower Limb*, Churchill Livingstone, Edinburgh

Lea Thomas, M., Fletcher, E. W. L., Cockett, F. B. and Negus, D. (1967) Venous collaterals in external and common iliac vein obstruction. *Clinical Radiology*, **18**, 403–411

May, R. (1979) *Surgery of the Veins of the Leg and Pelvis*, Georg Thieme, Philadelphia

May, R. and Thurner, J. (1957) The cause of the predominantly sinistral occurrence of thrombosis of the pelvic veins. *Angiology*, **8**, 419

Negus, D. (1970). The post-thrombotic syndrome. *Annals of the Royal College of Surgeons of England*. **47**, 92–105

Negus, D. and Cockett, F. B. (1967) Femoral vein pressures in post-phlebitic iliac vein obstruction. *British Journal of Surgery*, **54**, 522

Shull, K. C., Nicolaides, A. N., Fernandes, F. *et al.* (1979) Significance of popliteal reflux in relation to ambulatory venous pressure and ulceration. *Archives of Surgery*, **114**, 1304–1306

Taheri, S. A., Heffner, R., Meenaghan, M. A. *et al.* (1985) Technique and results of venous valve transplantation. In *Surgery of the Veins* (eds J. J. Bergan and J. S. T. Yao), Grune and Stratton, New York, pp. 219–231

Taheri, S. A., Nowakowski, P., Prendergast, D. *et al.* (1987) Iliocaval compression syndrome. *Phlebology*, **2**, 173–179

Tibbs, D. J. (1986) The intriguing problem of varicose veins. *International Angiology*, **5**, 289–295

Villavicencio, J. J., Collins, G. J., Youkey, J. R. *et al.* (1985). Nonsurgical management of lower extremity venous problems. In *Surgery of the Veins* (eds J. J. Bergan and J. S. T. Yao), Grune and Stratton, New York, pp. 323–345

Widmer, L. K., Zemp, E., Widmer, M. Th. and Voelin, R. (1986) Thromboembolic recurrence and post-thrombotic syndrome after deep vein thrombosis. In *Phlebology 85* (eds D. Negus and G. Jantet), John Libbey, London, pp. 556–559

Woodyer, A. B., Walker, R. T. and Dormandy, J. A. (1986) Venous claudication. In: *Phlebology 85* (eds D. Negus and G. Jantet), John Libbey, London, pp. 524–527

## Bibliography

Brightmore, T. G. J. and Smellie, W. A. B. (1971) Popliteal artery entrapment. *British Journal of Surgery*, **58**, 481–484

Chilton, C. P. and Darke, S. G. (1980) External iliac venous compression by a giant iliopsoas rheumatoid bursa. *British Journal of Surgery*, **67**, 641

Hudson, I. and Sadow, G. J. (1990) An unusual cause of femoral vein obstruction. *Journal of the Royal Society of Medicine*, **83**, 331–332

Inada, K., Hirose, M., Iwashima, Y. and Matsumoto, K. (1978) Popliteal artery entrapment syndrome: a case report. *British Journal of Surgery*, **65**, 613–615

# 10

# Complex patterns of venous disorder

In previous chapters (see Chapters 5, 8 and 9) complex patterns of venous abnormality have been referred to in which deep vein problems coexist with simple incompetence in the superficial veins and warning was given of the poor response to surgery for varicose veins if this combination is not recognized. In this chapter these complex states (Tibbs, 1986) will be viewed from the standpoint of the deep veins to explain further why confusing evidence of superficial vein incompetence may be found in the presence of a predominantly deep vein problem and to what extent this should affect decisions upon treatment.

## The significance of pubic and lower abdominal varicosities

Varicosities crossing the pubic area or winding upwards on the lower abdomen usually denote damage or occlusion to the underlying iliac veins or inferior vena cava and this is particularly true if there is an undoubted history of a deep vein thrombosis (see Chapter 9). However this is not invariably so.

## Cross-over simple superficial vein incompetence without deep vein abnormality (and see Chapter 5)

Typically the patient has had previous surgery for varicose veins and this has included high ligation of a long saphenous vein. The opposite limb has subsequently developed varicosities arising from the long saphenous system but on inspection a large varicosity is seen crossing the lower pubic region. This inevitably leads to suspicion that there is occlusion in the opposite common iliac vein, perhaps caused by the previous vein surgery. However, there is an alternative explanation that has to be weighed up. It is possible that the original operation ligated the termination of the long saphenous vein at too low a level so that the superficial epigastric and external pudendal

veins were left intact and a pathway of incompetence has now established itself through these veins and across the pubic region to the saphenous vein of the opposite side (Figure 10.1). This is most likely to arise when this vein is guarded by a competent valve in its uppermost part but there are no competent valves below this level. In this way blood can flow over from the common femoral vein of one side to the low pressure segment of saphenous vein beneath the competent valve on the opposite side and tumble down this vein, and via varicosities, to the area of slack veins in the lower part of the limb.

This unusual pattern of cross-over incompetence can be proved by:

1. Effective control of varicosities in the limb by selective occlusion of the pubic varicosities by finger pressure. This test will, however, fail if the uppermost saphenous valve is incompetent or a multiplicity of pubic veins defeats effective closure of the cross-over flow.
2. A directional flowmeter applied to the pubic varicosities whilst the patient exercises by rising onto the toes; this will show that the direction of flow is, say, from left to right (but beware of the difficulty of determining direction within a tortuous vein), and if the incompetent saphenous vein on the right side is occluded intermittently, flow in the pubic veins shows a corresponding series of interruptions.
3. Functional phlebography which can demonstrate flow from one side, across the tortuous pubic veins and spilling down the opposite long saphenous vein; at the same time the patency of the iliac veins can be confirmed.

With this evidence it is permissible to remove the source of incompetence, that is, the saphenous stump in the contralateral limb, and to eliminate its superficial epigastric and pudendal branches; on the affected side, flush ligation and stripping of the long saphenous vein is carried out. The evidence should be incontrovertible and a phlebogram is usually a necessary preliminary to ensure that the iliac veins are patent and that the pubic veins are not part of a collateral mechanism. Only a careful

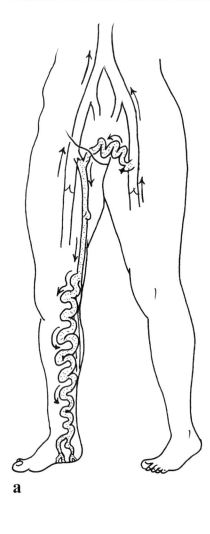

a

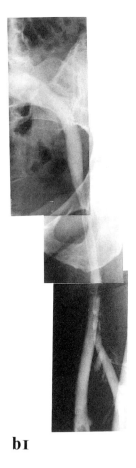

b1

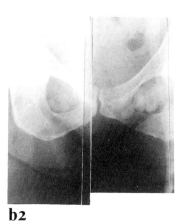

b2

**Figure 10.1** *Cross-over superficial vein incompetence without any deep vein abnormality; long saphenous varicosities on one side arising from a saphenous stump on the opposite side.*

*(a) Diagram of right-sided varicosities taking source from pubic varicosities arising from tributaries that have survived inadequate saphenous ligation on the left side.*

*(b) Clinical example of simple cross-over incompetence illustrated by functional phlebography in a female patient with right-sided varicosities 3 years after left long saphenous high ligation and stripping. Examination in near-vertical position, with opaque medium injected into a calf vein on the left side.*

> *1. Femoral and iliac deep veins outlined passively and showing them to be widely patent throughout.*
> *2. Immediately after three exercise movemements, flow through a large pubic varicosity crossing over to the right side where it descended down the long saphenous vein; original X-ray films show this clearly, but too faintly for reproduction. See also Figure 5.16.*

*(c) Cross-over incompetence in a woman, aged 36, with recurrent varicose veins on both thighs following bilateral high*

*ligation and stripping of the long saphenous veins, 18 years previously. Varicosities present in right and left pudendal regions and on both thighs could all be controlled by pressure over the right long saphenous stump; cross-over incompetence was suspected. Phlebography was performed and the illustrations show posterior views of two phases of filling with injection of medium into an inner thigh varicosity on the left side, with patient near upright.*

> *1. Medium travels across to the right side via pudendal and vulval varicose veins and outlines the stump of the previously ligated right long saphenous vein.*
> *2. With further filling, various interconnecting branches can be seen on both sides and the deep veins show faintly on the right. At operation it was confirmed that the right saphenous stump was joined by intact superficial epigastric and external pudendal veins; these communicated with the left thigh varicosities via the left external pudendal vein and, in addition, were the source of extensive varicose veins on the right thigh (right short saphenous vein incompetence was also present and gave rise to a separate set of varicose veins on the calf) (see page 197)*

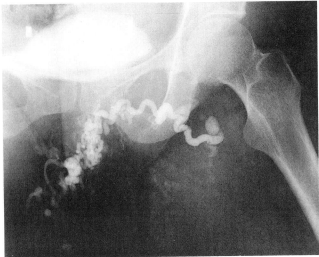

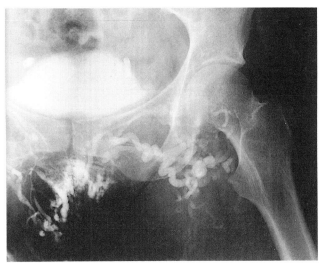

Left         Right    Left         Right

**CI**                    **C2**

**Figure 10.1** *(continued)*

examination will unravel a complex state of this sort and point to the correct course of action; pubic varicosities must be regarded as a contraindication to surgery until proved otherwise. Theoretically, a simple cross-over incompetence of this sort could also arise without any preceding surgery but the author has not yet seen this.

Apart from the exception given above, pubic varicosities denote occlusion in the underlying iliac veins but this does not preclude the possibility of extensive simple incompetence in superficial veins below this level.

## Superficial vein incompetence below iliac vein occlusion on the same side

The usual significance of pubic and lower abdominal varicosities is that they are acting as collaterals to occlusion in the iliac veins, most commonly on the left side. Below this level the pumping mechanism may be in good order so that it is returning blood upwards and creating a low pressure area of slack veins in the lower part of the limb. These are the circumstances which allow a pathway of superficial incompetence to develop, running from above a pumping mechanism to the low pressure area beneath it. Thus, it is quite possible for varicose veins, typical of a retrograde circuit of incompetence, to be present in such a limb and this is not rare. The commonest pattern is of typical simple incompetence in the long saphenous system below an occluded left common iliac vein (Figure 10.2). This is confusing to the examiner and the full diagnosis may not be recognized if the pubic varicosities have not been looked for. In these circumstances surgery to the long saphenous vein is likely to give an unsatisfactory result with no improvement in the symptoms caused by the unrecognized iliac vein occlusion and, more seriously, a decided deterioration in the limb because important collaterals arising from the

uppermost saphenous vein have been removed. Alternatively, the presence of pubic varicosities may understandably deter the surgeon from any form of surgery when, in fact, a complete evaluation might make it clear that the deep veins below the inguinal ligament are normal and the saphenous vein is not acting as a collateral and can be safely removed, provided its uppermost branches, which form part of the collateral circuit past the iliac occlusion, are left intact. The decision to do this should not be taken lightly however and caution is preferable to the risk of damaging collaterals to obstructed deep veins. In deciding on the form of treatment, a minimal requirement is that selective occlusion of the saphenous vein gives satisfactory control of the varicosities in the limb and a Doppler flowmeter shows downflow in it after exercise; a phlebogram should confirm healthy deep veins below the inguinal ligament with spillover from the common femoral down the saphenous vein. However, the operation cannot be regarded as satisfactory because it leaves intact the enlarged inferior epigastric and external pudendal veins, and the portion of saphenous stump they join, which will constantly threaten to provide the source of a new pathway of incompetence based on remnants of the old one. This is, of course, a common cause for recurrence after inadequate operations for uncomplicated long saphenous vein incompetence (see Chapter 5). Conservative management, with elastic support, may be the wisest course in the face of so many uncertainties.

## Iliac vein occlusion with cross-over incompetence in superficial veins of the opposite limb

Incompetence in superficial veins of the limb opposite to an iliac occlusion is not rare and one important cause for this is illustrated in Figure 10.3. Here, the source of

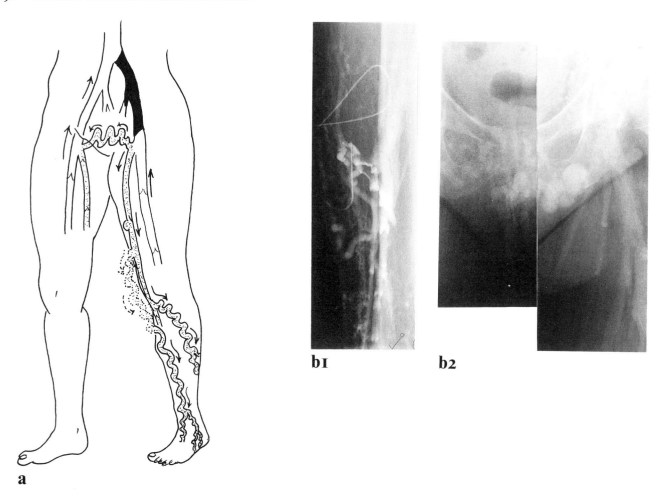

**Figure 10.2**  *Long saphenous incompetence in the limb below iliac vein occlusion on the same side.*

*(a) Diagram showing post-thrombotic occlusion affecting only the left iliac veins. The deep veins below the inguinal ligament are virtually undamaged so that development of left long saphenous incompetence and varicosities has proved possible or was present beforehand. These enlarged veins are not acting as collaterals but show the typical downflow after exercise of simple incompetence. Note the large pubic collateral vein taking outflow from the limb across to the right side. This pubic vein(s) arises from the uppermost tributaries of the long saphenous vein and will therefore be endangered by surgery to the long saphenous vein. Nevertheless, it is important to preserve it but this will mean that a source for incompetence flow persists and may give rise to recurrent varicosities.*

*(b) Clinical example illustrated by functional phlebography in a female patient, aged 57 years. Eighteen years previously she had developed left iliac deep vein thrombosis following hysterectomy. This limb had remained slightly swollen since that time and, more recently, varicosities had appeared in the thigh and calf. Phlebography performed with the patient near upright and opaque medium injected into a varicosity on the calf.*

*1. After 5 ml injection and one exercise movement, medium flows down and into normal, well-valved deep veins of the lower leg.*

*2. At a later stage, after injection of 80 ml and exercise × 2, normal well-valved deep veins are seen up to the inguinal ligament but the iliac veins do not fill. Typical collateral pubic varicosities are present taking flow across the pubic region to the right side. Spill-over flow is seen passing down the long saphenous vein which shows no valves. This vein has the characteristics of simple incompetence and is not acting as a collateral. Its removal, with preservation of its uppermost tributaries, would be permissible but prone to recurrent varicosities.*

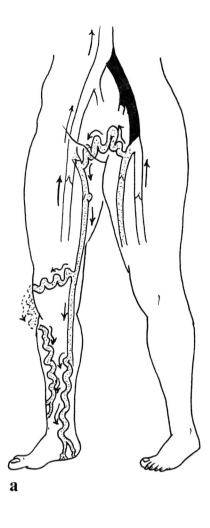

a

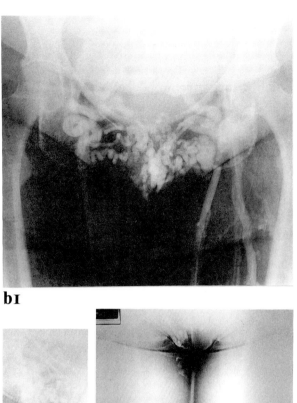

b1

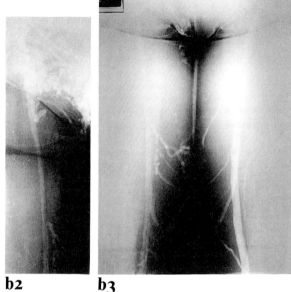

b2    b3

**Figure 10.3** *Cross-over superficial vein incompetence arising from pubic collaterals caused by iliac vein occlusion on the opposite side.*

*(a) Diagram showing left iliac vein occlusion causing a large pubic varicosity taking outflow from the left limb across to the right side. This acts as a source for downflow in an incompetent right long saphenous vein and varicosities arising from it.*

*(b) Clinical example illustrated by functional venogram in a female patient aged 58 years, who had sustained a 'white leg of pregnancy' 33 years previously. Her present complaint was of recurring phlebitis in varicose veins on the right leg and eczema in the overlying skin. The left limb had remained slightly swollen since the original deep vein thrombosis but otherwise symptom free. Examination confirmed typical simple incompetence on the right side which appeared to take its source from large pubic varicosities. Phlebography carried out with patient in near-upright position and medium injected into a vein on the left calf.*

    *1. View of upper thighs and pubic region after injection of 100 ml of medium and exercise × 3. The left saphenous vein shows strong preferential upflow; the femoral vein was occluded and deformed in its lower part (not shown here but see Figure 11.25(a)) and the left iliac veins could not be filled; venous outflow from the limb is by multiple pubic varicosities seen connecting with uppermost tributaries of the long saphenous vein of the right side. Downflow in the incompetent right long saphenous vein is clearly seen.*

    *2. Further view of the right side at slightly later stage to show downflow in the right saphenous vein through varicosities in the thigh.*

    *3. Later phase, showing both thighs. On the patient's left side, the long saphenous vein is enlarged with strong upward preferential flow; on the right side the long saphenous vein and varicosities have been outlined by incompetent downflow, with the cross-over pubic veins as the source of flow. These pictures give unequivocal evidence of opaque medium injected into superficial veins of the left calf travelling over to outline the right saphenous vein and varicosities. This circuit only occurred after brief exercise which created slack veins in the lower part of the right limb, thus causing downflow in the incompetent right saphenous system. For further details of this patient see Figures 5.17(a), (b) and 9.3(c). Prior Doppler flowmetry had indicated the probability of finding this cross-over phenomenon on functional phlebography. Conservative management was advised in this patient in order not to endanger the collateral venous outlet from the well-compensated left lower limb* incompetence is from large varicosities crossing the pubic region as collaterals to the obstructed iliac vein. It bears obvious similarity to the cross-over incompetence following inadequate surgery to the long saphenous system, described in the first section of this chapter and illustrated in Figure 10.1. The essential difference is that in iliac occlusion the pubic veins are valuable collateral vessels compensating for deep vein damage and must not be interfered with. The terminal branches of the long saphenous vein are likely to be important in this collateral mechanism and will be destroyed by the usual operation of flush ligation. The distinction between the two conditions may not be easy on clinical grounds. The collateral veins usually form multiple channels so that tests based on selective occlusion of pubic veins are unreliable; a further variable is the competence of the uppermost saphenous valve which may or may not prevent alternative filling from its own femoral vein. In simple cross-over incompetence below normal iliac veins, a Doppler flowmeter may show cessation of flow in pubic veins on compression of the saphenous vein in mid-thigh and this is a useful pointer, but the only reliable diagnosis is by functional phlebography demonstrating conclusively the state of the iliac veins and the associated collaterals.

When the condition is shown to be associated with iliac occlusion, surgery to relieve the simple superficial incompetence may still be permissible provided the terminal branches of the long saphenous vein, which form part of the collateral mechanism, are left intact. Caution is advised however and unless all aspects are clearly understood it is best to avoid surgery which is not essential rather than run the risk of aggravating problems caused by the deep vein occlusion. As expressed in the previous section, surgery sparing the collaterals may prove inadequate so that a new pathway of incompetence based on this source may soon appear.

## Simple superficial incompetence below femoropopliteal occlusion with or without iliac vein occlusion

It has been previously pointed out (see Chapter 8) that in a post-thrombotic state where the femoral and popliteal veins are deformed or occluded, varicose veins are seldom seen because the collateral flow in the superficial veins is in their natural direction; these veins become prominent but not tortuous and a Doppler flowmeter confirms strong upflow in them as would be expected of collaterals. Nevertheless, in some limbs well-developed varicose (tortuous) veins can be seen at various levels down the limb. A directional flowmeter placed over these veins may well show a component of strong downflow apparently counter to the expected collateral upflow. This apparent confliction is explained when it is recalled that incompetent veins become varicose due to gravitational down-

fall in them from above a pumping mechanism to below it. Any group of muscles in the leg can act as a pumping mechanism, and so can the foot itself, to form the basis of a retrograde circuit of this sort (Figure 10.4, and see Figure 5.19(b)–(d)) and many such groups will have escaped damage at the time of thrombosis. In the post-thrombotic limb, the principal superficial veins, such as the long saphenous and its major branches, will be conducting collateral upflow but an incompetent side branch may establish connection with an area of slack veins below a surviving pumping mechanism. In this way there is a general collateral upflow in the main superficial veins overlying occluded deep veins but with substantial spill-over down incompetent side branches. This is particularly marked immediately after the foot is raised off the ground

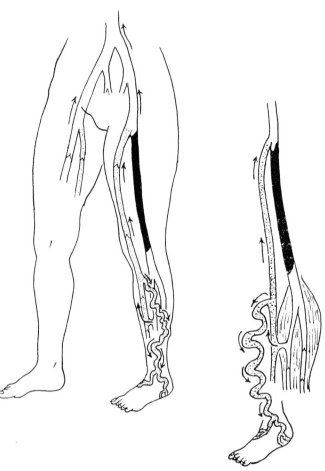

**Figure 10.4** *Incompetence with varicosities developing in branches of the principal collateral superficial veins past popliteal or femoral deep vein occlusion.*

*Diagram showing left femoropopliteal occlusion with strong upflow in the overlying long saphenous vein whilst acting as collateral to the obstructed deep veins. The pumping mechanisms in the deep veins below the knee, including those of the foot, are virtually undamaged and, in spite of abnormal flow patterns, are capable of creating low venous pressure under the foot and lower leg. This is sufficient to allow blood from the main collateral veins to spill down incompetent side branches to these low pressure areas. A good example of this phenomenon is illustrated in Figure 5.19(b)–(d)*

but when it is put down again there is a strong surge upwards as the venous pool on its underside is compressed by body weight. The veins involved respond to this surge back and forth by enlarging and becoming tortous; pre-existing varicosities will of course provide a readymade pathway for this pattern of failure. Clearly this retrograde flow will handicap the efforts of the undamaged venous pumps and diminish still further the overall ability of the limb to return its blood in the upright position; moreover, the upward surge from the foot will cause undesirable peaks of excessive pressure. Such varicosities do not have collateral function and the term 'secondary varicosities' is not really appropriate although it does at least indicate recognition of the underlying deep vein defect. The prominent true collateral veins are of course 'secondary' but will not have the tortuosity

**Figure 10.5** *Intricate pattern of superficial vein incompetence simulating deep vein incompetence. The patient, a man aged 46, presented with discomfort behind the left knee and a large varicose vein in the lower posterior thigh. His history included a fracture of the tibia at the age of 19 years, with 3 months in plaster and, recently, high ligation of the long saphenous veins on both sides, with a subsequent procedure to remove residual varicosities. Two years later further veins had appeared on the back of the thigh; these showed strong upflow with exercise and an initial diagnosis of post-thrombotic syndrome was considered.*

*(a) 1–4. Photographs to show the left lower limb with the varicosity running posteriorly from popliteal fossa obliquely to mid-thigh. The front view shows varicose veins meandering down the left thigh and knee, with large varicosities on the inner aspect below the knee, all of which are in keeping with a long saphenous origin. Doppler flowmetry showed strong upflow in the posterior thigh vein after exercise. A tapwave test confirmed that a large long saphenous vein was present from groin to ankle and Doppler flowmetry to this showed downflow simultaneous with the upflow of the posterior thigh varicose vein; both flows were controlled by finger pressure over the short saphenous termination. Photoplethysmography showed a short recovery time at 10 seconds but this improved to 20 seconds with finger occlusion of the posterior thigh varicose vein or the long saphenous at knee level.*

*(b) 1. Functional phlebography (see page 202). A composite picture (posterior view) is shown with a pair of posteriorly running varicose veins from popliteal fossa to mid-thigh where they can be seen joining an intact, oversized long saphenous vein. Flow in these veins was upwards on exercise but in the long saphenous vein it was downwards; at groin level the long saphenous ends blindly without any communication with the common femoral vein. Many varicosities, including those running across the front of the thigh, arise from the long saphenous and are especially large below the knee; 2 shows additional details of these in externally rotated view. The short saphenous vein is not separately identifiable but some gastrocnemius veins fill readily and a further communication with the long saphenous vein and its varicosities is present in the upper calf. At surgery, the posterior thigh varicose veins were found to unite to form a single large vein which passed through a well-formed aperture in the fascia high in the fossa. Within the popliteal fossa this vein, believed to be an upward extension of the short saphenous vein, ran downwards for several centimetres before merging with a branched gastrocnemius vein. These veins were ligated and removed; the long saphenous vein was stripped together with extensive removal of its varicosities. A good result was confirmed 6 months later.*

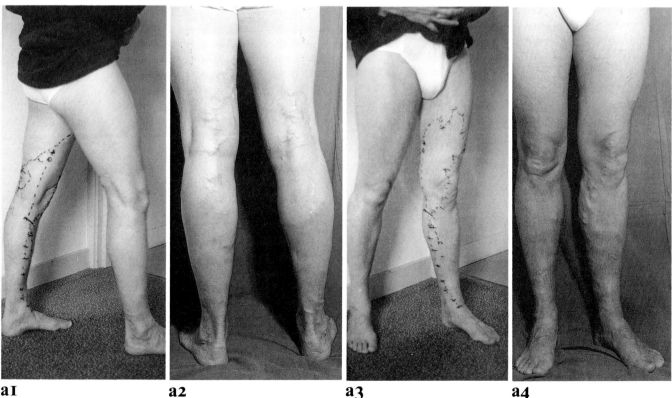

**aI**          **a2**          **a3**          **a4**

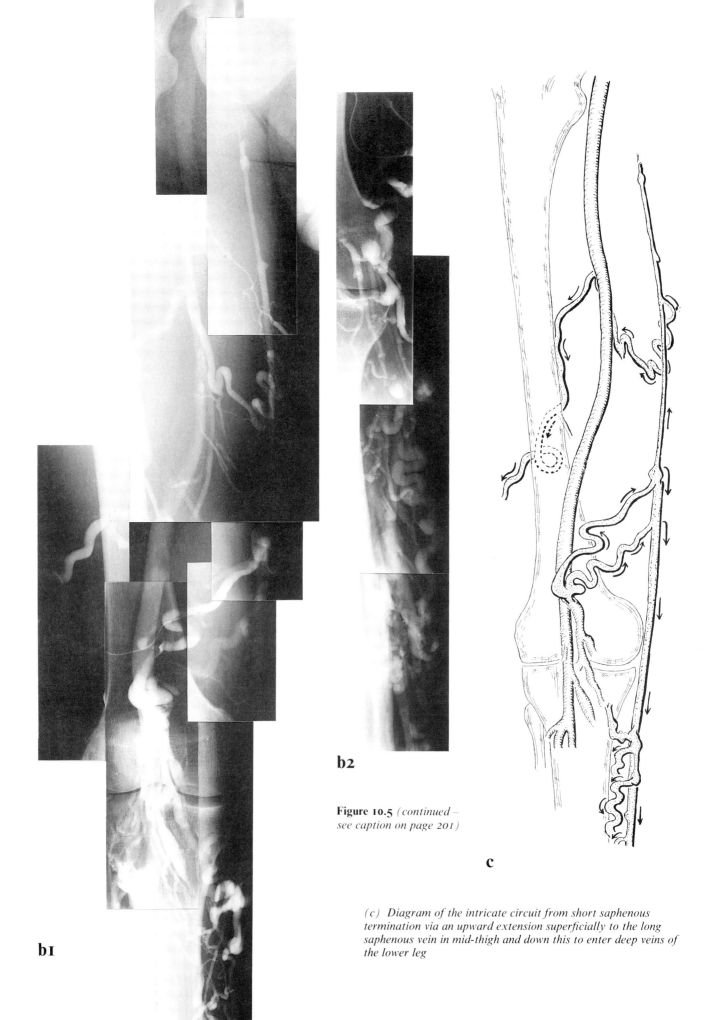

**b2**

**Figure 10.5** *(continued –*
*see caption on page 201)*

**c**

*(c)  Diagram of the intricate circuit from short saphenous*
*termination via an upward extension superficially to the long*
*saphenous vein in mid-thigh and down this to enter deep veins of*
*the lower leg*

**b1**

characteristic of varicose veins, unless pre-existing varicose veins have been utilized as collateral channels. This is perhaps being a little pedantic but it is important to understand the basic processes, with flow and counterflow, if the clinical signs, flowmeter observations and phlebographic findings are to be interpreted correctly and lead to the decision whether interfering with a vein is likely to be beneficial or damaging.

Localized treatment, by surgery or sclerotherapy, of varicose veins arising from collateral superficial veins, as described above, may be permissible if Doppler flowmetry and phlebography have both confirmed that they are not contributing to collateral return. An elastic support up to the knee may, however, be effective.

## Intricate patterns of superficial vein incompetence as a source of confusion with deep vein problems

An intricate pattern is a special variety of mixed superficial vein incompetence with strong upward flow in one varicose vein and simultaneous downward counterflow in a vein nearby. The vein with upward flow may be the most obvious feature and therefore mistaken for collateral flow past obstructed deep veins, as in the post-thrombotic syndrome. It is only likely to occur when inadequate surgery to one or both saphenous systems in a limb has disrupted the normal superficial vein anatomy. In the case illustrated in Figure 10.5 the long saphenous vein had been ligated at high level without stripping. A new pattern of incompetence was soon established, with flow up a vein connecting the short saphenous termination to the unstripped long saphenous vein in mid-thigh. This gave rise to an obvious varicose vein on the posterior thigh, with strong upflow in it detected by Doppler flowmetry after exercise. Since the patient's history included a fractured tibia on the same side 20 years earlier, the initial suspicion was of deep vein impairment and collateral flow in the vein. However, careful mapping out located the unstripped long saphenous vein which showed Doppler downflow simultaneous with the upflow in the posterior thigh varicosity but prevented by temporary occlusion of this by finger pressure. Full investigation, given in Figure 10.5, showed that, in fact, this was an intricate circuit of flow from the popliteal deep vein, via short saphenous termination and an upward extension to join the long saphenous in mid-thigh and from there flow down to re-enter the deep veins of the leg on muscle relaxation.

The author had seen several similar cases before and for this reason took care to document this case when it presented. Upward flow in incompetent superficial veins during exercise in an upright position is not rare and may occur in the following circumstances:

1. A varicose vein that is essentially downward running takes a meandering course, turning in an upward direction for several centimetres before turning down again. This is quite often seen on the front of the thigh.
2. When an incompetent short saphenous vein communicates with a competent long saphenous vein in the upper calf and fills this vein with its downflow to create appreciable distension and brief upflow in the long saphenous until pressures equalize. Again, this is quite common and may be viewed as manometric filling of the long saphenous at a pressure representing the full popliteal deep vein pressure; without the short saphenous connection its valves would prevent such filling. This is an occasional reason for misdiagnosis of long saphenous incompetence when, in fact, it is the short saphenous that is at fault. Proper mapping out, a selective saphenous occlusion test and use of the Doppler flowmeter should prevent this error.
3. The intricate pattern of incompetence, described above, is merely a special version of the manometric filling just referred to but with the interconnecting vein taking a long oblique course upwards before joining an incompetent, unstripped, long saphenous vein which cannot fill from its upper end because of previous surgery.

## Comment

It is clear that complex states may be encountered which will make a decision upon the possible role of surgery difficult. A valuable guiding rule throughout venous surgery in the lower limb is that no vein should be removed unless benefit is predicted by control of varicose veins with a selective saphenous occlusion test, a Doppler flowmeter shows downflow after exercise, or functioning phlebography shows spill-over and downflow in the vein in question; any one of these may provide acceptable evidence but preferably all three in cases of uncertainty.

## Reference

Tibbs, D. J. (1986) The intriguing problem of varicose veins. *International Angiography*, **5**, 289–295

# 11

# The role of the perforator

There are numerous perforating or communicating veins connecting the superficial and the deep veins in the lower limb at all levels (Figure 11.1). These perforating veins are valved to permit only inward movement of blood and it is generally agreed that their normal function is to allow flow from superficial veins into the deep veins as an essential preliminary to upward pumping, against gravity, towards the heart. The long saphenous vein has little effective pumping mechanism of its own and the many perforating veins that connect with it, directly or indirectly, take immediate advantage of any drop in deep vein pressure to disperse the long column of blood that would otherwise develop up its length. Thus, every time deep vein pressure drops, for example following calf muscle contraction, blood from superficial veins will drain inwardly to the deep veins just emptied (Figure 11.2). This is partly by direct flow into the principal deep veins but also by indirect entry to them through venous sinuses in muscle. The important role of the large venous sinuses in gastrocnemius, soleus and other muscles is to act as pump chambers propelling blood from muscular activity upwards and this has already been described in Chapter 2. However, it is commonplace to see these sinuses filling from the superficial veins during functional phlebography (Figure 11.2). In this way, at each footstep the saphenous vein is broken up into a series of low pressure segments between its valves (Figure 11.3). Even a small movement will forestall the build up of full venous pressure (a column from foot to heart) in the saphenous vein and its branches, and this is a process continually repeated when the patient is up and about. For it to be effective there must be a mechanism to prevent a reverse process of blood from the deep veins spilling over from, or being pumped into, the superficial veins.

A liberal supply of effective valves throughout the saphenous systems ensures that gravitational downflow in these veins cannot occur in the normal state. The upper end of a saphenous vein entering the common femoral deep vein is, in effect, a large perforator and normally well guarded by at least one valve; in the same way, perforating veins have their own valves to prevent

outward flow (Figure 11.4). In addition, as described below, it is likely that perforators are protected from unwanted outward flow by the arrangement of muscle fibres and fascial coverings; this may be as important as the valves are in the prevention of a forceful outward pumping when muscle contraction occurs. Clearly, if these mechanisms fail, the superficial veins will be exposed to considerable pressure by the forceful ejection of blood from the deep veins through the perforating veins at the moment of muscle contraction. This concept of 'perforator blowback', so well developed by Cockett in the 1950s (Cockett 1955) is typical of his papers and is an important contribution to the evolution of thought at that time), has fascinated surgeons for many decades but an undue preoccupation with this may lead to the overlooking of simpler and more easily cured states, such as massive concealed long saphenous incompetence (see Chapter 4). It seems likely that the role of the perforator has often been misunderstood in the past and this chapter is an attempt to put this into proper perspective.

## Valves and fascial gates in perforating veins

Many authors, including Linton (1938), Cockett (1956), Dodd et al. (1957), Dodd and Cockett (1976) and Thompson (1979), have emphasized that the perforating veins have valves which normally prevent outward flow. However, over the years, a few accounts have given evidence that this is not invariably so. Johnston and Whillis (in Gray's Anatomy 1938) state that valves 'are absent in the very small veins, i.e. less than 2 mm in diameter'; this is a general reference, not specifically related to perforating veins, but does raise the possibility that many lesser

**Figure 11.1** *Superficial veins and the principal sites for perforating veins (marked with small arrows); over sixty 'perforators' are normally present. (From Boileau Grant (1947) with permission.)*

*(a) Lower limb: anteromedial view.*
*(b) Lower limb: posterior view.*
*(c) Ankle and dorsum of foot: anterolateral view (see page 205)*

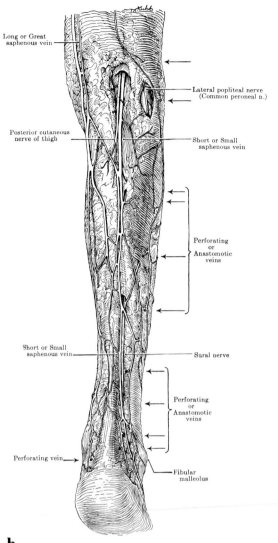

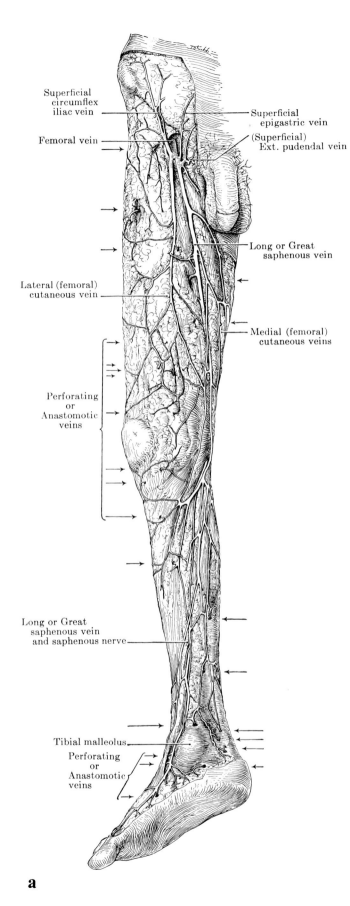

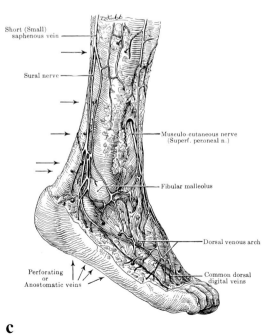

**Figure 11.1**

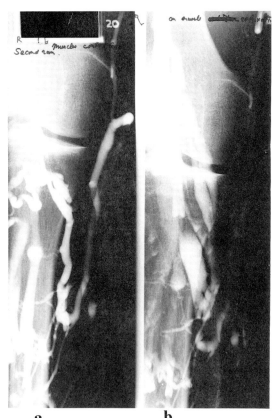

**a**　　　　**b**

**Figure 11.2** *Functional phlebogram of upper calf to show deep veins outlined:*

*(a) During muscle contraction by rising on toes*
*(b) Immediately after relaxation of muscle.*

*Contraction has emptied the pumping chambers (muscle sinuses) so that they are not seen but on relaxation they fill from the superficial veins which are no longer visible*

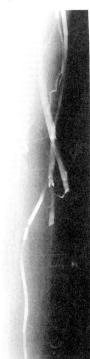

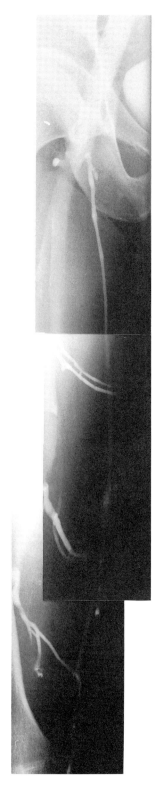

**Figure 11.3** *A normal long saphenous vein partially emptied by perforator inflow to deep veins following muscle contraction and relaxation; the column of blood has been broken into a series of low pressure segments separated by competent valves*

**Figure 11.4** *Normal thigh perforators allowing only inward flow. They are shown here with the patient horizontal so that opacified blood ran easily up the long saphenous vein and into the deep veins. Spillover outwards could not be demonstrated and these are normal competent perforating veins; the cause of the patient's venostasis was found below the knee. The upper pair of perforators cross behind the superficial femoral vein to join the profunda vein*

perforating veins are valveless and, collectively, a number of these could allow appreciable outward flow in certain conditions in the normal limb. Similarly, a study by Barber and Shatara (1925) found that perforating veins of less than 1 mm in diameter have no valves and that some of the larger ones have valves directing blood outwardly. Hadfield (1971) confirmed that small perforating veins have no valves and that valves in the larger ones often appeared insufficient; he concluded that the arrangement and oblique lie of perforating veins between muscle and the fascial aperture appeared to play an important role in preventing outflow and protecting superficial veins from excessive deep vein pressure on muscle contraction. In reviewing this subject, McMullin, Coleridge Smith and Scurr (1991) quote the authors just given and also a study by Raivio (1948) who found that when the valve of a perforating vein was positioned outside the deep fascia its cusps directed blood outward but when inside the fascia the valve was arranged to allow only inward flow.

It does appear that nature has made provision for flow in both directions so that pressure between superficial and deep veins can be continuously balanced and this fits the practical observations on normal and abnormal limbs referred to below. It is also a reminder that it is not justifiable to assume automatically that outward flow is abnormal, and observations on the limb only whilst muscles are relaxed (that is, fascial gates open), and especially when horizontal, may give a misleading impression of abnormality. But yet it is clear that normally the mechanism of valves and fascial gates is primarily adjusted to protect the superficial veins from the excessive deep vein pressure generated by muscle contraction. Perhaps the key to this is in the speed and volume of adjustment permitted in one direction as compared with the other. Thus, a large volume can be easily shifted rapidly inwards from superficial to deep veins but in the outward direction, from deep to superficial, only a much slower, restricted adjustment is possible (rather like free fall compared with fall slowed by parachute). This fits the known physiological and anatomical facts but requires experimental proof.

## The forces creating movement of venous blood

It is now recognized that flow in the various forms of failure of venous return against gravity is more complex than was originally thought. The advent of improved methods of radiology, especially use of the image intensifier, and the use of non-irritant osmolar opaque media, together with instrumental techniques, such as Doppler flowmetry and Duplex or colour flow imaging ultrasonography, have given a much clearer understanding of the patterns of flow and counter flow in the various disorders when the patient is upright and moving. In this there are two prime moving forces:

1. Muscle contraction and pressure on the underside of the foot, both of which give forceful upward pumping against gravity.
2. Gravity, which causes venous blood constantly to seek any avenue that will allow it to fall back down the limb; this becomes particularly evident if there is a deficiency or incompetence of valves.

In abnormal states considerable variation in direction and volume of flow through perforators may be found and often the question is whether the primary fault is a localized failure in the valvular mechanism of one or two identifiable perforators, or whether this is purely an incidental matter secondary to a more widespread failure.

## The distribution of perforating veins; variations in normal patterns of flow

Anatomists depict numerous perforators (Figure 11.1) throughout the limb and this is, of course, correct. Well over 60 such communications between superficial and deep veins are said to be present (Thomson, 1979). These veins are often paired and share the same fascial aperture with an artery emerging to nourish subcutaneous tissue and skin. In procedures removing the perforating veins, the destruction of this small artery can scarcely bring benefit but may increase any element of ischaemia in a skin that is already unhealthy. Venous surgeons, who are concerned with abnormal states, emphasize a limited number of perforators at well-defined sites (Linton, 1938; Cockett, 1955; May, 1979; May et al., 1981; Negus, 1985) which they believe to be especially important and many of these have been given eponyms (Figure 11.5). Attention is concentrated upon enlarged and abnormal veins that are often found in venous disorders and surgical descriptions are to do with the most common points of failure rather than detailed normal anatomical states. To understand the possible role of the perforator in any venous disorder it is necessary to be familiar with the different patterns of perforator flow that may be found and in the description that follows it is assumed that, in the ideal state, perforator flow is well governed by valves and fascial mechanisms so that it is predominantly inwards, from superficial to deep veins. However, exceptions can be found in apparently normal individuals, as well as in venous disorder. For example, if the popliteal deep vein is partially obstructed by firm pressure with the thumb, a Doppler flowmeter will often pick up an immediate upflow in the long saphenous vein whilst it acts as a collateral conducting blood past the semi-obstructed popliteal vein (Figure 11.6) (see also Figures 4.13, 4.14 and 5.1(a)). This must be the result of considerable collective perforator outflow and can quite easily occur in an apparently normal limb in certain conditions. In spite of this apparent defect in the perforator valvular control the outward flow ceases promptly when the popliteal

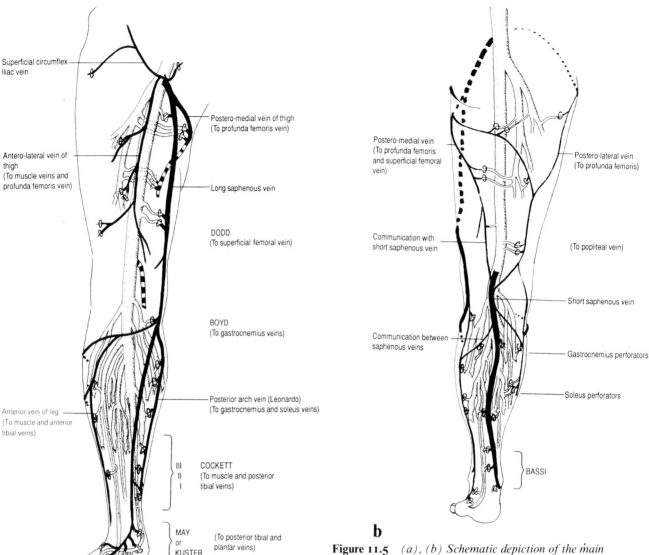

**a**

Superficial circumflex Iliac vein

Postero-medial vein of thigh (To profunda femoris vein)

Antero-lateral vein of thigh (To muscle veins and profunda femoris vein)

Long saphenous vein

DODD (To superficial femoral vein)

BOYD (To gastrocnemius veins)

Posterior arch vein (Leonardo) (To gastrocnemius and soleus veins)

Anterior vein of leg (To muscle and anterior tibial veins)

III
II    COCKETT
I     (To muscle and posterior tibial veins)

MAY or KUSTER    (To posterior tibial and plantar veins)

**b**

Postero-medial vein (To profunda femoris and superficial femoral vein)

Postero-lateral vein (To profunda femoris)

Communication with short saphenous vein

(To popliteal vein)

Short saphenous vein

Communication between saphenous veins

Gastrocnemius perforators

Soleus perforators

BASSI

**Figure 11.5** *(a), (b) Schematic depiction of the main perforating veins recognized by venous surgeons. Many connections between superficial veins and the deep conducting veins and muscle sinuses are shown but in reality these are far more numerous than is indicated. Some of the eponyms given to perforators considered to be of clinical importance are shown*

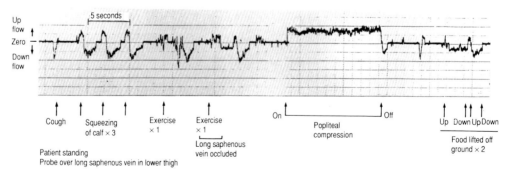

Up flow
Zero
Down flow

5 seconds

Cough
Squeezing of calf × 3
Exercise × 1
Exercise × 1
Long saphenous vein occluded
On    Popliteal compression    Off
Up  Down Up Down
Food lifted off ground × 2

Patient standing
Probe over long saphenous vein in lower thigh

**Figure 11.6** *Artificially created perforator outflow in a patient with simple varicose veins. Doppler flowmeter tracing of upflow induced in the long saphenous vein by moderate thumb pressure over the popliteal vein. This upflow is caused by perforator outflow due to slight venous congestion and ceases as soon as thumb pressure is released. Exercise will not cause this unless the deep vein is compressed and it illustrates why a constricting rubber tube should not be used for a Trendelenburg test*

compression is released and is not evident if the calf muscles are then repeatedly exercised. Pressure studies and observations made at phlebography confirm that widespread interchangeability of blood between superficial and deep veins in both directions is commonly found. The boundary between normal and abnormal in this respect is ill defined and there is a need for further study to clarify how much bidirectional interchange does occur in the normal and at what stage such interchange must be regarded as abnormal.

## The boundary between normal and abnormal perforator flow

During muscle contraction in the normal state all perforators in the vicinity are shut off by valves and fascial gates so that no flow in either direction occurs in them (Figure 11.2(a)). When the muscle has relaxed there is free interchange in both directions, depending upon local pressure gradients (Figure 11.2(b)). Thus, immediately after contraction the deep veins are slack, with empty muscle sinuses and superficial blood flows into them through perforators. If the subject now stands still, with muscles relaxed, deep vein pressure will rise steadily due to filling by arterial, transcapillary inflow. When this exceeds superficial vein pressure, flow will tend to move outwardly through multiple perforators until pressures equalize; perforator valves seem only partially effective in opposing this slow drift outwards. With renewed muscle contraction, valves and fascial 'shutters' combine to oppose outward ejection and this is the normal protective mechanism. By contrast, in some states of valve or fascial failure outward pumping is not controlled and this can be a most damaging form of venous failure (Figure 11.23); it may occur as a localized or widespread phenomenon and is considered further presently.

Even though it must be admitted that the boundary of

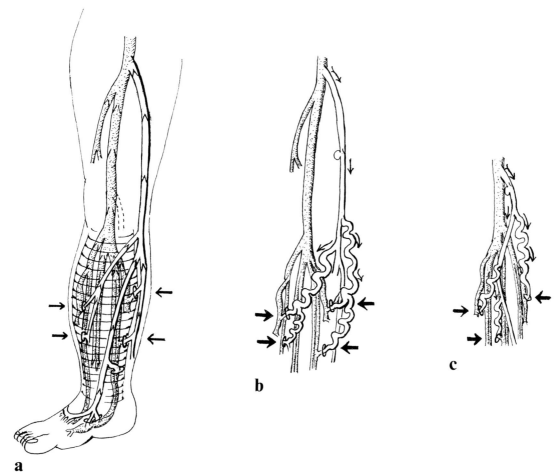

**a**

**Figure 11.7** *Diagrams of inward perforator flow.*

*(a) Normal multiple inward flow, small in amount and of short duration because downflow to each perforator is limited by valves in superficial veins.*

*(b) Long saphenous incompetence with abnormally increased inflow following muscle contraction-relaxation (systole and diastole); downflow in superficial veins is not limited by valves and perforator inflow continues until deep veins are filled to capacity.*

*(c) Short saphenous incompetence (posterior view) inflow is similar to (b)*

normality is ill defined, let us try to clarify the various patterns of perforator flow that may be seen in patients, ranging from mild to severe abnormality. All observations apply to the upright subject, exercising intermittently because, in these circumstances, nearly all venous disorders are related to some form of failure in the successful return of venous blood against gravity. The flow patterns will be described in three categories:

1. Abnormally increased inward flow.
2. Heavy outward flow.
3. A combination of the two as surge back and forth.

Perforators may be playing opposite roles at different levels in the same limb and the circumstances and significance of this are discussed below.

## Inward flow from superficial to deep veins

1. Inward perforator flow (Figure 11.7(a)) is a normal phenomenon following reduction in deep vein pressure caused by muscle contraction and relaxation, the release of weight from the underside of the foot or a change in the position of the limb. This inward flow is limited by the valves in the neighbouring superficial veins so that only the area of veins corresponding to each perforator will empty through it. Thus, inward flow is normally of short duration and superficial blood tends to be segmented into a series of cascades divided off by valves (Figure 11.3). However, the interconnecting network formed by the lesser superficial veins makes this a very flexible arrangement depending on the circumstances of the moment.

2. Unnaturally large inward perforator flow, in terms of volume or duration, will occur if one or more superficial valves allows unnatural downflow (Figure 11.7(b), (c)); usually a chain of incompetent valves has established a pathway of incompetence, which may be confined to a saphenous vein, or may take a more complex and tortuous route through its branches. This occurs by loss of competence in an otherwise normal

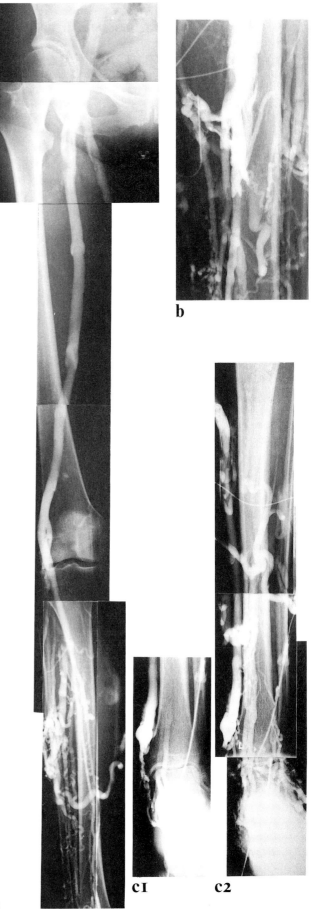

b

c1    c2

a

---

**Figure 11.8** *Phlebograms of downflow in simple long saphenous varicose veins after exercise, with patient in near-vertical position. Five different patients are shown.*

*(a) Composite phlebogram. Flow down long saphenous vein (largely off picture) passes through a large branch, crossing front of tibia, to a number of lesser branches and via multiple perforators to anterior tibial veins and muscle sinuses of the peroneal muscles. This is a common form of incompetence.*

*(b) Inflow from long saphenous varicosities by perforators on medial aspect of leg to enter posterior tibial veins and soleal sinuses; a varicosity crosses the front of the leg to fill anterior tibial venae comitantes.*

*(c) Long saphenous incompetence with inflow by perforators on inner leg and ankle to enter posterior tibial and plantar veins. Two phases of filling are shown. Also shown is a large varicose vein on the shin sending flow into anterior tibial veins.*

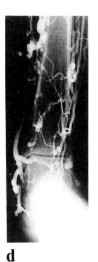

**d**

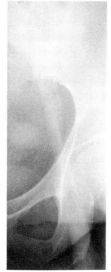

**eI**

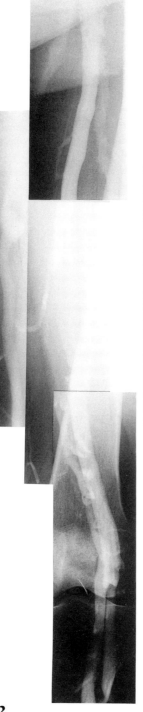

**e2**

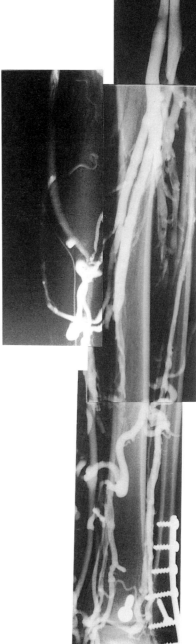

**e3**

**Figure 11.8** *(continued)*
*(d) Flow via long saphenous varicosities to foot perforators and by peroneal perforators into anterior tibial veins.*

*(e) This patient, a female age 53 years, was seen with varicose veins and slight swelling of the foot; all the features of simple long saphenous incompetence were present but there was a history of a severe fracture at the ankle many years before which had been screwed and plated. For this reason, a functional phlebogram was carried out and a composite picture from this is shown.*

*1. Vicinity of long saphenous termination before exercise.*
*2. Thigh region after exercise with flow down incompetent and sacculated long saphenous vein.*
*3. Composite view from lower thigh to ankle, showing inflow through mid-leg perforators to paired deep veins in the upper leg. It can be seen that the deep veins in the vicinity of the old fracture look very attenuated, in keeping with thrombosis at the time of injury. The long and short saphenous veins overlying this area appear to be acting as collaterals past occluded deep veins with flow from the foot re-entering undamaged deep veins by paired perforating veins in the mid-leg. However, during phlebography, it was evident that the perforators were also receiving substantial flow coming down the limb from the main part of the long saphenous vein, which was enlarged and sacculated. Thus, the perforators seemed to be acting as part of a collateral channel from the foot but also burdened by inward flow from the incompetent long saphenous vein above. Clearly it would have been unwise to remove the collateral vessels but equally it was desirable to take away the incompetent saphenous vein above this. High ligation and stripping of the saphenous vein down to mid-leg was carried out, with preservation of the perforating vein and the vein joining it from below. This removed the varicose veins and relieved discomfort, with some improvement in the swelling. Would obliteration of the perforators have caused increased swelling? They were not at fault and it was best not to chance it!*

set of valves or where there is an inborn inadequacy in the number of valves. The corresponding inflow will usually be spread between multiple perforators (Figures 11.8, 11.9) but not infrequently one perforator predominates and may be individually recognizable. There is great variation in the inward flow that will result and this will depend on two factors:

(a) The rapidity of leakage allowed by the incompetent superficial valves, which may vary from a trickle to a torrent.

(b) The effectiveness of the musculovenous pump in clearing the deep veins of blood to create 'slack' vein ready to accept inflow.

In its least form a small flow of prolonged duration may occur, detectable only by instruments and unnoticed by the patient (Figure 11.10). When maximal, the inward flow may be so heavy that the duration is quite brief (Figure 11.11) because of the rapidity with which pressures between superficial and deep veins will equalize. In the latter circumstances a weak musculovenous pumping mechanism may be overwhelmed so that there is a sustained, unrelieved high venous pressure in superficial and deep veins, leading to the venotensive changes of lipodermatosclerosis and ulceration (see Chapter 5).

Increased perforator inflow, as just described, arising from superficial valve incompetence, is an essential part of 'simple' or primary varicose veins, by far the commonest of the venous disorders and with the characteristic features of superficial downflow, saccules in the saphenous vein and tortuosity in the branch veins. One-fifth of these patients will show mild to severe venotensive skin changes.

In most states where an abnormally large single perforator develops due to inflow from superficial incompetence, the perforator is playing an incidental role and treatment directed solely towards its elimination, without removal of the incompetent superficial veins, is unlikely to give long-term benefit. The characteristic of this group of patients is downflow in the superficial veins following exercise, and an unequivocal control of varicosities by a Trendelenburg test; this should be performed by fingertip

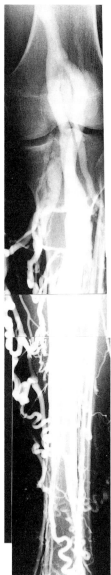

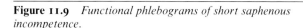
a1

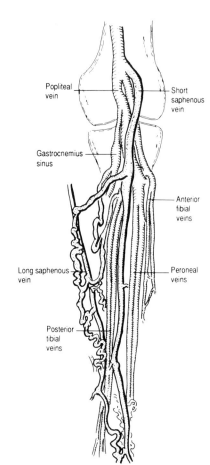
a2

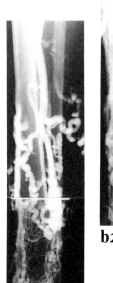
b1

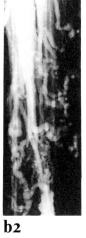
b2

**Figure 11.9** *Functional phlebograms of short saphenous incompetence.*

*(a) Composite phlebogram (posterior view). With patient in near-vertical position, medium has been injected into a varicose vein on the back of the calf and has filled not only the short saphenous vein but, by perforators, has entered a gastrocnemius sinus, and peroneal and tibial veins to fill popliteal and femoral veins. A varicosity runs off the picture to the foot where inflow will pass by foot perforators to the plantar veins.*

*(b) Another patient with multiple entry by perforators from short saphenous varicosities to tibial and peroneal veins, and soleal sinuses; other varicose veins descend to plantar veins in the foot. Two phases of filling are shown*

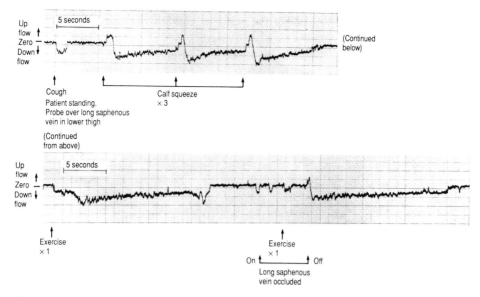

**Figure 11.10** *Minor incompetence in the long saphenous vein. Doppler flowmeter tracing of prolonged, slow downflow through valves allowing only slight leakage. This continues for nearly 20 seconds before pressure between superficial and deep veins equalizes and flow ceases*

pressure localized to the suspected pathway of incompetence because any form of tourniquet may congest the deep veins and actually cause a misleading, artificial perforator outflow to fill the varicose veins.

Doppler flowmeter studies show that many of these patients have a brief component of perforator outflow at the moment of muscular contraction (Figure 11.11) but this is small compared with the inflow that follows relaxation of the muscle. Its presence does not prevent a good result after removal of incompetent superficial veins but flowmeter examination in these patients will usually show the interesting artefact (Figure 11.6; see Figures 4.13, 4.14, 5.1(a)2) already described above in normal subjects. Partial obstruction of the popliteal vein by compression with a thumb (not a tourniquet) causes strong upflow in the saphenous vein due to free perforator outflow whilst venous blood is re-routed collaterally to the superficial

veins. However, when popliteal compression is released and a selective Trendelenburg test using fingertip control (not a constricting band) is carried out, and the patient exercised whilst control of saphenous incompetence is maintained, there will be little or no filling of the superficial veins (Figure 11.12). This implies that the perforators, in spite of their demonstrated ability to allow outward flow, do not permit it to occur when there is unrestricted normal return in the deep veins. It seems unlikely, in circumstances of proven superficial incompetence with increased perforator inflow, that a small component of outflow at the moment of muscle contraction has any great significance. Thus, in the majority of patients with superficial incompetence, with or without skin change, perforator outflow plays little part and is insufficient to have any adverse effect.

In most cases special search for perforators, often small

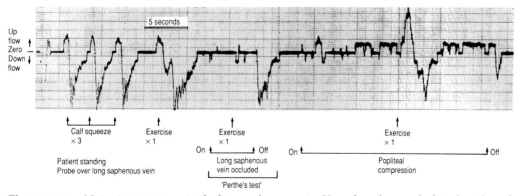

**Figure 11.11** *Major incompetence in the long saphenous vein. Here the valves are leaking heavily and downflow is at first swift but soon dwindles as the pressures equalize by perforator inflow. Such rapid perforator inflow strongly conflicts with the efforts of the musculovenous pump to reduce pressure and a weak pump may be easily overwhelmed. (Note: Doppler tracing, such as this, shows only the velocity of flow and is not necessarily a good indication of the flow volume.) This tracing also shows the characteristic spurt of upward flow at the actual moment of muscle contraction*

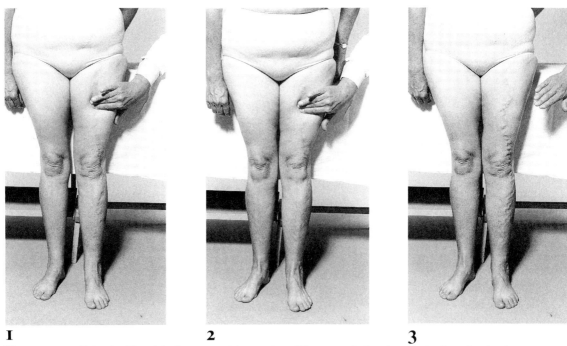

I                                   2                                   3

**Figure 11.12**   *Selective Trendelenburg test with exercise whilst control of varicose veins is maintained.*

*1. The limb has been elevated to empty the varicosities, the incompetent veins controlled by localized finger pressure and the patient asked to stand.*

*2. The patient has been exercised by rising on toes three times whilst control is maintained; the varicose veins remain empty and there is no evidence of perforator outflow.*

*3. Control is removed and varicosities immediately fill by flow from above*

and multiple, need not be made but when a large individual perforator is known to be present then this is best eliminated. Bjordal (1972, 1974, 1977, 1981) showed by electromagnetic flowmeter that the flow in large mid-leg perforators beneath long saphenous incompetence showed a small outward flow on contraction but a far larger inflow on muscle relaxation; with repeated contractions while walking the overall inward flow far exceeded the outward flow. If the saphenous vein was now occluded the inward flow ceased but the component of outward flow increased, apparently because it was now unopposed by saphenous downflow. Bjordal advised that when a large perforating vein was present this should be removed together with the incompetent saphenous vein since otherwise its ability for outflow may persist and actually increase, so continuing the venous stasis in the lower leg. This advice is certainly in keeping with our own views expressed elsewhere in this book. It is likely that the present day operation removing the peripheral varicosities through multiple small incisions is likely to achieve this in any case.

Observations on this are easily confused by the effect of the foot pump which may cause a strong surge upwards in both superficial and deep veins whenever the foot is put to the ground after raising it (Figure 11.13). This is particularly marked when incompetent veins, usually enlarged and tortuous, run to the foot and here Doppler flowmetry will detect a substantial downflow on raising

the foot (see Chapter 5). To confuse matters still further, it is certainly possible for different patterns of abnormality to coexist so that, in addition to superficial incompetence, some form of valve failure in the leg is also present and capable of giving heavy perforator outflow of the types described below. In such mixed patterns elimination of both components, the superficial incompetence and a heavy outward leakage from a perforator, may be necessary for successful treatment. The characteristic Doppler surge back and forth, usually found in these patients, is valuable in giving warning of this possibility.

### Perforator surge back and forth between superficial and deep veins

In this state a strong component of perforator outflow is present at the time of muscle contraction but followed by a sudden reversal on muscle relaxation with inflow from superficial to deep veins. The volume of blood moving in each of these phases is roughly equal so that blood surges back and forth without achieving any purposeful upward flow (Figure 11.14(a)) and venous hypertension develops. Surge will occur when there is a combination of the following circumstances:

1. Superficial incompetence is present to provide unlimited inflow whenever the opportunity presents, i.e. on muscle relaxation.

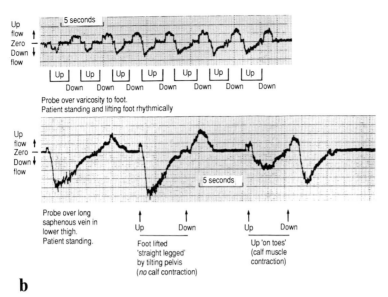

**b**

**Figure 11.13** *(a) Doppler tracing with probe over a large varicosity running to underside of the foot. Strong surge occurs with rhythmical foot raising; as pressure to its underside is released there is downflow and this is reversed when the foot is placed down again.*

*(b) Simple lifting of the foot usually causes substantial downflow in an incompetent saphenous vein at thigh level when varicosities run to the foot, as shown in this tracing. This may confuse the effect of muscle contraction when rising on the toes*

**Figure 11.14** *Patterns of surge in incompetent leg perforators.*

*(a) Between tibial and incompetent superficial veins.*

*(b) Between muscle sinus (e.g. gastrocnemius or soleus) and surface veins. Such leakage may be solitary and suitable for surgery or sclerotherapy, or multiple and widespread so that surgical cure is impracticable*

2. Although damage to the pumping mechanism may be present it still has sufficient capacity to shift deep venous blood upwards with muscle contraction to give a short phase of reduced pressure in the deep veins and thus allow perforator inflow.

3. There is some form of failure in the control of perforator outflow at muscle contraction. This may be the result of:

    (a) An inborn deficiency of valves, either localized or widespread (see Chapter 7).

    (b) Weak vein syndrome leading to early development of defective valves in deep veins and perforators (see Chapter 7).

    (c) Local damage by thrombosis and subsequent recanalization in deep veins, including those within

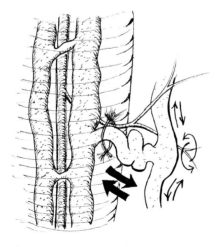

**a**

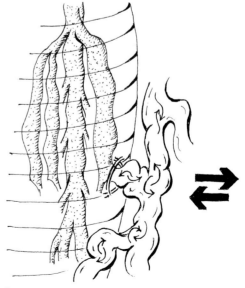

**b**

the muscles, and the perforating veins. Direct trauma, such as blows or kicks sustained in various sports, may have the same effect. Similarly medical procedures such as an intravenous drip into a saphenous vein during childhood may cause local damage.

(d) The persistence of collateral channels established as a temporary need during deep vein thrombosis which has subsequently recanalized.

(e) The presence of unnaturally large communications between muscle veins, such as the gastrocnemius or soleus sinuses, and the superficial veins (Figures 11.14(b), 11.22). These may be caused by developmental errors which enlarge as the years go by or by persistence of collateral channels established at the time of local venous thrombosis or injury as described above.

(f) There is also some evidence that a haematoma caused by an injury rupturing veins, common enough in the leg, may organize into a valveless venous spongework connecting between deep and superficial veins.

Convincing examples of these conditions will be regularly seen in a typical venous clinic. Their presence is first suspected by unsatisfactory control with a selective Trendelenburg test and confirmed by a Doppler flowmeter showing substantial surge back and forth. A careful history may give clear evidence of some form of injury or thrombosis many years before and functional phlebography may identify one or more perforators through which surge is occurring. Often one enlarged perforating vessel predominates. The more extreme state of widespread absence of valves thoughout the limb is considered at the end of this chapter and in Chapter 7.

If functional phlebography shows that the deep veins are widely open and in good order, and a large perforator connecting with an incompetent saphenous system is allowing obvious surge (Figure 11.15), then it is advisable to remove the perforator together with the saphenous vein. In the presence of satisfactory deep veins, this is unlikely to do harm and may well bring real benefit to the patient; it may also prevent the persistence after operation of a foot circuit based on the perforator as described below. It should be noted that the Doppler flowmeter seldom localizes a perforator precisely, because the surge affects superficial veins over a wide area and usually functional phlebography is necessary to give its exact position. Similarly, confusion may arise in many cases of superficial incompetence because enlarged veins to the foot give substantial surge, picked up by the Doppler flowmeter as the foot is raised and put down again.

Perforator surge caused by a combination of superficial and perforator incompetence is seen only in a minority of varicose vein patients and corresponds with Cockett's perforator 'blowout' syndrome (Cockett and Elgan, 1953; Cockett, 1955). However, it is important to distinguish

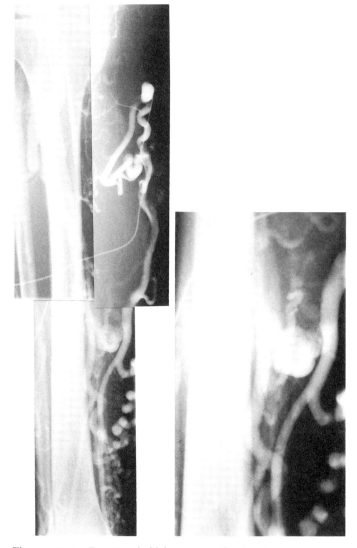

**Figure 11.15** *Functional phlebogram confirming strong surge via a large perforator connecting with an incompetent long saphenous branch. An enlarged view of the varicosed perforator is also shown. Although relatively valveless, the deep veins were shown to be widely open throughout; surgical removal of perforator and saphenous vein was therefore permissible and benefited the patient*

this from the much more serious state of outward pumping due to deep vein impairment with the perforators being forced to act as essential components of a post-thrombotic collateral mechanism returning blood past deformed or obstructed deep veins. Here the perforator is not causative but incidental to a more widespread process. Its surgical removal may take away a valuable compensatory mechanism and this, together with other categories of perforator outflow, will now be considered.

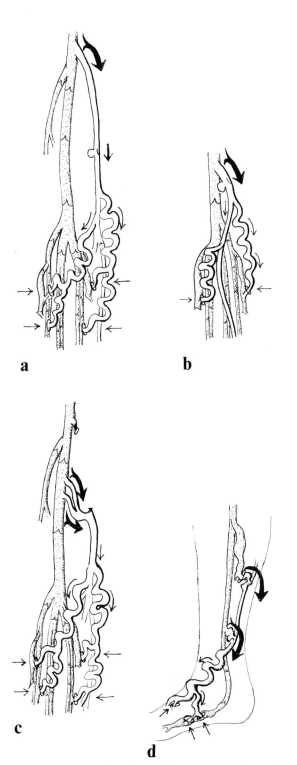

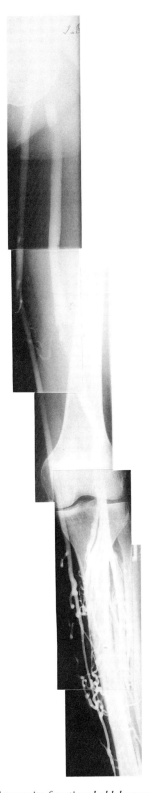

**Figure 11.16**  *Outward perforator flow allowing spillover from deep to superficial veins and gravitational downflow.*

*(a), (b)  From the upper end of incompetent long or short saphenous systems.*

*(c)  In recurrent varicose veins after removal of the uppermost long saphenous vein; a pair of incompetent mid-thigh perforators have established outflow into the remaining saphenous system with reappearance of varicose veins and venostasis.*

*(d)  Spillover through a perforator from a venous sinus in muscle or a tibial vein, with downflow to the foot*

**Figure 11.17**  *Composite functional phlebogram showing spillover from the common femoral vein down the saphenous vein and varicosities to re-enter the deep veins below the calf muscle pump. Flow outwards from a high-level 'perforator', in this example the termination of the long saphenous vein, and downwards to re-enter deep veins again by perforators below a pumping mechanism is the basic pattern of simple (primary) varicose veins*

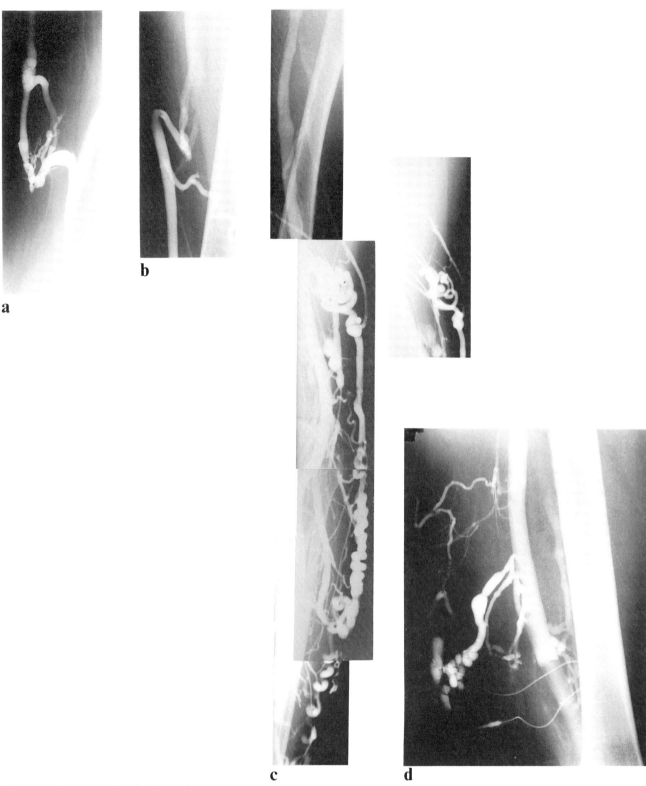

**Figure 11.18**   *Examples of spillover from mid-thigh perforators and the cause of recurrent varicose veins below this level.*

*(a)  Shown by functional phlebography in upright patient.*

*(b)  Shown by 'upward trace' used to give more detail of spillover seen briefly on screening.*

*(c)  Spillover in lower thigh to a varicosity running down to enter a gastrocnemius muscle sinus. The smaller picture is by 'upward trace' in a different rotation to give additional detail; this shows various connections but the veins are partially collapsed by near-horizontal positioning and fail to demonstrate the actual source of spillover; this was probably from an upward extension of the short saphenous vein.*

*(d)  Mid-thigh perforator as the source for recurrent varicose veins following inadequate stripping of the long saphenous vein 4 years previously*

## Perforator outflow from deep to superficial veins

This will occur in several widely differing circumstances, the first relatively innocuous and easily cured but the others potentially far more injurious and difficult to eliminate.

### I. High-level spillover and gravitational downflow. Foot circuits

This is, of course, the characteristic pattern in simple varicosities where incompetent superficial veins allow gravitational flow to occur from above a deep vein pumping mechanism to below it (Figure 11.16(a), (b)). The upper termination of a saphenous vein is no more than a particularly large perforator and incompetence in

this vein provides a special example of perforator outflow from a deep vein, falling down the saphenous vein and its varicose branches to re-enter the deep veins by perforators at various points below such pumping

**Figure 11.19** *(a) Phlebograms outlining peroneal perforators, which are the origin of spillover down varicosities to the foot. Various stages of filling are shown; the narrowing in one varicose vein is due to abortive needle puncture; the paper-clip marker is at the point of clinical control of the varicosities.*

*(b), (c) Spillover from gastrocnemius and soleus muscle sinuses to the foot.*

*(d) Spillover from posterior tibial veins at the ankle and running to the foot.*

*All these examples are suitable for local surgery (or by sclerotherapy but great caution is needed near ankle because of proximity to artery)*

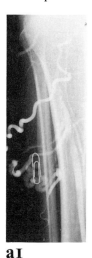

**a1**

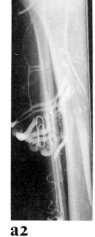

**a2**

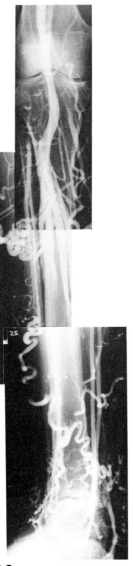

**a3**

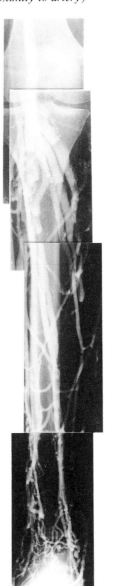

**b**

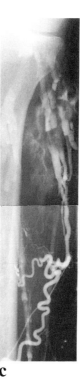

**c**

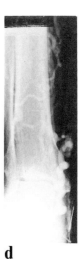

**d**

mechanisms as the calf muscles and the foot (Figure 11.17; see Chapter 4). Exactly the same phenomenon can occur through incompetent perforators in the thigh (Papadakis *et al.*, 1989) or in the leg below the knee (Figures 11.16(c), (d), 11.18, 11.19). Doppler flowmetry or functional phlebography readily demonstrate the downward flow occurring after each muscle contraction. Where this arises from leg perforators (Figures 11.16(d), 11.19), such downward flow will usually run to the underside of the foot and will occur every time the foot is raised. If correctly identified, surgical removal or obliteration by injection will bring the patient considerable benefit but,

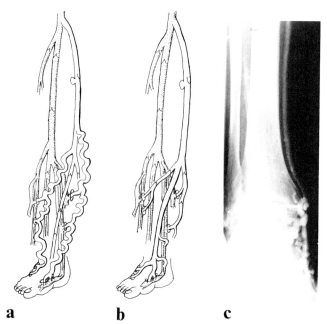

**a**          **b**          **c**

**Figure 11.20**  *Concealed or 'straight through' incompetence.*

*(a), (b) Diagrams comparing: long saphenous incompetence accompanied by varicosities (a) and concealed or 'straight through' incompetence of the long saphenous system (b) in which there are no obvious varicose veins intervening between an incompetent saphenous vein and perforators running to deep veins. This can give rise to severe venous hypertension and ulceration. It is not uncommon but is easily overlooked or attributed to perforators.*

*(c) Phlebogram of the lower end of a long saphenous vein incompetent throughout its length, with no more than ankle varicosities running to the foot, but yet the cause of threatened ulceration*

**Figure 11.21**  *Diagrams of spillover to the foot from deep veins in the leg evident after surgery removing incompetent veins above this level.*

*(a) Long saphenous vein before and after stripping down to the upper calf but leaving an incompetent perforator which allows spillover to foot varicosity.*

*(b) Incompetence to foot before and after long saphenous stripping is continued by connection with unsuspected short saphenous incompetence.*

*(c) Short saphenous varicosities to foot before and after short saphenous stripping, taken over by a gastrocnemius perforator not previously recognized*

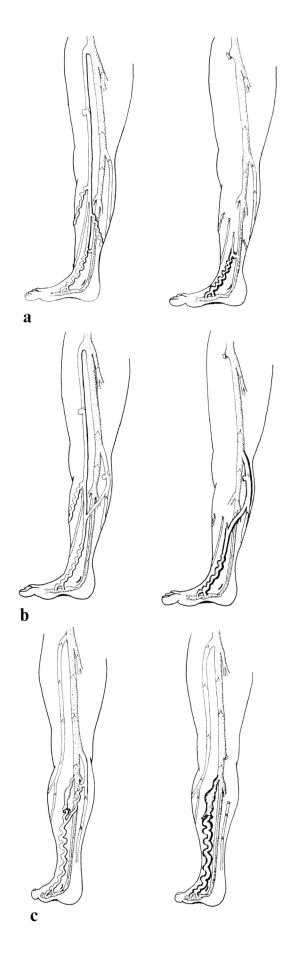

**a**

**b**

**c**

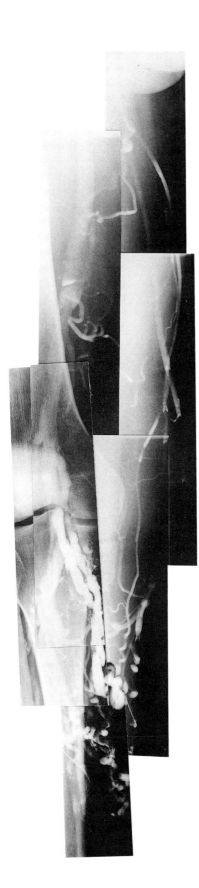

**Figure 11.22** *Gastrocnemius incompetence uncovered by surgery for short saphenous incompetence. The original state was one of short saphenous incompetence with calf varicose veins and threatened ulceration; the varicose veins were well controlled by selective short saphenous occlusion, Doppler flowmetry and phlebography confirmed a valveless short saphenous vein with downflow after exercise. Short saphenous ligation and stripping brought some improvement but varicose veins persisted on the inner calf and venotensive changes continued. A composite phlebogram 3 months after surgery is shown. Varicosities are present on the inner calf and their origin from a gastrocnemius perforator is clear. The stump of ligated short saphenous vein can be seen. Note that the long saphenous vein is well valved and most unlikely to be at fault*

again, precision in diagnosis is not always easy. One common cause of error is a concealed long saphenous incompetence (Figure 11.20) with varicosities running to the foot and only evident in the lower part of the leg (Figure 11.20(c)). It is all to easy to conclude that the origin of this downflow is from a mid-leg perforator. Alternatively, quite often a saphenous incompetence flows into an enlarged perforator in the mid-leg but also connects on to foot varicosities so that if the saphenous vein is removed without taking away the perforator then the foot circuit may persist but now being fed by perforator outflow in the mid-leg (Figure 11.21(a)). This may be sufficient to cause continuing venous stasis (Bjordal, 1972, 1977). In the same way a latent incompetence in the short saphenous vein, or perforators communicating with it, may take over a foot circuit once the dominant downflow of the long saphenous vein has been removed but leaving the hitherto unsuspected alternative source of supply to a foot circuit (Figures 11.21(b), (c), 11.22). In clinical practice it is not always possible to foresee such events and a second operation may be necessary to complete treatment. However, in any case of varicose veins, particularly when venous stasis and the threat of ulceration is present, it is important to look for foot veins and for evidence of any enlarged leg perforator; possible continuity with the short saphenous vein must be checked upon by the tapwave test. A Doppler flowmeter placed over an incompetent saphenous vein or a major tributary will show heavy downflow on raising the foot if substantial pooling on its underside is occurring, and this is a valuable indicator.

At operation any obvious varicosities going to the foot should be eliminated and if there is good reason to believe that there is a large perforator in the leg this should be identified and removed at the same time. It will often arise from the posterior arch vein but this is the sort of case where stripping of the long saphenous vein down to the mid-leg or ankle (but beware of the saphenous nerve) may be desirable and is considered further in the chapter on the surgical treatment of varicose veins (see Chapter 20).

## II. Perforator outflow pumping upwards

This is a very different category, difficult to cure and in which injudicious surgery may do considerable harm. It is seen typically in the post-thrombotic (postphlebitic) syndrome (see Chapters 8 and 9) where previous thrombosis has severely damaged major deep veins so that deformity or actual obstruction is causing resistance to venous return (Figure 11.23). There is usually widespread

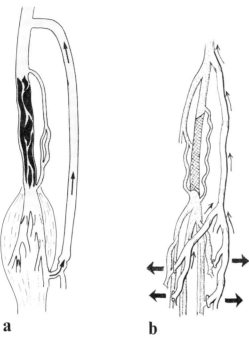

**Figure 11.23**  *Diagrams of perforator outflow as part of an upward running collateral mechanism past obstructed or deformed deep veins in post-thrombotic syndrome.*

*(a)  Dominant perforator in the lower leg taking collateral outflow to the long saphenous vein or its posterior arcuate branch.*

*(b)  Multiple perforators from venous sinuses of calf-peroneal muscles and tibial veins*

accompanying valvular damage so that effective musculovenous pumping is severely impaired. The deep veins are no longer adequate to meet the requirements of venous return created by muscular activity and return by collateral veins is essential. This usually occurs by outflow through multiple leg perforators and via branch veins into short or long saphenous veins, whichever will allow the blood to flow most easily back into deep veins somewhere above the obstruction (Figure 11.24(a)–(c)), or, in case of iliac occlusion (Figure 11.25), into lower abdominal varicosities acting as collaterals and taking flow to the opposite side. This state of affairs must always be suspected if there is a history of previous deep vein thrombosis and where there is no satisfactory control by a selective Trendelenburg test, without use of any constricting band. Doppler flowmetry gives a characteristic picture of continuous upflow in the long saphenous vein

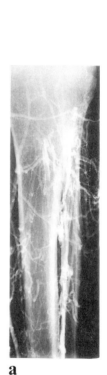
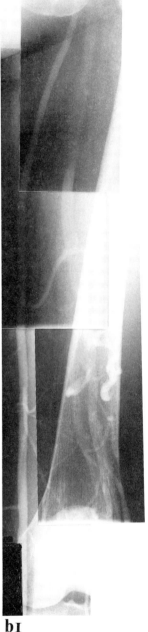

a         b1

**Figure 11.24**  *Collateral mechanisms with perforator outflow in deep vein obstruction by recent thrombus and by post-thrombotic fibrotic changes.*

*(a)  Acute thrombosis obstructing deep veins. Multiple perforators have taken on a collateral role with outflow to superficial veins.*

*(b)  The above-knee (1) and below-knee (2) portions of a composite phlebogram in a post-thrombotic limb. Preferential flow up long and short saphenous veins takes blood past an obstructed popliteal vein (and see page 223).*

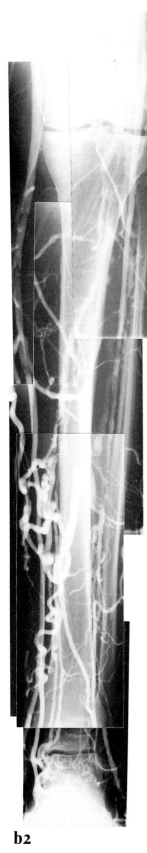

**b2**

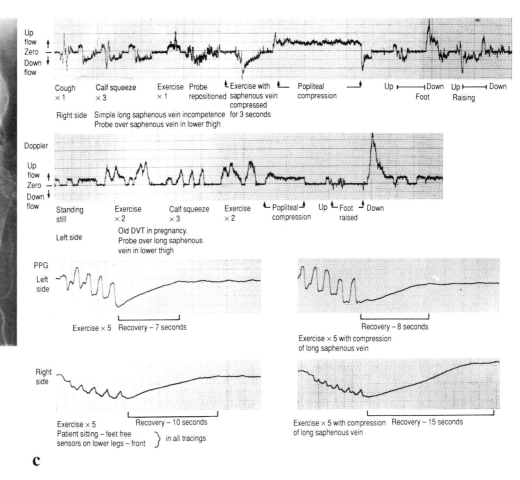

Up flow / Zero / Down flow

Cough × 1    Calf squeeze × 3    Exercise × 1    Probe repositioned    Exercise with saphenous vein compressed for 3 seconds    Popliteal compression    Up Down Foot    Up Down Raising

Right side    Simple long saphenous vein incompetence
Probe over saphenous vein in lower thigh

Doppler

Up flow / Zero / Down flow

Standing still    Exercise × 2    Calf squeeze × 3    Exercise × 2    Popliteal compression    Up Foot raised Down

Left side    Old DVT in pregnancy.
Probe over long saphenous vein in lower thigh

PPG
Left side

Exercise × 5    Recovery – 7 seconds

Recovery – 8 seconds
Exercise × 5 with compression of long saphenous vein

Right side

Exercise × 5    Recovery – 10 seconds
Patient sitting – feet free
sensors on lower legs – front  } in all tracings

Exercise × 5 with compression    Recovery – 15 seconds
of long saphenous vein

**c**

**Figure 11.24** *(continued)*
*(c)  In the same patient as (b), Doppler flow patterns showing upward collateral flow on the left side but downflow in simple saphenous incompetence on the right side. Plethysmography showing a shortened recovery period on the left side but no improvement with saphenous compression; on the right side with simple incompetence a reduced recovery period is improved by saphenous occlusion*

and its branches and this is accentuated when the leg muscles contract (Figure 11.26). Functional phlebography will show preferential upflow in saphenous veins (Figure 11.27) and, by appropriate techniques, deformity or obstruction in the deep veins may be confirmed.

*Removing perforating veins in the post-thrombotic syndrome*

Regrettably, in the past, a saphenous vein acting as a collateral to an obstructed deep vein may have been removed so that lesser branches are compelled to take over collateral function but, even so, the same diagnostic features will be present although in a more haphazard anatomical arrangement (Figure 11.28 (a)). A long saphenous vein, acting as collateral, may have good valves and, although considerably enlarged, provide a reasonably satisfactory conduit for venous return with

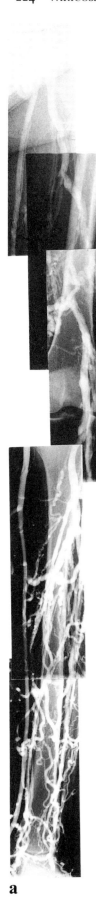

a

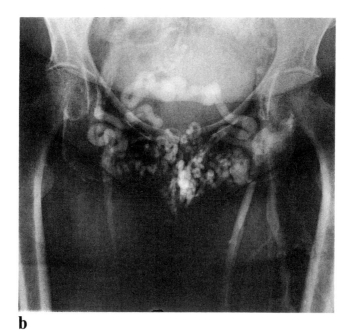

b

**Figure 11.25** *Perforator outflow in post-thrombotic syndrome.*

*(a)  Composite functional phlebogram showing multiple perforators in the collateral role. The femoral vein is deformed and occluded; the popliteal vein communicates with the profunda femoris but this is insufficient outlet and flow is driven, via perforators, preferentially up the long saphenous vein. Iliac vein occlusion is also present so that pubic varicosities pass flow over to the opposite side.*

*(b)  The pubic collateral varicosities in greater detail; these arise from the uppermost branches of the long saphenous vein*

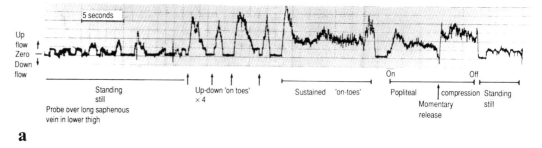

a

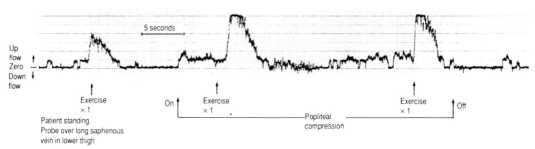

b

**Figure 11.26** *Collateral upflow in post-thrombotic deep vein impairment diagnosed by Doppler flowmetry.*

*(a)  Doppler flowmeter tracing from lower-thigh long saphenous vein in a post-thrombotic limb (postpartum), showing continuous upflow accentuated by exercise; patient is standing.*

*(b)  Similar tracing from the right long saphenous vein in a male patient following bilateral tibial fractures with deep vein thrombosis some years previously*

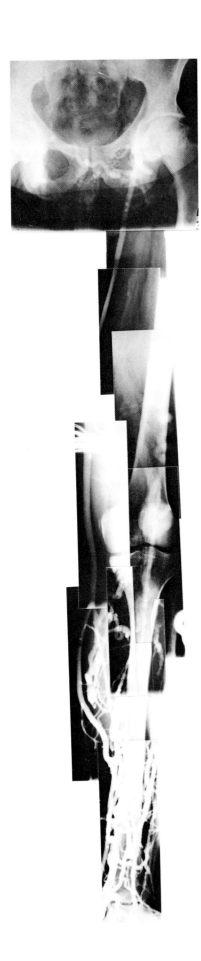

**Figure 11.27** *Composite functional phlebogram showing preferential upflow in the long saphenous vein in a post-thrombotic limb, with obstruction and deformity in deep veins. The iliac veins did not fill and pubic collateral veins are present*

effective valves to give a most valuable substitute for the deep veins (Figure 11.28(b)). Removal of this vein cannot improve the patient and a most careful assessment by functional phlebography is necessary in all these patients before any surgery is contemplated. In some circumstances where there is intractable ulceration it may be permissible to remove an individual perforator identified on phlebography while leaving a well-valved long or short saphenous vein substantially intact. This is done in the belief that removal of the perforator will lead to a redistribution of collateral outflow to multiple leg perforators so that the main impact of forceful ejection of blood to the surface is not concentrated in one small area to cause the ulcer; intense local venous hypertension is converted to a more generalized but benign hypertension (Figure 11.29). This decision requires particular care and should be backed by plethysmographic tests to make sure that shutting off the perforator with localized finger pressure does not cause an adverse response.

The very specialized operations of vein reconstruction may depend upon using the long saphenous vein, perhaps by re-routing it, and this is an additional reason for not sacrificing it without good reason, based on detailed investigation. However, it must be said that venous reconstruction of this sort is not a regularly practised skill and has yet to be shown of proven value. It is not easy to improve upon natural collateral arrangements!

## III. Local defects in perforator valve control

Local defects in perforator valve control, particularly below the knee, may cause substantial outflow from one or more perforators but not as part of a collateral mechanism. When there is accompanying superficial incompetence this may cause substantial surge back and forth through perforators and this had been considered above. However, it may be occasionally a primary cause for venous problems in the leg or foot. Here, unnaturally large veins communicating between gastrocnemius or soleus sinuses and the surface veins may well be at fault (Figures 11.14(b), 11.22, 11.30) and a list of possible causes for this has already been given in the previous section upon surge. Phlebography will be necessary to demonstrate this and to confirm that the deep veins are normal. With proper selection, surgical treatment can be successful and this is considered further in Chapter 20. The subject of gastrocnemius perforator incompetence has been well reviewed by Hobbs (1988) and includes studies by phlebography and ultrasonography.

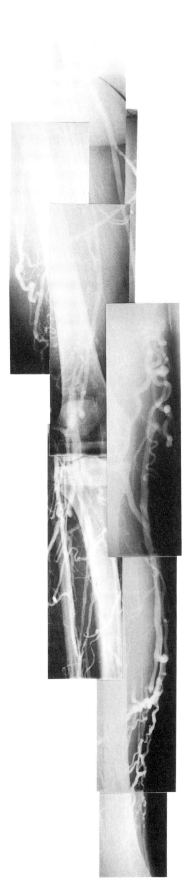

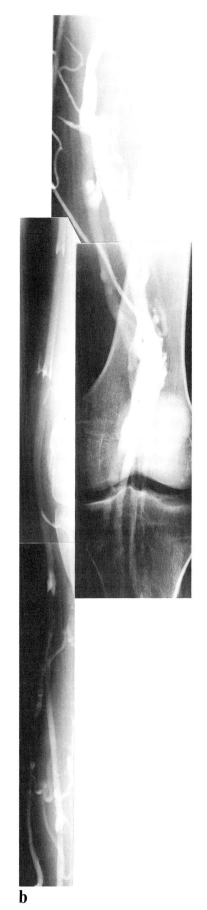

**Figure 11.28** *The collateral saphenous vein as an asset to be preserved.*

*(a) Composite functional phlebogram of a patient, aged 32 years, who sustained postpartum deep vein thrombosis of right side, 4 years previously, with persisting swelling and ulceration over the last 2 years. The ulcer had been made worse by saphenous ligation and removal of 'varicose veins' in the mid-thigh. There is extensive failure of the deep veins to fill and strong preferential flow up the superficial veins, in particular the long saphenous which is interrupted in the thigh. The dependence of this limb on the superficial veins for collateral venous return is clear. In such a limb, enlarged veins are likely to be compensatory and not causative; a collateral saphenous is an important asset. See Figure 24.7 for recordings on this patient*

*(b) A well-valved long saphenous vein acting as the main collateral vein in a post-thrombotic limb. This vein is fulfilling a valuable function and its removal, or an extensive assault on perforators, could further damage the limb*

**a**

**b**

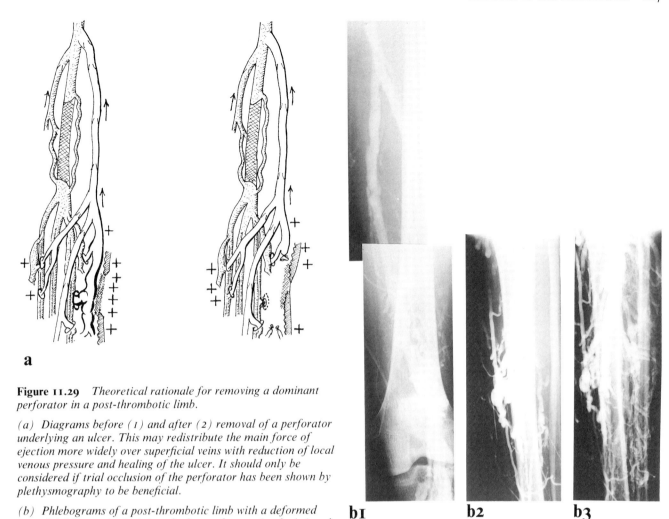

**a**

**Figure 11.29** *Theoretical rationale for removing a dominant perforator in a post-thrombotic limb.*

*(a)  Diagrams before (1) and after (2) removal of a perforator underlying an ulcer. This may redistribute the main force of ejection more widely over superficial veins with reduction of local venous pressure and healing of the ulcer. It should only be considered if trial occlusion of the perforator has been shown by plethysmography to be beneficial.*

*(b)  Phlebograms of a post-thrombotic limb with a deformed superficial femoral vein (1) and a leg perforator (early (2) and late (3) filling) which could be removed with possible advantage*

**b1**            **b2**            **b3**

## IV.  Widespread deficiency of valves

Widespread deficiency of valves is probably inborn, and gives rise to a state that we have called the valveless syndrome (primary valve failure; see Chapter 7). In this, multiple perforators seem to allow flow freely in either direction entirely at the dictates of superficial and deep venous pressures of the moment (Figure 11.31). There is no history of deep vein thrombosis and no deep vein obstruction but the overall musculovenous pumping mechanism is grossly defective and, at the time of muscle contraction, widespread outward flow under pressure from multiple perforators occurs. These patients present with venotensive changes, often with severe ulceration. Warning of this state is given by inability of the clinical tests to confirm any obvious pathway of superficial incompetence. Doppler flowmetry will show heavy surge in the superficial veins, plethysmography confirms an inadequate response to exercise with a very reduced recovery period which cannot be improved by any manipulation; functional phlebography will show widely open deep veins but fails to reveal satisfactory valves (Figure 11.32). This emphasizes the importance of systematic assessment of all patients, especially when venotensive changes are present. Such widespread perforator outflow in the valveless syndrome can scarcely be improved by surgery, but removal of massive varicose veins or individual perforators is permissible (Figure 11.33) as this is unlikely to have the same damaging consequences as ill-considered surgery in deep vein obstruction. Conservative management by external support to the leg and elevation at every possible opportunity (see Chapter 7) may be all that can be offered to the patient.

## Ligation of perforators in venous ulceration

Discussion on perforators would not be complete without reference to the influence of Cockett and others in the

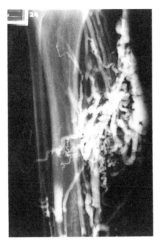

**a**

**Figure 11.30** *Misleading appearances caused by filling of gastrocnemius vein during functional phlebography in a man aged 54, 20 years after unsuccessful surgery for long saphenous varicose veins and now threatened with venous ulceration.*

*(a) Initial phlebogram shows massive intercommunication between superficial varicose veins and a leash of gastrocnemius venous sinuses. It might be concluded that the cause was gastrocnemius vein incompetence.*
*(b) However, the complete set of phlebograms shows recurrent incompetence from the groin downwards; an unstripped long saphenous vein is joined by a large communicator from the femoral vein in mid-thigh (also shown in Figure 11.18(a)). Doppler flowmetry and phlebography both showed substantial post-exercise downflow in the saphenous remnants and into the gastrocnemius veins; this is not in keeping with gastrocnemius incompetence, nor is the slender appearance of the gastrocnemius veins. Surgery removing the long saphenous remnants and the varicose veins brought considerable benefit but, because the phlebograms had shown an additional source of incompetence from profunda femoris vein, the patient was advised to wear a one-way-stretch stocking up to the knee. When reviewed one year later the limb was remaining stable in good condition. Ultrasonography with colour flow imaging would be particularly helpful in determining the role of the gastrocnemius veins in an intricate case such as this.*

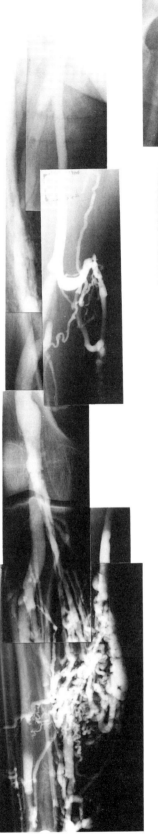

**b**

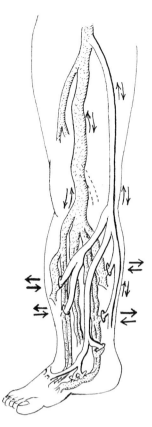

**Figure 11.31** *Diagram of the valveless syndrome in which there is a widespread deficiency of valves. This leads to surge back and forth in the deep veins and perforators without any purposeful upward pumping. It is a cause for severe venostasis and ulceration*

**Figure 11.32** *Composite functional phlebogram of the valveless syndrome with ulceration. No satisfactory deep vein valves could be demonstrated and, on exercise, heavy surge was seen in the perforator shown medially in the lower leg. The widely open deep veins make it clear that this perforating vein has no collateral function and that removing it would be permissible. However, the ulcer healed with conservative management and external support*

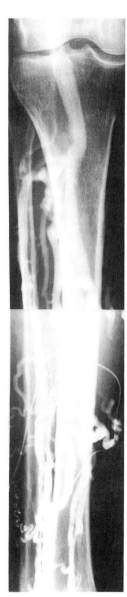

**11.32**

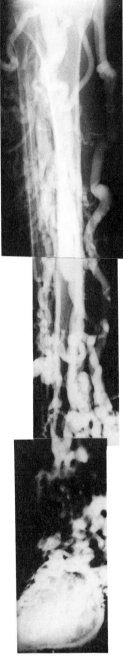

**11.33**

**Figure 11.33** *Composite functional phlebogram of the weak vein syndrome in a female aged 65 years, with venotensive change and ulceration. Both superficial and deep veins are expanded in width and length; massive varicosities run to the foot and widespread surge between deep and superficial veins was seen. The deep veins are enlarged and slightly baggy but with no evidence of occlusion; removal of any obvious perforators, the saphenous veins and their varicosities is permissible but recurrence is likely. Control of the varicosities was possible by selective occlusion of the long saphenous vein and so this was removed surgically, combined with instructing the patient in conservative management of venous hypertension. With this*

*regimen the ulcer healed and, if the patient is conscientious in elevating the limb and in using elastic support, may not recur.*

Note. *The opposite limb of this patient had obstruction of the popliteal vein with large collateral veins but without any clinical history of deep vein thrombosis; this is shown in Figure 8.6(b). A combination of thrombotic occlusion on one side and severe non-thrombotic venous insufficiency on the other, such as this, is not rare and it is uncertain whether the limb described above is the result of minor thrombotic episodes without occlusion, or whether a similar weak vein syndrome present on the opposite side made it prone to thrombosis*

1950s because, for a while, perforators in the leg came to dominate much of the thinking upon venous disorders. At that time, the link between venous ulceration and a previous deep vein thrombosis was well established (Bauer, 1948; Lockhart-Mummery and Smitham, 1951; Linton, 1953; Cockett, 1955; Dodd *et al.*, 1957) and it was accepted that when the deep veins recanalized widespread damage to their valves remained, with the resulting incompetence and reflux causing high venous pressure in the lower leg. It was argued that this high pressure, conducted to the surface by enlarged perforators, was the main cause for overlying ulceration and that ligation of such perforators could heal the ulcer, although not curing the background post-thrombotic state. This line of thought was extended to explain why venous ulceration develops in some cases of saphenous incompetence, attributing this to incompetence in perforating veins and believing that removing these was the key to curing the ulcer. However, since the incompetent saphenous vein was to be removed at the same time, it was difficult to know whether a successful outcome was due to removal of perforator or the saphenous vein, or required both to be done.

In the post-thrombotic state attempts to eliminate the damaging component of deep vein reflux were taken further by reports of successful treatment of ulceration by ligation of incompetent popliteal or superficial femoral deep veins (Bauer, 1948; Linton and Hardy, 1948; Linton 1953) and supported by favourable comment from Lockhart-Mummery and Smitham (1951). Cockett (1955), after carrying out deep vein ligation in 22 cases, concluded that it failed to improve the ulcer unless accompanied by ligation of perforating veins under the ulcer. By 1970 disillusionment had set in amongst many surgeons who found that they were unable to reproduce the reported successes and were troubled by the persistent swelling, aching calf and recurrent ulceration following deep vein ligation; often perforator ligation was not successful but, in part, this was due to misinterpretation of the views expressed by Cockett and failure to use the careful selection he advocated. Deep vein ligation was soon abandoned and perforator ligation less enthusiastically practised but dispute still continues upon the role of the perforator in the causation of venous ulcer (and, for that matter, of simple varicose veins). Much of this can now be seen in better perspective, aided by the means for accurate investigation available today. Recently, Cockett (1988) restated his indications for ankle perforator ligation, essentially those he has used since the 1950s and it is interesting to compare these with present practice. He gives three groups of patients in whom ankle perforators may play a major role in producing ankle ulceration and these will be considered in turn.

The first group of venous ulcers is those found in long or short saphenous vein incompetence without previous deep vein thrombosis and here perforator ligation is strongly indicated. Cockett states, 'High ligation, stripping [of saphenous vein] and extrafascial ankle perforator ligation produce an absolute cure in these cases, as there is no deep vein obstruction.' Present opinion is in full agreement with this and recognizes that about 50% of ulcers arise from simple superficial vein incompetence and are curable by adequate removal of the pathway of incompetence, including any enlarged perforator that is known to be present; emphasis is on the superficial incompetence rather than the perforators.

The second group described by Cockett is defined as those 'who have suffered a peripheral calf thrombosis in the past, and now have simple perforator incompetence but without any serious deep vein obstruction' and these patients 'can also get excellent curative, long-term results from ankle perforator ligation, particularly if done before serious skin deterioration sets in'. However, this is an ill-defined group likely to include a variety of venous disorders, uncertain in their response to perforator ligation and requiring investigation by the best of modern techniques to demonstrate if the venous disorder is suitable for surgery and not likely to be harmed by it. Clinical judgement alone will not be sufficient here. Without scrutiny by Doppler flowmetry, ultrasonography and functional phlebography, superficial vein incompetence from concealed saphenous incompetence or by mid-thigh perforator may go unrecognized when treatment should include removal of the source and pathway leading down to the perforator; primary valve failure (valveless syndrome) should be recognized as perforator surgery is likely to be ineffective; clinically unsuspected post-thrombotic states may be found where perforator ligation may sacrifice important collateral vessels. This group of 'localized thrombotic damage will require careful appraisal if a reasonable success rate is to be safely achieved. Surgical exploration for enlarged perforators (Linton, 1938, 1953; Cockett, 1955, and see Chapter 20) of uncertain causation is seldom necessary now and should be replaced by identification of the perforator at phlebography and its elimination through a small incision.

The third group referred to by Cockett is one in which perforator ligation is strongly contraindicated and consists of patients who have had an extensive iliofemoral thrombosis. A particular warning is given of the poor results to be expected from perforator surgery in this group. In such patients extensive deformity and obstruction is present in the deep veins so that venous hypertension in the leg is due to a combination of this together with widespread incompetence in the valves. Perforating veins in the leg are part of a compensatory mechanism contributing to venous return and not to be sacrificed lightly, but at the same time they are conducting high pressure from the deep vein to the surface. Present opinion agrees that an ulcer in iliofemoral or any other pattern of severe post-thrombotic deep vein damage will seldom benefit by removing such perforators, or even less likely, by removing a saphenous vein, possibly well valved, thereby sacrificing a valuable collateral channel.

To distinguish this from the favourable circumstances found in superficial incompetence is crucial but easily achieved by the investigations referred to above. Operations reconstructing deep vein or valves (see Chapter 21) may be possible but in most cases conservative treatment is all that can be offered to this iliofemoral group. However, as mentioned earlier, there is an occasional exception when an intractable ulcer has a large perforator under it which is thought to be giving an unusual concentration of pressure to this area. It is possible that the ulcer will heal if the perforator is removed so that collateral flow is redistributed to a number of perforators elsewhere but it is essential to assess the flow patterns by phlebography beforehand and to test the response to plethsymography caused by temporary occlusion of the perforator whilst the patient exercises.

In this third group, Cockett's warning against perforator ligation is in full accord with present day thinking. His advice of 40 years ago was not for the wholesale destruction of perforators but only in selected circumstances and if this is heeded good results can be obtained and indeed many surgeons continue to support his original views, for example, Negus (1985, 1991). Perhaps the greatest difference is in the first group in which Cockett laid emphasis on the role of the perforator, whereas now it is on the causative role of the superficial incompetence with the perforator an incidental feature best eliminated if it shows enlargement and surge. As regards the other groups, the undesirability of large exploratory operations to remove perforators in post-thrombotic states is now widely recognized, together with an increasing awareness of the value of the ever-improving means for precise diagnosis available to us.

## Conclusion

It is hoped that the discussions on perforator flow given above have made it clear that the mere identification of an enlarged perforator does not justify its removal. The significance of that perforator must be determined and a decision made appropriately from this. In arriving at this decision the clinical tests may not be sufficient and it is here that additional investigation by Doppler flowmetry, plethysmography, functional phlebography and ultrasonography can prove so valuable. The role of the perforator in venous disorders is the most frequently misunderstood aspect of all. The questions must always be, is it incidental, is it causative or is it possibly fulfilling a useful collateral role?

## References

Barber, R. F. and Shatara, F. I. (1925) The varicose disease. *New York State Journal of Medicine*, **25**, 162–166

Barker, W. F. (1978) The postphlebitic syndrome: management by surgical means. In *Venous Problems* (eds. J. J. Bergan and J. S. T. Yao), Year Book Medical Publishers, Chicago, pp. 383–393

Bauer, G. (1948) The etiology of leg ulcers and their treatment by resection of the popliteal vein. *Journal of International Chirurgica*, **8**, 937

Bjordal, R. I. (1972) Circulation patterns in incompetent perforating veins in the calf and in the saphenous system in primary varicose veins. *Acta Chirurgica Scandinavica*, **138**, 251

Bjordal, R. I. (1974) Circulation patterns in the saphenous system and the perforating veins of the calf in patients with previous deep vein thrombosis. *Vasa supplementum*, **3**.

Bjordal, R. I. (1977) Haemodynamic studies of varicose veins and the post-thrombotic syndrome. In *The Treatment of Venous Disorders* (ed. J. T. Hobbs), MTP, Lancaster, pp. 37–55

Bjordal, R. I. (1981) Circulation patterns in incompetent perforating veins of the calf in venous dysfunction. In *Perforating Veins* (eds R. May, P. Partsch and J. Staubesand), Urban & Schwarzenberg, Munchen, pp. 71–88

Boileau Grant, J. C. (1947) *Atlas of Anatomy*. Balliere, Tindall and Cox, London

Cockett, P. B. (1955) The pathology and treatment of venous ulcers of the leg. *British Journal of Surgery*, **43**, 260–278

Cockett, F. B. (1956) Diagnosis and surgery of high-pressure leaks in the leg. *British Medical Journal*, **2**, 1399–1413

Cockett, F. B. (1988) Indications for and complications of the ankle perforator exploration. *Phlebology*, **3**, 3–6

Cockett, F. B. and Dodd, H. (1976) *The Pathology and Surgery of the Veins of the Lower Limb*, Churchill Livingstone, Edinburgh

Cockett, F. B. and Elgan Jones, D. E. (1953) The ankle blowout syndrome. *Lancet*, **i**, 17–23

Dodd, H., Calo, A. R., Mistry, M. and Rushford, A. (1957) Ligation of ankle communicating veins in the treatment of the venous-ulcer syndrome of the leg. *Lancet*, **ii**, 1249

Green, N. A., Griffiths, J. D. and Lavy, G. A. D. (1958) Venous drainage of anterior tibio-fibular compartment of leg, with reference to varicose veins. *British Medical Journal*, **1**, 1209–1210

Hadfield, J. I. H. (1971) The anatomy of the perforating veins in the leg. In *The Treatment of Varicose Veins by Injection and Compression*, Stoke Mandeville Symposium

Haeger, K. (1977) Leg ulcers. In *The Treatment of Venous Disorders* (ed. J. T. Hobbs), MTP, Lancaster, pp. 272–291

Hobbs, J. T. (1988) The enigma of the gastrocnemius vein. *Phlebology*, **3**, 19–30

Johnston, T. B. and Whillis, J. (1938) *Gray's Anatomy*, Longmans Green, London, p. 666

Linton, R. R. (1938) The communicating veins of the lower leg and the operative technic for their ligation. *Annals of Surgery*, **107**, 582–593

Linton, R. R. (1953) The post-thrombotic ulceration of the lower extremity: its etiology and surgical treatment. *Annals of Surgery*, **138**, 415–433

Linton, R. R. and Hardy, I. B. Jr (1948) Postthrombotic syndrome of the lower extremity. Treatment by interruption of the superficial femoral vein and ligation and stripping of the long and short saphenous veins. *Surgery*, **24**, 452–468

Lockhart-Mummery, H. E. and Smitham, J. H. (1951) Varicose ulcer. A study of the deep veins with special reference to retrograde venography. *British Journal of Surgery*, **38**, 284

McMullin, G. M., Coleridge Smith, P. D. and Scurr, J. H. (1991) Which way does blood flow in the perforation veins of the leg? *Phlebology*, **6**, 127–132

May, R. (1979) *Surgery of the Veins of the Leg and Pelvis*, Saunders, Philadelphia

May, R., Partsch, P. and Staubesand, J. (eds) (1981) *Perforating Veins*, Urban & Schwarzenberg, Munchen

Negus, D. (1985) Perforating vein interruption in the post-phlebitic syndrome. In *Surgery of the Veins* (eds J. J. Bergan and J. T. Yao), Grune & Stratton, New York, pp. 191–204

Negus, D. (1991) *Leg Ulcers*, Butterworth–Heinemann, Oxford

Papadakis, K., Christodoulou, C., Christopoulos, D. *et al.* (1989) Number and anatomical distribution of incompetent thigh perforating veins. *British Journal of Surgery*, **76**, 581–584

Raivio, E. (1948) Untersuchungen uber die venen der unteren extremitaten mit besonderer berucksichtigung der gegenseitigen venen bindungen zivischen den oberflachlichen und tiefen venen. *Ann. Med. Exp. Biol. Fenniae*, **26**

Thomson, H. (1979) The surgical anatomy of the superficial and perforating veins of the lower limb. *Annals of the Royal College of Surgeons of England*, **61**, 198–205

# Bibliography

Akesson, H., Brudin, L., Cwikiel, W. *et al.* (1990) Does the correction of insufficient superficial and perforating veins improve venous function in patients with deep venous insufficiency? *Phlebology*, **5**, 113–123

McMullin, G. M., Scott, H. J., Coleridge Smith, P. D. and Scurr, J. H. (1990) A reassessment of the role of perforating veins in chronic venous insufficiency. *Phlebology*, **5**, 85–94

Vandenriessche, M. (1989) The association between gastrocnemius vein insufficiency and varicose veins. *Phlebology*, **4**, 171–184

Zukowski, A. J., Nicolaides, A. N., Szendro, G. *et al.* (1991) Haemodynamic significance of incompetent perforating veins. *British Journal of Surgery*, **78**, 625–629

# 12

# Congenital venous disorders

This chapter is concerned with the angiodysplasias, that is, abnormalities in the development of veins, arteries and lymphatics. Neighbouring embryonic tissue such as bone may participate and the malformations vary from insignificant to massive involvement of an entire limb to a degree that affects the patient's way of life and ultimately may cause loss of the limb. For descriptive purposes they are divided here into:

- Localized vascular abnormalities (angiodysplasia).
- Extensive venous, arterial or lymphatic abnormalities.
- Mixed or complex vascular abnormalities (mixed angiodysplasias).

The lymphatic states are referred to because they are often present in combination with the other abnormalities, or are important in the differential diagnosis, but for a complete account specialist works should be consulted (Kinmonth, 1972).

## Localized angiodysplasia

### Lesions of venous origin

*Simple angiomas (also known as haemangiomas or phlebangiomas)*

These arise from abnormal development of the small blood vessels and two types are usually described, the capillary and the cavernous, according to the type of blood vessel that predominates, although in fact both types may be present to some extent.

**Capillary naevus** This lesion is a common cutaneous birthmark and is composed of tissue filled with an unnatural excess of capillary-type vessels (Figure 12.1). The main feature is a disfiguring, flat area of red discolouration and hence such terms as port wine naevus. Another variety is the strawberry naevus which forms a compressible bulge just beneath the skin and mottled red in colour. This distinctive swelling, present at birth, usually disappears within a year or two. Other more diffuse types persist and may become more obvious as the child grows. They are, however, non-malignant ham-

artomas (tumours caused by developmental errors) and harmless in spite of apparent spread.

*Treatment* For small lesions treatment by plastic surgery, micro-injections of sclerosant or repeated application of an argon laser may be successful. Treatment of the more extensive lesions is often impracticable.

**Cavernous naevus** This is composed of a spongework of blood-filled caverns or sinuses (Figure 12.1) and often accompanies abnormalities in the development of veins. It has no regard for the usual tissue boundaries and may often spread in continuity across skin, subcutaneous fat and muscle. Almost any structure in the body may be

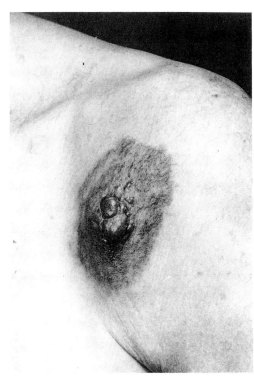

**Figure 12.1** *A mixed angioma on the shoulder. It was deep red in colour and the raised centre portion composed of large irregular blood-filled spaces typical of cavernous angioma. The surrounding area was of capillary angioma made up of numerous small calibre vessels of regular outline*

233

affected, usually without any ill effect and unknown to the patient. It is most commonly recognized in the subcutaneous tissues where it is clearly visible as a bluish swelling which varies in prominence. Besides being a visible blemish, it may cause discomfort when maximally distended or by virtue of its position, such as on the underside of the foot or hand (Figure 12.2). If near the surface quite severe bleeding may occur with injury. Spontaneous thrombosis may occur and occasionally cause regression.

**Possible relationship of cavernous angioma to trauma in childhood**  Occasionally an adult patient with a sub-

stantial cavernous haemangioma on an extremity gives a clear history of trauma by crushing of the affected area in infancy and an example is given in Figure 12.3. The peculiarly well defined lesion, together with the account passed on by the parents, is very persuasive but equally it is fully understandable that parents who had not previously noticed an abnormality might attribute a persisting swelling to the injury. It is conceivable that a haematoma in an infant might organize to form an angiomatous structure. In this case it has similarities to the revascularization (neovascularization) that has been shown to re-establish flow following interruption of a vein and a probable cause for one form of recurrence

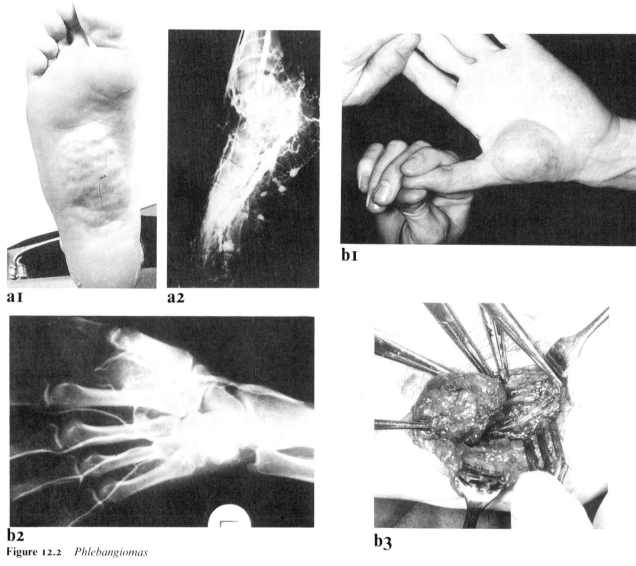

**a1**  **a2**  **b1**

**b2**  **b3**

**Figure 12.2**  *Phlebangiomas*

*(a)*  *1. Cavernous angioma on the underside of the foot. This was causing discomfort on standing and was relieved by surgical resection which proved relatively easy.*
*2. Venous phase of arteriogram showing patchy filling of the same angioma on the sole of the foot.*

*(b)*  *Cavernous angioma of the hand.*
*1. Before operation.*
*2. Angioma outlined by arteriography. Filling of angioma by this means is not always successful; direct injection is often more informative.*
*3. During operation, with the main bulk of the angioma separated*

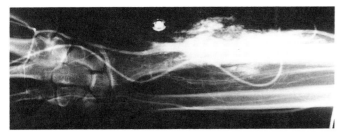

**Figure 12.3** *Angioma within the forearm, first observed after crush injury as an infant of 2 years. This arteriogram is of an angioma in a man who complained of swelling in the right forearm which became tense and caused discomfort with manual work. At operation it was found to be well defined and completely enveloping the radial artery. In other respects it seemed a typical cavernous haemangioma and was comparatively easy to remove, with preservation of the artery, giving a good result. Whether trauma in childhood can ever cause a form of cavernous angioma is not known but some cases, such as this, suggest this possibility*

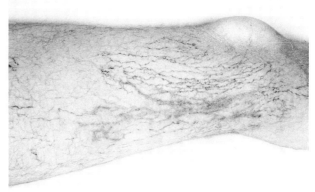

**Figure 12.4** *Hereditary telangiectasia with numerous small veins running in the skin of the thigh; both sides were similarly affected and there was a family history going back several generations. The dark areas are veins successfully sclerosed by a trial injection but the patient declined further treatment because the veins troubled him so little (see Figure 19.8(b)1 for close-up view)*

after ligation of a saphenous vein; this is discussed with illustrations in Chapter 5.

*Treatment* Localized angiomas are often suitable for surgical removal by meticulous dissection, separating the vascular spongework from the normal neighbouring tissues and structures (Figure 12.2(b)3). The blood within is at low pressure and although during operation bleeding can be copious it is easily controlled by light pressure or by use of a tourniquet. There is no surrounding capsule or clear boundary and inevitably outlying areas of angioma have to be cut across and left behind rather than risk damage to important anatomy. Postoperative haematoma formation may be troublesome because of the numerous apertures in divided remnants, each capable of bleeding so that effective haemostasis is difficult. This difficulty is increased by the deceptive way in which the vascular spongework may collapse down, especially under tourniquet, so that its potential for bleeding later, when it refills, is underrated; it is helpful to lift up tissue with forceps to see if this reveals the gaping spaces lined with shining endothelium that characterize cavernous angiomas. If approached with proper respect, surgery is perfectly feasible in the circumscribed lesions but the more diffuse states can provide formidable problems.

**Hereditary telangiectasia** This is a rare condition that runs in families to give numerous irregular venules, about 1 mm across, on the skin of the lower limbs (Figure 12.4). Although these may bleed with mild trauma this is not an undue problem. It is an unwelcome blemish and treatment by injection of dilute sclerosant to each vein is possible but tedious. This is a separate condition from hereditary haemorrhagic telangiectasia (Osler–Weber–Rendu disease) which can cause troublesome bleeding from the nose, mouth and intestinal tract as well as the skin.

Telangiectasia may also occur as a small birthmark which persists but may be treated by sclerotherapy or surgical excision. Other varieties of localized or widespread telangiectasia are usually acquired, often as a harmless manifestation of advancing years, but may have diagnostic importance, for example, in lupus erythematosis or in liver disease.

## Lesions of arterial origin

### Localized arteriovenous fistula

An arteriovenous fistula is most frequently seen as a localized lesion causing a swelling, perhaps pulsatile as in the cirsoid aneurysm, often with a thrill or bruit and prominent veins leading from it. In the congenital variety (Figure 12.5(a)–(c)) surrounding structures, including bone, show hypertrophy (Figure 12.14). Treatment is by surgical excision if the lesion is suitable, or by occluding the artery of supply by a technique of embolism through an arterial catheter. This condition is discussed more fully in the section upon diffuse arteriovenous fistulas later in this chapter.

## Lesions of lymphatic or mixed origin

### Localized congenital lymphatic abnormalities

The lymphatic abnormalities will be described in this chapter only in so far as they relate to other vascular changes. Localized lymphatic states include cysts and cystic hygroma, lymphangioma, lymph fistula, and lymphangioma circumscriptum (Browse *et al.*, 1986). They are often intermingled with haemangioma to produce complex lesions. The most comprehensive account on lymphatic disorders is by Kinmonth (1972).

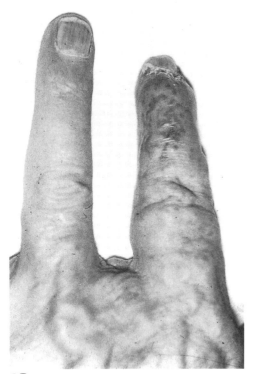

**a1**

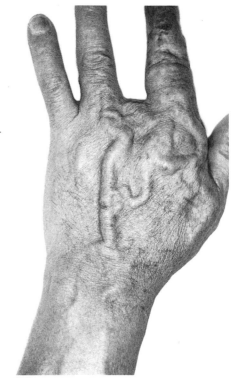

**a2**

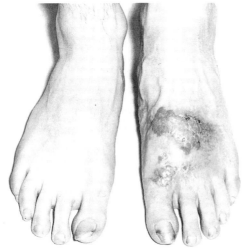

**b**

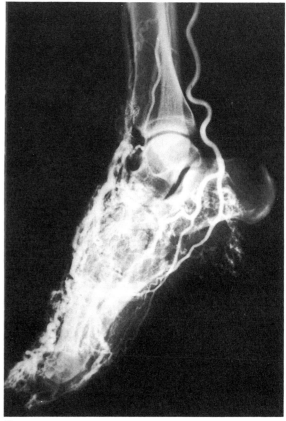

**c**

**Figure 12.5** *Localized congenital arteriovenous fistula.*

*(a) 1, 2. The hand of a man aged 40 years. The first and second fingers showed changes that had increased through childhood and were only temporarily relieved by amputation of the second finger. The enlarged veins are typical and denote high venous pressure and flow; the index finger shows characteristic venous ulceration. Amputation of the index finger brought relief from ulceration and haemorrhage, but remaining fistulous areas in the palm may cause trouble in the future.*

*(b) Arteriovenous fistulous lesion confined to the foot of a boy aged 12 years. Enlarged veins are evident and the skin is showing brown pigmentation with the threat of ulceration to come, typical of the changes caused by venous hypertension. The fistulous area ramified through deeper structures of the foot so that local excision was not possible. A policy of external support was* followed but it is possible that amputation may become necessary sooner or later.

*(c) Arteriogram of a similar arteriovenous lesion in the foot of a young woman*

# Widespread, diffuse or regional angiodysplasia

## Classification

The vascular system of a limb can develop abnormally in various ways to produce extensive venous lesions which may be divided broadly into the following categories (adapted from Malan and Puglionsi, 1964):

1. Abnormal or aberrant anatomical arrangement of the major veins which are displaced and perhaps malformed in some fashion.
2. Venous dysplasias, that is abnormal development of vein structure and composition of which there are several forms:
   (a) Phlebectasia, an unnatural and irregular enlargement or varicosity, recognized most easily in the superficial veins but it may also affect deep veins.
   (b) Phlebangiomatosis, a mainly cavernous, diffuse angiomatous state in place of capillary beds, venules, and lesser veins. It may involve superficial and deep tissues, including bone.
   (c) Hypoplasia or agenesis, an underdevelopment, atresia or total failure, most significant when affecting deep veins.
3. Mixed angiodysplasia, where any of the states given above combine with lymphatic and other tissues; various complex forms may occur with other congenital malformations, such as spina bifida or incomplete development of a hand or foot.
4. Arterial dysplasias, the most important of which is the formation of arteriovenous fistula. This may be localized, as previously described, or multiple and diffuse.
5. Lymphatic dysplasia, which may be obscured by the venous lesions but is commonly present and may take various forms.

Any of the states above may be accompanied by increased bone growth with corresponding change in the length of limb. There appears to be two forms of bone overgrowth related either to venous lesions or to arteriovenous fistulas and this is discussed presently.

*Anatomical anomalies of the major veins*

*Note.* Varicose veins from simple superficial incompetence are quite frequently seen in young patients and may well be due to an inherited insufficiency of valves, but, once a major underlying disorder has been excluded, it is best to view them as acquired varicose veins of early onset rather than a congenital anomaly. This will not be considered further in this chapter except in connection with differential diagnosis.

When true anomalies arise, one dominant pattern is based on persistence of the embryonic axial vein as a 'sciatic' vein similar to the well-recognized arterial anomaly (Figure 12.6), but not necessarily occurring concurrently with it. This aberrant deep vein terminates in the profunda femoris vein or accompanies the sciatic nerve into the pelvis to join the internal iliac vein (Figure 12.7(a)). The superficial veins may share in the abnormal development, for example, by persistence of an external marginal vein usually absorbed, to form a large lateral channel running subcutaneously up the outer aspect of the limb (Figures 12.7(b), 12.8) giving branches to the aberrant deep vein. In its lower part this deep vein is usually in continuity with the popliteal vein and often appears to substitute for the normal superficial and common femoral veins which are separate from it, smaller than usual (hypoplastic), or even absent (agenetic). In fact the main venous return from the limb may be largely dependent upon the abnormal vein which may be large

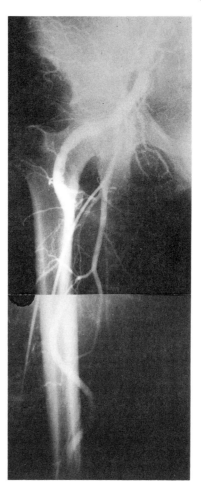

**Figure 12.6** *An example of a persistent sciatic artery to show the course taken in this anomaly, extending from the internal iliac artery, through the sciatic notch, and down the thigh alongside the sciatic nerve. It was present bilaterally and revealed by chance when investigating claudication caused by thrombosis of the aberrant artery of the opposite side. Note the course running parallel with the neck of the femur when viewed anteroposteriorly. A sciatic vein may terminate by taking a similar course but the anomalous artery and vein are not necessarily both present in the same patient*

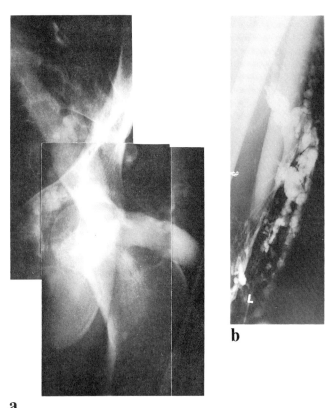

**a**

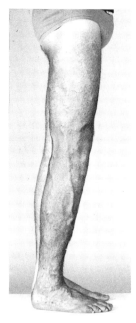

**Figure 12.8** *Persistent lateral vein in a patient with Klippel–Trenaunay syndrome*

**Figure 12.7** *Phlebograms of sciatic vein and accompanying subcutaneous vein. This was associated with extensive angiomatosis and phlebectasia in a boy of 16 years. (See Figure 12.16 for clinical photograph of this patient.) The femoral vein was hypoplastic but there was no discrepancy in the length of the limbs.*

*(a) Upper part of sciatic vein following a similar course to the artery in Figure 12.6 and joining the internal iliac vein.*

*(b) Communications between a subcutaneous lateral vein and the thigh portion of the anomalous sciatic deep vein illustrated in (a)*

and valveless so that an unwary surgeon may be tempted to ligate or even remove it together with the superficial lateral vein. This can cause a surgical disaster by precipitating venous gangrene and loss of the limb. When a congenital anomaly of the venous system is suspected careful evaluation by phlebography is essential before any form of venous ablation is carried out, no matter how undesirable the abnormal veins may seem to be; they may have the indispensible virtue of being the main pathway of venous return. The valveless veins are perhaps the source of considerable inconvenience to the patient but this is manageable by an appropriate way of life and external support. There can be no justification for putting the limb in danger by removing abnormal veins without knowledge of the alternative venous return.

The anomalies described above have many variants in actual form and extent. The lateral superficial venous channel referred to above may develop without any abnormality in the deep vein and is an example of phlebectasia; it is a common feature of Klippel–Trenaunay

syndrome (see below) but not necessarily accompanied by this.

*Phlebectasia and phlebangiomatosis*

These changes are often diffuse and extensive, without following any fixed pattern. In the same limb it may be possible to identify the typical spongework of cavernous angiomas alongside massively enlarged superficial veins, such as the lateral venous channel described above. The changes are not uniform; in parts of the limb massive, often tortuous, superficial veins may predominate with normal overlying skin, whilst in other parts the skin is extensively affected by a mixed capillary and cavernous angiomatosis communicating freely with ectatic veins beneath (Figures 12.7(b), 12.16). Aberrant major deep veins may accompany this but not necessarily so. Any combination of abnormalities can occur and perhaps are all representative of the similar fault in the development of the venous system.

The enlarged veins and cavernoangiomatous tissue form a series of channels and provide a pathway, however unsatisfactory, of venous return. This is a very important point because it is possible that there has been an accompanying failure of the deep veins to develop (agenesis) and the extensive abnormal superficial veins are the only channels of venous return. Extensive surgical attack upon the massive venous lakes, for cosmetic reasons or for fear of haemorrhage, could well lead to loss of the limb in these circumstances (Figure 12.9). Thus the point must be made once again that with congenital venous abnormalities it is essential to visualize the deep veins by phlebography before any ablative treatment is contemplated.

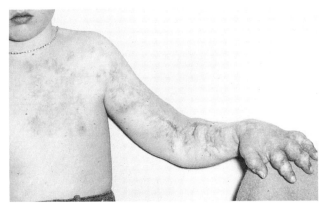

**Figure 12.9** *Severe phlebangiomatosis and phlebectasia present from birth and affecting the left upper limb and shoulder. At the time of this illustration the patient was a boy of 8 years and extensive removal of cavernous angiomas had been carried out in the forearm. A further operation removing only enlarged superficial veins and angiomatous tissue caused venous gangrene, with loss of the limb, because of aplasia of the deep veins*

### Mixed and complex dysplasias

This group (Kinmonth *et al.*, 1976) includes mixed venous and lymphatic angiomas which are commonly combined. Complex states may arise where there are accompanying dysplasias in other tissues, such as bone, or neurofibromatosis, or if there are further congenital lesions elsewhere in the body.

### Multiple or diffuse arteriovenous fistula

Although the malformations described on the venous side may be unsightly and troublesome to the patient, they do not have the unpleasant complications and significance of the main arterial abnormality, arteriovenous fistula. In this state there is a communication between arteries and veins without a normal intervening capillary bed. Instead, multiple channels allow substantial shunting of blood virtually directly into the veins. An arteriovenous fistula may arise from trauma but here the communication is usually by a single large opening; in the congenital form, the shunt is by many small channels forming a spongework (arteriovenous angioma or arterial cavernous angioma) over an area of tissue. This may be limited to a few centimetres across, for example, part of a foot, or involve a whole limb (Parkes-Weber's syndrome), with adverse consequences both for the limb and for the heart. This distinctive angiodysplasia is described more fully later in this chapter.

### Distinguishing acquired varicose veins from congenital venous disorder

Unnaturally positioned and enlarged veins in a young person should always give rise to suspicion of venous or arterial dysplasia. The veins may appear so typically varicose that they are interpreted as being simple (primary) varicose veins due to saphenous incompetence in, say, a teenager. Such simple varicosities should appear in the usual sites familiar in adults and, above all, be well controlled by a selectively applied Trendelenburg test. In the absence of such positive recognition, no 'varicose vein' in a young person should be subjected to surgery without careful thought and, if in doubt, backed by phlebography confirming normal deep veins.

The surgeon must be aware of the patterns of congenital abnormality that may first present as 'varicose veins', such as the Klippel–Trenaunay (1900) and Parkes-Weber's (1907, 1918) syndromes. Not only may unwitting surgery to, say, the prominent veins of the latter syndrome cause alarming difficulties but there are other aspects to consider, such as possible inequality of limb length. These syndromes are considered in more detail later in this chapter.

### Ulceration in the congenital vascular disorders

Ulceration commonly occurs sooner or later in extensive congenital venous and arterial disorders. Both are caused by sustained high venous pressure just as in acquired incompetence of superficial and deep veins. In the congenital venous states this is due to venous reflux in large, abnormal valveless superficial or deep veins; in arteriovenous fistula, however, the mechanism is different and it is the arteriovenous shunt transferring arterial pressure across to the venous side that causes venous hypertension, the common denominator between these conditions.

The various changes described above may be only one aspect of extensive developmental errors in the limb. A well-known example of this is the Klippel–Trenaunay syndrome in which vascular changes, not necessarily severe, are associated with bone overgrowth so that the limb becomes progressively longer than the normal side as the child grows. This must be specifically looked for in any young patient with vascular blemishes because the bone changes may pass unnoticed in the early years. Correspondingly when the presenting manifestation is inequality of the limbs due to overgrowth on one side then a search for vascular and other tissue abnormalities should be made. A description of these states follows.

## Patterns in clinical presentation of congenital vascular abnormalities in the limbs

The clinical presentation of the various forms of angiodysplasia, described above, may be grouped into several broad categories. It has already been pointed out that alteration in the length of the affected limb may accompany vascular abnormality and this is a distinguishing feature used in the grouping. The following categories occur:

1. Venous dysplasia *without* change in the limb length.
2. Venous dysplasia *with* change (usually lengthening) in the limb length, known as Klippel–Trenaunay syndrome. Confusion has been caused in the past because some descriptions failed to distinguish between this and the separate condition of limb lengthening due to arteriovenous fistulas.
3. Mixed or complex tissue dysplasia with or without alteration in the length of the limb.
4. Arteriovenous fistulas, usually accompanied by overgrowth of bone and lengthing of the limb (Parkes-Weber's syndrome), depending on the extent of fistula formation. Venous angiomatosis seldom accompanies this category but discolouration due to underlying arteriovenous fistulous spongeworks may be mistaken for it. In some past descriptions, the Klippel–Trenaunay syndrome, a venous dysplasia, has not been distinguished from this separate entity.
5. Overgrowth of the limb without any vascular abnormality; usually seen in orthopaedic rather than vascular clinics.

*Note 1.* 'Limb overlengthening' is a much more specific term than hypertrophy which implies increase in bulk as well as length. Many of these limbs do have a considerable increase in bulk, but in some it is slight and indeed some arteriovenous fistulous limbs may be more slender than the normal side. The bone change has its own significance as regards the patient's welfare and management. It is an aspect separate from the vascular changes which are usually closely related to the general bulk of the soft tissues. Angiomatous tissue, especially when filled with blood, is bulky and, together with any associated lymphatic dysplasia and consequent oedema, accounts for much of the increase in size.

*Note 2.* Howell (1978) reports hypostatic ulceration in six cases of XXY chromosomal abnormality with Klinefelter's syndrome. All were associated with varicose veins, chronic oedema and pigmentation; in three there was no history of deep vein thrombosis. All were above average height, 1.77 m (approximately 5 ft 9¾ in.) or more. It seems likely that, perhaps, one in three patients with this syndrome will have defective veins leading to ulceration. It is of interest that a chromosomal abnormality should be linked with defective veins and unusual length of the limbs but the relevance of this to the overgrowth of limbs discussed in this chapter is uncertain.

## Relationship of overlengthening of the limb to angiodysplasia

In the past there has been confusion caused by failure to distinguish between the lengthened limb in Klippel–Trenaunay syndrome, a purely venous dysplasia, and Parkes-Weber's syndrome, a phenomenon of arteriovenous shunting. The original authors describing these syndromes gave clear descriptions, one without any suggestion of arteriovenous fistulous manifestations (except bone lengthening), and the other with all the features now recognized as characteristic of arteriovenous fistula. Although these two syndromes have some similarities they are in fact very different in prognosis and in their management. The purely venous syndrome is relatively harmless and usually requires only conservative treatment, but the arteriovenous state can present severe problems, progressive deterioration, an increasing burden to the heart and possibly a threat to life, forestalled only by losing the limb. For this reason the eponymous titles given to these syndromes are retained as obvious markers in describing two clinically separate conditions.

The shared feature of bone lengthening gave rise to the confusion between them. However, when it had been established that Parkes-Weber's syndrome was a phenomenon of arteriovenous shunting with vascular involvement of the epiphyses as the cause of bone overgrowth, and this was reproducible experimentally, many attempts were made to demonstrate a hidden hyperaemia in Klippel–Trenaunay syndrome. However, no really convincing evidence of this has yet been found; the typical appearances of arteriovenous fistula have not been demonstrated by arteriogram and, for example, Baskerville, Ackroyd and Browse (1986) found only slight increase in the overall blood flow through the limb, whilst Partsch, Mostbeck and Wolf (1986) could not find any evidence of arteriovenous shunts by labelled microspheres injected into the arteries. A different aetiology for the bone lengthening in Klippel–Trenaunay syndrome must be considered but yet, for reasons given presently, it is hard to believe that there is not some relationship.

If hypervascularity is not the cause, does Klippel–Trenaunay syndrome relate to any other state giving similar changes in the length of a limb? Bone overgrowth and overlengthening is also well recognized as an orthopaedic condition without any vascular abnormalities (McCullough and Kenwright, 1979; Clarke, Tibbs and Kenwright, 1986). Although the cause here is unknown it does indicate that bone overgrowth is possible without hypervascularity, but there is no evidence that this relates to Klippel–Trenaunay. It is theoretically possible that a factor causing venous abnormality might also affect the rate of growth in a limb, but these two states occur independently too often for this explanation to be likely.

Returning to the possibility of a relationship between Klippel–Trenaunay and Parkes-Weber's syndromes, one does see the occasional disturbing case with the features of both conditions and Figure 12.10 shows one example. This boy was aged 7 years when first seen, with his right upper limb 1 inch (2.54 cm) longer than the left side and slightly larger; widespread but faint cutaneous vascular markings were visible, with very prominent veins showing strong 'arterial' pulsation easily identified by a Doppler

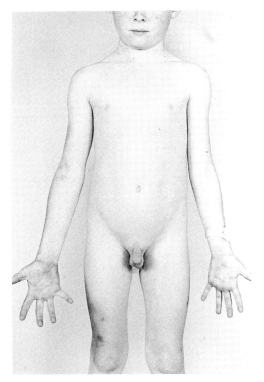

**Figure 12.10** *The right upper limb of this boy of 7 years was 2.5 cm longer than the left side and it showed obvious hypervascularity, with pulsatile flow shown on Doppler flowmetry to the enlarged superficial veins (Figure 12.11). On the back of the arm and shoulder there was a faint but definite vascular mottling. Arteriography failed to demonstrate arteriovenous fistulas so that there is uncertainty whether this should be classified as Parkes-Weber's or Klippel–Trenaunay syndrome*

flowmeter (Figure 12.11) and not present on the normal side. No bruits were present and there were no abnormal changes on arteriography except that the veins were quickly opacified. Seen again at the age of 11 the discrepancy between the two limbs was more pronounced but causing no disability. In this patient the absence of unequivocal arteriovenous fistula places him in the Klippel–Trenaunay group, but perhaps this is using its definition too rigidly and a state of diffuse arteriovenous microfistulas, not revealed by the usual techniques, is present. Other features, such as high flow rate, may give better criteria than radiographically outlined fistulas. Positive demonstration of arteriovenous shunts by angiography is absolute proof but failure to show them may

not be sufficient evidence that they do not exist. As additional evidence, Baskerville *et al.* (1985) used calf blood flow as a method to exclude arteriovenous fistulas from their series of patients with Klippel–Trenaunay syndrome and Partsch, Mostbeck and Wolf (1986) recommend the use of radioactively labelled microspheres injected into the artery to identify or exclude the presence of arteriovenous shunts. To summarize the present view, in one group there is a hyperdynamic circulation causing bone overgrowth; in the other there is a venostatic circulation and the cause of bone overgrowth is uncertain.

The division into the two syndromes is a reasonable working policy in the light of present knowledge but many questions remain unanswered and sooner or later ideas may have to be revised. In the meantime it is intriguing to watch the evidence assemble, year by year, so that eventually the jigsaw puzzle may fit together.

*Summary*

In brief there are at least four circumstances in which overgrowth of a limb, determined by congenital factors, may occur:

1. In association with venous angiodysplasia.
2. In association with arteriovenous fistula.
3. As an orthopaedic condition in its own right, without other known abnormalities.
4. In association with neurofibromatosis.

The two main syndromes will be described in detail presently but, first, it is perhaps relevant to give the combined experience of the Vascular Clinic, John Radcliffe Hospital, Oxford and the Nuffield Orthopaedic Centre, Oxford in respect of limbs showing bone overgrowth and lengthening (Clarke, Tibbs and Kenwright, 1986). This is in keeping with much larger series, published with excellent discussions, and included in the references at the end of the chapter (Gomes and Bernatz, 1970; Lindenauer, 1971; Askerkhanov, 1972; Dodd and Cockett, 1976; Gloviczki *et al.*, 1983; Young, 1983; Baskerville *et al.*, 1985; Hollier, 1985; Browse, Burnand and Lea Thomas, 1988; Mulliken and Young, 1989). These conditions are comparatively rare and the Oxford experience is summarized below:

1. A total of 59 patients with overgrowth and lengthening in a limb, with and without congenital vascular abnormalities, were seen over a 15-year period; patients

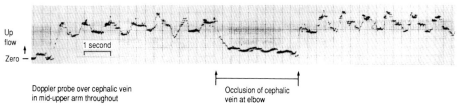

**Figure 12.11** *Doppler flowmeter tracing from the cephalic vein of the patient illustrated in*

equally of both sexes, varying from childhood to young adults on first attendance.

(a) Limbs with bone lengthening but WITHOUT vascular change:

(i) Seventeen were segmental hypertrophy (Figure 12.12), that is, lengthening confined to one limb; two of these showed extensive neuro-fibromatosis.

(ii) Ten were included in hemihypertrophy (Figure 12.13) of entire one side of the body (head, trunk, limbs).

(iii) One limb was on the opposite side to hemi-hypertrophy (crossed segmental).

(b) Limbs with bone lengthening and WITH vascular change:

(i) Six limbs with multiple arteriovenous fistula (Parkes-Weber's syndrome) all had increase in bone length but not necessarily in bulk (Figures 12.14, 12.24).

(ii) Seventeen limbs with venous and angiomatous changes typical of Klippel–Trenaunay syndrome and without any evidence of arteriovenous fistulas (Figure 12.15).

(iii) One limb (arm) with minor vascular changes and undoubted hypervascularity but with no

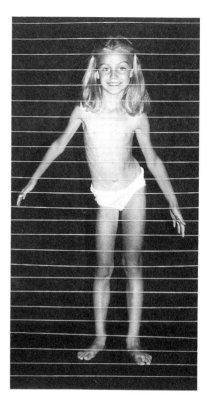

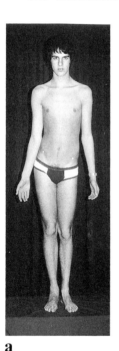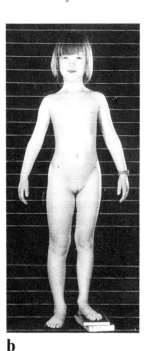

**a**          **b**

**Figure 12.12** *Overlengthening of a limb without any vascular abnormality. Both the patients illustrated show 'segmental hypertrophy', that is to say, lengthening of one limb only.*

*(a) The anterior superior spines have been marked to indicate the degree of pelvic tilt. Marking the iliac spines in this way gives rapid recognition of pelvic tilt due to discrepancy in lower limb length in the standing patient.*

*(b) A child with gross inequality in the lower limbs: here a platform under the shorter side has levelled the pelvis*

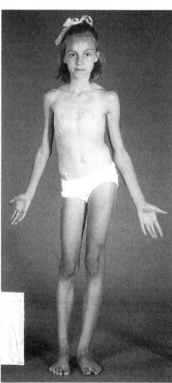

**Figure 12.13** *Overgrowth of the entire body on one side, without vascular abnormality. These two photographs, of the same girl at the age of 3 years and at 9 years, illustrate 'hemihypertrophy', that is where one-half of the head and trunk, and both the limbs on that side, show overall enlargement and lengthening*

detectable arteriovenous fistulas (Figure 12.10): classified as Klippel–Trenaunay syndrome.

(c) Limbs WITH extensive vascular change but NORMAL in LENGTH:

Seven limbs with extensive venous and angiomatous changes similar to those seen in Klippel–Trenaunay syndrome but without any overlengthening of the limb and with normal bone structure (Figure 12.16).

2. Conclusions

(a) Extensive venous and angiomatous change can occur without bone overgrowth and limb lengthening; this suggests that this form of vascular change is not in itself a stimulus to bone overgrowth.

(b) All arteriovenous fistulas seen were associated with bone overgrowth and limb lengthening; this suggests arteriovenous fistula is causative or that a common origin is shared.

(c) Bone overgrowth and limb lengthening can arise without arteriovenous fistulas or venous angiomatous changes being present; this orthopaedic variety may be a process unrelated to the vascular ones.

3. General prognosis and treatment

(a) Limbs without vascular change:

Limb overlengthening, on its own, carried a good prognosis. Simple raising of the shoe was sufficient for most of these patients. The main increase in limb length occurred before the age of 10 years and by adult life the length was not so great as earlier predictions suggested. An annual check was made on velocity of growth and in seven cases epiphysiodesis was performed because of a rapid increase in the discrepancy in length. In other patients it appeared best to wait until skeletal maturity and then to correct any severe residual discrepancy by subtrochanteric femoral bone shortening.

(b) Limbs with vascular change:

The worst problems arose in patients with vascular change, particularly arteriovenous fistulas, and included ulceration, which was intractable and painful, and, in one patient, disseminated intravascular coagulation due to clotting within an extensive venous malformation. Pulmonary embolus is a recognized complication of Klippel–Trenaunay syndrome but was not seen in this series. Two arteriovenous fistulous limbs and one Klippel–Trenaunay upper limb came to amputation for reasons directly related to the vascular abnormalities.

## Klippel–Trenaunay syndrome

In 1900 Klippel and Trenaunay from Paris described a congenital syndrome affecting a limb and consisting of essentially three features: angiomas, varicose veins and hypertrophy in soft tissues and bone, with lengthening of the limb. This syndrome is the commonest of the

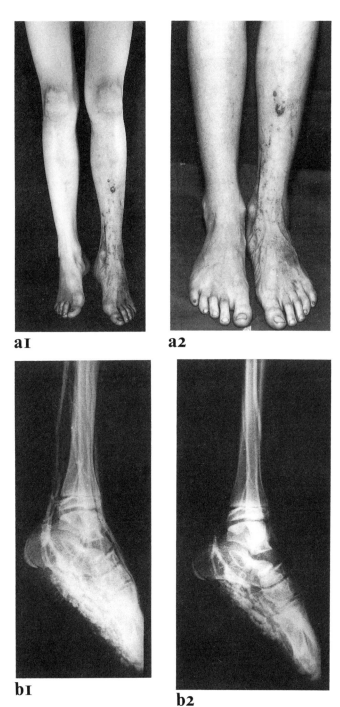

**a1**　　　**a2**

**b1**

**b2**

**Figure 12.14**　*An example of Parkes-Weber's syndrome in a boy aged 9 years*

*(a) 1, 2. Two views showing areas of pigmentation and threatened ulceration caused by arteriovenous fistulas in the leg and foot. The tibia is about 2 cm longer than the normal side and there is a corresponding increase in the size of the foot. In Figure 12.24 a much more extensive example of this condition is shown.*

*(b) 1, 2. Arteriograms showing rapid perfusion of vascular spongework in the foot*

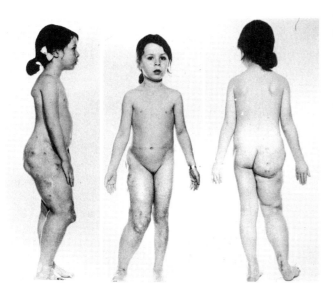

**Figure 12.15** *Examples of Klippel–Trenaunay syndrome.*

(a) *Three views of a child, aged four, with the lower limb showing massive hypertrophy and lengthening. There was extensive phlebectasia and phlebangiomatosis but no evidence of arteriovenous fistulas. It is likely that widespread lymphatic changes were present as well.*

(b) *1–3. A young woman whose left lower limb was 3 cm longer than the normal side and had an area of brown pigmentation with recurring ulceration at the ankle. There were no superficial vascular abnormalities but phlebography showed the deep veins to be deficient and grossly abnormal. No evidence of arteriovenous shunting could be found. Minor vascular abnormalities were present elsewhere, including the right side of the face.*

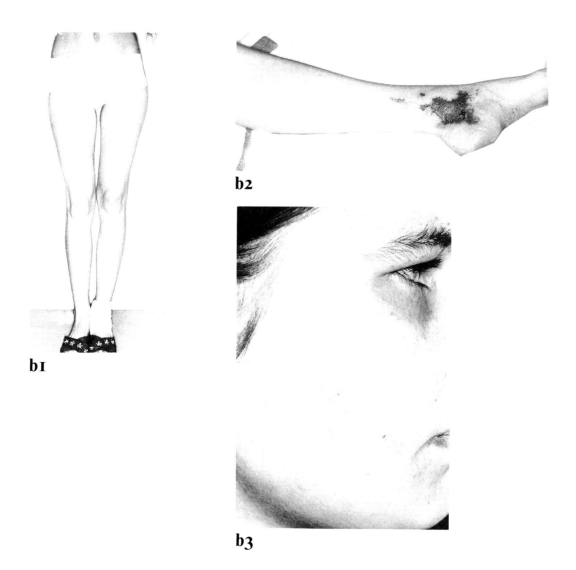

**b1**

**b2**

**b3**

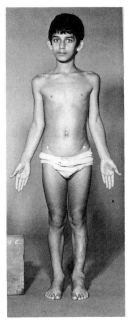
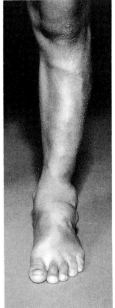

**cI**     **c2**

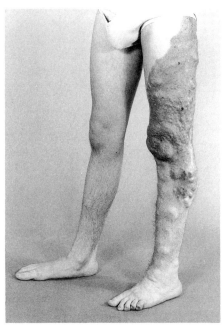

**Figure 12.15** *(continued)*

*(c) 1, 2. A boy, aged 9 years, with a massive phlebectasia on the outer aspect of the foot and leg but with no cutaneous angiomatosis; only the tibia was lengthened by 2 cm and no other bones showed this change.*

*3. A phlebogram outlining the massive lateral vein confined to the leg in this patient. Above knee level all veins appeared normal. Normal deep veins were identified below the knee so that it was permissible to remove surgically the worst of the subcutaneous veins and this was successful*

**c3**

**Figure 12.16** *Extensive venous abnormality (phlebectasia and phlebangiomatosis) without any lengthening of the limb. A youth of 16 years with extensive angiomatous change, both capillary and cavernous, in the thigh and buttock. Massive phlebectasia was present from the foot to the knee and this communicated with a lateral subcutaneous channel and with the sciatic vein illustrated in Figure 12.7. Strong elastic support to the upper thigh allowed this boy to lead an active life, including playing football. Surgery to the lateral channel at a younger age had brought temporary improvement. The phlebectasia below the knee, where the skin was normal, was treated by surgical excision and injection, with success; in the thigh similar treatment through the angiomatous skin created quite large areas of necrosis and the attempt at this level was discontinued. The femoral vein was hypoplastic so that the sciatic vein was, in fact, the main venous drainage and care was taken not to interfere with this*

congenital vascular states, being about three times more frequently seen than either similar congenital vascular changes without lengthening of the limb, or multiple arteriovenous fistulas (Parkes-Weber's syndrome). It is not necessarily evident at birth, although most are, and will tend to increase in apparent severity as the child grows. It is not hereditary and occurs equally in the sexes; no history of provoking circumstances such as birth trauma, maternal illnesses or teratogenic drugs during pregnancy has been identified. A lower limb is affected about six times more commonly than an upper limb; in about one in ten patients it may be bilateral or affecting an upper and a lower limb on the same side but occasionally on different sides (crossed segmental). The vascular features are very variable and are summarized below:

### Large aberrant veins (phlebectasia)

The most characteristic is the lateral superficial channel or trunk (Figure 12.17) and the sciatic vein (Figures 12.7, 12.18), described in a previous section of this chapter. When present these veins are almost diagnostic but these aberrations may not be evident in some cases that have all the other features.

### Hypoplasia or agenesis of principal deep veins

Lindenauer (1971) reports abnormality in the deep veins in all of 14 patients having venograms and, in 13 of these, absence of popliteal and superficial femoral deep veins. However, Baskerville *et al.* (1985) carrying out phlebography in 49 Klippel–Trenaunay limbs found a high incidence of abnormal lateral superficial embryonic channels with 60% having normal deep veins and only 18% with deep vein atresia, but 45% had evidence of incompetent communicating veins. Whatever the exact

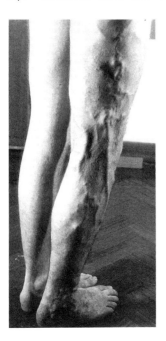
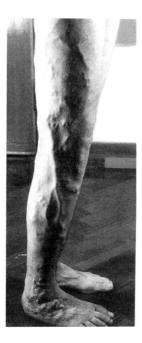

**Figure 12.17** *Klippel–Trenaunay syndrome. This illustrates the lateral superficial channel that is common in this syndrome or, indeed, in any limb with extensive venous abnormalities. Two views show the extensive anomalous subcutaneous veins in the same patient*

incidence it is clear that at least some degree of deep vein, perforating vein and valvular abnormality is likely to be present even if hypoplasia or agenesis of deep veins has not occurred. This is in accord with the authors own experience. It is important because of its surgical implications and explains the venous ulceration these patients are prone to in adult life, even when massive aberrant deep veins or lateral superficial channels are not present. Incidentally, phlebography can only outline vessels through which flow takes the opaque medium and large, stagnant malformations may fail to be visualized, or the reverse may happen and abnormal vessels divert blood stream from normal deep veins so that they appear to be absent; the reliable demonstration of valves is notoriously difficult. For these reasons negative findings on phlebography are treacherous to interpret and these limitations may account for wide differences in reported series, for example, Lindenauer's high proportion of deep vein aplasia was presumably based on the negative finding of deep veins failing to fill.

**Figure 12.18** *Phlebogram of a patient with a lateral subcutaneous channel very similar to that shown in Figure 12.17 and communicating with a sciatic deep vein which terminates in the profunda femoris. Other views showed normal popliteal and superficial femoral veins but preferential flow up the abnormal channel made this difficult to demonstrate so that only faint outlines were obtained; it would have been easy to miss this and draw the erroneous conclusion that the normal deep veins were absent. 1. Below knee. 2. Knee level and above*

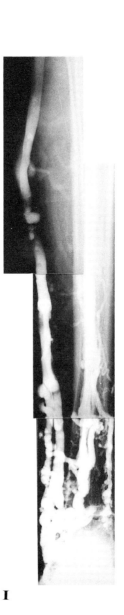
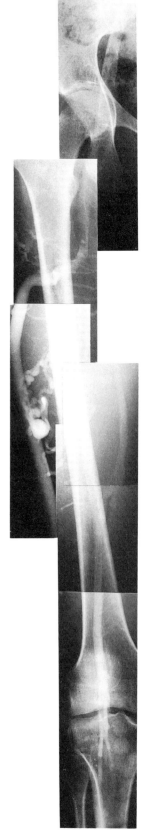

**1**　　　　**2**

## Angiomatous change

This may be in the form multiple discrete angiomas, mainly in the superficial tissues, or confluent, diffuse changes in superficial and deep layers. The angiomas are usually of the cavernous type but often intermingled with capillary angiomas especially if the skin is involved.

## Lymphatic abnormalities

Lymphangiomas mixed with haemangiomas commonly occur. Lymphatic hypoplasia with resultant lymphoedema is present in greater or lesser degree in many patients. Lymph cysts and fistulas to the skin surface may also occur.

## Bone overgrowth, giving rise to lengthening

This is, of course, by definition, an essential feature of this syndrome. However, shortening of bone may occur occasionally with the same type of vascular changes. The author has seen one patient with a typical Klippel–Trenaunay limb in which the tibia showed approximately 4 cm overlengthening but the femur was shortened by almost the same extent so that the overall length in the limb was virtually normal although the knee joint was, inevitably, displaced upwards (Figure 12.19).

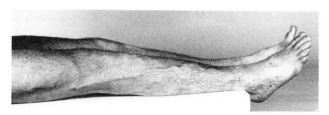

**Figure 12.19** *The same patient as shown in Figure 12.17 positioned to show the increase in length in the right tibia and upward displacement of the knee joint. The femur, however, was slightly shortened so that the overall length of the limb was little changed from the normal side*

## Abnormalities elsewhere

About 15% of patients will show angiomatous involvement elsewhere, in the head and neck or in the trunk where it may be subcutaneous, intra-abdominal or intrathoracic; rectal or urinary tract angiomas may cause bleeding. Associated birth deformities are quite common and include syndactaly, dislocation of the hip, partial agenesis of metatarsus or phalanges.

## Tendency to ulceration

Because the venous anomalies are usually valveless it is difficult to know whether gross enlargement of the veins is a result of this, or is due to an inherent weakness in abnormal veins. Their progressive enlargement as the child grows suggests that, without the protection of valves, the raised pressures and surge of blood within the system are an important factor. Although they are adequate venous conduits they allow heavy reflux in the upright position, and counteract upward pumping against gravity so that their presence can lead to venous hypertension and ulceration. Nevertheless, the performance of the musculovenous pump is often near normal because sufficient calf deep veins are in good order and able to provide a strong pumping mechanism even though this is partly invalidated by the valveless neighbouring veins. Baskerville *et al.* (1985) in a study of 32 Klippel–Trenaunay limbs, using foot volumetry, found that only five of these had obvious impairment of the musculovenous pumping mechanism but 27 had a very shortened recovery time in keeping with heavy reflux caused by valvular incompetence.

It is uncommon to see overt venotensive changes (venous stasis) and ulceration until adult life is reached and even then there may be a surprising absence of skin changes for some years in spite of extensive venous abnormality. In childhood this may be due to the adaptability of young tissues or the lower venous pressures (depending on distance from foot to heart level). Surgery taking out carefully selected veins may be successful in some cases but as there is virtually no means of effective reconstructive surgery to veins and valves, the patient must be urged to follow a protective policy from an early stage, usually by elastic support and high elevation whenever possible. It is often difficult to persuade a young patient to follow such a policy conscientiously until problems actually arise.

## Symptoms and complications

Discomfort or pain may arise to a variable degree. Ulceration, which may be accompanied by bleeding, is likely to occur sooner or later, caused by venostasis or atrophy of poor quality skin involved in angiomatous change. Haemorrhage from minor trauma is always a danger; episodes of thrombosis in the enlarged veins or in the cavernous angiomas are fairly common and occasionally extend to cause pulmonary embolism. Depending on the degree of lymphatic involvement and skin oedema, cellulitis may occur; hyperhydrosis may be a problem. The overlengthened limb will cause inequality between the two sides, with tilting of the pelvis and secondary effects upon the spine in adult life.

## Prognosis

This congenital syndrome shows a considerable variation between patients so that in some it may be no more than a somewhat awkward limb with relatively inconspicuous vascular change, allowing the patient to lead a reasonably active life. At the other extreme the limb may show gross, irregular enlargement, vividly discoloured by cutaneous angiomatosis, vulnerable to minor injury and clearly a most troublesome burden for the patient; other congenital deformities and angiomas elsewhere may increase the patient's disability and even shorten life. Fortunately most are only of moderate severity and, in spite of the few extreme cases, the approach should be optimistic, for much can be done to improve the limb, avoid complications and give general encouragement to the patient.

### Investigation and management

When the condition is first recognized the patient should come under the long-term care of a vascular unit, a paediatric unit (to look for other possible congenital lesions), and an orthopaedic unit (to advise upon problems relating to the overlengthened limb). The child should be encouraged in all normal activity as far as possible and there should be an annual follow-up by orthopaedic and vascular surgeons.

### Phlebography

Investigation should include phlebography, but this may be postponed for some years if the limb is not unduly troublesome. When problems arise or if treatment to superficial phlebectasia is contemplated then it is essential that phlebography should be carried out to identify the deep veins. These may be absent or underdeveloped and their role taken over by the very veins being considered for surgical removal. In the authors own experience an upper limb was lost due to extensive removal of superficial cavernous angiomatosis which was in fact the main pathway of venous return (Figure 12.9). Phlebography must also be directed to identifying any major aberrant vein, such as a sciatic vein. Phlebography in Klippel–Trenaunay syndrome is well described by Lea Thomas and Macfie (1974) and Lea Thomas (1982).

### Arteriography

Arteriography does not usually provide much useful information but should be carried out if there is serious suspicion that arteriovenous fistulas are present, using an appropriate technique of serial exposures.

### Lymphangiography

Lymphangiography is seldom necessary but is indicated when surgery is contemplated on a lymphatic lesion. This may give warning of a deficiency in lymphatics that could be aggravated by surgical interference; radioactive colloid uptake is simpler to use and usually proves an adequate alternative.

## Treatment of extensive venous lesions and Klippel–Trenaunay syndrome

For extensive venous and angiomatous lesions involving most of a limb, one or more of the following three principles of treatment may be required:

- Containment of the huge venous spaces by external support.
- Segmental removal by surgery, or obliteration by compression sclerotherapy.
- Correction of orthopaedic abnormalities.

### Conservative treatment by external support

In the less severe examples the child may be allowed to lead a normal life for many years but sooner or later external support may become desirable or necessary. If it is apparent that the varicosities are progressively enlarging into massive venous sinuses or if cavernous angiomas are forming protruberant masses under the skin then this process should be controlled, usually by a strong elastic stocking. This will prevent excessive filling of the venous spaces and, of course, give considerable protection from injury. A young person may at first not like this but will soon come to welcome having the unsightly veins and angiomas reduced in size and concealed by the stocking. It will require fitting by an expert orthotist, with renewal and adjustment for size at regular intervals.

Another reason for elastic support will be actual or threatened ulceration caused by venous stasis, usual in these patients sooner or later. The support may improve the efficiency of the venous pumping mechanism and help to keep ulceration at bay. Good results here are often obtained using a one-way-stretch stocking up to the knee. At this level it is more likely to be tolerated by the young patient and stay in place in the upper calf because there is no downward pull, but may have to extend higher if extensive angiomatous lesions are present in the thigh. If ulceration is not responding to treatment, inelastic external support, as with other forms of venous ulceration, is always more effective than elastic support and should be used in the form of a paste bandage, applied while the limb is elevated. This is ideal because it restrains the venous spaces as soon as they start to fill when the limb is put down, but allows free circulation when it is elevated. There are dangers in elasticity, especially in a bandage with the additive effect of successive turns, because it exerts pressure unnecessarily when the limb is raised with venous spaces collapsed and, in treating ulceration, this may actually oppose the benefits of elevation by impairing arterial flow.

The patient must understand the importance of putting the limb in high elevation whenever possible so that a considerable part of the day is spent in the position where gravity is assisting rather than opposing venous return.

## Ulceration and haemorrhage

The patient must of course be warned against the consequences of even minor injury that may damage the skin and start an ulcer that will prove very difficult to heal. Similarly heavy haemorrhage can occur from the large blood-filled spaces just beneath the skin and the patient must be given precautionary instruction on the control of this by elevation of the limb and firm pressure on the bleeding point. An additional advantage of external support is the protection this gives against the unavoidable knock. The patient must also be aware of the significance of deterioration in the skin as a forerunner to ulceration, and if this arises, of the need to meet this threat by increasing the efficiency of external support, perhaps by use of an inelastic paste bandage, and increased periods of elevation. The price of a pain-free and fully functioning limb is vigilance and preparedness to meet any threat by extra care. It is far easier to forestall an ulcer than to heal it once established. However, if the worst happens most ulcers can be healed eventually by the usual principles of elevation and external support; in this respect the limb with congenital vascular malformation is not very different from the other venous states (see Chapter 13).

Haemorrhage from an established ulcer is always worrying since prolonged firm pressure to control the bleeding by pad and bandage may cause local damage by ischaemia and exacerbate infection so that the ulcer deteriorates. A culture should be obtained from the ulcer at the earliest opportunity and, if a destructive pathogen such as staphylococcus is found, an appropriate antibiotic given. The limb should be elevated continuously and pressure bandage avoided as soon as haemorrhage has ceased; a bland non-adherent dressing is used on the ulcer. During this period of elevation the patient must be urged to follow a system of exercise to combat the ill effects of immobilization in bed. As soon as the ulcer enters a healing phase, trial may be given to applying a paste bandage and mobilizing the patient in stages. When healing is complete the patient may return to the usual form of external support. Conservative management along these lines is usually the best policy for ulceration and haemorrhage but in some circumstances more active treatment by surgery or sclerotherapy may have to be considered.

## Active intervention by surgery

**Excision of angiomatous tissue** Surgery has a valuable role to play in some of these patients but must never be a decision lightly taken. Haemorrhage during or after surgery may be a problem and angiomatous skin tends to heal badly and certainly will not tolerate undermining. Operation is indicated only when the surgeon can see a clear opportunity for improving the limb and is satisfied that adequate deep veins are present. This may be by removal of massive varicosities or localized angiomas under normal skin and can be relatively easy; where the skin is angiomatous it must be recognized that skin coverage following removal of the underlying lesion may be a problem, with necrosis of skin edges and likely failure of skin grafts to take. A pedicle graft may prove an answer in certain positions, such as over joints, but it must always be born in mind that the patients own angiomatous skin, given proper care, can usually serve well and the patient should not be exposed to possible risk of prolonged difficulties due to skin deprivation. Other aspects are discussed in the section on treatment of local angiomas above. In suitable cases surgery can be repeated at intervals to give staged removal of adjoining areas; heroic massive single operations would seem unwise in view of the unpredictability of healing in some cases.

**Attempted control of venous reflux** The other reason for surgery is to remove large valveless channels thought to be playing a major part in venous stasis. The care needed to confirm the presence of adequate deep veins has already been emphasized; an enlarged valveless vein may be infinitely preferable to no adequate vein for venous return. Much can be learned about the possible benefits of removing a particular varicosity by the usual clinical tests (control of filling from above by localized compression, as in a selective Trendelenburg test), by use of the Doppler flowmeter (favourable if it shows predominant downflow after exercise) or by functional phlebography (favourable if showing downflow caused by exercise and demonstrating good venous return in other vessels). Usually however these tests do not give an unequivocal response because the venous channel under investigation is only part of a much more widespread state of incompetence, and practical experience shows that the difficulties encountered, such as poor healing, are not often justified by the benefits obtained. Lindenauer (1971) reporting 25 cases found that 13 out of 14 cases were made worse by removal of large varicosities; Gloviczki et al. (1983), however, reported improvement in 10 out of 11 carefully selected cases. Taheri et al. (1988) describe improvement in a young woman with Klippel–Trenaunay syndrome following transposition of an incompetent superficial femoral to a valved profunda femoris vein (see Figure 21.8) and discuss the role of this procedure.

Each case must be judged upon its own merits but it is indefensible to carry out a major removal of enlarged veins without proper investigation and understanding. One final cautionary word, surgery to an unrecognized case of multiple arteriovenous fistulas is a misfortune which should not arise with proper forethought!

## Injection sclerotherapy

This may give limited benefit but often only temporarily.

It can be followed by necrosis of overlying skin if this is angiomatous, with prolonged difficulties in healing the consequent ulceration. For this reason injection through heavily angiomatous skin is not advised but where it is felt that a reduction of large veins and angiomas beneath reasonably healthy skin may bring advantage then it is permissible to give this trial using 3% sodium tetradecyl sulphate. The total amount is limited to 3 ml, distributed over several sites, with the actual delivery of sclerosant made into a vein emptied by elevation of the limb, and followed by the application of a pad and compression bandage (and see Chapter 19). If an initial trial of injection gives an encouraging response then treatment may be continued, segment by segment, over a period of some months and in this way a useful measure of success can be achieved.

### Treatment of the orthopaedic defects

This aspect is best under orthopaedic supervision. In the upper limb the excessive length causes no significant problem. In the lower limb, tilting of the pelvis, with consequent arthritis of the lumbar spine in early adult life, is the main problem and correction should be started as soon as inequality is detected. Usually it is sufficient to raise the shoe on the normal side to equalize the two sides. If it becomes apparent at annual examination that the discrepancy in length is increasing excessively then epiphysiodesis can be very successful (Figure 12.20). However it is usually best to wait until bone maturity has been reached in young adult life and then, if the disability is severe, carry out subtronchanteric femoral shortening to the affected side (McCullough and Kenwright, 1979); only a minority of patients will require this and most continue satisfactorily with a raised shoe.

## Arteriovenous fistulas: Parkes-Weber's syndrome

In this disorder (Parkes-Weber, 1907, 1918) multiple communications between arteries and veins have developed without normal intervening capillary beds. This is not a direct connection of the two systems but through a spongework of vascular tissue capable of transferring heavy flow from one side to the other. The basic pattern is of a well-developed single artery breaking into multiple branches to feed the spongework, with a number of veins taking away the outflow, perhaps coalescing into one or more large veins. Even in the widespread states it is usually possible to pick out numerous 'units' of this sort, each with its own feeding artery. This gives opportunity for treatment by therapeutic embolization (plugging) of the artery. As is the rule with congenital vascular defects the condition may be very localized, perhaps with only one unit a few centimetres across and a single feeding artery, or, at the other extreme, numerous arteriovenous fistulous units are present, widespread throughout an entire limb and beyond.

### Clinical features

A comparatively small lesion will produce a swelling with enlarged veins running from it, perhaps slightly blue if near the surface, usually showing soft pulsation, possibly with a palpable thrill, and emitting a 'to and fro' bruit. It is compressible by finger pressure and refills rapidly upon release; ulceration of overlying skin, particularly in the hand or foot, is often present by adolescence (Figure 12.5(a), (b)). In a more extensive lesion other effects dependent upon arteriovenous shunting will become increasingly evident according to its size. The main artery leading down to the defect will enlarge considerably and give a characteristic humming note on auscultation; the veins in the vicinity, and perhaps widely through the limb, will enlarge and a Doppler flowmeter will show pulsatile upward flow in them. The heart reponds to the haemodynamic changes created by the arteriovenous shunt by tachycardia and hypertrophy; in the more extreme cases heart failure may eventually occur. In lesions sufficiently large to set up tachycardia, Branham's sign (Branham, 1890) may be observed; this is a slowing of the pulse rate when the main artery is compressed and the arteriovenous shunt temporarily diminished in its effect.

**Parkes-Weber's syndrome** Another very distinctive feature of the arteriovenous fistula is overgrowth of neighbouring bones. This and the other features of arteriovenous fistulas were described by Parkes-Weber in 1907 and the syndrome is still known by his name. If the lesion is confined to part of the hand or foot (Figure 12.14) only the corresponding part of the bone structure will enlarge but if the fistulas are widespread the bone structure of the entire limb may be affected to give considerable overgrowth in length (Figure 12.24) and this becomes more evident as the child grows. The bone overgrowth is thought to be a direct response to the high blood flow through the limb and particularly at the epiphysises.

**Ulceration and haemorrhage with arteriovenous fistulas** A further feature in the older child, or as an adult, is the development of pigmentation and ulceration in the extremity. The mechanism of this is of considerable interest to the venous surgeon because of its similarity to the skin changes caused by sustained venous hypertension (stasis) found in the various venous disorders described in earlier chapters. There is little doubt that the high venous pressure created by arteriovenous fistula is the cause of the same manifestations occurring in Parkes-Weber's syndrome. Indeed, a number of cases have now been reported of similar pigmentation and ulceration in the hand below an arteriovenous shunt created for access in repeated renal dialysis. These changes soon go if the arteriovenous fistula is dismantled (Figure 12.21). A tendency to ulceration is, of course, also seen in Klippel–

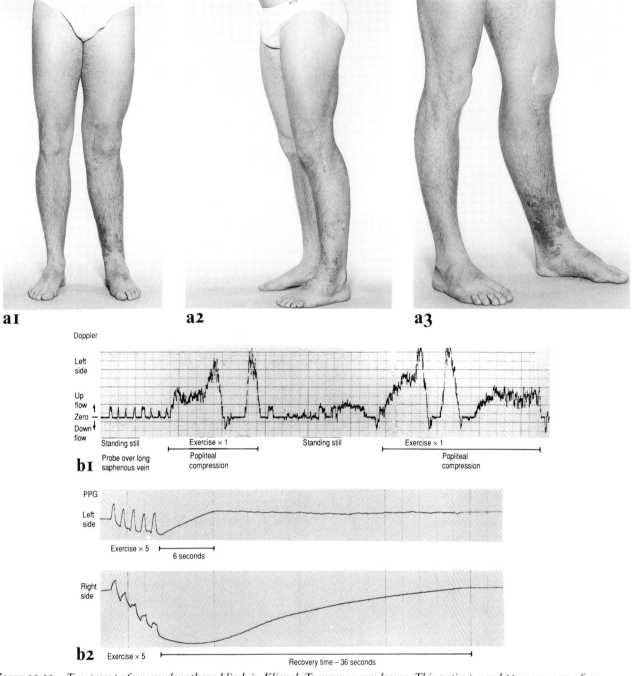

**Figure 12.20**    *Treatment of an overlengthened limb in Klippel–Trenaunay syndrome. This patient, aged 22 years, came from abroad; epiphysiodesis had been carried out to control excessive lengthening of the left limb as a boy. This gave a good result and enabled him to play hockey in a national team.*

*(a)   1–3. The general appearance of the limbs are shown in these photographs. The scars of the operation on left femoral and tibial epiphyses can be seen and there is reasonable equality of length between the limbs; marked venotensive skin change and threatened ulceration at the left ankle are present; there are no varicose veins and cutaneous angiomatosis is not evident.*

*(b)   1. Doppler flowmetry tracing showing upflow in the long saphenous vein, accentuated by exercise. This indicates that it is acting as an important channel of venous return; compression of the popliteal fossa accentuates this, suggesting that there are further veins carrying upflow crossing the fossa.*
*2. Photoplethysmography confirmed a severely impaired venous pumping mechanism on the left side but normal on the right. Phlebography was not carried out as the patient was travelling on. It is not known whether the venous changes are the result of deep vein thrombosis caused by the limb operations or, more likely, whether they are due to congenital abnormality of the deep veins accompanied by overgrowth of limb, that is, Klippel–Trenaunay syndrome*

*Epiphysiodesis is usually reserved for patients where the velocity of growth shows excessive increase. In many cases, at bone maturity, the limb discrepancy may not be as severe as earlier changes might have suggested. In others, correction of length by subtrochanteric femoral shortening can be carried out in the young adult if necessary*

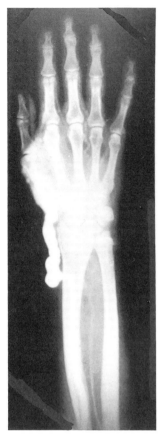 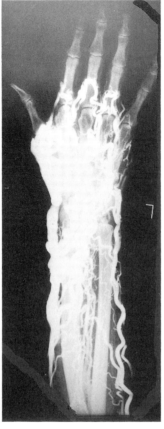

**Figure 12.21** *Arteriovenous shunt created to facilitate access in repeated renal dialysis. Two stages of filling during arteriography are shown. At the time these arteriograms were obtained, 2 years after construction of the shunt, the patient had developed pigmentation and ulceration in the fingers. This receded, with healing of the ulcers, soon after the arteriovenous shunt was closed*

Trenaunay syndrome, and has caused confusion in the past, but here the common denominator, high venous pressure, is due to venous incompetence by valveless channels and *not* by transfer of arterial pressures to the venous side as in arteriovenous shunt. In Parkes-Weber's syndrome veins are usually well valved throughout and defective veins are not a feature; capillary and cavernous angiomatous lesions are not usually seen in combination with angiographically proven arteriovenous fistulas and in some descriptions it is not easy to be certain of the strictness of the criteria used in the diagnosis of multiple arteriovenous shunts.

Haemorrhage, which may be severe, is likely to occur from the highly vascular tissue underlying a persistent ulcer and eventually the state of the limb may become so distressing to the patient that amputation has to be considered. It would not be correct, however, to regard this as inevitable as many of these limbs may be maintained indefinitely in a useful state by external support and selective therapeutic embolization to the arteries supplying the fistulas. Moreover, amputation does not necessarily offer an 'easy' solution because the fistulous communications may extend well above the highest levels of amputation and the process will continue in the amputation stump (Sako and Varco, 1970).

**Heart failure due to massive arteriovenous shunting** The loss of peripheral resistance on the arterial side and the effect of immediate transfer of cardiac output across to the venous side causes a considerable burden upon the heart in maintaining a normal blood pressure and in dealing with the unnaturally large venous return. At first it responds by hypertrophy but eventually it may prove unequal to the task and cardiac failure will occur so that the patient's life is threatened as a young adult. The surgeon watching over the patient must always be aware of this possibility and a clear warning of the increased burden on the heart is provided by a tachycardia that is temporarily relieved by compressing the main artery to the affected limb (Branham's sign). In these circumstances the patient should be placed under the supervision of a cardiologist and eventually it may become essential to find some way of reducing the degree of arterial to venous shunting.

*Prognosis*

In giving any prognosis to the parents of a child with an arteriovenous fistulous limb any emphatic statement of disaster ahead should be avoided. Few of these limbs need come to amputation and with care good function can be preserved throughout the patient's life. Moreover, our understanding and techniques for ameliorating the harmful effects of this vascular abnormality have improved steadily over the years and are likely to continue to do so. An ill-considered amputation may produce formidable difficulties and fail to eliminate the arteriovenous fistulas in the amputation site (Sako and Varco, 1970). At the outset it is best to explain that with special care and supervision it should be possible to preserve a useful limb, and it is best to watch the pattern of events as the child grows so that decisions can be made at appropriate stages. The author has seen great distress caused to parents of children with comparatively harmless vascular abnormalities, particularly in Klippel-Trenaunay syndrome, when an inexpert opinion has been given that the limb will have to be removed at an early age. This is seldom the case, even with extensive arteriovenous fistulas. Advice of this severity should only be given by those who have the experience and understanding of congenital vascular abnormalities to justify their opinion. Our approach must be that if the limb has reasonable function and is not causing distress then it can probably be preserved indefinitely and every effort must be made to ensure that this is so. However, it must be admitted that an appreciable number of Parkes-Weber's syndrome will eventually cause severe problems which may compel desperate remedies but this minority will reveal themselves all too clearly as the child grows.

## Investigation

**Arteriography** When the clinical examination has lead to diagnosis of extensive arteriovenous fistulas, and there is usually little doubt about this, then by far the most important investigation is by arteriography. This should be carried out by some form of serial or video technique which will display the entire limb, and the portion of trunk above it, at the various phases of flow by opacified blood through the arteries, fistulous tissue and into the veins. This may require more than one run and where there are areas of special concern arterial catheterization to selected branches can give more detailed information. The direct evidence given by arteriography, demonstrating the fistulous formations, is far superior to any other investigation (Figure 12.22), and measurement of secondary effects, such as oxygen saturation of the venous blood, add little useful information. In a child it is an examination only to be repeated at long intervals but it seems justifiable to have arteriography soon after the initial clinical diagnosis has been clearly established. This will act as an important baseline for further examinations in years to come and will also give information upon the extent and pattern of the abnormality so that likely forms of intervention can be provisionally identified. Phlebography is not usually of any value in arteriovenous fistula unless it is used under tourniquet to run the opaque medium retrogradely through the fistulous areas. This is a technique appropriate for a single acquired fistula rather than the diffuse congenital form.

**Cardiology** Another baseline to be established is that of the cardiac state. This should include a chest X-ray for heart size and observations on the pulse rate in response to temporary occlusion of the main artery leading to the limb. When the lesions are extensive the child should be seen regularly by a cardiologist.

**Orthopaedic aspects** The orthopaedic consequences of Parkes-Weber's syndrome will become more apparent as the child grows and this aspect is best supervised by an orthopaedic clinic. Certainly limb measurements should be carried out annually, with radiographic checks at longer intervals.

## Treatment

Indications for treatment are:

- Protection of the limb, if possible, from deterioration.
- Discomfort or pain, usually caused by ulceration.
- Ulceration and haemorrhage.

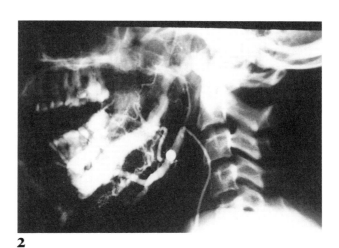

**I**

**2**

**3**

**Figure 12.22** *Congenital arteriovenous fistulas involving bone elsewhere in the body. Arteriograms showing various phases of filling in the left lower jaw of a young person, who presented with intermittent bleeding and a diffuse, pulsatile swelling in the mouth. Blood opacified from a catheter into the lingual artery rapidly transits to a massively enlarged inferior dental vein. The process was largely confined to the bone which was resected and successfully replaced with a bone graft. (Mr J. Raines' case)*

- Heart failure, threatened or actual.
- Inequality in the length of the limb.

The principles of treatment are:

1. Containment of the limb by strong external support which resists overexpansion of the blood vessels and diminishes flow through the arteriovenous shunts.
2. Surgical removal of localized arteriovenous fistulas, where this is practicable.
3. Surgical ligation of arteries carefully selected by arteriography.
4. Transluminal occlusion (embolization) of selected arteries.
5. Compensation or correction for orthopaedic abnormalities.

These will now be discussed.

**Containment by external support** When the arteriovenous fistulous limb is upright the swift flow of blood fills vascular spaces and veins more quickly than it can be removed. Thus the veins rapidly fill to maximal capacity and high venous pressure. If the patient then lies horizontally with the limb elevated, venous return can outpace the arterial inflow so that capillaries, vascular spaces and veins all collapse and the harmful high venous pressure in the limb falls away. At the same time the volume of the limb shrinks considerably, especially in the more vascular parts. If an *inelastic* external support is applied around the limb in elevation, then as soon as the patient stands this support will resist expansion of the vessels and will maintain them in a narrowed state.

Two important considerations arise from this:

1. Elevation is likely to be beneficial to the arteriovenous fistulous limb by keeping it in a state of minimal venous pressure. Aspects related to high arterial to venous shunting, such as overloading the heart, will not however be benefited by this.
2. External support with an inelastic bandage applied to the elevated limb provides an unyielding encasement that constricts the arteriovenous shunts and reduces flow through them when an upright position is assumed.

A paste bandage, applied to the elevated limb, forms an ideal inelastic support, giving a close, firm encasement. Experience has shown that an inelastic paste bandage is the most effective method in the healing of ulcers in these patients. Presumably its constricting effect on the arteriovenous shunts reduces the flow through them, lowers the high venous pressure and allows healing to occur. It is effective when the patient is up and about and, because it is not elastic, it cannot exceed the natural hydrostatic pressure in the limb at any level; similarly it does not exert any damaging elastic compression when the limb is elevated.

The technique of applying a paste bandage is described in Chapter 13 and the discussion there emphasizes the undesirability of using a strong elastic bandage unless this is most skilfully applied. Successive turns of an elastic bandage can easily build up an excessive pressure continuously exerted whether the limb is vertical or horizontal; this may cause ischaemia with pain and deterioration in the ulceration. Although superior in effect, a paste bandage is tedious to apply, somewhat unsightly and does need skilful application, not easy for the unassisted patient. To avoid these disadvantages, a well-fitted elastic stocking may be used when the limb is in a favourable state without any threat of ulceration. This needs to be expertly fitted so that it gives minimal elastic compression to the limb in elevation but immediate resistance to any filling of the blood vessels caused by the upright position. If ulceration threatens then inelastic support by a paste bandage should be used.

In a child, when the limb is causing no problems and the skin is in good condition it is debatable whether there is any advantage in external support and it is reasonable to postpone this until such time as skin changes, such as pigmentation or threatened ulceration, start to appear. At this stage, an elastic stocking up to the knee may help to protect the limb from deterioration and also from knocks and minor injuries which may not heal well. If the limb is in good condition and causing no symptoms the young patient will be unwilling to use the elastic stocking and may only be persuaded when problems appear; it would seem unwise to insist upon its use without evident reasons.

**Conservative management of ulceration and haemorrhage** Ulceration can eventually cause haemorrhage and for this reason should not be allowed to continue unchecked. For active ulceration an initial spell of high elevation, with brief walks each hour to maintain muscles and joints in good condition, may be necessary. When the ulcer commences healing then trial may be given to use of a paste bandage applied up the knee and renewed each week; the patient is encouraged to increase mobility but always returning to a position of high elevation when not actively walking about. At a suitable stage the patient may return to a relatively normal life but should always take care to elevate the limb at every possible opportunity. When the ulcers are completely healed the paste bandage may be discarded and replaced with an elastic stocking but the patient should be fully prepared to revert to a paste bandage if ulceration should reappear.

*Haemorrhage* This can usually be controlled without undue difficulty by elevation and firm pressure to a pad over the site of bleeding. Initially the pressure may have to be by hand but, as opportunity allows, a non-adherent dressing should be put in place with a pad of folded gauze over this and a bandage from the foot up to the knee firmly applied. When there has been no haemorrhage for some days a paste bandage may be substituted with a non-adherent dressing over the ulcer, and cautious mobility resumed. If there are repeated episodes of haemorrhage without any sign of healing some form of intervention, probably by embolization through an arterial catheter, will have to be attempted and this is discussed below.

**Surgical removal of localized arteriovenous shunts**  Where the lesion is comparatively small, perhaps involving part of the hand or foot, some form of surgical removal of the effected part may be the most practical treatment. It is likely, however, that the process will re-emerge and further surgery will be needed sooner or later. It has already been pointed out above that amputation of an entire limb may in itself be a formidable undertaking and may only give temporary respite before active arteriovenous shunting becomes evident in the amputation stump (Sako and Varco, 1970). However, this may have achieved a great reduction in the arteriovenous shunting and removed the patient from danger of progressive heart failure, or taken away a limb with extensive, painful ulceration with persistent repeated haemorrhages. Needless to say any surgery attempting to remove arteriovenous fistulous tissue, either by partial amputation in hand or foot, or by a major amputation, should be preceded by a most careful assessment of the arterial supply and pattern of arteriovenous shunting so that the operation may be planned accordingly. Except for well-defined local lesions it is always best to exploit fully treatment by transluminal embolization before resorting to major surgery.

If major amputation is necessary the indications are likely to be repeated haemorrhage, incurable painful ulceration or gross loss of function. For the operation itself provision must be made to control the main arterial supply to the limb at a high level. This can be done by a tourniquet, if amputation is to be low enough to permit this, or by a small separate exposure to the common iliac artery so that it may be temporarily clamped. Alternatively a suitably sized Fogarty catheter may be used, passed upwards from the main artery exposed at the site of amputation or separately in the groin; the balloon is inflated in the common iliac artery. Great care must be taken with haemostasis, particularly in the bloodless field given by a tourniquet.

**Treatment of arteriovenous fistulas by control of the arterial supply**  To the unwary it must seem obvious that reducing the arterial supply to an arteriovenous limb will improve all the problems arising from arteriovenous shunting. In the past many attempts have been made to help the patient by ligating the main artery and relying upon the collateral circulation to maintain viability of the limb. This invariably brings disappointment or disaster. If the limb remains viable, the collateral circulation quickly expands so that within a few weeks all the arteriovenous manifestations are as obvious as ever; alternatively extensive gangrene is precipitated. Surgical methods ligating a main artery or even selected branches are difficult to regulate and either produce only a tem-

porary improvement or a dramatic loss of blood supply to the limb, and the margin between these two extremes is narrow. These limbs show an extraordinary capacity to utilize the abnormal arterial system to generate a collateral circulation compensating for the the vessels that are shut off, but the immediate danger of reducing arterial supply in the presence of extensive fistulas is that it abruptly reaches a critical level inadequate to perfuse tissues. Presumably this is because the input has become insufficient to meet the wastage through the fistulas and at the same time perfuse capillary beds opposed by high venous pressure on the other side. With transluminal occlusion by arterial catheterization (Figure 12.23) it is possible to carry out repeated procedures each occluding no more than one or two selected arteries and in this way to stage the process until sufficient has been achieved yet, hopefully, stopping short of the critical point causing ischaemia. Although surgical ligation of a branch artery clearly indentified as the supply to an arteriovenous fistulous area is still permissible, multiple staged procedures by arterial catheterization, with the great advantage of little disturbance to the patient, have superseded the various forms of surgical ligation. However, one form of surgical approach, preserving the main artery but ligating the branches along its length (Cotton and Sykes, 1969), known as skeletalization of the artery, has achieved some successes, although the proportion of failures is not known. The same effect should certainly be obtainable by catheter-directed embolization with far less disturbance and risk to the patient. However, no method is perfect and in the case history presented below a Gianturco coil, inserted into a major branch of the popliteal artery, shifted to cause occlusion of the lower popliteal and upper tibial arteries. This certainly brought relief from cardiac failure and healing of ulceration in the lower leg, but the limb came perilously close to gangrene. The arterial pressure at the ankle dropped to about 50 mmHg and elevation of the limb caused pallor and rest pain but yet Doppler flowmeter examination showed rapid flow of blood in the main arteries at the ankle. Clearly, an arterial pressure adequate to perfuse normal capillary beds only built up when the limb was in a dependent position and arteriovenous shunting was opposed by venous pressure. In elevation arterial blood loss through the shunts, unopposed by venous pressure, took away the reduced arterial inflow so rapidly that it was insufficient to perfuse the capillary beds. Nevertheless the patient soon acquired a protective policy towards her limb and continued an active life bringing up her two children. This does however illustrate the fine balance between arteriovenous shunting and viability of the limb if occlusion of a main artery occurs. We have yet to learn a technique that eliminates multiple arteriovenous fistulas but preserves adequate arterial perfusion of the capillary bed. Other techniques may be developed and, for example, Riche *et*

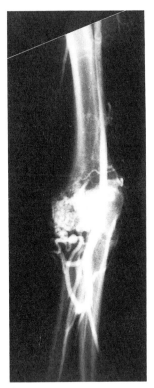

a

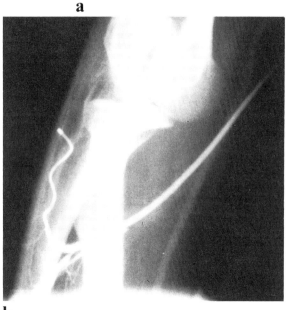

b

**Figure 12.23** *Treatment of a congenital arteriovenous fistula by embolization of the feeding artery through a transarterial catheter. Here, a 5 cm pulsating swelling at the elbow was successfully treated with a Gianturco coil introduced by catheter down the brachial artery.*

*(a) Arteriogram outlining the feeding artery and fistulous area beyond.*

*(b) After introduction of the coil with the artery now occluded*

al. (1986) describe the injection of liquid polymer into the veins of the fistulous area whilst the circulation is arrested by tourniquet, so that the material runs back to block the fistulas.

*Case history.* This case history is included because it illustrates so many important aspects of Parkes-Weber's syndrome and its treatment, and includes two successful pregnancies.

Patient S.D. was first seen as a girl aged 14, complaining of enlargement of the left lower limb, undue prominence of the veins and brown discolouration near the ankle (Figure 12.24). Examination confirmed that she had typical Parkes-Weber's syndrome with the left lower limb longer than the right side, all the superficial veins very prominent and brown areas of discolouration, similar to those seen in venous stasis, present in the lower leg and on the foot. The main arteries were clearly enlarged and giving augmented pulsation; on auscultation the common femoral artery emitted a continuous humming which could be heard widely over the left iliac fossa. Over the thigh, leg and foot, at varying strengths, could be heard the typical machinery bruit of arteriovenous shunts. In several areas on the inner calf and thigh diffuse pulsation could be felt. Branham's sign of slowing of the pulse on compression of the main artery of supply, the left common femoral, was not present, and on X-ray there was no cardiac enlargement. The enlarged superficial veins showed continous high flow and strong pulsation in time with the heart beat (Figure 12.25).

Arteriography confirmed considerable enlargement of the main arteries from common iliac level downwards, with similar enlargement of many branches. In a number of places throughout the limb and left pelvis diffuse areas of arteriovenous shunts could be recognized, often with enlarged arteries leading into them (Figure 12.26). The opacified blood appeared almost immediately in the main superficial and deep veins which were clearly outlined.

A conservative policy was adopted and the patient given thigh-length elastic support, which she often omitted to wear at first, and was encouraged to lead a normal life. On orthopaedic advice the right shoe was raised to equalize the limb lengths. She was seen annually and found to be handicapped very little so that she was able to train successfully as a nurse and enjoyed dancing amongst other activities.

At the age of 22 she married and within a year became pregnant. The world literature gave no guidance upon this situation and it was viewed with some misgivings, particularly as the left side of the pelvis was extensively involved with arteriovenous fistulas. After consultation between surgeons, cardiologist and obstetrician it was decided, fortunately, to accede to the patient's wishes and allow pregnancy to continue on a month-by-month basis. In the event pregnancy (Figure 12.27) and childbirth caused no difficulties; the cardiologist kept a watchful eye throughout and although the heart showed some

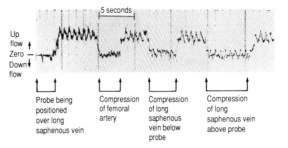

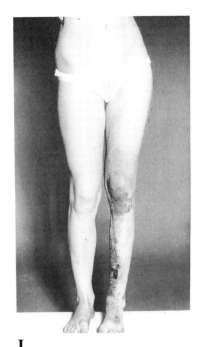

1

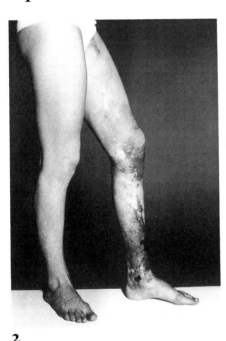

2

**Figure 12.25** *Parkes-Weber's syndrome, patient S.D. Doppler tracing to show the strong arterial pulsation detectable in the superficial veins*

**Figure 12.24** *Parkes-Weber's syndrome, patient S.D. Photographs of the patient at the age of 18 years The left limb shows obvious lengthening and the veins are unduly prominent. Pigmentation and scarring of past ulceraton, due to high venous pressure, are extensive over the lower limb and at the knee. Loud bruits could be heard throughout the limb and pulsation of tissue masses could be felt in many areas (see text and Colour Plate 7 for further details)*

hypertrophy this was considered to be within acceptable limits. About 2 years later she become pregnant again and was so keen to have a further child that no attempt was made to dissuade her and once more pregnancy and childbirth were uneventful and there was no perceptible deterioration in the limb.

By the age of 26 the patient, now a busy mother and housewife, did begin to show signs of renewed deterioration in the limb and decompensation in the heart state; at this stage Branham's sign had become positive (Figure 12.28) and ulceration became more extensive. The cardiologist expressed concern at the heart state and the matter of major amputation was seriously discussed with the patient. It was her wish that every alternative measure should be tried first and at this time the technique of embolization by arterial catheter had become available. This was carried out, occluding several major branches supplying large areas of fistulous tissue, and brought about a marked improvement in the cardiac state which has remained stable since then. However the ulcerated areas in the lower leg had not shown any great response and later caused two episodes of quite alarming haemorrhage. These were controlled without undue difficulty by elevation and a pressure pad. Further embolization was then carried out by arterial catheter to selected branch arteries in the upper calf. This brought considerable improvement to the leg and foot with progressive healing of the ulcers but it was noticed that the ankle pulses had disappeared and subsequent arteriogram showed that a Gianturco coil used for arterial occlusion had moved back into the lower popliteal artery and caused its occlusion. Since that time the patient has retained good function in the limb but has to be very protective towards it. If the limb is elevated the foot becomes pale and numb; similarly numbness and rest pain are set up by firm bandaging or strong elastic compression. The patient now avoids raising the leg above the horizontal and, if there is a tendency for ulceration to recur, can heal this by keeping the leg in a horizontal position so that venous pressure is minimal but yet perfusion is maintained. The haemodynamic significance of this has been discussed in the previous section. This patient is now aged about 30 and bringing up her children successfully with no great limitation on her mobility. It is perhaps expecting too much for this now precarious limb to be preserved indefinitely; undoubtedly the cheerful courage shown by this patient has been an inspiration

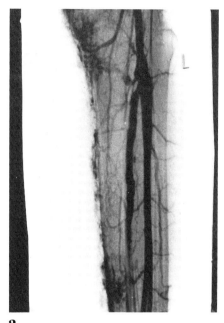

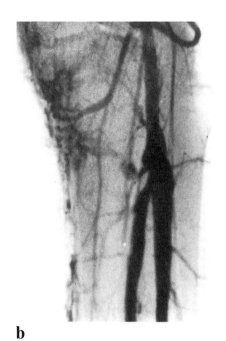

**a**                                                                          **b**

**Figure 12.26**  *Parkes-Weber's syndrome, patient S.D.*

*(a)  Arteriogram showing areas of arteriovenous fistulous tissue with feeding arteries down the inner side of the leg.*

*(b)  Close-up view of a fistulous lesion and feeding artery in the upper leg. This was subsequently occluded by a Gianturco coil (see text)*

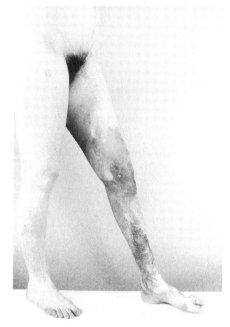

**Figure 12.27**  *Parkes-Weber's syndrome, patient S.D. Patient in the fourth month of pregnancy with the leg in a very favourable state*

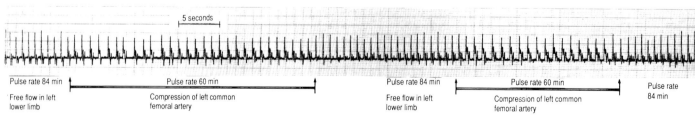

**Figure 12.28**  *Parkes-Weber's syndrome, patient S.D., showing positive Branham's sign. Pulse rate recorded by Doppler over the right radial artery while the common femoral artery to the arteriovenous fistulous limb (left) is occluded for 14.5 and 9.5 seconds. Each time, the pulse rate slows from 84 to 60 per minute in response to shutting off the arteriovenous shunts*

to her medical attendants and a major factor in the preservation of the limb so far. It could be argued that amputation should have been carried out at an early stage but the achievements of this patient have justified the decisions taken and at all times a watchful policy has been followed, with patient and surgeons fully prepared to carry out amputation if this becomes necessary. (Principal medical attendants; D. J. Tibbs and J. Webster, Surgeons. E. W. Fletcher, Radiologist.)

*Management of the orthopaedic aspects*

As with Klippel–Trenaunay syndrome, the young patient should be placed under orthopaedic supervision so that overlengthening of the limb is compensated for by raising the shoe on the normal side. This will restore symmetry and bring the pelvis to a horizontal position. However, unlike Klippel–Trenaunay syndrome, it is unlikely that the orthopaedic surgeon will be willing to carry out epiphysiodesis or, at a later stage, shortening of the femur, because of the unknown difficulties from haemorrhage that major surgery might cause during and after operation. Reviewing the world literature, there do not seem to be any reports of these operations being carried out successfully for Parkes-Weber's syndrome although there are many favourable references in its use in the venous dysplasias and, of course, for overgrowth of the limb without vascular changes. The disadvantages of a limb one or two inches longer than the normal side are easily compensated for by raising the shoe and any undue risk to avoid this does not seem justified.

Having given warning that few surgeons do corrective surgery to shorten the hypervascular limb one does recognize how much the alternative of somewhat ungainly footware is disliked by the patient and that in some cases correction of bone length may be justifiable. This might be so where bone lengthening and vascularity are confined to the tibial region and the proposed operation is to the subtrochanteric femur. In this case the vascular state in the vicinity should be assessed beforehand by serial arteriography. If there is no evidence of arteriovenous fistulous tissue in the area then the operation would seem justifiable. However, provision for temporary control of the main artery of supply at high level should be made. This will probably be the common iliac artery and it should be exposed through a muscle-splitting lower abdominal, extraperitoneal incision; alternatively the common femoral artery could be exposed so that if problems arose a Fogarty balloon catheter could be passed up to occlude the common iliac artery. The exceptionally vascular state of these limbs must not be underrated because the main arteries and their branches are much larger than normal and the collateral circulation is formidable. As an example, shutting off only the external iliac artery might well make no appreciable difference to bleeding in the subtrochanteric region via the uncontrolled internal iliac artery and the cruciate anastomosis. It would seem a safe rule to avoid major orthopaedic surgery if enlarged arteries (or bruits) extend up to, and certainly above, the level of intended operation.

## References

Askerkhanov, R. P. (1972) Clinical aspects and treatment of arterio-venous fistulae. *Khirurgiia (Moskva)* **48**, 98–102 (English abstract)

Baskerville, P. A., Ackroyd, J. S., Lea Thomas, M. and Browse, N. L. (1985) The Klippel–Trenaunay syndrome: clinical, radiological and haemodynamic features and management. *British Journal of Surgery*, **72**, 232–236

Baskerville, P. A., Ackroyd, J. S. and Browse, N. L. (1986) Is the Klippel–Trenaunay syndrome a mesodermal abnormality? In *Phlebology 85* (eds D. Negus and G. Jantet), John Libbey, London, pp. 767–769

Branham, H. H. (1890) Aneurismal varix of the femoral artery and vein following gunshot wound. *International Journal of Surgery*, **3**, 250–251

Browse, N. L., Whimster, I., Stewart, G. et al. (1986) Surgical management of 'lymphangioma circumscriptum'. *British Journal of Surgery*, **73**, 585–588

Browse, N. L., Burnand, K. G. and Lea Thomas, M. (1988) *Diseases of the Veins*, Edward Arnold, London, pp. 603–625

Clarke, P. J., Tibbs, D. J. and Kenwright, J. (1986) Bone overgrowth and vascular anomalies in the limbs; combined experience of an orthopaedic centre and a vascular clinic. In *Phlebology 85* (eds D. Negus and G. Jantet), John Libbey, London, pp. 798–800

Cotton, L. T. and Sykes, B. J. (1969) The treatment of diffuse congenital arterio-venous fistulae of the leg. *Proceedings of the Royal Society of Medicine*, **62**, 245–247

Dodd, H. and Cockett, F. B. (1976) *The Pathology and Surgery of the Veins of the Lower Limb*, Churchill Livingstone, London, pp. 160–170

Gloviczki, P., Hollier, L. H., Telander, R. L. et al. (1983) Surgical implications of Klippel–Trenaunay syndrome. *Annals of Surgery*, **197**, 353–362

Gomes, M. M. R. and Bernatz, P. E. (1970) Arteriovenous fistulas: a review and ten-year experience at the Mayo Clinic. *Mayo Clinic Proceedings*, **45**, 81–102

Hollier, L. H. (1985) Surgical treatment of congenital venous malformations. In *Surgery of the Veins* (eds J. J. Bergan and J. S. T. Yao), Grune and Stratton, London, pp. 275–284

Howell, R. (1978) Hypostatic ulceration and Klinefelter's syndrome. *British Medical Journal*, **2**, 95–96

Kinmonth, J. B. (1972) *The Lymphatics: Diseases, Investigation and Treatment*, Arnold, London

Kinmonth, J. B., Young, A. E., Edwards, J. M. et al. (1976) Mixed vascular deformities of the lower limbs, with particular reference to lymphography and surgical treatment. *British Journal of Surgery*, **63**, 899–906

Klippel, M. and Trenaunay, P. (1900) Du Noevus Osteo-hypertrophique. *Archives of General Medicine*, **3**, 641–647

Lea Thomas, M. (1982) *Phlebography of the Lower Limb*, Churchill Livingstone, Edinburgh

Lea Thomas, M. and Macfie, G. B. (1974) Phlebography in the Klippel–Trenaunay syndrome. *Acta Radiologica*, **15**, 43–56

Lindenauer, M. S. (1971) Congenital arteriovenous fistula and the Klippel–Trenaunay syndrome. *Annals of Surgery*, **174**, 248–263

Malan, J. B. and Puglionsi, A. (1964) Congenital angiodysplasias of the extremities. I: Generalities and classification, venous dysplasia. *Journal of Cardiovascular Surgery*, **5**, 87

McCullough, C. J. and Kenwright, J. (1979) The prognosis in congenital lower limb hypertrophy. *Acta Orthopaedica Scandinavica*, **50**, 307–313

Mulliken, J. B. and Young, A. E. (1989) *Vascular Birthmarks, Hemangiomas and Malformation*, Saunders, Philadelphia

Parkes-Weber, F. (1907) Angioma formation in connection with hypertrophy of the limbs and hemihypertrophy. *British Journal of Dermatology*, **19**, 231

Parkes-Weber, F. (1918) Haemangiectactic hypertrophy of limbs – congenital phlebarteriectasis and so-called congenital varicose veins. *British Journal of Childhood Diseases*, **15**, 13

Partsch, H., Mostbeck, A. and Wolf, C. (1986) AV shunts in congenital vascular malformations of the limbs. New approaches to diagnosis. In *Phlebology 85* (eds D. Negus and G. Jantet), John Libbey, London, pp. 791–794

Riche, M. C., Melki, J. P., Laurian, C. *et al.* (1986) Le role de l'hyperpresson veineuse dans les malformations arterioveineuses des membres. In *Phlebology 85* (eds D. Negus and G. Jantet), John Libbey, London, pp. 801–803

Sako, Y. and Varco, R. L. (1970) Arteriovenous fistula: results of management of congenital and acquired forms, blood flow measurements, and observations on proximal arterial degeneration. *Surgery*, **67**, 40–61

Taheri, S. A., Williams, J., Bowman, L. and Pisano, S. (1988) Superficial femoral vein transposition in Klippel–Trenaunay syndrome. *Phlebology*, **3**, 123–127

Young, A. E. (1983) Maldevelopments of the vascular system: clinical conundrums. In *Development of the Vascular System* (Ciba Foundation Symposium 100), Pitman Books, London, pp. 222–243

## Bibliography

Carruth, J. A. S. (1984) Argon laser in the treatment of port wine stain. *Journal of the Royal Society of Medicine*, **77**, 722–724

Friedman, E. I., Taylor, L. M. and Porter, J. M. (1988) Congenital venous valvular aplasia of the lower extremities. *Surgery*, **103**, 24–26

Gorenstein, A., Katz, S. and Schiller, M. (1988) Congenital angiodysplasia of the superficial venous system of the lower extremities in children. *Annals of Surgery*, **207**, 213–218

Greenhalgh, R. M., Rosengarten, D. S. and Calnan, J. S. (1972) A single congenital arteriovenous fistula of the hand. *British Journal of Surgery*, **59**, 76–78

Haughton, V. M. (1975) Hemoclip-Gelfoam emboli in the treatment of facial arteriovenous malformations. *Neuroradiology*, **10**, 69–71

Kheterpal, S. (1991) Angiodysplasia: a review. *Journal of the Royal Society of Medicine*, **84**, 615–618

Lawler, F. and Charles-Holmes, S. (1988) Uterine haemangioma in Klippel–Trenaunay–Weber syndrome. *Journal of the Royal Society of Medicine*, **81**, 665–666

Lendorf, A., Struckmann, J., Strange-Vognsen, H. H. and Nielsen, S. L. (1988) Congenital angiodysplasia of the lower limb: the Klippel–Trenaunay syndrome and arteriovenous fistulae. *Phlebology*, **3**, 31–39

Lodin, A. and Lindvall, N. (1961) Congenital absence of valves in the deep veins of the leg. A factor in venous insufficiency. *Acta Dermato-Venereologica (Stockholm)*, **41**, (Suppl. 45), 7–91

Rabe, E. (1987) Acute and chronic venous insufficiency in infancy and childhood. *Phlebology*, **2**, 249–255

Schwartz, R. S., Osmundson, P. J. and Hollier, L. H. (1986) Treatment and prognosis in congenital arteriovenous malformation of the extremity. *Phlebology*, **1**, 171–180

Tibbs, D. J. (1953) Metastasizing haemangiomata. *British Journal of Surgery*, **XL**, 465–470

van der Stricht, J. (1988) Classification of vascular malformations. *Phlebology*, **3**, 203–206

# 13

# Ulceration

## Part 1 Venous ulcers: the surgeon's viewpoint

In patients with a chronic ulcer on the leg or foot it is important not to assume too readily that venous insufficiency is the cause. This is an easy assumption to make because some 90% of ulcers in western communities have this origin. Alternative causes should always be considered, particularly if there is not strongly positive evidence of a venous origin. The problem is common (Widmer, Mall and Martin, 1977; Callam *et al.*, 1985; Cornwall, Dore and Lewis, 1986; Franks, Wright and McCallum, 1989) and 1% of the adult population suffers from leg ulcers at some time in their lives (Callam *et al.*, 1987b).

### Venous ulceration: an overall view

Venous ulceration is a phenomenon of high venous pressure and is seen typically in the vicinity of the ankle (Cockett, 1955). The usual cause for this is some form of venous disorder but any condition giving rise to venous hypertension can cause the same response, for example, arteriovenous fistula, whether multiple congenital lesions, or a single acquired variety with, say, ulceration in the hand below an arteriovenous fistula created for access in renal dialysis (see Figure 12.21). A venous ulcer will always be accompanied by other evidence of venous hypertension, that is, surrounding pigmentation, induration and swelling; veins in the vicinity are likely to be unduly prominent, if not grossly varicosed, when standing, and, on elevation of the limb, will collapse into deep grooves and hollows. Additional evidence of venous disorder is given by the clinical and special tests or, when necessary, by functional phlebography. The different patterns of venous abnormality that may cause ulceration and their assessment by clinical means and special investigations are given in detail in Chapters 2, 6, 8, 12, 24 and 25 (and see Colour Plates 1–7); only the general aspects will be summarized here.

### Causes of venous ulceration

#### Inadequate venous return against gravity – the cause of venous hypertension and ulceration

*Failure of the musculovenous pump*

The fundamental cause of venous ulceration is venous hypertension, that is to say, a sustained high venous pressure in the lower part of the limb, unrelieved by exercise, when the patient is upright and moving. However, ulceration may take many years to develop and the time of onset is probably related to the severity of the hypertension and a continuing deterioration in the musculovenous pump with the passage of time. A determining factor is thought to be the gradual development of cuffs of fibrin around the capillaries due to excessive transudate from the overdistended vessels and reduced fibrinolysis (Colour Plate 16). This forms a nutritional barrier (Browse and Burnand, 1978; Burnand *et al.*, 1982; Leach, 1984) which eventually gives rise to liposclerosis, as discussed in Chapters 6 and 8.

The chain of events leading to venous ulcer is summarized in Figure 13.1. The effect of venous hypertension will be aggravated by a peak of excessive pressure, repeated each time the foot is put to the ground and the dilated veins on its underside are forcibly emptied. All these events arise when the musculovenous pumping mechanism is proving inadequate in its task of returning venous blood from the foot and lower leg against gravity. There are two basic causes for this:

1. Massive downflow in incompetent superficial veins which overwhelms the collective efforts of the musculovenous pumps, particularly if they are less effective than normal. This state can certainly be greatly improved, if not cured, by surgical removal of the pathway of incompetent superficial veins, usually including the long or short saphenous veins (see Chapter 6).

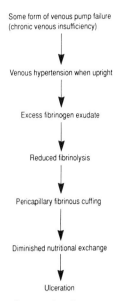

Figure 13.1 *Chain of events leading to venous ulceration.*

2. Insufficiency of the musculovenous pump itself, caused either by previous thrombotic damage to deep veins and valves (see Chapter 8) or an inborn deficiency of valves within the deep veins which often appears to deteriorate progressively through life (see Chapter 7). Surgery removing veins in these states may not be beneficial and, in the post-thrombotic limb, may actually cause harm by removing valuable collateral veins. With these patients, treatment will usually have to be by conservative means, following a policy of support bandage and elevation of the limb whenever possible. Skin grafting to the ulcer will not prove successful unless it is backed by an appropriate regimen of this sort. It is this group that produces the intractable venous ulcer that can only be controlled by constant vigilance. Included in this category of pump inadequacy is a localized form, the incompetent perforator, but this state, beset with misinterpretations, is a topic returned to later in this chapter and is fully discussed in Chapter 11.

Additional factors may aggravate a venous ulcer, for example, anaemia, or locally, ischaemia due to arterial disease; infection of the ulcer with a pathogen, such as *Staphylococcus aureus* or a beta-haemolytic streptococcus, may be the cause of pain and failure to heal.

### Arteriovenous fistula

Arteriovenous fistula causing ulceration has already been referred to and may be regarded as a special case of venous hypertension caused by copious arteriovenous shunting. The fistula may be congenital, or traumatic, in origin and is seldom difficult to diagnose once this possibility comes to mind. The surrounding skin will show the brown discolouration typical of ulceration caused by raised venous pressure. The most distinctive

feature is the presence of a bruit easily heard with a stethoscope, and a Doppler flowmeter will find pulsatile flow in the prominent veins running from this area. An arteriogram with serial films will confirm the diagnosis. Arteriovenous fistula is more fully discussed in Chapters 12 and 17 (and see Colour Plate 7).

Before considering further the recognition and treatment of venous ulcer, the range of ulcers in the leg from other causes will be considered.

## Other causes of chronic leg ulcer

The list of possible causes for ulceration is long and only some of the more important ones will be considered here.

### Ischaemic ulcer

This is usually due to atherosclerotic occlusion in the main arteries of the limb. It is mentioned first because it is quite common and failure to recognize it may lead to

**Figure 13.2** *Ischaemic ulceration.*

*(a) An ischaemic ulcer on the front of the leg, 10 cm above the ankle, in a woman aged 71. Ischaemia was caused by atherosclerosis with occlusion of superficial femoral and anterior tibial arteries. The ulcer is 'dry' and its base is sparsely lined with inactive granulation tissue; there is no sign of any epithelial ingrowth. The surrounding tissues do not show the stigmata of venous ulceration, that is, pigmentation, induration or enlarged veins. The scaly discoloured skin is the result of accumulation of skin debris under protective dressings; it is wrinkled by recent subsidence of oedema. Arterial reconstruction was feasible and brought about healing of the ulcer. However after 18 months the ulcer reappeared and it was found that the reconstruction had closed; amputation became necessary because of rest pain in the foot.*

*(b) Ulceration of a toe in an ischaemic foot. The patient was admitted for nocturnal rest pain which he had been relieving by hanging the foot out of the bed all night. A Doppler flowmeter was just able to detect an ankle pulse with a pressure index of 0.3, that is to say, at a level of critical ischaemia. On brief elevation the forefoot and toes showed obvious pallor; the dorsum of the foot was markedly oedematous and tender due to prolonged dependency and streptococcal infection. Initial treatment was given by adequate analgesia, antibiotics and positioning the limb slightly below horizontal, with active movement encouraged. After 48 hours, as shown in the photograph, the foot shows generalized wrinkling due to recent subsidence of oedema; the tip of the second toe is mummified due to gangrene of several weeks' duration. An ulcer is present over the bony prominence at the proximal interphalangeal joint; this had allowed entry of streptococcal infection to the dorsum of the foot but ischaemia has prevented any inflammatory response. Arterial reconstruction was not feasible and amputation was advised in order to relieve rest pain. Venous ulceration on the toes is a rarity and the commonest cause for ulcer here is a diabetic neuropathy and/or ischaemia from arterial disease. In such cases there is abundant evidence of the true cause (see Chapter 17) so that confusion with venous ulceration should not arise*

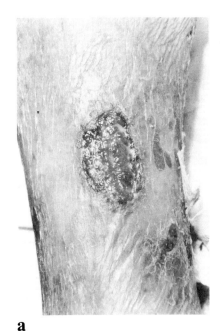

**a**

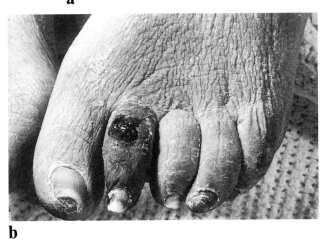

**b**

In any ulcer the arterial supply in the limb should be checked upon by confirming adequate pulses and this is of especial importance if the patient is in considerable pain. In its most severe form the ischaemic patient sits in a knee-up position (Figure 13.3 and see Colour Plate 12)

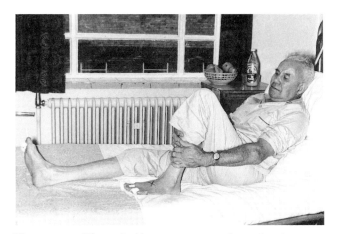

**Figure 13.3**  *The typical knee-up posture of a patient in great misery from ischaemic rest pain*

much unnecessary suffering with eventual loss of the limb (Callam *et al.*, 1987a). This important state is discussed in Chapter 17. An ischaemic ulcer can be several centimetres across and if it is positioned near the ankle may be mistaken for a venous ulcer (Figure 13.2). This is a bad error as the principles of treatment needed for a venous ulcer (elevation and firm bandaging) are in direct conflict with the requirements of an ischaemic ulcer. Elevation can only reduce the blood supply further (see Colour Plates 10 and 11) and, indeed, may put the foot at risk of being lost; similarly any form of pressure bandage will further impede the precarious arterial blood supply (see Colour Plate 17). Such measures will increase the patient's pain and cause the ulcer to deteriorate. In cases of uncertainty, it is best to avoid raising the leg above the horizontal and to not use any form of compression bandaging. Expert arterial assessment is, of course, particularly important if any form of surgery is contemplated and there are no easily recognized ankle pulses, or if the foot does not maintain good colour in elevation.

or with the limb hanging over the side of the bed and clearly in great misery. The ulcer may be only quite small, or of considerable size with a sloughing base which may eventually progress to exposing necrotic tendon or muscle (Figure 13.4). It does not show the pigmented, indurated surroundings that are so typical of the venous ulcer (unless ischaemia is superimposed upon a longstanding venous disorder and this is not a rare combination in the elderly). The ischaemic ulcer may occur on the front of the shin without any evident lesion of the foot. Another favourite site is over a bony prominence, such as a malleolus, and an ulcer here should always arouse suspicion of ischaemia or diabetic neuropathy, or both. It is important to realize that an ischaemic ulcer will not be able to react to infection with the usual inflammatory response or purulent exudate and may show no more than blue, dying skin edges with steady deterioration when, in fact, it is heavily invaded by *Staphylococcus aureus* or a similarly destructive organism. An ischaemic limb must not be elevated, but given a slight down position with frequent active movement and hourly short walks; only loose dressings should be applied and an appropriate antibiotic given. An arteriogram will be needed to determine if arterial reconstruction is feasible. If rest pain is severe this will only be relieved by restoration of the blood supply by arterial surgery or by amputation. The latter measure should never be resorted to without arteriogram because many of these patients will prove suitable for successful balloon angioplasty or arterial surgery. Clearly, in the assessment of any patient with ulceration it is necessary to be adept at feeling ankle pulses but, since these may be remote because of induration and swelling, it is also necessary to be skilled in the use of a

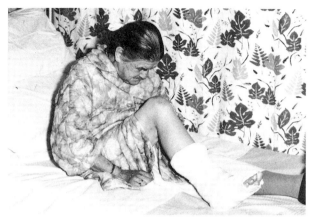

**a**

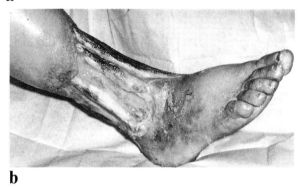

**b**

**Figure 13.4** *Ischaemic rest pain and massive ulceration of the leg.*

*(a) For 3 months prior to this photograph the patient had refused to come into hospital for treatment (see also Figure 17.7(b)). She has the typical posture adopted to relieve pain in an ischaemic foot and the bandages cover an ulcer.*

*(b) With the bandages removed massive ulceration is revealed. Necrotic muscle and tendon are easily recognizable. A venous ulcer does not cause a patient to sit in this knee-up position or to hang the leg out of bed, nor does it expose necrotic muscle or bone. In a limb with this severity of change, confirmation of ischaemia is readily obtained by the clinical and special investigations described in Chapter 17*

Doppler flowmeter in detecting the pulses and measuring peripheral arterial pressure.

Martorell's ulcer is the name given to ulceration appearing in older patients known to have arterial disease but yet with a reasonable overall arterial supply to the leg and foot. The origin is uncertain but may be by localized arterial thrombosis or microembolism from aortic disease. The ulcer may persist for many months but eventually heal.

### Diabetic ulcers

These are mainly due to neuropathy but ischaemia is often an additional factor. A diabetic peripheral neuropathy causes diminished sensation, with inability to feel pain in the affected parts, so that the protective reflexes are lost and any point of prolonged pressure to the skin may ulcerate without the patient being aware that anything is amiss. Thus a painless ulcer, often disregarded by the patient, may develop under a metatarsal head or over a malleolus. Ulcers over the bony prominences of foot or ankle should arouse immediate suspicion of diabetes (Figure 13.5 and see Colour Plate 8). Arterial insufficiency, without accompanying neuropathy, causes a different form of vulnerability in the skin, and, as previously stated, on its own may cause similar ulcers over malleoli or joints of the toes; in combination with a diabetic neuropathy it will accelerate the tendency to ulceration. A diabetic ulcer exposes the surrounding tissue to a constant threat of bacterial invasion which typically creates a progressive but painless cellulitis that may eventually destroy the foot (see Colour Plate 9). In this way, diabetes is a threat to the foot as well as to the patient's general health and it is a bad error to misdiagnose its characteristic lesions on the foot or ankle as venous in origin. All new patients with ulcer should have a routine check of the urine or blood to exclude diabetes.

### Neuropathic ulcers

These ulcers also arise from various other neurological states including spina bifida, tabes dorsalis, syringomyelia and injuries to spinal cord or peripheral nerves (Figure 13.6). As with diabetes these ulcers will be painless. The ulcers of certain forms of leprosy are in part neuropathic.

### Specific infection

Specific infection may be a cause of ulceration either as an expression of systemic illness or as a localized infection. The range of possibilities, including syphilis and tuberculosis, as rarities, will not be considered further here but in every case the possibility of a generalized cause for ulceration of the leg should never be too far from mind, epecially with the present increasing frequency of the acquired immune deficiency syndrome (AIDS) which takes many forms, including Kaposi's sarcoma. Appropriate serology may be important.

*Bacteriological note.* All ulcers become colonized by harmless commensal organisms but, as stated above, specific pathogens may complicate ulceration of any type and must not be overlooked. Culture for the prevailing organisms is a necessary routine at the outset. It is important to realize that the ischaemic ulcer will not be able to show the normal inflammatory response to infection, so that it may go unrecognized, with the ulcer surrounded by an area of blue, dying skin.

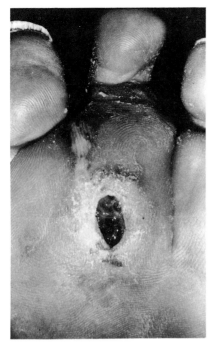

**a**

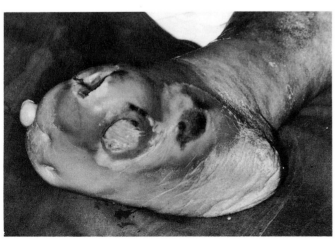

**d**

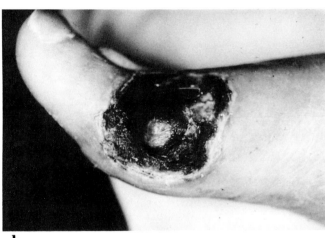

**b**

**c**

**Figure 13.5**   *Ulceration in diabetes. The cause is diabetic neuropathy with loss of pain sensation and protective reflexes; this may be aggravated by accompanying arterial disease. The ulcer typically occurs by pressure necrosis over bony prominences against which the skin may be crushed for prolonged periods without any warning pain.*

*(a)   Perforating ulcer on the the sole of the foot, overlying the head of the second metatarsal bone. This ulcer is painless and may remain unchanged for many months but is unstable because eventually infection will enter through it to invade the surrounding tissues (and see Colour Plates 8 and 9).*

*(b)   A similar lesion exposing the first metatarsophalangeal joint.*

*(c)   The final outcome after many years in a diabetic foot in which four metatarsal heads and corresponding toes have been successively amputated to allow perforating ulcers to heal. Further ulceration has now occurred on the sole of the foot and allowed entry of infection, with a cellulitis spreading painlessly from it. This has caused extensive necrosis of tendons and ligaments within the foot and ankle. There is comparatively little swelling and the overlying skin shows little discolouration. This process has simmered for many weeks without the patient being aware that the foot was being steadily destroyed by the tunnelling infective gangrene to which diabetic patients are particularly prone.*

*(d)   Diabetic ischaemic gangrene of a toe with a painless but destructive cellulitis spreading from it to the dorsum and underside of the foot. This was far more extensive than the obvious skin changes would suggest and amputation was necessary.*

*Diabetic ulceration and complications arising from it are insidious and very damaging. On the foot it is unlikely to be confused with venous ulceration but over a malleolus it may be unless the examiner is alert to this possibility (see Chapter 17)*

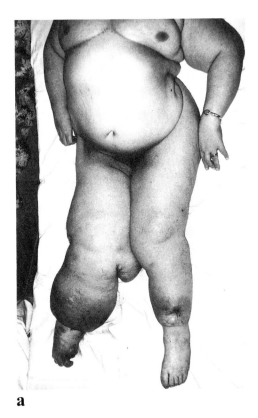

**a**

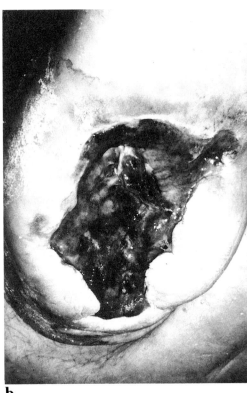

**b**

**Figure 13.6** *(a), (b) Neuropathic ulceration at the heel in a young woman with spina bifida and lymphatic dysplasia in the right lower limb*

*Neoplastic ulcers*

Neoplastic ulcers, such as melanoma (Figure 13.7) or epithelioma, are always possible although usually with recognizable malignant features. Raised, everted edges are characteristic of epithelioma but this clinical feature may not be evident in a malignant melanoma. Brown to

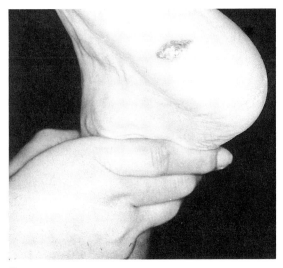

**a**

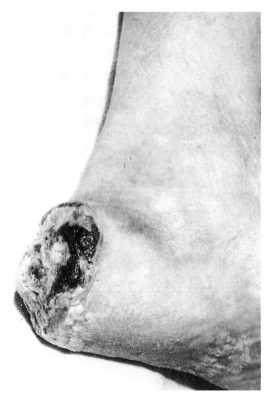

**b**

**Figure 13.7** *Malignant ulcers on the foot.*

*(a) Malignant melanoma on the underside of the heel. This lesion showed variegated pigmentation, irregular outline and commencing ulceration near its centre.*

*(b) Epithelioma of the heel (squamous carcinoma) (by courtesy of S. Rose)*

black discolouration usually accompanies a melanoma and may spread into the tissues round it, but this is unlikely to be confused with venous pigmentation. Danger signals with a pigmented lesion or mole are: itching or pain; size greater than 8 mm or progressive increase in size; variegation in the shades of brown to black within the lesion; irregular outline; inflammation or a reddish edge; bleeding or exudation, perhaps forming a crust; ulceration (Which? Consumers Association, 1988). Malignant change in any longstanding ulcer is a well-recognized cause for a venous ulcer failing to heal (Marjolin's ulcer) (Figure 13.8(a),(b)). This is usually a squamous cell carcinoma but sarcoma is possible, although very rare (Berth-Jones et al., 1989). If there are any doubts about the nature of an ulcer then biopsy is essential; if melanoma is suspected, excision of the entire lesion with a generous margin is the best form of biopsy. The development of rodent ulcer (basal cell carcinoma) in an area of venotensive change must be rare (McQueen 1980) but an example of this is illustrated in Figure 13.8(c).

## Chronic leg ulcers in the tropics

The tropics bring their own distinctive varieties of ulcer on the leg and foot. The term 'tropical ulcer' (Naga sore) is used for a particular ulcer on the lower leg, commonly occurring in Africa, South Asia and tropical America, and probably the result of infection, nutritional deficiency and trauma (or insect bite). The organisms *Fusobacterium fusiforme* and *Borrelia vincenti* are usually present and considered causative, but other bacteria such as proteus and pseudomonas are possible contaminants (Manson Bahr and Bell, 1987). It develops within a few weeks and quickly breaks down to a large painful ulcer that persists indefinitely unless it is treated. Many other infective ulcers occur, including yaws, leprosy, acquired immune deficiency syndrome, fungus infections and cutaneous leishmaniasis (also known by a variety of names such as oriental sore or Aleppo boil, caused by the same organism as kala-azar and occurring mainly in North Africa, the Middle and Far East and South America). Many of these ulcers will have features in common with venous ulceration but will lack the essential evidence of an accompanying venous insufficiency. Moreover, in most, positive identification is possible by microbiology, serology or biopsy.

This is a large topic (well covered by Manson-Bahr and Bell, 1987) and will not be considered further here. However, it must be pointed out that with present widespread international travel and holidays in exotic places an appreciable number of ulcers from the tropics are now being diagnosed in temperate countries, so that this possibility cannot be ignored.

## Blood dyscrasias

Any severe anaemia, sickle cell anaemia (see Colour Plate 23), thalassaemia, hereditary spherocytosis or leukaemia can provide obscure forms of chronic leg ulceration. It is wise to carry out a routine blood examination at an early stage as this proves to be an occasional pitfall in a condition which may be treatable or has important general implications.

## Nutritional and metabolic disorders

Vitamin and nutritional deficiencies, uraemia and other metabolic disorders may cause or aggravate chronic ulceration.

## Skin sensitivity or allergy

Skin sensitivity or allergy to materials used at work, applied medicinally or for cosmetic reasons, can either cause or aggravate ulceration (see Colour Plates 18–21). It is commonplace for leg ulcers to be exacerbated by inappropriate ointments, particularly antibiotics, cortisone and antiseptics, and this possibility must be considered at intervals in the long-term management of ulcers (Figure 13.9). A wide range of drugs taken internally for other conditions may cause skin reactions and eventually ulceration but these are likely to be widespread and not confined to the one limb.

## Trauma

Trauma as a single episode commonly sets off an ulcer in the presence of venous stasis, ischaemia and in many of the generalized states listed in this section. The skin of patients on heavy dosage of corticosteroids will become fragile and be especially vulnerable to any form of minor trauma so that extensive separation of skin may occur and be very difficult to heal.

**Trauma by injection of chemical or by insect bite** Subcutaneous, or worse, intradermal injection of venosclerosant can cause necrosis and prolonged ulceration (see Chapter 19). Many chemicals used medically and industrially can have the same effect. High pressure injection of grease, as used in servicing automobiles, can cause widespread destruction of subcutaneous tissue and the overlying skin. Many insect bites inject a necrotoxin to which may be added infection and so cause unpleasant, prolonged ulceration. Insect bite may also implant parasitic or protozoal (e.g. leishmaniasis) organisms to cause chronic lesions but this is uncommon in temperate climates.

**Repeated trauma** either caused at work or self-inflicted in psychiatric disorders or malingering (dermatitis artefacta) can be an occasional but puzzling cause for ulceration. Injury to the skin may also be thermal, from

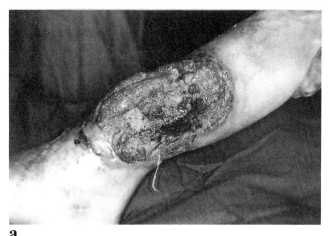

**a**

**Figure 13.8** *Malignancy complicating venous ulceration.*

*(a) Malignant change in longstanding ulceration (Marjolin's ulceration), thought to be venous in origin. This had been present for many years and it is not known when malignant change commenced. At the stage shown the neoplasm had invaded deeply to expose underlying muscle and bone, which had fractured (squamous cell carcinoma).*

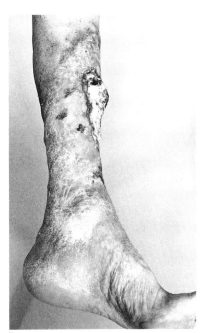

**b1**

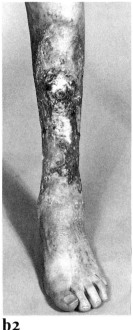
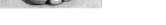

**b2**

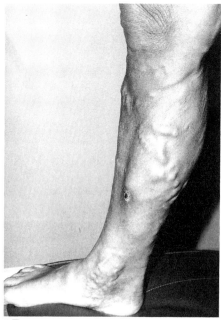

**c1**

**c2**

*(b) 1, 2. Another example of Marjolin's ulcer in longstanding 'venous ulceration'. The heaped-up tissue in its upper part was hard and irregular to touch; this should always arouse suspicion that malignant change has occurred and biopsy should be carried out. Marjolin's ulcer has usually invaded the underlying deep tissues and bone by the time it has been recognized, so that amputation is often the only realistic treatment (squamous cell carcinoma).*

*(c) An unexpected finding of rodent ulcer (basal cell carcinoma) masquerading as a venous ulcer.*

*1. A 1 cm scabbed ulcer with a small area of pigmentation and induration surrounding it, present for 2 years in a female patient aged 57. Massive varicosities due to long saphenous vein incompetence were present and all tests*

*indicated substantial venous hypertension (see Figure 6.6 for further details). Surgical treatment to the veins was carried out and it was confidently expected that the ulcer would heal over the coming weeks.*

*2. When reviewed 1 year later treatment of the venous state had given an excellent result with no remaining veins and the photoplethysmogram now normal. However the ulcer, shown here, had persisted and somewhat increased in size. Every few weeks it shed the crust on its surface but this soon reappeared and the edge was slightly beaded; rodent ulcer was suspected. Surgical excision confirmed that it was a basal cell carcinoma. This is a rare combination and it is not known whether it was a rodent ulcer from the outset or a development in a small venous ulcer. The patient said that it all started with an insect bite*

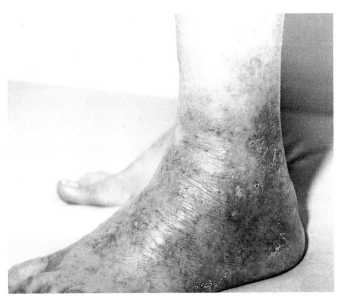

**Figure 13.9** *Skin sensitization or allergy to materials used in treatment of venous ulceration. In this patient an area of active venotensive change, with threatened ulceration, had been treated by a preparation containing neomycin. Over the next few weeks a reactive dermatitis developed, with multiple breaks in the skin exuding fluid. This soon cleared on ceasing to apply neomycin; the venotensive skin changes subsided with elevation and subsequent mobilization in an inelastic (paste) bandage*

radiation or from chemicals, possibly unsuspected by the patient.

### Rheumatoid arthritis

This may be accompanied by a diffuse vasculitis and is a not uncommon cause for intractable ulceration, sometimes mistakenly treated as venous ulcer (see Colour Plate 22).

### Systemic, autoimmune and microvascular diseases

Systemic, autoimmune and microvascular diseases (see Colour Plates 14 and 15) such as systemic lupus erythematosus, erythema nodosum due to pulmonary sarcoidosis (Figure 13.14) and polyarteritis are rare but potent causes for ulceration.

**Microvascular disorders** Chilblains can give prolonged, painful ulceration on the back of the lower legs, foot and toes (and the hand), lasting through the winter months. They occur especially in teenage girls with acrocyanotic limbs (erythrocyanosis fridiga) and by adult life they usually cease, but the acrocyanosis and tendency to oedema persists and Raynaud's phenomenon may be troublesome. In cases of recurring distress lumbar sympathectomy by surgery or phenol injection can give great benefit but should not be resorted to without strong cause in young people. The condition is independent of varicose veins but if a venous disorder does arise the limb tends

to react more severely than one without acrocyanosis. Undoubted varicose veins should be treated in the usual way but the patient warned that the acrocyanotic trait is a separate matter and may continue to cause an unsatisfactory appearance and tendency to oedema.

This list of causes for leg ulceration is by no means complete but emphasizes the need to be aware of the many possibilities, all too easily overlooked because venous ulcers predominate. When first seen, and at intervals afterwards, alternative diagnoses and a wide range of aggravating factors must be considered. Figure 13.10 outlines a diagnostic approach.

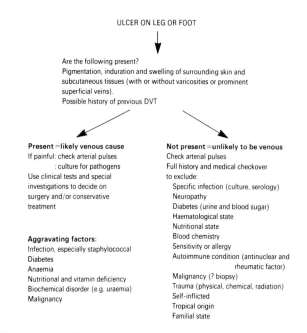

**Figure 13.10** *Diagnostic approach to ulcers of the leg*

## Identifying the venous ulcer

The foregoing section has indicated the wide range of diagnostic traps to be avoided before deciding on a policy of treatment. Fortunately, the venous ulcer usually has easily identifiable features that distinguish it from other forms of ulceration in the leg or foot and these may be summarized as follows:

### Occurrence

Venous ulceration occurs nearly equally in the two sexes, and is seen through a wide age group. It is seldom seen in childhood, and is then due to arteriovenous fistula, but thereafter it arises with increasing frequency throughout adult life. It may be seen in young adults after deep vein thrombosis caused by injury or pregnancy, or in congenital defects of the venous system in the lower limbs, as in Klippel–Trenaunay or Klinefelter syndromes (see Chapter 12). Age and sex are therefore of little diagnostic value, nevertheless, venous ulceration is by far the commonest cause of ulceration in western communities and in any patient with ulceration on the leg it is the first diagnosis to consider further or reject.

## Site

The commonest site is on the inner aspect of the lower leg just above the ankle. However, it is also found on the posterior or outer aspect of the leg and occasionally on the foot, so that although no site below the knee can be said to exclude it, an ulcer in the most characteristic position just above the ankle does considerably increase the probability of a venous origin. Ulceration on the weight-bearing areas under the foot is most unlikely to be venous in origin.

## Appearance and accompanying features

The ulcer itself is relatively non-specific in appearance and the best identifying features are in the surrounding tissues.

*Venotensive changes in surrounding and underlying tissues: lipodermatosclerosis*

It is here that the most characteristic visible and palpable changes of venous ulceration are to be found. They provide the evidence of venous disorder and, by implication, the likelihood that this is the cause of ulceration. The same changes without ulceration give warning that it is impending. The skin shows brown pigmentation; this is very variable in extent and density but is almost always present to a recognizable degree (Figure 13.11(a)–(e) and see Colour Plates 2–6). The subcutaneous layers are indurated and thickened by fibrosis and oedema (lipodermatosclerosis or liposclerosis). These changes again vary greatly and may be no more than a small area around and under the ulcer, or any size up to a massive encirclement of the leg (Figure 13.12). Lying intermingled with the indurated tissue are one or more enlarged veins which protrude when the patient stands and collapse into hollows or grooves, easily palpated, when the limb is elevated. In dark-skinned patients in whom venous pigmentation may be difficult to recognize the characteristic induration and grooving on elevation provides clear evidence of venotensive change.

**Cellulitis in the surrounding tissues** Invasion of the tissues around a venous ulcer by pathogenic organisms will cause the usual inflammatory reaction of pain, heat, redness and swelling (unlike the ischaemic ulcer where lack of blood supply may not allow these changes to appear). The intensity of inflammation will depend on the virulence of the pathogen involved and will vary from a chronic low grade change to an acute severe reaction possibly accompanied by lymphangitis (which may be mistaken

for superficial phlebitis). Culture and antibiotic treatment will be necessary in most cases showing inflammatory changes.

The surrounding skin may show the following additional changes:

**Eczema** This is a common accompaniment to pigmented venous hypertension and, hence, venous ulceration. It may overlie varicosities in a patchy fashion, following their course (Figure 13.13(a)), or, in a more widespread fashion, in an area of venotensive change (Figure 13.13(b)). The skin is often thickened and lichenified by constant rubbing and scratching in response to itching (lichen simplex). When eczema is seen on the lower limbs together with obvious varicose disorder it is likely to have been caused by this and if surgical cure of the venous condition is possible this will be followed by a gradual subsidence of the eczema. It is a form of sensitization and is easily reawakened if the venous hypertension has not been satisfactorily controlled. Its presence may considerably complicate treatment as it may become infected or, not infrequently, be severely aggravated by sensitivity to material applied to the ulcer by way of treatment, particularly antibiotics (see Part 2 in this chapter). Skin

---

**Figure 13.11** *Threatened and early venous ulceration; some unexpected causes and the need for comprehensive assessment (see page 271).*

*(a) Massive concealed long saphenous incompetence causing venotensive changes at the ankle, with pigmentation, liposclerosis and commencing eczema. Unless this is treated it will certainly progress to ulceration.*

*(b) Further example of venotensive changes from simple superficial vein incompetence. The only evident varicosity is comparatively small and at knee level, but the long saphenous vein is heavily incompetent.*

*(c) Another example, with early ulceration 1 cm across, again due to concealed saphenous incompetence.*
    *1. Before operation (and see Figure 6.7(b)2 for Doppler and photoplethysmogram).*
    *2. Six weeks after operation and immediate mobilization; the ulcer has healed, pigmentation is less intense, the surrounding skin more settled in appearance and discomfort has subsided. Because the patient was overweight and had a standing occupation as a bartender, he was advised to wear elastic support up to the knee whilst at work.*

*(d) Venotensive changes and recurring ulceration at the right ankle. The limb should always be fully inspected in the diagnosis of venous ulceration and in this patient the varicosities seen at the right groin suggest deep vein problems extending to the iliac vein. However, this is an example of cross-over simple incompetence arising from inadequate ligation of the left long saphenous termination (see Chapters 5 and 10).*

*(e) Area of venotensive change with recurring ulceration in a girl of 15 years. At this age, congenital venous abnormalities must be considered. Checking on the limb length showed that the left side was 4 cm longer than the right side and phlebography confirmed gross abnormality in the deep veins; these features are characteristic of Klippel–Trenaunay syndrome (see Chapter 12)*

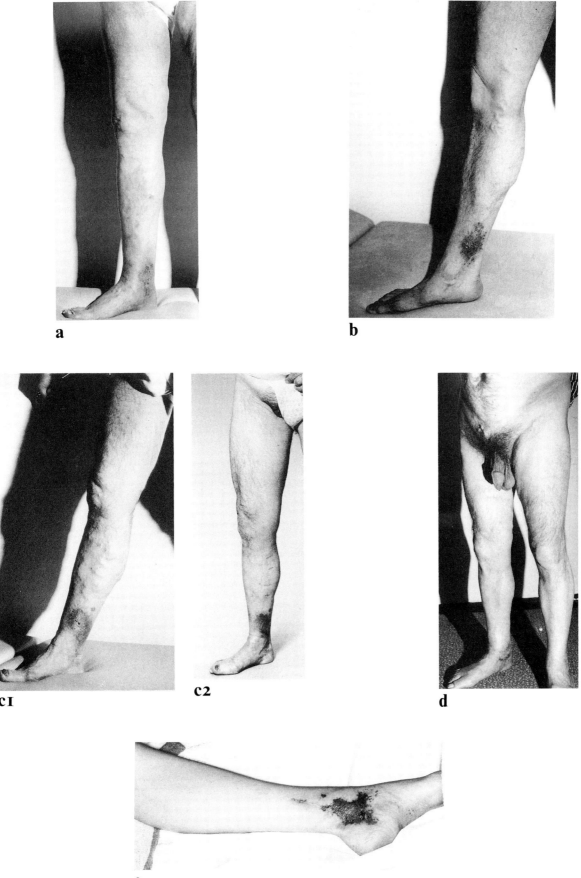

Figure 13.11

**Figure 13.12** *The changes accompanying venous ulceration and some points in diagnosis and management.*

*(a) An ulcer present for some months and showing pigmentation in the surrounding skin. Underlying this the tissues were indurated and grooved by enlarged veins, here collapsed because the limb is horizontal.*

*(b) Venotensive change and active ulceration due to incompetence in the long saphenous system, with a massive varicosity taking retrograde flow to the foot (and see Figure 4.8(b) for Doppler and photoplethysmogram). This patient could not find time to have treatment by surgery but was successfully treated by sclerotherapy to the foot varicosity.*

*1. Before treatment.*
*2. Three weeks after treatment. The foot vein is a firm cord and no longer an active pathway of incompetence. The skin changes have diminished, the ulcer is healing and the original discomfort has gone. The patient was urged to wear elastic support up to the knee and advised to have treatment completed by surgery when his commitments allow this.*

*(c) An actively deteriorating ulcer caused by chronic venous insufficiency. The ulcer is up to 8 cm across with blackened, necrotic edges and unhealthy looking granulation tissue; the surrounding area is indurated and pigmented. The foot shows multiple venous flares even though the limb is horizontal (see page 273).*

*(d) Extensive venotensive change with pigmentation and induration encircling the entire lower part of the leg. Several small areas of ulceration are present near the front. Massive concealed saphenous incompetence was an important factor in causation but phlebography showed there was a deficiency of deep vein valves. Surgical removal of the long saphenous vein gave considerable improvement but the patient was advised to wear elastic support up to the knee and to elevate the limb whenever possible as a permanent protective measure. When seen 2 years later the skin was in a settled state without ulceration or discomfort. The patient was urged to continue with protective measures (see page 273).*

*(e) 1, 2. Massive ulceration; aggravation of venous ulceration by simultaneous arterial disease. This elderly patient had massive bilateral ulceration and was found to have gross incompetence in the long saphenous veins together with bilateral occlusion of the superficial femoral arteries. Surgery, first to one side and then the other, was carried out, using each saphenous vein as a reversed vein graft, bypassing the occluded arteries. On the right side this gave an excellent long-term result with healing of all ulceration. On the left side the ulceration at first improved but after a few months relapsed to its original state (shown in the illustration). After a further 2 years of continuing ulceration and pain, amputation to the left side was advised; the arterial reconstruction remained open throughout but there was extensive occlusion of tibial arteries on that side which may explain this failure to thrive. The right limb remained healed and in good condition. Simple superficial vein incompetence alone is most unlikely to cause such extensive ulceration as seen in this patient and when encountered an additional factor, such as arterial disease, should be looked for. This is an unusual case with puzzling features but in less extreme cases a moderate sized ulcer due to combined venous and arterial insufficiency can be cured by using the saphenous vein to reconstruct the main artery and in this way the two conditions are treated by a single procedure (see Chapter 17) (see page 273).*

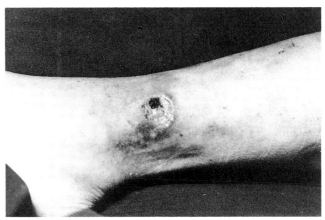

a

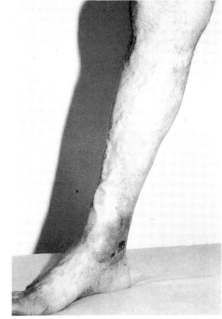

b1

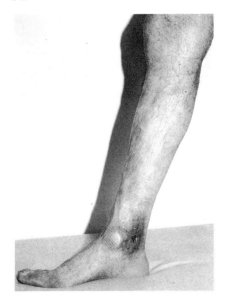

b2

There are several further points to note:

*(i)* The care of a limb with an occluded main artery directly conflicts with the requirements of venous ulceration. It is most unwise to use compression bandage or elevation if there is any degree of arterial insufficiency.

*(ii)* A patient with massive ulceration may become very anaemic and possibly deficient in proteins. Full blood examination is necessary and if need be a blood transfusion given. No ulcer, or skin graft, will heal satisfactorily in severe anaemia.

*(iii)* A large area of granulation tissue with widespread bacterial colonization will cause toxic absorption and considerable protein loss in exudate. As with burns, skin grafting can make a dramatic improvement but at the same time the process causing ulceration must be corrected.

*(iv)* Some of the largest and most puzzling ulcers the author has seen have been caused by self-inflicted injury in hysteria. These ulcers heal quickly with correction of anaemia, appropriate antibiotics and skin grafting, but it is essential to encase the limb in a protective shell of some sort. However, this does not cure the cause and relapse may soon occur on leaving hospital unless psychiatric treatment has been successful. Although such cases do occur they are rare and this diagnosis must only be made after most careful exclusion of all other possible causes and then only when strongly positive evidence of self-infliction has been obtained.

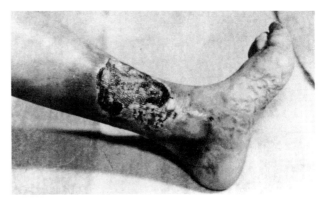

c

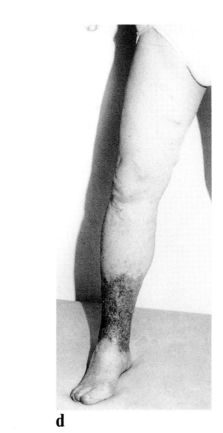

d

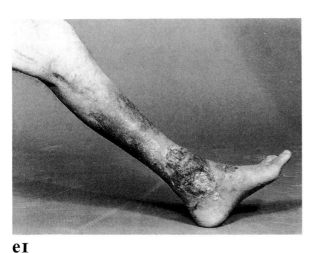

e1

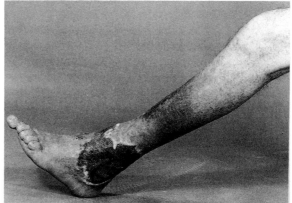

e2

**Figure 13.12** *(continued)*

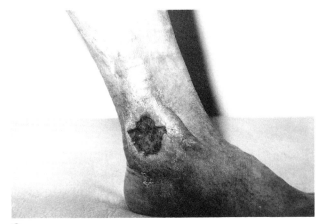

**f1**

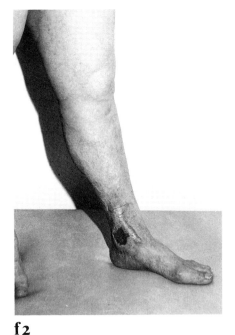

**f2**

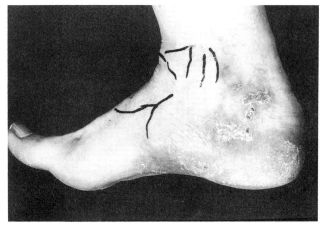

**a**

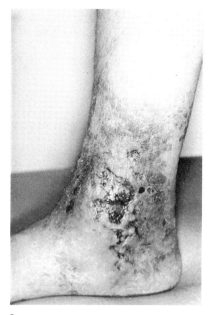

**b**

**Figure 13.12** *(continued)*

*(f)  1, 2. Chronic venous ulceration due to previous deep vein thrombosis (post-thrombotic syndrome). The ulcer shown in this illustration had been present for several years. Light pigmentation, with underlying induration, is present extensively in surrounding skin; there is no eczema. The scar is due to previous unsuccessful surgery to 'long saphenous vein and perforators'. In this limb the superficial veins are acting as collaterals past deformed and occluded deep veins and further surgical interference to them is contraindicated. This ulcer was healed by a spell of elevation and the patient mobilized with elastic support up to the knee and urged to elevate the limb whenever possible. He was able to prevent recurrence by these means*

**Figure 13.13**  *Eczematous skin changes in venous hypertension.*

*(a)  Eczema following the distribution of saphenous varicosities extending down to the foot but with no other evidence of hypertension.*

*(b)  An actively deteriorating venous ulcer with scattered irregular satellite ulcers which will soon coalesce unless  venous hypertension is relieved. In addition the surrounding skin shows marked eczema making it even more vulnerable. These changes arose from combined saphenous incompetence and valve deficiency in the deep veins (see Figure 7.2 for further details); it was evident that the patient was in urgent need of a spell of elevation to prevent rapid enlargement of the ulcer. With conservative treatment the ulcer healed and subsequently the saphenous vein was stripped in order to remove a major cause of venous hypertension. It was hoped this would reduce the tendency to ulcerate sufficiently for simple measures by the patient to prevent recurrence. An eczema such as this can be improved by corticosteroid cream but an eczematous skin has increased sensitivity to allergens, so that preparations containing antibiotic or other common allergens should not be used; steroid application to the ulcer itself prevents healing and care should be taken to avoid this (see text)*

manifestations of systemic disease may be mistaken for venous eczema (Figure 13.14) and although usually little harm is done if varicose veins are treated on this assumption, it does mean that an important diagnosis may be delayed. In some unrelated skin diseases, such as psoriasis, varicose veins may be an aggravating factor, so that their removal is beneficial and recommended for that reason (Figure 13.15).

The patient may also develop eczematous areas at distant sites, such as the trunk or upper limbs, but here there is always a possibility that the venous disorder in the lower limbs is not the cause but incidental to a generalized eczema developing for other reasons. The venous specialist must be alert to the possibility of eczema having a separate cause from an evident venous disorder, or that the 'eczema' is, in fact, some other skin disease, possibly an expression of potentially serious systemic disease. The index of suspicion must be high if the eczema does not follow the distribution of varicosities (usually below the knee but occasionally on the thigh) or is not in areas affected by venous hypertension, or when distant parts of the body are affected.

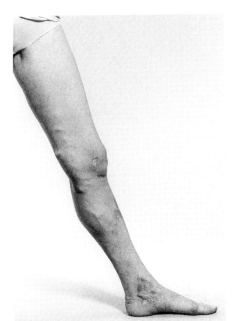
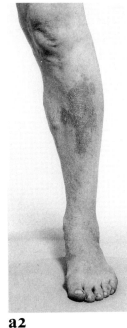

a1          a2

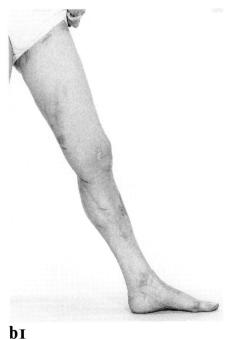
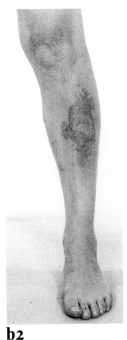

b1          b2

**Figure 13.14**  *Other skin conditions may be mistaken for those with a venous origin.*

*(a)* *1, 2. This skin eruption was attributed to venous eczema caused by long saphenous varicosities which were treated surgically.*

*(b)* *1, 2. Six weeks later the varicosities had gone but the skin lesion showed no improvement. Further investigation showed that this was, in fact, an erythema nodosum due to pulmonary sarcoidosis treated 5 years previously*

**Figure 13.15** *Other skin conditions, correctly diagnosed, may be aggravated by venous hypertension.*

*(a), (b) Views of the leg of a patient with extensive psoriasis particularly troublesome in this limb where substantial incompetence in the long saphenous system was also present. This was thought to be an aggravating factor and was treated surgically. The patient subsequently reported a decided improvement in the psoriasis of that limb*

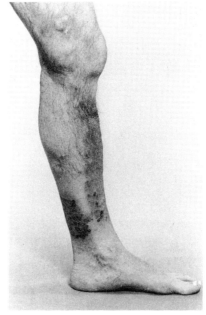 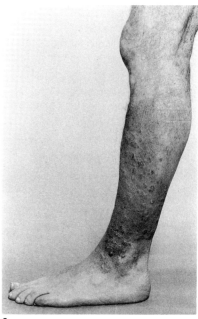

a                              b

**Atrophie blanche** This is not uncommon in venous hypertension and may be seen set amongst venous pigmentation or the scarring of past ulceration. The affected skin is white, thinned and often surrounded by fine vascular marking due to compensatory proliferation of capillaries (see Colour Plate 13); the area may vary from a few millimetres to several centimetres or more across (Figure 13.16). However, it is not specific to venous disease and its nature is not fully understood. It appears to be the result of thrombosis and obliteration of stressed capillaries in venous hypertension, or, in other cases, due to vasculitis and capable of causing extensive necrosis of skin (see Colour Plates 14 and 15). Whatever the origin, its presence is a warning of a vulnerable skin unable to respond to minor trauma or, more seriously, the forerunner of a destructive vasculitis. In the treatment of this there may be no response to any medication until the limb is put in high elevation and this suggests that venous pressure is an important factor in its occurrence (T. Ryan, personal communication).

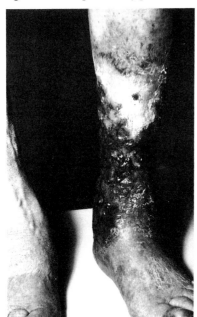

**Figure 13.16** *Other features seen in threatened or recurring ulceration. This patient, an elderly lady with a longstanding post-thrombotic syndrome (see Figure 9.5(a)), had struggled for many years to control extensive ulceration above the ankle. In mid-leg, above the ulcer, a white area of intense scarring and thin atrophic skin can be seen, left by repeated episodes of ulceration and healing. This is know as atrophie blanche and is found in longstanding venous hypertension, with or without ulceration*

**Venous flares** These are formed from overdistended venules and small veins in and immediately under the skin, often arranged in radiating or parallel lines (corona phlebectatica), and caused by prolonged hypertension (Figure 13.17). They will be particularly evident around the ankle and extending onto the inner aspect of the foot. With this manifestation there appears to be considerable variation in the individual response to venous hypertension, possibly due to such factors as inherent tissue strength, age, or excessive peaks of pressure change, and in some patients in whom extensive venous flares might be expected this is not found. When present it is a strong pointer to the presence of venous disorder and the possibility of venous ulceration; however, absence of venous flares at the ankle or foot must not be regarded as excluding hypertension.

**Sensitization reaction** The skin surrounding an ulcer may show dermatitis, which may be severe, caused by medical

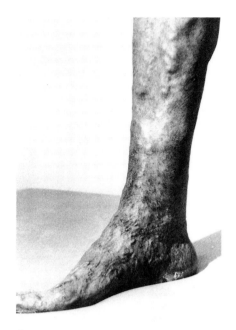

**a**

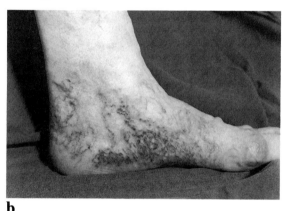

**b**

**Figure 13.17** *(a), (b) Venous flares or corona phlebectatica. In many patients with venous hypertension, flares of veins are seen in the lower leg and foot due to distension of small veins in, and immediately beneath, the skin. These may occur with venous hypertension from any cause but are not always present. They are also seen in the thinned atrophic skin of the elderly without other evident venotensive changes. However, their presence is always a warning that significant venous hypertension may be present. Both photographs are from elderly patients with substantial incompetence in the superficial veins*

applications and materials used in treatment of the ulcer (Figure 13.18).

*Features within a venous ulcer*

**Size of ulcer** This varies from a few millimetres to massive, perhaps even encircling the leg. There may be a central ulcer with small satellite ulcers around it, particularly when active deterioration is occurring (Figures 13.13(b), 13.19(a)).

**Edges** In a phase of active deterioration the edges are abrupt and irregular (Figures 13.13(b), 13.19(a)); in a

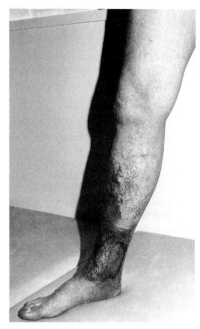

**Figure 13.18** *Sensitization reaction to medical applications in venous ulceration. This patient shows severe reaction in the skin around an ulcer treated by tulle gras impregnated with sodium fusidate. After several weeks of this treatment there was a severe deterioration, shown in the photograph, with a large area of exuding dermatitis. The original venotensive changes were caused by massive, and relatively concealed, incompetence in the long saphenous system. The condition improved quickly upon ceasing to use gauze and the veins were treated surgically*

healing phase the edges slope smoothly into a thin line of grey, newly grown epithelium (Figure 13.21(b)). The edges are never heaped up or everted and, if present, this suggests either a primary neoplasm (epithelioma) or malignant change in a longstanding ulcer; proliferating granulation tissue may at times simulate this.

**The ulcer base** There is great variation here depending upon the phase of the ulcer. In a healing phase the base will be of clean granulation tissue but in a phase of deterioration it will show sloughing tissue, from grey to black in colour, intermingled with areas of fibrin. A venous ulcer in a dormant phase may be covered completely with a thick dark-coloured crust or scab so that the underlying ulcer cannot be seen (Figure 13.20); here the characteristic surroundings, described below, will be most helpful. Thus there is no characteristic appearance for the base but there are some appearances which are certainly *not* characteristic:

Appearances of the base *not* in keeping with venous ulceration:

- Destruction through deep fascia exposing muscle and tendon strongly suggests ischaemic origin; this will cause severe pain provided it is not diabetic in origin.
- Exposed bone is not characteristic of venous ulcer but very typical of the (painless) diabetic ulcer which occurs at pressure points over bony prominences and,

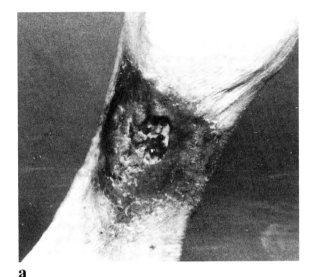

a

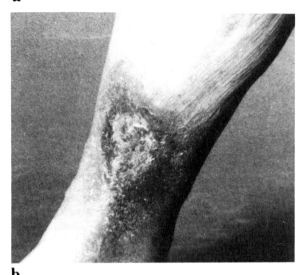

b

**Figure 13.19** *Venous ulceration in a phase of active deterioration, and after healing (see Figure 6.1 for further details of this patient).*

*(a) A 3 cm ulcer which has deteriorated rapidly and causing increasing pain. The edges are abrupt and irregular; small satellite ulcers are appearing at the lower part. The base shows inactive granulation tissue and some necrotic material; surrounding tissue is deeply pigmented.*

*(b) The cause of the ulcer, simple incompetence in the saphenous vein, has been removed by surgery, and now, 6 weeks later, the ulcer has healed (and see Colour Plates 2 and 3)*

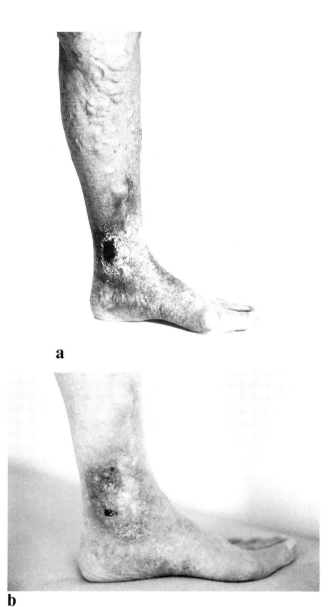

a

b

**Figure 13.20** *Scabbed or crusted ulcers.*

*(a) This ulcer was caused by long saphenous incompetence and showed typical features, including venous flares on the foot. However, the ulcer has formed a thick, hard protective crust and cannot be seen. It appears to be in a dormant phase, often well tolerated by the patient, but nevertheless it is unstable and may deteriorate at any time.*

*(b) Appearance 2 months after surgery to the long saphenous system, with removal of the crust from the ulcer and gentle curettage to the underlying granulation tissue. This has given a good result with healing of the ulcer except for a small scab which was shed soon after. The skin anterior to healed ulcer shows atrophie blanche*

under the foot, is characteristically punched out in appearance.

- A heaped-up, irregular, hard base should strongly suggest malignancy and the need for biopsy, but may be mimicked by excess granulation tissue to some extent.

A venous ulcer causes loss of skin and varying degrees of exposure of subcutaneous tissue and it sits on an area of indurated and oedematous tissues; it neither generates bulk (but malignancy does) nor exposes deep tissues such as tendons or bone (but ischaemia, diabetes or occasionally malignancy may do so).

**Discharge from the ulcer** This varies from a slight watery exudate in the clean ulcer through to heavy purulent

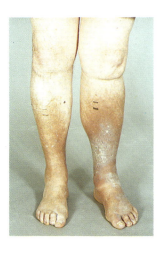

**1.** *The typical pigmentation of venous hypertension, and oedema, in post-thrombotic syndrome following multiple injuries. This is bilateral but the left side is more severely affected due to iliofemoral thrombosis (and see Figure 8.8(d))*

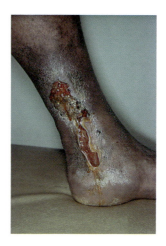

**6.** *Longstanding ulceration, induration and skin pigmentation in post-thrombotic syndrome. This was not in any way suitable for surgery but the patient conscientiously followed a regimen of elevation and support bandage. The ulcer slowly healed over the next 4 months (and see Figures 8.5(a) & 13.22)*

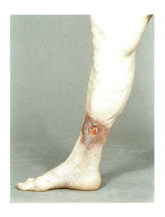
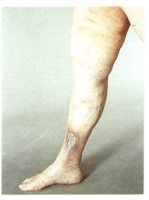

**2 and 3.** *Ulcer healing when venous hypertension is treatable. **2.** Pigmentation and ulceration at the ankle caused by superficial (long saphenous) vein incompetence. **3.** Six weeks after surgery and early mobilization; the ulcer has healed well (and see Figures 6.1(b) and 13.19)*

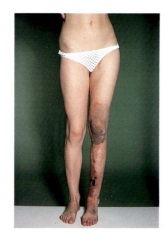

**7.** *The venous hypertension in congenital multiple arterio-venous fistulas is another cause for skin pigmentation and ulceration, as shown in this patient; the overlengthening of the limb is also characteristic (Parkes-Weber's syndrome) (and see Figure 12.24)*

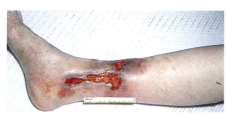
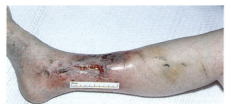

**4 and 5.** *To illustrate the speed of epithelial ingrowth when main cause (venotension from long saphenous incompetence) is removed. **4.** Ulcer before surgery and early mobilization. **5.** Three weeks later the ulcer has been greatly reduced by epithelial ingrowth, and healed within 2 months (and see Figure 13.21). Skin grafting offers little advantage here*

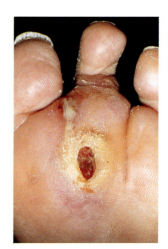

**8.** *Diabetic neuropathy causing ulceration by pressure necrosis of skin under head of second metatarsal bone. Healing occurred quickly after this bony prominence was excised (and see Figures 13.5(a) & 17.9(a))*

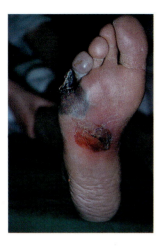

**9.** *Tunnelling gangrene in untreated diabetes. Over some weeks infection has tracked painlessly from an open lesion on a toe, and now the sole of the foot is filled with pus and a mass of necrotic tendons, even though the plantar skin is still intact. Amputation of foot is unavoidable (and see Figure 17.10(b))*

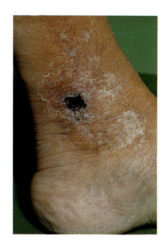

**13.** *Patches of atrophie blanche in an area of venotensive change. Such skin is vulnerable to injury and may undergo necrosis*

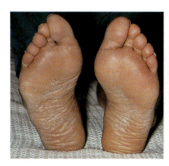 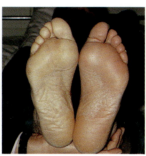

**10 and 11.** *Testing for ischaemia.* **10.** *With feet down – both show good colour.* **11.** *The feet have been raised 18 in. (45 cm) and blanched by hand pressure to forefoot and toes; the colour recovers quickly on the left side but the right side remains pale and will only recover colour slowly when put down (and see Figure 17.6)*

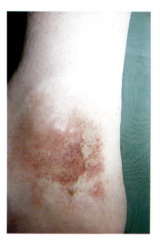 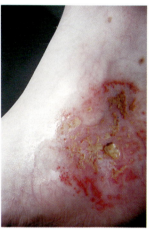

**14.** *Skin at ankle in early stage of necrosis due to vasculitis. Many small vessels are thrombosed and others are dilated.* **15.** *The same patient, now with multiple confluent points of necrosis as the skin breaks down to form a large ulcer*

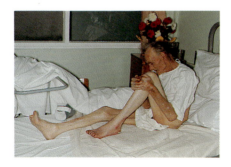

**12.** *The typical posture of ischaemic rest pain; note tobacco-stained fingers. A leg with skin lesions and pain of this severity must always be suspected of ischaemia; no limb should be treated by elevation without checking adequacy of arterial supply (and see Figure 17.7(a))*

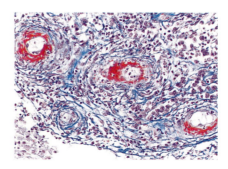

**16.** *Pericapillary cuffs of fibrin (stained red) in venous hypertension*

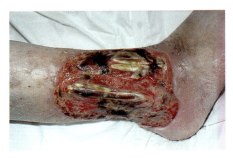

**17.** *An ischaemic ulcer that was mistreated and greatly exacerbated by elevation and compression bandage. A venous ulcer does not expose necrotic tendon in this way and the severe pain of this patient was typical of ischaemia. Amputation was necessary*

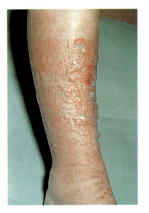 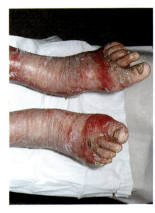

**18.** *Skin reaction to elastic adhesive bandage applied directly to skin is not uncommon, as shown here.* **19.** *An underlying layer of cotton or paste bandage can protect the skin from an outer layer of rubberized adhesive bandage but here it was allowed to overlap the toes, creating strong reaction*

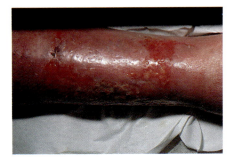

**20.** *Unsuitable adhesive tape used to retain dressing may strip away the surface layers, as in this example caused by sellotape*

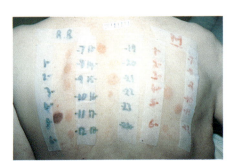

**21.** *A series of reactions to patch tests for sensitivity. The most important here are to lanolin, parabens and neomycin*

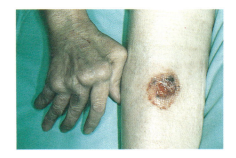

**22.** *Pyoderma gangrenosum due to vasculitis in a patient with rheumatoid arthritis*

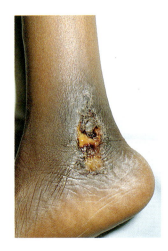

**23.** *Ulceration in a young woman with sickle-cell anaemia. This should always be excluded in a young patient with a leg ulcer*

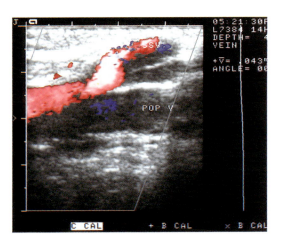

**24.** *Ultrasonic colour flow imaging (see Chapter 23). The upper popliteal vein and short saphenous termination are visualized and shown here immediately after release of calf compression. Flow towards the heart, coloured blue, has largely ceased but the short saphenous vein shows immediate reflux, coloured red – away from heart – indicating its incompetence. (Scanner used – Acuson 128 XP/10. By courtesy of Mr P. D. Coleridge Smith FRCS and Vincent Medical Ltd, Slough, UK)*

discharge in the infected ulcer. In the latter much depends on the prevailing organism and it may be blood stained, coloured yellow or green; in these circumstances bacteriological culture (including anaerobic) is highly desirable. There may be an offensive odour if longstanding necrotic tissue is present and this is best remedied by physical removal of the sloughs. None of these changes is specific to venous ulceration but do indicate an urgent need to reverse the processes that have caused them.

### Other features implying likelihood of venous disorder

In leg ulcers a history of previous deep vein thrombosis is especially relevant and should always be enquired for. In women this is most likely to have occurred during pregnancy or immediately after childbirth and often the patient refers to it as 'white leg of pregnancy'. In both sexes, major fracture of bones in the pelvis or lower limbs is very likely to have caused deep vein thrombosis which may occur without the patient being aware of it. Serious illness, surgical operations and the tell-tale accompaniment of pulmonary embolus or anticoagulant treatment are valuable pointers. If significant deep vein damage has persisted there is likely to be at least some oedema in the limb which in severe cases extends up to the groin.

The patient may well give a story of simple varicose veins, slowly enlarging over the years, and more recently giving rise to skin irritation and discoloured skin changes in the area now ulcerated. However, simple (primary) varicose veins are commonplace and it is always possible for an ulcer of completely different origin to be superimposed upon them. The true venous ulcer is a late development in the changes caused by venous hypertension and is always preceded by at least some of the premonitory changes given above and seen in the vicinity of the ulcer. Without such changes the presence of varicosities alone is insufficient to make a firm diagnosis of venous ulcer.

### Diagnosis by clinical response to treatment

The venous ulcer is often also referred to as a 'gravitational ulcer' because its activity is profoundly influenced by the position of the limb. Prolonged downward positioning will aggravate the ulcer, but if the limb is elevated continuously the ulcer will commence to heal within a few days because in this position there is free venous return without any venous hypertension. If it fails to do so, then there must be strong suspicion that the diagnosis is at fault and a full reappraisal is necessary. Nevertheless, there are other circumstances which may prevent a venous ulcer from healing, however favourable the treatment is otherwise, and these will include the following aggravating factors:

1. The limb also has ischaemic arterial disease; this combination is quite common in the older patient and ischaemia may predominate; this is especially deceptive if the patient had oedema when first seen, which was in fact due to hanging the limb out of bed to relieve ischaemic rest pain.
2. Poor general health caused by diabetes or liver, renal and other systemic disease, including malignancy.
3. Anaemia and blood dyscrasias generally.
4. Malnutrition and vitamin deficiency.
5. Uncontrolled infection in the ulcer, especially by *Staphylococcus aureus* and beta-haemolytic streptococcus.
6. The presence of necrotic tissue.
7. Unsuitable local applications to the ulcer, especially those to which the patient is sensitive.
8. Self-inflicted trauma in psychiatric states.
9. Simple lack of cooperation by the patient in following instructions.

Having established that the ulcer is venous in origin then the next stage in its management is to decide what form of venous disorder is present so that treatment appropriate for this may be decided on. This aspect of investigation should give further proof of a venous disorder consistent with venous ulceration. If it does not, then the nature of the ulcer is unsubstantiated and renewed thought must be given to its diagnosis. A systematic approach to ulceration of the leg or foot is illustrated in Figure 13.10.

## Management of the venous ulcer

### Recognizing the curable venous ulcer: the role of surgery

A venous ulcer, either longstanding or an ever-recurring one, is potentially curable if the venous hypertension that causes it can be corrected. This should certainly be possible when the primary cause is the overwhelming of the pumping mechanism by heavy downward flow in incompetent superficial veins. A typical example would be in a massive incompetence in a long saphenous system (Figure 13.21(a), (b)), either with easily visible varicosities, or of the 'concealed' variety without obvious varicosities (see Chapter 4). Surgical removal of this pathway of incompetence relieves the musculovenous pump of the excessive load upon it so that its ability to reduce venous pressure is restored and the ulcer will heal (Figure 13.21(c)–(e)). In our experience nearly 50% of new patients presenting with actual or threatened ulcer fall in this category and it is therefore a very important group to recognize reliably. This has been considered in Chapters 4–6 and the method of examination will only be summarized here:

1. With patient standing, the enlarged veins are mapped out by the tapwave technique; this will locate the likely

pathway of incompetence, including a 'concealed' saphenous vein.

2. A selective Trendelenburg test is applied by finger pressure to the suspected pathway of incompetence to see if this gives good control even when the patient exercises during the test. A Perthes' test similarly applied by finger pressure will usually give strong additional evidence but may be less certain in its interpretation and an equivocal result does not invalidate unequivocal control by a selective Trendelenburg test.

3. Clearly positive control by a selective Trendelenburg test is usually sufficient evidence that removal of the pathway of incompetence will bring benefit to the patient and operation is indicated. If there is any doubt then additional investigations will be needed.

4. The directional Doppler flowmeter should show downflow in the pathway of incompetence or its branches after calf muscle contraction or raising the foot (Figure 13.21(a)1).

5. With superficial incompetence of sufficient severity to cause an ulcer, photoplethysmography (or other forms of plethysmography, volumetry or direct venous pressure measurement) should show an abnormally shortened recovery time after exercise. This reverts to near normal when the pathway of incompetence is temporarily occluded by finger pressure (not by a constricting band) (Figure 13.21(a)2). A positive result is very meaningful and gives firm reassurance that operation will be beneficial; it also confirms that the pathway of incompetence has been correctly identified, but a negative result cannot be relied upon to exclude simple incompetence in the suspected vein.

6. If there are still doubts or if there is a history of possible deep vein thrombosis then functional phlebography must be used.

## Functional phlebography in diagnosis of causative venous disorder

### Superficial vein incompetence

If ulceration is caused by superficial vein incompetence there is usually no need to resort to phlebography but when it is used it will show the following features (and see Chapter 22):

• Downflow in superficial veins after exercise, with opacified blood entering the deep veins at low level.

• Further injection of medium will outline widely open deep veins, without deformity up the length of the limb.

• Exercise at this stage will cause spillover from the source at high level and down the pathway of incompetence (see Chapter 4).

• Rapid change from near vertical to near horizontal and back again (swill test) will display deep vein valves.

These findings represent a clear demonstration of superficial incompetence, with satisfactory deep veins; surgery to remove the pathway of incompetence is indicated and very likely to benefit the ulcer. A swill test may demonstrate a deficiency of deep valves in keeping with a weak musculovenous pump easily overwhelmed by downflow in superficial veins. This is a common accompaniment of venous ulceration caused by superficial incompetence and not a contraindication to surgery.

**Perforating veins seen at functional phlebography** An enlarged perforating vein seen at functional phlebography in conjunction with typical simple superficial incompetence, as outlined above, is often found; its predominant flow is in an inward direction but may be accompanied by some outward surge on muscle contraction. Provided all other tests are in keeping with simple incompetence this vein is to be viewed as part of

---

**Figure 13.21** *Response to surgical treatment in an ulcer caused by gross saphenous incompetence on right side.*

*(a) Clinical diagnosis of the cause of ulceration is confirmed by:*

> *1. Doppler flowmetry showing the characteristic downflow after exercise of simple saphenous incompetence.*
> *2. Photoplethysmography before and after temporary saphenous occlusion; this reverts to a normal recovery time when retrograde flow in the saphenous vein is prevented.*

*(b) Appearance of the ulcer in an early phase of healing after 10 days' elevation at home as a preliminary to admission into hospital (and see Colour Plate 4). Towards the ankle, most of the ulcer edge slopes down to active epithelial ingrowth; the edges furthest from the ankle are abrupt and show little sign of healing; the ulcer base shows good granulation tissue. At this stage surgery to the incompetent veins was carried out. Next day the patient was asked to walk for 5 minutes every hour and to elevate the limbs between walks. On the third day she was sent home with light elastic support up to the knee and encouraged to return to normal activities.*

*(c) Three weeks after surgery, the ulcer is closing satisfactorily with edges sloping down to epithelial ingrowth (and see Colour Plate 5).*

*(d) At 2 months, most of the ulcer has healed except for a crusted area in the upper part.*

*(e) One year later the patient returned with signs of breakdown in the healed area. She had ceased taking any protective measures and was urged to return to a policy of elastic support and elevation whenever possible. With this renewed care the skin soon became healthy again. Many patients with venous ulcer caused by saphenous incompetence have a relatively poor musculovenous pump and, after operation, it is important to explain that time must be found for spells of elevation during the day and that the elastic support must be used conscientiously. The operation has made the leg much less prone to ulceration but the balance is still precarious and unfair stress, such as prolonged standing, may cause the ulcer to return*

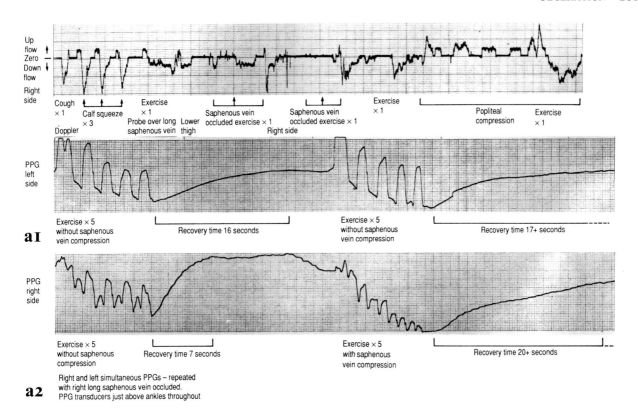

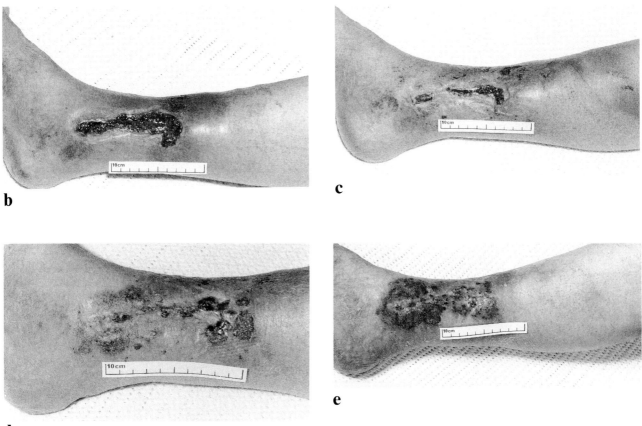

**Figure 13.21**

the pathway of incompetence and should be removed at the time of surgery. When ulceration is present nearby it is particularly desirable that this perforator should be eliminated because it may form the basis of a recurrent pathway of incompetence and, moreover, its component of outflow may persist and cause surge back and forth to the foot with local peaks of high pressure (see Chapter 11).

**Other perforating veins for which surgery is indicated** Special mention must be made of particular types of perforating veins seen at functional phlebography where surgical removal is indicated:

- Veins which are the high-level source of superficial vein incompetence, as is often the case in recurrent varicose veins. These perforators can only be adequately demonstrated at phlebography in the near-upright position. This will fully distend the veins and allow gravitational downflow. In these circumstances an incompetent perforator will show unnatural enlargement and some tortuosity, with outflow from it spilling down the pathway of incompetence. It is commonplace to see normal perforators at varicography; in the horizontal position, with collapsed veins, the distinction between normally and abnormally (incompetent) functioning perforating veins is not possible. The mere outlining of a perforating vein in the thigh is not adequate proof that it is at fault.
- Certain perforators from the big muscle sinuses in the calf region may eject blood to the superficial vein with some force. Provided it is clear that these are not fulfilling a collateral role, their surgical removal may be beneficial.

**Deep vein impairment (post-thrombotic limb) at functional phlebography** Preferential upflow in the superficial veins and evidence of deformed deep veins is a clear indication that the superficial veins are acting as collaterals past impaired deep veins. This upflow will have emerged through multiple perforators, but one or more may show obvious enlargement on phlebography. This is part of a collateral mechanism and such outward flowing perforating veins should only be removed in special circumstances (see below and Chapter 11). Removal of enlarged perforating veins should not be an automatic response and the role of these veins must be carefully evaluated by the full range of special tests before any decision upon surgery (or sclerotherapy).

**Policy with an ulcer caused by deep vein impairment: the ulcer that can be treated but not cured**

If superficial vein incompetence is not the cause of venous hypertension and deep vein impairment is present then the role of surgery is much more problematical. In some cases, a perforating vein underlying an ulcer may be creating a localized high pressure by forceful collateral

outflow. It may be possible to redistribute this by removing the vein and in this way lower the venous pressure in the vicinity sufficiently to enable the ulcer to heal. The benefits of such a procedure can to some extent be predicted by plethysmographic or volumetric studies beforehand and this is discussed in Chapter 11. In other cases a true cure would require reconstruction of the deep veins and their valves, but this form of surgery is still under development and not yet generally accepted. This is considered further in Chapter 21. Patients with ulceration in this category are usually treated by a conservative regimen which will now be considered.

## The intractable venous ulcer: principles in management

When those ulcers that are likely to respond to surgery removing incompetent superficial veins have been identified, and ulcers not caused by venous disorder have been separated off, there remains a sizeable number of patients with venous ulcers that can be controlled but not cured; these may heal in response to treatment but soon return if there is any failure in care of the limb (Figure 13.22). The patient will have to learn a way of life that mitigates the effects of venous hypertension and to realize that the price of relief from the miseries of ulceration is perpetual vigilance. This need not however be unduly burdensome for the patient.

**Figure 13.22** *Treatment of chronic venous ulceration in a post-thrombotic limb. This patient had sustained a popliteal occlusion many years previously and his clinical details and the findings by Doppler flowmetry, photoplethysmography and functional phlebography are given in Figure 8.5. The superficial veins were acting as collaterals and surgery to remove them was contraindicated. Conservative management was commenced with several weeks of high elevation and a programme of exercise, with progressive mobilization in the later stages of ulcer healing.*

*(a) The ulcer before treatment. It has abrupt irregular edges without any sign of healing; poor, inactive granulation tissue covers the base and there is a trickle of thin pus from its lower part. The surrounding area shows widespread pigmented liposclerosis (and see Colour Plate 6).*

*(b) The ulcer at 2 months and showing that it has largely healed, with the surrounding skin looking much healthier. At this stage the limb was given inelastic support by a paste bandage up to the knee and the patient encouraged in free mobility but still spending a good proportion of the day in high elevation.*

*(c) The appearance at 4 months, with the ulcer now fully healed and the surrounding skin looking healthy. The patient has been given a one-way-stretch, graduated, elastic stocking up to the knee and encouraged to return to work; the limb was to be elevated at every opportunity, particularly at home in the evening. This patient followed the regimen of treatment conscientiously and now knows the principles that enable the ulcer to heal and that must continue to be used to prevent recurrence. The lessons of his treatment are important if he is to remain independent of continuing medical care*

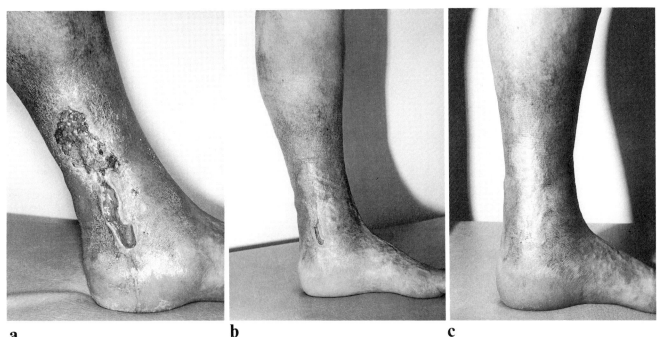

**a**       **b**       **c**

**Figure 13.22**

Previous unsuccessful surgery does not exclude the need to assess each patient carefully before deciding that the ulcer can only be managed by conservative means. Sometimes there are pleasant surprises such as the discovery of an inadequately performed saphenous ligation and stripping, with a simple incompetence re-established. However, with or without previous surgery, most patients in this group will have deep vein impairment resulting from an old deep vein thrombosis or have a valveless syndrome of inborn deficiency in valves. Even when the pumping mechanism is severely impaired venous hypertension can be relieved by simple high elevation of the limb (but first check upon the pulses to exclude ischaemia) to give simple gravitational drainage towards the heart (Figure 13.23). The greater the proportion of the day that is given to this, the more effective it will be; at night the same process continues by raising the foot of the bed. This is the most fundamental way of improving the patient's existing state and of controlling the ever present tendency for ulceration to recur. Each patient has to learn by experience for how long and to what height elevation is needed. It depends upon the severity of the pump failure and the state of the ulcer; when the ulcer is active and must be healed, then elevation almost continuously, day and night, will be necessary, with only short breaks, perhaps 5 minutes each hour, for walking and visits to the bathroom. The policy is not one of bed rest but one of *limb elevation* and the patient must be encouraged to exercise the limbs and the body repeatedly so that physical deterioration does not occur. Hourly walks for a few minutes will keep the antigravity muscles in good condition without materially setting back the ulcer and will avoid a total dependence upon others. However, the patient must be given strict rules not to have more than, say, 5 minutes' liberty. Firmly applied crepe bandages worn whilst in bed will give sufficient support to the veins during the brief excursions out of bed; strong elastic support continuously compressing the elevated limb and interfering with arterial supply is undesirable, may cause pain, and should be avoided.

The true venous ulcer will almost invariably improve and heal with this regimen and failure to respond must put the diagnosis of 'venous' in doubt; it is a diagnostic test in itself. Increased pain in elevation calls for urgent reassessment of the arterial supply but the infected ulcer can respond this way and appropriate antibiotics may be needed. Once the ulcer has healed the patient can give an increasing proportion of the day to being up and about but always elevating whenever nothing purposeful is being done. In this way the patient is introduced to active life again and can eventually return to work. This will depend upon the nature of employment and the tolerance of the ulcer to the standing required. In some cases return to former employment may not prove possible and another occupation must be found. Once the patient is up and about, the smaller the proportion of time given to elevation, the greater the need for an effective pumping mechanism and all thought must be given to ways of improving the defective mechanism that has proved inadequate in the past. This is the second key principle in the control of the intractable ulcer. Unfortunately, although elevation is very effective it is a severe restriction to ordinary life but other methods of improving the pumping mechanism and allowing mobility are relatively feeble measures. They all depend on providing external support up to various levels in the limb and this can be by elastic or inelastic bandages and stockings.

When a normal person rises from lying to standing

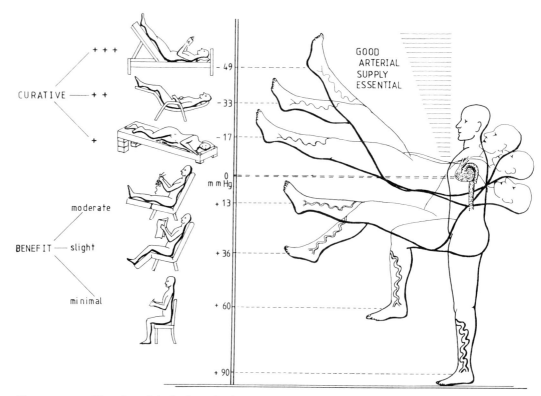

**Figure 13.23** *Elevation of the limbs is, by far, the most important measure in treating venous ulcer. This is only truly effective when the limb is raised above the level of the heart because then there is no venous pressure in the extremity. This diagram shows various positions of elevation related to heart level and the resulting venous pressures in the lower leg. Elevation is only curative, for example in healing an ulcer, when it is well above heart level and maintained there for prolonged periods with minimal interruption. Lesser elevation brings some benefit and may be sufficient to protect a healed ulcer from recurrence. Always assess arterial supply before advising a policy of elevation*

there is a substantial increase in the volume of the limb, particularly in its lower part and the foot. This is largely due to filling of the veins and in the patient with abnormally enlarged veins the increase is much greater and represents venous blood pooled in the lower part. In most ulcer patients the veins of the leg and foot are unnaturally distended and form a massive unwanted reservoir upon which the enfeebled pumping mechanism expends itself. Thus, with exercise, blood may surge back and forth between deep and superficial veins with little effective upward pumping and the weak effort of the damaged pump is further reduced. Equally damaging is the fact that these patients often develop a vast spongework of veins on the underside of the foot which fill immediately the foot is raised from the ground. At the very moment the blood should be available for upward pumping it is sequestered in the foot spongework; moreover, when the foot is put down, blood is forced upwards from its underside to cause a sharp peak of excessive pressure. With these factors in mind it is not hard to understand that external support limiting this unwanted pooling of venous blood will improve the effectiveness of the pump.

External support will be at its most effective in massive simple superficial vein incompetence because here the pump is at least adequate and external compression will

close off the downflow which is overwhelming the pump. In fact, if an ulcer heals quickly in response to no more than elastic support then it is almost certainly caused by superficial incompetence (and hence curable by surgery). In all other circumstances external support can only give limited improvement to the pump and may on its own be inadequate to promote healing of an ulcer.

*Elastic support*

Elastic support has the advantages of conforming well to a limb, with good appearance and, as a stocking, allowing it to be drawn over the heel. However, it has the disadvantage that at all times it gives continuous compression even when the limb is elevated and this may actually reduce blood supply to the limb. In some circumstances, such as in a post-thrombotic limb with deformity of deep veins, it may interfere with a long saphenous vein acting as a collateral, to the disadvantage of the limb. A stocking giving graduated compression is designed to minimize this but not infrequently the patient prefers to avoid wearing the elastic support because the limb is more comfortable and does better without it. Wearing elastic support does not bring automatic improvement in a limb and each patient has his own pattern of abnormality which may or may not be suited by one or other style of elastic support. Advice upon this is given in Chapter 18.

## Inelastic support or containment

This is usually applied to the foot and leg as a paste bandage which is put on with the limb elevated so that the veins are collapsed. The bandage sets to form a firm shell closely applied, but not compressing the limb; when the patient stands the veins are restrained by the inelastic shell but fill to the hydrostatic pressure corresponding with their level below the heart. Thus the compressive force is never more than this venous pressure and immediately falls away as the limb is elevated; there is no elastic compression that may embarass local blood flow. The pooling of blood in the spongework of superficial veins is greatly reduced so that a defective pump does not waste its limited efforts trying to shift a large pool of stagnant blood that rushes back after each movement. This is the most effective method of improving pumping efficiency in the post-thrombotic limb and experience confirms this because it gives the best rate of healing in ambulatory treatment of ulcers. However, it has the drawback that self-application is difficult and the appearance is poor so that it tends only to be used in treatment of active ulceration or at times of threatened recurrence. The wise patient will use it whenever it is apparent that the ulcer is becoming active and continue until control is re-established.

## Elastic webbing bandage

Elastic webbing bandage requires a special word because it has certain dangers and can be used either to give elastic or inelastic support. The experienced patient with recurring ulceration finds that if it is applied lightly with the limb elevated, then, on placing the limb down, the bandage is strong enough to resist distension of the veins in the same way as a paste bandage. The appearance is unwieldy but the patient accepts this because of the comfort and security from recurrence it gives. It can, of course, be stretched on firmly to give elastic compression but here a word of warning must be given. Layer upon layer of firmly stretched elastic bandage exerts great compression so that it may severely impair blood flow and cause the patient great pain. Even worse, if an error of assessment of the ulcer has been made and it is, in fact, ischaemic, the limb may be lost. The patient is unlikely to apply the bandage in this fashion but an inexperienced medical attendant may. Compression above a certain strength (perhaps 50 mmHg) does not bring increasing benefits and soon passes into a stage of causing damage. The object is external support and not tight compression: tissues cannot thrive or survive compression that approaches or exceeds that of the arterial supply. No one should be permitted to apply elastic webbing bandage without proper instruction.

Bandages without strong elastic recoil are safer, less bulky and just as successful. Any bandage support should be applied with the limb elevated so that when it is put to the ground the veins fill within the support until hydrostatic pressure to heart level has been reached and no more; in this way a nicely regulated support, preventing overdistension of the veins, is provided. A strong but relatively inelastic bandage is ideal. It should be sufficiently flexible to conform to the limb contours, yield little and, as the veins fill within the bandage, provide no more compression than the hydrostatic pressure caused by the position of the limb. Chapter 18 gives further details of the various types of external support available.

## Summary

For the active ulcer, several weeks of elevation, with active movements and brief walks each hour, is usually needed and is the quickest way to heal it. When the ulcer is substantially healed the patient is mobilized progressively with external support to the leg, preferably by inelastic bandage; between activity the limb is elevated. Later the support can be changed to a well-fitted graduated elastic stocking up to the knee and a policy of elevation whenever possible followed (see Chapter 18). For recent, and not too severe ulceration, ambulatory treatment, well supervised, and using an inelastic bandage (paste), applied to the leg in elevation, can be very successful; when the ulcer has healed, recurrence is prevented by use of elastic support and elevation whenever possible.

## Applications to the ulcer

The types of preparation that can be used and the principles behind their use are considered here and are further discussed in the second half of this chapter giving the dermatologist's viewpoint. It must always be remembered that healing and long-term prevention of ulceration depends on control of the underlying cause, venous hypertension, and this is the fundamental of treatment. Applications to the ulcer can, however, make a most valuable contribution in cleansing it, controlling infection and subduing eczema. However, ill-chosen materials applied to the ulcer may do great harm and there must be constant awareness of possible adverse reactions caused by sensitivity or severe allergic responses to which these patient are so often prone. Deterioration in the ulcer usually calls for prompt reappraisal and complete change of treatment since otherwise, if the warning is not heeded, severe reactions can occur. Some of the ulcers causing most distress to the patient have been exacerbated in this way. The worst offenders in this respect are antibiotic or antiseptic ointments and creams, particularly when the deterioration is attributed to mounting infection and persisted with. Corticosteroids used in excessive strength or over a prolonged period are often at fault and can prevent healing. Highly coloured dyes of any sort are best avoided, partly because of sensitivity reactions but also because they conceal the true state of the ulcer and surrounding skin.

### Bacterial culture

At the initial dressing, a swab should be taken and sent off in transport medium for culture; this is the best opportunity to identify pathogens before various applications interfere. Perhaps the most damaging common organism is *Staphylococcus aureus*, but culture should also make special provision to look for beta-haemolytic streptococci and anaerobic organisms (Schraibman, 1987). Harmless commensal organisms are inevitable and should be ignored, but in the ulcer that is clearly unhealthy the presence of known pathogens may be an indication for using antibiotics systemically.

### Cleansing agents

Saline or hydrogen peroxide are non-sensitizing and usually sufficient when used every day or two. Various proprietary materials and hydrocolloids are available, bland in nature, and absorbing exudate so that, when lifted away they leave the ulcer cleaned of much of its debris (and see Part 2 in this chapter).

### Controlling infection

Because of the risk of skin sensitivity reaction it is usually best to avoid local antibiotics and antiseptics. If culture has shown a damaging pathogen to be present then their use is permissible but it is preferable to give the appropriate antibiotic systemically to ensure a full response. Some patients become so easily sensitized that it is not wise to use these agents indiscriminately or to waste their possible benefits by failing to use simultaneous control of venous hypertension. Surface applications on their own will seldom be sufficient, and in the meantime the difficulties may be compounded by losing through sensitivity or bacterial resistance yet another potentially valuable antibiotic with little achieved. Infection will not be controlled in the presence of necrotic tissue or encrusted exudate, and a physical debridement may achieve far more than antibiotics alone even if this requires an anaesthetic.

### Use of corticosteroid applications

Used sparingly and at weak strength these are permissible if the skin around the ulcer shows marked eczema. It must be remembered that an unpleasant skin reaction may be the result of sensitivity to another preparation previously used and which should be withdrawn. Moreover, an eczematous skin is more vulnerable to sensitization and the actual ingredients of a steroid preparation can be a potent cause of reaction and deterioration in the very condition it is intended to treat. These substances include antibiotics, lanolin, paraben preservatives and accompanying fragrances that are normally well accepted by the skin (Which? Consumers Association, 1986). Steroids applied to the ulcer itself can prevent healing and should not be used (Buxton, 1987).

### The dressing in contact with the ulcer surface

The main requirement here is for the dressing to be absorbent and easily removed painlessly, without sticking. Surgical gauze moistened with saline easily dries out and sticks tenaciously unless a layer of gel (e.g. Scherisorb) is interposed. Proprietary materials made from rayon or polyester (e.g. N-A knitted viscose dressing and Melolin perforated film mounted on absorbent dressing – both supplied sterile) may be used in combination with creams, ointments or gels and are useful for most ulcers; if used on their own they can allow the ulcer to dry which may be most unfavourable, especially in ischaemic ulcers where drying causes further death of exposed surface layers and increased pain. Tulle gras, often combined with other agents, such as antibiotics, is widely used but can stick painfully and is best avoided. Various absorbent granules, films and sachets, taking exudate and debris away with them on removal, are available (e.g. Granuflex hydrocolloid dressing and Geliperm film or paste of polyacrylamide-agar gel, supplied in sterile packs: both these preparations are non-adherent and designed to provide an ideal moist environment for the healing of ulcers; the importance of this is fully reported by Ryan *et al.* (1985) and Cherry, Ryan and McGibbon (1984)). If odour is a problem, activated charcoal is helpful but here surgical debridement may be a better answer. Dressings of prepared porcine skin may be of value in some circumstances.

### Skin grafts

Split skin or pinch grafts (which may be taken and applied under local anaesthetic in many cases) can be very helpful in speeding up the epithelialization of an ulcer but only when it has reached the right stage of healing in response to measures controlling venotension. It should never be done unless the ulcer has reached a 'healing phase' as shown by its edges shelving in gently to a definite grey line of new epithelium, with a base of healthy, clean looking granulation tissue and an absence of pathogens on culture; the graft will otherwise soon be shed. Skin grafting on its own cannot cure an ulcer but is a valuable supportive measure for the large ulcer, perhaps 5 cm or more across; a lesser ulcer, if capable of taking grafts, will heal almost as quickly on its own; in both cases continued control of venotension is essential and must be maintained in some fashion indefinitely. At this procedure it is best to remove the outer spongy layer of granulation tissue with a blunt instrument, such as the handle of a scapel, and to dissect away any remaining dead tissue.

A variation on this is to excise the entire ulcer area, down to, or including the deep fascia, and then apply a split skin graft; this allows for simultaneous removal of underlying veins, if indicated. It should perhaps be reserved for the very indurated ulcer which has not responded satisfactorily to the simpler method with split skin outlined above. Both methods will require continued care by the patient to prevent eventual breakdown and recurrent ulceration.

No skin grafting procedure will succeed if the underlying cause is ischaemia. This must always be suspected in a dry, painful ulcer which fails to develop a good base of granulation tissue and commencing ingrowth of epithelium in response to preliminary treatment.

**Myocutaneous free graft by microvascular surgery** This can certainly bring a block of well-vascularized tissue and skin to replace the excised ulcer. In the presence of simple venous incompetence, healing is easily obtained without this complex surgery so that it is not indicated. In the patient with severe venous hypertension from other causes it can give the ulcerated area a fresh start but the basic problem of impaired venous return remains and ulceration will eventually reappear if the patient does not conscientiously follow a policy of elevation whenever possible and use of external support. Failure is likely when a venogram shows severe post-thrombotic damage to the deep veins below the knee. It is doubtful if the valves in the principal vein of the myocutaneous flap can prove an effective substitute for a severely impaired pumping mechanism in the leg. The role of this recently evolved technique has yet to be fully evaluated. Similar considerations apply to the older method of a pedicle flap.

## Pharmacological therapy in post-thrombotic syndrome and venous ulceration

### Fibrinolytic enhancement

In the belief that the pericapillary cuffs of fibrin are a significant cause for the manifestations of venous hypertension in the post-thrombotic syndrome, Burnand et al. (1980) suggested the use of stanozolol (Stromba) in order to enhance fibrinolysis and reduce the fibrin cuffs. Initial trial has not indicated any striking benefits but in the small numbers so far reported (Layer et al., 1986) its use does appear to confer some advantage in the healing of recurrent ulceration. However. 'Which' Consumers' Association (1985), concludes 'Stanozolol does not con-

vincingly benefit patients with the skin changes that may precede venous ulceration of the leg, or with established ulceration. Its prolonged use carries various hazards'. Certainly stanozolol can have adverse affects but the proponents of this therapy claim that the dosage required for fibrinolytic enhancement is below that likely to cause harm.

### Reducing capillary permeability

It is well established in the laboratory that hydroxyethylrutosides can reduce capillary permeability. Since increased permeability is regarded as an important adverse consequence of venous hypertension, this preparation (Paroven) has been given extensive trial, particularly on the continent. Opinions are divided upon its clinical efficacy but, amongst many other published works, Belcaro (1986), de Jongste, ten Cate and Huisman (1986) and Pulvertaft (1986) report favourably upon its use in venous hypertension and the post-thrombotic syndrome.

### Improving flow within capillaries

Haemorheological studies have shown the improved flow within small vessels that follows the use of drugs capable of improving the deformability of red cells (Braasch, 1971; Reid et al., 1976; Dormandy, 1979). Pentoxifylline (Trental) is effective in this respect but the clinical benefits are not easy to recognize. Weitgasser (1983) found improved healing of venous ulcers using this preparation, which also retards platelet aggregation. The scarcity of other reports upon this perhaps indicates that few workers have been favourably impressed by its advantages. The field of haemorheology in respect of liposclerosis and venous ulceration have recently been advanced by the observation (Thomas, Nash and Dormandy, 1988) that white cells accumulate in the capillaries of dependent lower limbs. This causes damage to endothelium, with increased permeability, and may silt up the capillaries sufficiently to stop flow (and see Chapter 8). Possible developments from this are awaited.

## References

Belcaro, G. V. (1986) Treatment of chronic venous hypertension of the lower limbs by O-(b-hydroxyethyl)-rutoside and elastic compression. In *Phlebology '85* (eds D. Negus and G. Jantet), John Libbey, London, pp. 834–836

Berth-Jones, J., Graham-Brown, R. A. C., Fletcher, A. *et al.* (1989) Malignant fibrous histiocytoma: a new complication of chronic venous ulceration. *British Medical Journal*, **298**, 231–232

Browse, N. L. and Burnand, K. G. (1978). The postphlebitic syndrome: a new look. In *Venous Problems* (eds J. J. Bergan and J. S. Yao), Year Book Medical, Chicago, pp. 395–405

Braasch, D. (1971) Red cell deformability and capillary blood flow. *Physiological Review*, **51**, 679

Burnand, K., Clemenson, G., Morland, M. *et al.* (1980) Venous lipodermatosclerosis: treatment by fibrinolytic enhancement and elastic compression. *British Medical Journal*, 1, 7–11

Burnand, K. G., Whimster, I., Naidoo, A. and Browse, N. L. (1982) Pericapillary fibrin in the ulcer bearing skin of the lower leg. The cause of lipodermatosclerosis and venous ulceration. *British Medical Journal*, 285, 1071–1072

Buxton, P. K. (1987) Leg ulcers. *British Medical Journal*, 295, 1542–1545

Callam, M. J., Ruckley, C. V., Harper, D. R. and Dale, J. J. (1985) Chronic ulceration of the leg: extent of the problem and provision of care. *British Medical Journal*, 290, 1855–1856

Callam, M. J., Harper, D. R., Dale, J. J. and Ruckley, C. V. (1987a) Arterial disease in chronic leg ulceration: an underestimated hazard. *British Medical Journal*, 294, 929–931

Callam, M. J., Harper, D. R., Dale, J. J. and Ruckley, C. V. (1987b) Chronic ulcer of the leg: clinical history. *British Medical Journal*, 294, 1389–1391

Callam, M. J., Ruckley, C. V., Dale, J. J. and Harper, D. R. (1987c) Hazards of compression treatment of the leg from Scottish surgeons. *British Medical Journal*, 295, 1382

Cherry, G. W., Ryan, T. and McGibbon, D. (1984) Trial of a new dressing in venous leg ulcers. *Practitioner*, 228, 1175–1178

Cockett, F. B. (1955) The pathology and treatment of venous ulcers of the leg. *British Journal of Surgery*, 43, 260–278

Cornwall, J. V., Dore, C. J. and Lewis, J. D. (1986) Leg ulcers: epidemiology and aetiology. *British Journal of Surgery*, 73, 693–696

Dormandy, J. A. (1979) Clinical importance of blood viscosity. *Viscositas*, 1, 5

Franks. P. J., Wright, D. and McCollum, C. N. (1989) Epidemiology of venous disease: a review. *Phlebology*, 4, 143–151

de Jongste, A. B., ten Cate, J. W. and Huisman, M. V. (1986) The effectiveness of O-(*b*-hydroxyethyl)-rutosides in the post-thrombotic syndrome. *Phlebology '85* (eds D. Negus and G. Jantet), John Libbey, London, pp. 837–839

Layer, G. T., Powell, S., Pattison, M. and Burnand, K. G. (1986) Early results of a trial of adjuvant fibrinolytic enhancement therapy in the healing of venous ulcers. In *Phlebology '85* (eds D. Negus and G. Jantet), John Libbey, London, pp. 587–590

Leach, R. D. (1984) Venous ulceration, fibrinogen and fibrinolysis. *Annals of the Royal College of Surgeons of England*, 66, 258–263

Loudon, I. S. L. (1981) Leg ulcers in the eighteenth and early nineteenth centuries. *Journal of the Royal College of General Practitioners*, 31, 263–273

McQueen, A. (1980) The skin. In *Muir's Textbook of Pathology* (ed. J. B. Anderson), Edward Arnold, London, pp. 1049–1085

Manson-Bahr, P. E. C. and Bell, D. R. (1987) *Manson's Tropical Diseases*, Ballière Tindall, London

Pulvertaft, T. B. (1986) General practice treatment of symptoms of venous insufficiency with oxerutins: results of a 660-patient multicentre study in the UK. In *Phlebology '85* (eds D. Negus and G. Jantet), John Libbey, London, pp. 853–856

Reid, H. L., Dormandy, J. A., Barnes, A. J. *et al.* (1976) Impaired red cell deformability in peripheral vascular disease. *Lancet*, i, 666

Ryan, T. J. (ed.) (1985) *An Environment for Healing: The Role of Occlusion* (Royal Society of Medicine International Congress and Symposium Series No. 88), Royal Society of Medicine, London

Schraibman, I. G. (1987) The bacteriology of leg ulcers. *Phlebology*, 2, 265–270

Thomas, P. R. S., Nash, G. B. and Dormandy, J. A. (1988) White cell accumulation in dependent legs of patients with venous hypertension: a possible mechanism for trophic changes in the skin. *British Medical Journal*, 296, 1693–1695

Weitgasser, H. (1983) The use of pentoxifylline ('Trental' 400) in the treatment of leg ulcers: results of a double-blind trial. *Pharmatherapeutica*, 3, 143–151

Which? Consumers' Association (1985) Does Stanozolol prevent venous ulceration? *Drug and Therapeutics Bulletin*, 23, 91–92

Which? Consumers' Association (1986) Skin sensitisers in topical corticosteroids. *Drug and Therapeutics Bulletin*, 24, 57–59

Which? Consumers' Association (1988) Malignant melanoma of the skin. *Drug and Therapeutics Bulletin*, 26, 73–75

Widmer, L. K., Mall, Th. and Martin, H. (1977) Epidemiology and socio-medical importance of peripheral venous disease. In *The Treatment of Venous Disorders* (ed. J. T. Hobbs), MTP, Lancaster, pp. 3–11

## Bibliography

Adair, H. M. (1977) Epidermal repair in chronic venous ulcers. *British Journal of Surgery*, 64, 800–804

Allen, S. (1991) Venous ulceration in drug abusers: an important physical sign. *Phlebology*, 6, 47–48

Backhouse, C. M., Blair, S. D., Savage, A. P., Walton, J. and McCollum, C. N. (1987) Controlled trial of occlusive dressings in healing chronic venous ulcers. *British Journal of Surgery*, 74, 625–627

Baker, S. R., Stacey, M. C., Jopp–McKay, A. G., Hoskin, S. E. and Thompson, P. J. (1991) Epidemiology of chronic venous ulcers. *British Journal of Surgery*, 78, 864–867

Beaconsfield, T., Genbacey, O. and Taylor, R. S. (1991) The treatment of long-standing venous ulcers with an extract of early placenta – a pilot study. *Phlebology*, 6, 153–158

Blair, S. D., Wright, D. D. I., Backhouse, C. M., Riddle, E. and McCollum, C. N. (1988) Sustained compression and healing of chronic venous ulcers. *British Medical Journal*, 297, 1159–1161

Burnand, K. G., Whimster, I., Clemenson, G., Lea Thomas, M. and Browse, N. L. (1981) The relationship between the number of capillaries in the skin of the venous ulcer-bearing area of the lower leg and the fall in foot vein pressure during exercise. *British Journal of Surgery*, 68, 297–300

Cheatle, T. R., McMullin, G. M., Farrah, J., Coleridge Smith, P. D. and Scurr, J. H. (1990) Skin damage in chronic venous insufficiency: does an oxygen diffusion barrier really exist. *Journal of the Royal Society of Medicine*, 83, 493–494

Cheatle, T. R., Stibe, E. C. L., Shami, S. K., Scurr, J. H. and Coleridge Smith, P. D. (1991) Vasodilatory capacity of the skin in venous disease and its relationship to transcutaneous oxygen tension. *British Journal of Surgery*, 78, 607–610

Coleridge Smith, P. D., Thomas, P., Scurr, J. H. and Dormandy, J. A. (1988) Causes of venous ulceration: a new hypothesis. *British Medical Journal*, 296, 1726–1727

Colgan, M., Dormandy, J. A., Jones, P. W., Schraibman, I. G., Shanik, D. G. and Young, R. A. L. (1990) Oxpentifylline treatment of venous ulcers of the leg. *British Medical Journal*, 300, 972–974

Dickson Wright, A. (1929) The treatment of varicose ulcer. *Proceedings of the Royal Society of Medicine*, XXIII, 1032

Dickson Wright, A. (1931) The treatment of indolent ulcer of the leg. *Lancet*, i, 457–461

Durable, M. and Ouvry, P. (1991) Haemodilution in venous disease. *Phlebology*, **6**, 31–36

Efem, S. E. E. (1988) Clinical observations on the wound healing properties of honey. *British Journal of Surgery*, **75**, 679–681

Gilliland, E. L., Dore, C. J., Nathwani, N. and Lewis J. D. (1988) Bacterial colonisation of leg ulcers and its effect on the success rate of skin grafting. *Annals of the Royal College of Surgeons of England*, **70**, 105–108

Grimaudo, V., Gueissaz, F., Hauert, J., Sarraj, A., Kruithof, E. K. O. and Bachmann, F. (1989) Necrosis of skin induced by coumarin in a patient deficient in protein S. *British Medical Journal*, **298**, 233–234

Hughes, L. E., Horgan, K., Taylor, B. A. and Laidler, P. (1985) Malignant melanoma of the hand and foot: diagnosis and management. *British Journal of Surgery*, **72**, 811–815

Irwin, S. T., Gilmore, J., McGrann, S., Hood, J. and Allen, J. A. (1988) Blood flow in diabetics with foot lesions due to 'small vessel disease'. *British Journal of Surgery*, **75**, 1201–1206

Lucarotti, M. E., Morgan, A. P. and Leaper, D. J. (1990) The effect of antiseptics and the moist wound environment on ulcer healing: an experimental and biochemical study. *Phlebology*, **5**, 173–179

Marsden, P. D. (1990) Cutaneous leishmaniasis. *British Medical Journal*, **300**, 1716–1717

Negus, D. (1991) *Leg Ulcers*, Butterworth-Heinemann, Oxford

Owens, C. W. I., Al-Khader, A. A., Jackson, M. J. and Prichard, B. N. C. (1981) A severe 'stasis eczema', associated with low plasma zinc, treated successfully with oral zinc. *British Journal of Dermatology*, **105**, 461–464

Partsch, H. (1991) Treatment of resistant leg ulcers by retrograde intravenous pressure infusions of urokinase. *Phlebology*, **6**, 13–21

Pflug, J. J. and Davies, D. M. (1985) Chronic swelling of the leg and stasis ulcer. *British Medical Journal*, **290**, 1273–1276

Prassad, A., Ali-Khan, A. and Mortimer, P. (1990) Leg ulcers and oedema: a study exploring the prevalence, aetiology, and possible significance of oedema in venous ulcers. *Phlebology*, **5**, 181–187

Rasmussen, L. H., Karlsmark, T., Avnstorp, C., Peters, K., Jorgenson, M. and Jensen, L. T. (1991) Topical human growth hormone treatment of chronic leg ulcers. *Phlebology*, **6**, 23–30

Rivlin, S. (1951) *The Treatment of Varicose Veins and their Complications*, Heinemann, London

Rivlin, S. (1958) Gravitational leg ulcer in the elderly. *Lancet*, **i**, 1363–1367

Schraibman, I. G. and Stratton, F. J. (1985) Nutritional status of patients with leg ulcers. *Journal of the Royal Society of Medicine*, **78**, 39–42

Senapati, A. and Thompson, R. P. H. (1985) Zinc deficiency and the prolonged accumulation of zinc in wounds. *British Journal of Surgery*, **72**, 583–584

Stacey, M. C., Burnand, K. G., Layer, G. T. and Pattison, M. (1990) Transcutaneous oxygen tension in assessing the treatment of healed venous ulcers. *British Journal of Surgery*, **77**, 1050–1054

Stacey, M. C., Burnand, K. G., Pattison, M., Lea Thomas, M. and Layer, G. T. (1987) Changes in the apparently normal limb in unilateral venous ulceration. *British Journal of Surgery*, **74**, 936–939

Stringer, M. D., Melcher, D. and Stachan, C. L. J. (1986) The lower limb as a presenting site of malignant lymphoma. *Annals of the Royal College of Surgeons of England*, **68**, 8–11

Zumla, A. and Lulat, A. (1989) Honey – a remedy rediscovered. *Journal of the Royal Society of Medicine*, **82**, 384–385

# Part 2   Vascular factors in the management of leg ulcers: the dermatologist's viewpoint

Terence J. Ryan DM, FRCP
Consultant Dermatologist, Oxford

Leg ulcers are common, disabling and mostly badly managed. They are also costly, because they require frequent dressings and visits from medical and nursing attendants, especially if healing is delayed or never achieved and if there is recurrence. To have a leg ulcer is a handicap: the patient cannot walk far, there is pain and disfigurement, often an unpleasant odour, and the patient suffers loss of confidence and impaired performance. The burden on the family may be considerable and the demands of those who are in pain and who are also immobile is one of the larger burdens on the community. A large range of factors may cause or aggravate leg ulcers and some of these are summarized in Table 13.1 and Colour Plates 1–23. In the section that follows the three vascular systems which may be diseased and ten essential points of management are described.

## Three diseased systems

The three vascular systems to be considered are venous, arterial and lymphatic. Each of these may be separately affected but a mixed picture is common. The management, which depends on posture, movement and support, may have to be modified depending on the degree of impairment and the contribution of each system to the disease (Ryan, 1987).

Ulceration is essentially a break in the surface continuity of epithelium. It is commonly initiated by a minor knock or abrasion. The background of a diseased vascular system then ensures that a small wound does not heal and the inflammation and ischaemia result in a gradual increase in the size of the wound. In the age groups most commonly affected, that is over the age of 40 for venous ulceration and over the age of 80 for arterial disease, the capillary bed can be grossly abnormal (Ryan and Wilkinson, 1986). The clinical manifestation of these abnormalities is initially a very small purpuric spot or a cayenne pepper or brown discolouration

The rise of intracapillary pressure consequent on venous disease is the commonest reason for these abnormal capillary forms. Factors which predispose to this are the dependent limb and the failure of the venous system to return blood and empty the venous compartment in the leg. The tendency for blood to collect in the leg and to dilate capillaries is normally counteracted by the vasoconstrictor response in the arterioles when the leg is dependent. This combination of venous hypertension and

**TABLE 13.1**   Causes and aggravating factors in chronic leg ulcer

Arterial insufficiency ⎫
Venous insufficiency    ⎬ The vascular factors
Lymphatic insufficiency ⎭

In Western countries venous ulcers are by far the commonest, caused by previous deep vein thrombosis or severe superficial vein incompetence. Arterial ulcers are a not uncommon trap in diagnosis and to treat as venous can be disastrous. Lymphoedema is mostly an aggravating factor but prone to recurring cellulitis from stagnant crevices

**External injury**: laceration; contact dermatitis; decubitus, inoculation (including drug addicts and insect bites)
**Metabolic**: Diabetes mellitus
**Neuropathic**: Diabetes mellitus; neurological disorders; syringomyelia; spina bifida; alcoholic neuropathy; leprosy; nerve injury
**Blood disease**: Anaemia will aggravate, and be aggravated by, an ulcer; sickle-cell anaemia; thalassaemia; leukaemia; polycythaemia vera; thrombocythaemia; hereditary spherocytosis (acholuric jaundice)
**Infection**: Specific, tuberculosis; syphilis; acquired immunity deficiency syndrome

In tropical countries: amoebiasis, leishmaniasis, yaws (and see a specialized work on tropical diseases)

**Infection plus nutritional deficiency**: 'Tropical ulcer'; maltreated prisoners; the neglected elderly
**Nutritional deficiency**: Protein; vitamins
**Allergy and unsuitable medical applications**: Materials in ointments, dressings or elastic stockings, including antibiotics, lanolin and rubber; steroids can prevent healing of an ulcer
**Inflammatory**: Vasculitis from variety of causes including rheumatoid arthritis; pyoderma gangrenosum (ulcerative colitis)
**Neoplasm**: Squamous carcinoma (Marjolin's ulcer); malignant melanoma; basal-cell carcinoma (rodent ulcer); rarely sarcoma
**Congenital**: Deficiency of veins and valves (Klinefelter and Klippel–Trenaunay syndromes); arteriovenous fistulas; connective tissue (elastic and collagen fibres) defects

arterial vasoconstriction is rarely under perfect control, except in youth, and human beings have only recently evolved a lifespan longer than 40, before which leg ulceration is rare. As described elsewhere in this book the most common reasons for failure of the venous system are a previous deep venous thrombosis, gross incompetence in superficial veins or a chronic overexpansion of the venous system leading to inefficiency in the valves and incompetence of the communicating veins which join the deep to the superficial venous system. Normally the superficial venous system drains into the deep system but in venous disease it is not uncommon for reversal to occur.

The condition of lipodermatosclerosis as delineated by Browse and Burnand (1978, 1982) is the microvascular consequence of such venous disease in which blood components collect in the wall of the small vessels producing a cuff of fibrin (Figure 13.24 and Colour Plate 16) and other materials. This increases the distance required for the diffusion of oxygen and may also be a barrier to

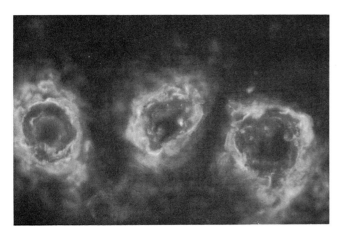

**Figure 13.24**  *Fibrinogen pericapillary cuffs shown by immunofluorescent stain in tissue near a venous ulcer*

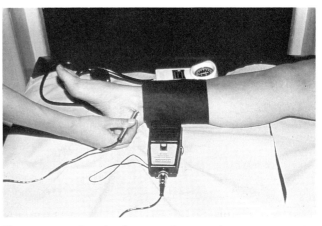

**Figure 13.25**  *Doppler flowmeter being used to assess arterial perfusion near ankle. The sphygmomanometer cuff pressure required to arrest flow in the posterior tibial artery is being measured*

diffusion. It also stiffens the vessel wall so that it is narrowed and cannot dilate in response to the demands of wound healing. While arterial ulcers usually develop in a much older age group and are associated in particular with atherosclerosis (Kulozik, Cherry and Ryan, 1986), poor perfusion of the tissues may result not only from obstruction of the larger arteries but in many patients because of sclerosis of the capillary bed. This is due to gradual sclerosis or fibrosis of the walls of the microvascular system, particularly proximally, where blood pressure is highest. It is a feature of not only hypertension itself but also diabetes mellitus and collagen diseases. Diseases of the lymphatic system also contribute to fibrosis. This is because when the lymphatic system is impaired the deposition of macromolecules such as proteins and lipids in the tissues and especially in the vessel walls contributes to the gradual impairment of blood flow. Dermatosclerosis is thus a complex phenomenon.

## Ten essential points of management

The first and most important test is to examine the arterial system. This is followed by an examination of the venous system and finally of the lymphatic system.

### 1. Arterial assessment

The arterial system is examined by taking the blood pressure of the leg using a sphygmomanometer in the same way as one takes the blood pressure in the arm (Ryan and Cherry, 1985). The only difference is that it is necessary to use a Doppler stethoscope (Figure 13.25). Such a stethoscope should be present in every health centre and the nurses should be familiar with its use. It is not much more expensive to include a small microphone so the patients can hear the flow in their own

arteries and understand some of the problems they themselves have to overcome. It is usual to use the 'arterial index', the ratio of arm to leg blood pressure, to decide whether there is a major arterial component in the disease. Because of calcification, complete compression of the arteries in the lower leg may be difficult to obtain with the sphygmomanometer cuff, and the ratio may be above 1. If, however, the pressure in the leg is below 60% of that in the arm then a severe degree of arterial perfusion impairment must be recognized and the vascular surgeon's opinion is imperative, because it may be treatable.

### 2. Venous assessment

Examination of the venous system consists of an assessment of the long and short venous systems, which should not be dilated, should empty proximally and should not fill from above when the leg is dependent. Similarly in healthy limbs the superficial saphenous veins will not fill when the muscle pump is activated by ankle movements. The simple examination of the venous system as a screen for venous disease is described in Chapters 2 and 4.

### 3. Lymphatic assessment

Examination of the lymphatic system includes the recognition of oedema and fibrosis. Such oedema almost invariably involves the foot, and the toes in particular, leading to stiffening of the skin so that folds of skin cannot be picked up between the fingers (Figure 13.26). Stiffening of the skin is associated with increased deep furrows at the base of the toes, and chronic oedema and fibrosis lead to a square rather than a rounded circumference of the toe. Lymphoedema is often present on the dorsum of the foot. Around the ankle the tissues become extremely thick and cobblestoned with hyperkeratosis. Lymphoedema results from lymphatic failure

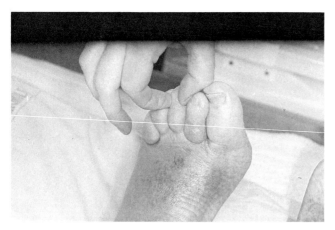

**Figure 13.26** *A foot with early lymphoedema, with fibrotic toes and deep crevices at their base; the skin cannot be picked up when pinched*

and this in turn frequently results from continual dilatation of lymphatics due to venous hypertension and constant flooding of the tissue with an excess of tissue fluid, lipid and protein, which overwhelms the ability of normal lymphatics to cope (Ryan, 1987).

Having assessed whether there is an arterial or lymphatic disorder, it is now possible to make a decision about the appropriateness of different regimens of therapy for venous disease. In practice about a third of all patients have mixed arterial and venous disease probably related to the chronicity of their disease. After determining the need for and availability of surgical procedures a variety of conservative measures may be employed. The importance of elevation, exercise and compression or support bandaging cannot be over-emphasized. Those who ignore this and rely simply on a hundred and one different forms of local dressing or other therapeutic agents are unlikely to heal any ulcer. The reason for the emphasis on assessment of the leg is that it is an unfortunate fact that adequate elevation or compression is undesirable in the leg suffering from severe arterial disease (see Colour Plate 17). In such patients one has to be aware that keeping the leg on the level is about the best that one can do and understand that patients often feel more comfortable with their legs in a dependent position (see Figures 17.1, 17.2, 17.6, 17.7 and 17.8). Such patients have to be encouraged to get their legs on the level during the night. In the presence of severe arterial disease poor perfusion is likely to prevent healing. A policy of doing no harm to a very vulnerable system includes the use of bland agents and careful avoidance of firm compression or constricting bands. Acceptance that this is an ulcer that may not heal is often better than determined efforts at trying to heal it at all costs. Those who suffer from claudication should 'stop smoking and keep walking' (Housley, 1988). There are now so many social as well as medical reasons why smoking should be discouraged that the patient should be left in no doubt

that everything that the medical profession can offer will have been wasted if smoking is continued. Finally, in the assessment, thought must be given to the possibility of some other cause or aggravating factor, summarized in Table 13.1.

## 4. Elevation

If there is no arterial disease the management of venous and lymphatic disease must include high elevation. The management of the 'venous' ulcer, if pure, is that much easier provided one can persuade the patient to elevate the leg adequately (Figures 13.23, 13.27 and 18.1) and to exercise as much as possible after compression bandaging or support stockings have been applied. It must be emphasized that a surgeon can cure some forms of venous disease and thus eliminate the cause of leg ulcers. This is especially so when there is pure superficial venous incompetence.

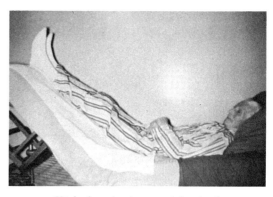

**Figure 13.27** *High elevation is essential to heal a venous ulcer but only after confirming a good arterial supply is present. An upturned chair, used as shown, is very effective*

## 5. Exercise

Exercise is good for all three vascular systems. The importance of recognizing a lymphatic element underlying disease of the leg is that elevation is not enough for the control of lymphoedema: lymphatics require movement in the tissues for macromolecules to pass into the lymphatics, and movement triggers spontaneous lymphatic pulsation so that materials pass along the lymphatics. Massage of the thigh and the abdomen may disperse the pool of oedema which impedes emptying of tissue fluids lying more distally in the limb (Stewart *et al.*, 1989).

## 6. Compression or support

Any compressive bandages which, due to the shape of the leg, swelling of the leg or poor bandaging techniques, result in a constrictive or garter effect around the leg will impair lymphatic drainage still further. Bandaging has to be firm around the foot and a gradient of gradually decreasing pressure is essential if obstruction to lymphatics is not to occur. Some legs are like inverted champagne bottles (Figure 13.28) and have a markedly greater circumference near the knee, and bandaging has to be that much less constrictive at that site. The skills of bandaging can only be learnt in the clinic. Self-adherent (cohesive) bandages such as Secure Forte (Johnson & Johnson) are an advantage because when applied around a swollen calf with less tension than around the foot and ankle, they are less likely to fall down. Various bandaging techniques can be recommended (Ryan, 1987) and a recently published sustained compression technique has been of proven value (Blair, 1988). Bandaging and support stockings are discussed further in Chapter 18.

Before discussing the ideal dressing one must consider problems which may make the management of the leg ulcer more difficult.

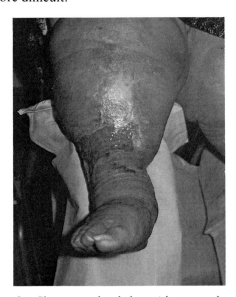

**Figure 13.28**   *Champagne-bottle leg, with venous ulcer*

## 7. Control of infection

It is naive to try and make a leg ulcer sterile (Ryan, 1987). One's aim is to eliminate dangerous bacteria such as the beta-haemolytic streptococcus Lancefield Type A, and to reduce excessive bacterial contamination (Figure 13.29). The estimate of excess can only be made by a partnership between those who take the bacterial swab and those who plate it and interpret it. It is by no means certain that bacteria in themselves are harmful except, perhaps, to newly grafted skin and a slight or moderate bacterial component may not be a good reason to worry. However, it is a reasonable assumption that a very heavy growth is less desirable, in which case a temporary attempt at reducing the excess by the use of antiseptics for a short period only may be an advantage. It is our practice to use the ancient remedies of eusol, 0.5% aqueous silver nitrate or 0.5% aqueous acetic acid on ulcers in which a heavy growth of bacteria has been ascertained and in which granulation tissue is not yet clearly apparent. There

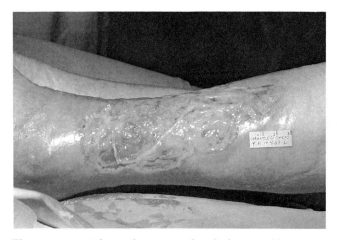

**Figure 13.29**   *A large ulcer, covered in thick pus and heavily infected by pseudomonas. The patient was severely anaemic, a factor preventing healing but also itself aggravated by the infection. The ulcer healed quickly when the anaemia and infection were treated. The aetiology of this ulcer was uncertain but later events suggested that it was self-inflicted*

is, of course, a stage of ulceration in which much slough, including black necrotic skin, is present. At this stage surgical debridement is desirable (Figure 13.30). When the slough is covered only with a yellow or greenish exudate, and no pink is seen, antiseptics may be valuable. Several recent studies have shown that antiseptics mostly are cytotoxic and they should not be used liberally when granulation tissue or epithelialization is to be encouraged. However, at the early stage of necrosis and exudate in excess the value of wet dressings which discourage infection justify their use.

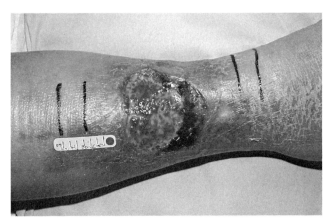

**Figure 13.30**   *A venous ulcer with a black slough of necrotic skin. An ulcer like this will not respond to treatment until the slough is removed, by surgical debridement if necessary. The skin marks are for girth measurement*

## 8. Avoidance of allergy and irritation

Contact dermatitis is most likely to occur in those patients who have had leg ulcers for a long time and in whom numerous agents have been used in an attempt to cure the ulcer without sufficent attention to the background needs of elevation, exercise and compression. Patients easily become sensitive to constituents of ointments, such as lanolin, and preservatives, such as parabens and chlorocresol – constituents not always clearly indicated in the data on the dressing (see Colour Plates 18–21). Most commonly patients become sensitive to antibacterial agents such as neomycin and the related soframycin or framycetin. As in all aspects of dermatitis, one must recognize that irritants can cause more problems than allergens. The patient's own exudate plus bacterial contamination may damage surrounding healthy skin.

Once the skin has become oedematous then it is necessary to soak up all the exudate and bacteria so that the skin is not irritated. Old-fashioned butter muslin in adequate amounts is still a very good way of absorbing exudate, but there are other more refined systems such as the charcoal dressings (Actisorb) and, most recent of all, the hydrocolloid dressings (Granuflex) (Ryan, 1985, 1988).

## 9. Appropriate dressings

There is no ideal dressing but two systems are currently preferred. One is the hydrocolloid dressing mentioned above and the other is the paste bandage (see Chapter 18). Both these dressings promote healing, have a low incidence of sensitization and discourage bacteria growth. One desirable feature of a healing ulcer is granulation tissue, which provides the bed for epithelium to migrate across the ulcer and is in itself an antibacterial covering for the ulcer and a contractile bed which seems to stimulate healing. To develop granulation tissue there seems to be a need for a moist environment and possibly an hypoxic one. This is encouraged by the occlusive hydrocolloid dressing (Ryan, 1985). There is a stage at which granulation tissue becomes proud and at this stage it may outgrow its blood supply, particularly if there is poor arterial perfusion or an excessive fibrin cuff preventing adequate dilatation of the capillary bed. Such granulation tissue can, in itself, become infected and necrotic. Wet saline dressings may be helpful at this stage. There is also a stage at which granulation tissue, instead of producing a sticky fibrin surface required for the migration of epithelium, actually is fibrinolytically overactive. It is at this stage that a little drying out or coagulation may be desirable. Currently, for the small ulcer, in which the bed seems unable to encourage final migration of epithelial cells, I apply a little Ster-Zac powder or allow the paste bandage direct contact with the ulcer surface rather than covering the ulcer with non-adherent materials.

Once it has entered a healing phase, with epithelial ingrowth at the edges, a very large ulcer may be healed most quickly by grafting with the patient's own skin (Figure 13.31), but it must be remembered that the very circumstances that enable a skin graft to succeed will also promote rapid healing without need of a graft.

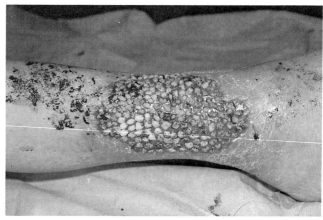

a

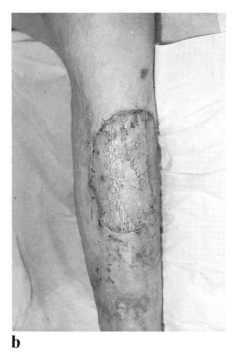

b

**Figure 13.31** *A large ulcer may be healed most quickly by skin grafting once the causative factors have been eliminated, but will not remain healed if they are allowed to return. Two types of graft are shown, both applied only when the ulcer edges showed commencing epithelial ingrowth.*

*(a) Pinch-grafts taken from thigh under local anaesthetic.*
*(b) A split skin graft, expanded by a mesh of multiple slits to increase its effective size*

## 10. Adequate follow-up to prevent recurrence

Unless surgery to the arterial system has been effective, continual problems from arterial ulcers are likely. In the case of ulcers due to venous disease, some are surgically curable, but in the others recurrence is virtually inevitable unless the patient is intensively educated and encouraged to wear support stockings or bandages (see Chapter 18), learn to elevate and to exercise as much as necessary. The physician should continue to take an interest in the patient to make sure that the stockings are renewed and the patient is not being neglected simply because he is now well.

# References

Blair, S. D. (1988) Sustained compression and healing of chronic venous ulcers. *British Medical Journal*, **297**, 1159–1161

Browse, N. L. and Burnand, K. G. (1978) The postphlebitic syndrome: a new look. In *Venous Problems* (eds J. J. Bergan and J. S. Yao), Year Book Medical, Chicago, pp. 395–405

Browse, N. L. and Burnand, K. G. (1982) The cause of venous ulceration. *Lancet*, **ii**, 243–245

Housley, E. (1988) Treating claudication in five words (Leader). *British Medical Journal*, **296**, 1483

Kulozik, M., Cherry, G. W. and Ryan, T. J. (1986) The importance of measuring the ankle brachial systolic pressure ratio in the management of leg ulcers. *British Journal of Dermatology*, **115**, 26

Ryan, T. J. (ed) (1985) *An Environment for Healing – The Role of Occlusion* (Royal Society of Medicine International Congress and Symposium Series No. 88), Royal Society of Medicine, London

Ryan, T. J. (1987) *The Management of Leg Ulcers*, 2nd edn, Oxford Medical Publications, Oxford, p. 101

Ryan, T. J. (ed.) (1988) *Beyond Occlusion: Wound Care* (Royal Society of Medicine International Congress and Symposium Series No. 136), Royal Society of Medicine, London, p. 141

Ryan, T. J. and Cherry, G. W. (1985) The assessment of vascular abnormalities of the leg. In *Recent Advances in Dermatology* (ed. R. H. Champion), Churchill Livingstone, Edinburgh, pp. 87–101

Ryan, T. J. and Wilkinson, D. S. (1986) Diseases of the veins and arteries: leg ulcers. In *Textbook of Dermatology* (eds F. J. G. Ebling, A. Rook and D. S. Wilkinson), Blackwell, Oxford, pp. 1187–1227

Stewart, J. B., Cherry, C. A., Cherry, G. W. and Ryan, T. J. (1989) Lymphatic function in patients with venous leg ulcers. *Journal of Investigative Dermatology*, **92**, 523

**TABLE 13.2**   *Leg ulcer allergens*

---

### A. OINTMENT BASES AND PRESERVATIVES

1. Wool alcohols (lanolins)
2. Probens
3. Propylene glycol
4. Chlorocresol
5. Ethylene diamine

### B. ANTIBACTERIAL AGENTS

6. Sodium fucidate
7. Gentamicin sulphate
8. Neomycin
9. Soframycin
10. Quinoline mix (Vioform)

### C. ADDITIVES IN BANDAGES

11. Ester gum resin
12. Azo disperse yellow no. 3
13. Colophony
14. Mbt thiuram (rubber)

### D. SELF-MEDICATION

15. Caine mix (local anaesthetics)
16. Antihistamine creams
17. Dettol
18. Germolene

---

# 14

# Oedema of the lower limb: differential diagnosis and treatment

The question whether a patient's oedema has a venous origin is a common one. To overlook this cause could be a bad error and, equally, to ascribe oedema incorrectly to the veins will lead to disappointing results in treatment, possibly at some risk to the patient. An understanding and recognition of the wide range of conditions causing oedema is essential for the successful management of venous disorders.

The total water content within the body of an adult weighing 70 kg is about 42 litres, of which 30 litres are intracelluar and 12 litres are extracellular. The extracellular fluid is composed of 3 litres within the vascular system (intravascular plasma) and 9 litres of interstitial fluid lying within the 'tissue space' outside the cells. The interstitial fluid is low in proteins but relatively high in electrolyte concentration to compensate for the low colloid osmotic pressure of the proteins. Oedema is due to accumulation of excess tissue fluid in the interstitial space. The interstitial fluid is not a static pool but an ever changing flow of transudate from the 'arterial' portion of capillary bed into the tissue space and its reabsorption back by the 'venous' portion of the capillaries and by the lymphatics. The lymphatics remove only about one-tenth of the reabsorbed fluid but at the same time have the essential role, not possible for capillaries, of removing large protein molecules and particulate matter from the interstitial space. Figure 14.1 summarizes the main factors determining this flow of interstitial fluid and the circumstances that upset normal balance to cause excess of fluid to collect so that oedema becomes evident. The conditions under which one or more of these factors predominates or recedes to give oedema is summarized below.

## Increased capillary transudation

The main causes for this are listed below:

### I. Raised intracapillary pressure due to increased venous pressure

This is perhaps the commonest cause for oedema and has two main causes:

#### Venous obstruction

1. Intrinsic causes: This may arise from active thrombosis (see Figure 16.3) or persisting occlusion caused by it. Occasionally tumour masses, such as hypernephroma, may proliferate within vein.
2. Extrinsic causes: Compression of a vein from without. Examples: by a tumour (Figure 9.11); a constricting band around a limb (provided the arterial supply is not also cut off) and giving either a sustained, if the band remains on, or a transitory oedema.

#### Increased venous pressure without venous obstruction

1. A generalized increase in venous pressure from heart failure is a common cause for bilateral oedema but salt retention is often an additional factor here.
2. An increase in pressure localized to one or both lower limbs caused by prolonged dependency.
3. Valvular insufficiency in the veins of a limb from any cause may lead to sustained venous hypertension in the upright position and consequent oedema.
4. Arteriovenous fistula is an occasional cause for a localized increase in venous pressure and may be a single communication, usually traumatic in origin but occasionally occurring spontaneously (see Figure 17.24(a)), or may involve a whole limb in multiple congenital fistulas (see Chapters 12 and 17).

Raised arterial pressure may be a contributory cause in major oedema, but seldom the only one.

## FORMATION OF TISSUE FLUID

## RE-ABSORPTION OF TISSUE FLUID

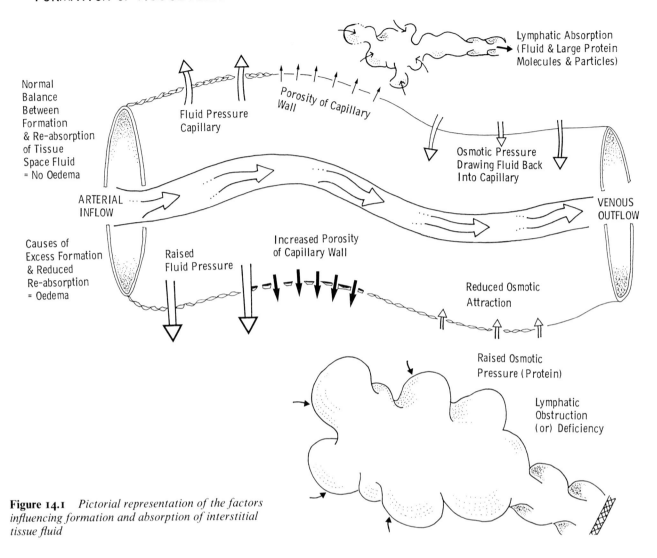

**Figure 14.1** *Pictorial representation of the factors influencing formation and absorption of interstitial tissue fluid*

### II. Increased capillary permeability

A variety of agents, either localized or generalized, may cause an increase in the porosity of the capillary membrane so that there is an outpouring of fluid and, in extreme cases, large protein molecules or even particulate matter. The main causes are:

1. Response to various stimuli within acceptable physiological limits, such as warmth or female hormones.
2. During inflammation, in response to injury by bacterial toxins or as an allergic reaction.
3. Overdistension of the capillaries by increased venous pressure as considered above.
4. Physical injury by trauma, burns, freezing or radiation.
5. Chemical injury either by exogenous poisons and drugs or endogenous electrolyte abnormalities.
6. Injury by lack of physiological requirements, such as oxygen.

7. Allergic response to foreign protein.

### III. Diminished reabsorption of interstitial fluid: changed osmotic pressure

The change causing reduced reabsorption, and hence oedema, is: *reduced osmotic pressure within the capillary.* The main force drawing fluid back from the tissue space into the capillary is the osmotic pressure of the circulating proteins. These will be reduced in any of the following conditions:

1. Renal disease, especially a protein-losing nephropathy.
2. Malnutrition causing reduction in plasma proteins, for example, famine oedema.
3. Prolonged protein loss in gastrointestinal states such as ulcerative colitis.

4. Severe protein loss due to extensive burns to the skin.
5. Hypoproteinaemia due to cirrhosis or other liver disease.
6. Haemodilution by excessive intravenous fluid.

### IV. Increased osmotic pressure in the tissue fluid

A raised osmotic pressure tending to retain or increase fluid in the interstitial space will be caused by:

1. Generalized states of salt retention that accompany hypertension, heart failure and renal disease; hormonal influence by pituitary and adrenal glands may initiate this.
2. Excessive intravenous saline.
3. A localized state, often one limb, of lymphatic obstruction causing a build up of large molecule proteins unable to escape (see below).
4. Increased capillary permeability allowing excessive escape of fluid, electrolytes and proteins, as described above.

### V. Lymphatic obstruction or insufficiency

These states are described later in this chapter. Failure of lymphatics to remove large molecule proteins will raise the osmotic pressure in the interstitial space so that fluid is retained and oedema forms. Fluid returned by lymphatics is not a critical factor because capillary reabsorption can easily compensate for this if the osmotic pressure is not raised.

### Combined states causing oedema

Two or more of the conditions described above may combine to cause oedema.
**Example 1** A mass of malignant glands in the groin may obstruct the lymphatics and also compress the underlying deep vein.
**Example 2** Prolonged dependency in a limb with severe ischaemic rest pain will combine with anoxia and increased capillary permeability to cause oedema.

### Factors in generalized oedema

Any generalized tendency to oedema will be first shown in the dependent parts, particularly the lower limbs, for example, in the renal failure of acute glomerulonephritis. Similar retention may also be caused by pituitary and adrenal response to 'stress', and is an added factor in heart failure. Other natural hormones play an important role in water retention often seen as a mild oedema of the lower extremities in premenstrual states and in pregnancy. Hormonal therapy can certainly cause water retention, sometimes severe, so that steroids, androgens, oestrogens and certain oral contraceptives all may cause

this. Various drugs, for example phenylbutazone and a range of drugs given for hypertension, are well recognized as being causes for water retention and oedema in the lower limbs. Excessive use of diuretics, possibly used to control oedema, may lead to electrolyte inbalance and consequent aggravation of oedema.

### Local factors that may influence development of oedema in a limb

Local circumstances in a limb, such as varicose veins or habitual prolonged standing, which would not ordinarily cause oedema, may do so if there is a background of mild water retention.

Ischaemia by occlusion of a main artery to a limb may reduce and conceal oedema that would otherwise be present; for example, a generalized oedema may not be recognized as such because an ischaemic limb may not reflect this and be regarded as the good limb with a troublesome oedematous opposite limb! Conversely, failure of an arterial reconstruction may be first evident by the sudden reduction in a postoperative oedema.

### Diagnostic approach to oedema of the lower limbs

The distinction between pitting and non-pitting oedema is a useful, but not entirely reliable, method of recognizing lymphoedema. A longstanding lymphoedema, which may well be bilateral, gives rise to oedema in the skin as well as subcutaneous tissue and causes a characteristically brawny swelling which does not pit easily on pressure and with a coarse 'orange skin' texture to the skin. These appearances are easily recognizable in the chronic case but in one of recent origin, such as the first onset of lymphoedema praecox, may not be so easily distinguished. This will be considered in more detail under a separate section on lymphatic oedema and for the moment will be put to one side so that the problem of bilateral pitting oedema may be considered.

### Bilateral pitting oedema

This is likely to signify a generalized state but not necessarily so; if the vena cava is thrombosed or there is an extensive, simultaneous process in both lower limbs, then a bilateral oedema may occur; it may have a simple explanation, for example following prolonged dependency during an air flight, or the elderly person who habitually sleeps sitting in an armchair. Bilateral pitting oedema of the lower limbs as part of a generalized state will arise in the conditions detailed in Table 14.1

**TABLE 14.1** Causes of bilateral pitting oedema from systemic disease

| Cause | Supporting signs | Investigations |
|---|---|---|
| Heart failure | Sacral oedema<br>Neck veins up<br>Liver enlarged and tender<br>?Ascites<br>(Salt and water retention)<br>Response to digoxin and diuretics | Chest X-ray<br>ECG |
| Renal disease | Oedema of face | Blood urea/creatine |
| Acute and chronic | Proteinuria | Serum proteins<br>Albumin/globulin ratio |
| Liver disease<br>Cirrhosis | Alcohol problems<br>Palpable liver<br>Other manifestations of liver disease | Liver series |
| Malignant ascites<br>Carcinomatosis peritonei | Obstructs vena cava by weight of fluid, but may have obstruction of lymphatics or thrombosis of vena cava as well<br>Secondaries or enlarged lymph glands elsewhere | Chest X-ray and CAT scan |
| Famine or nutritional oedema | Widespread in famine areas but may occur in land of plenty in the elderly living alone | |
| Generalized salt and water retantion | Other causes beside those given above include various forms of therapy by hormones, drugs or excessive intravenous drip. Oedematous states, perhaps hormone related, occur during the menstrual cycle, pregnancy and in other less well defined conditions | |

*Painful unilateral pitting oedema*

Unilateral oedema accompanied by pain may be caused by:

1. Any rapid recent accumulation of oedema which certainly causes discomfort if not actual pain.
2. Deep vein thrombosis. Discomfort is very variable in the early stages or in the less extensive thrombosis. It may be the first manifestation but in other cases a fairly extensive thrombosis may remain silent throughout; this is probably determined by the position, the extent and the rate of development of the process. An extensive deep vein thrombosis will cause considerable pain and swelling.
3. Superficial phlebitis may cause painful oedema but this is localized to one area of the limb, although in some cases it may be so extensive that it is mis-diagnosed as a deep vein thrombosis.
4. A widespread inflammatory condition, such as cellulitis, may mimic a deep vein thrombosis.
5. Any injury, especially when accompanied by a fracture, may cause oedema. The history usually makes the diagnosis clear but a spontaneous fracture, such as a 'march fracture' of a metatarsal, may be overlooked.
6. The chronically ischaemic limb with rest pain may show pronounced oedema due to the patient sleeping with the leg hanging out of bed to obtain some measure of relief. It is not uncommon for this to be mis-interpreted as a venous problem requiring treatment by elevation and compression bandaging, an error which can cause unnecessary loss of the limb.

*Note.* Oedema in a limb is not a feature of acute ischaemia (unlike some cases of chronic ischaemia). At an early stage, the acute onset of deep vein thrombosis may be mistaken for arterial embolism (acute ischaemia) because the rapid formation of oedema causes the limb to look pale and the pulses difficult to feel. This phase of clinical uncertainty will soon resolve as the oedema becomes more obvious. A Doppler flowmeter to identify arterial pulses at the ankle is valuable in the early diagnosis and in deciding whether to obtain a phlebogram or an arteriogram.

The list given above is not comprehensive but covers some of the more ususal problems.

*Painless unilateral oedema*

This may be caused by:
**Venous causes**
1. Post-thrombotic state.
2. External compression of the common iliac, external iliac, femoral or popliteal veins.
3. Valve deficiency in the deep veins.
4. Massive incompetence in superficial veins can certainly cause oedema, but usually not severe and often only a contributory cause aggravating a more general tendency to oedema; this is particularly so in the elderly with whom there should be caution over the expectation of relieving oedema when surgery to the veins is advised.

The positive recognition of venous abnormality, sufficient to cause oedema, is considered in Chapters 4–9.
**Lymphoedema** In the early stages lymphoedema may show pitting upon pressure and this sign cannot be entirely relied on to differentiate from other forms of oedema, especially in the young person.

**Hysteria (oedeme bleu)** Here the swelling is a response to the limb being kept hanging down without movement, or the secret application of a constricting band.

**Immobility** In a paralysed limb which is dependent for prolonged periods.

Again, this list is not comprehensive and a range of soft tissue, rheumatic and musculoskeletal conditions may be associated with lesser degrees of oedema with or without pain. This is discussed further under the section on obscure and troublesome minor oedema later in this chapter. The main clinical categories of oedema, and the possible causes, are summarized by diagram in Figure 14.2

**Longstanding severe oedema of whole limb or moderate oedema up to knee level: unilaterally or bilaterally:**

History of DVT  
Pigmentation } Venous cause likely. Confirm with:  
Ulceration } Doppler; phlethysmography;  
Enlarged sup. veins } phlebography; ultrasonography

Brawny and non-pitting } Lymphoedema. Photoplethysmography  
Peau d'orange } is normal. Radioactive uptake and  
Crevices in skin } Gamma camera can prove diagnosis.  
} Lymphangiogram only if essential

**Painful unilateral pitting oedema:**

Painful } One of following: Deep vein thrombosis;  
Recent onset } superficial phlebitis; cellulitis; diabetes;  
Acute process } lymphangitis; injury; ischaemia (due to hanging  
} leg out of bed because of rest pain); arterio-  
} venous fistula of acute onset.

**Painless unilateral pitting oedema (but some discomfort when oedema is maximal):** one of the following: Venous (superficial incompetence (varicosities), deficiency or absence of deep vein valves, previous DVT (post-thrombotic limb), subacute deep vein thrombosis); early lymphoedema; venous obstruction (tumour or popliteal cyst); suppressed bilateral state (one limb severely ischaemic); combined states (more than one cause); arteriovenous fistula; tight bandaging in mid or upper limb; hysterical manifestation (oedeme bleu due to prolonged dependency or constricting band); paralysed limb.

**Painless bilateral pitting oedema (but some discomfort when oedema maximal):** one or more of the following: Central cause, including heart failure, renal disease, liver disease, protein deficiency; malnutrition; unsuitable drug administration or undesirable response; excessive intravenous fluid and electrolyte therapy; obstruction to inferior vena cava or iliac veins by thrombosis, tumour or ascites; overt or hidden malignancy; arteriovenous (aorto-vena caval or iliac) fistula; symmetrical 'unilateral' state, that is, bilateral localized defects in lower limbs; ill-defined hormonal imbalance; prolonged dependency e.g. air travel, habitual sleeping in chair or paralysis; inborn or acquired (menopausal) tissue changes with increased capillary permeability.

**Figure 14.2** *The causation of oedema*

## Treatment of oedema of venous origin

The treatment of a venous oedema is often incidental to treatment of an ulcer and this is considered in Chapters 8 and 9. When the problem is purely one of oedema without any accompanying venotensive changes the surgeon must proceed with caution because venous disorder sufficient to cause even localized oedema will usually give other clear evidence of its presence. When obvious venous disease is present it must not be assumed that any enlarged superficial veins present are at fault and should be removed; these may, in fact, be collateral veins compensating for underlying deep vein occlusion in a post-thrombotic limb (see Chapters 6, 8 and 9). The circumstances in which surgery is likely to be appropriate in the treatment of oedema are summarized below.

### The role of surgery to the veins in treatment of oedema: guiding rules

Before considering surgery in the treatment of oedema it is essential to show that venous disease of sufficient severity to cause oedema is present and that the venous state is suitable for surgical treatment. The evidence for this is summarized in ascending order:

1. The oedema is unilateral and does not extend very far above the ankle.
2. Other non-venous causes have been consciously excluded, for example, lymphoedema.
3. The presence of substantial simple superficial vein incompetence; this may be accompanied by obvious varicose veins or take the form of a 'concealed' or 'straight-through' incompetence. The clinical tests must give full support to this diagnosis.
4. Supporting evidence of venous hypertension, viz. pigmentation and induration, possibly with ulceration as well.
5. Supporting evidence of substantial simple incompetence by Doppler flowmeter and/or by plethysmography showing a shortened recovery time that reverts to near normal with occlusion of the superficial veins under suspicion.

If these conditions are fulfilled then it is reasonable to treat the venous state by simple surgery removing incompetent superficial veins, in the belief that this may benefit the oedema. However, the following circumstances give warning that the oedema may not have a venous origin or that simple surgery will not improve matters, indeed may do harm, and only specialized surgery by vein or valve reconstruction has any possibility of bringing benefit:

1. If the oedema is bilateral. The many causes for bilateral oedema have been considered earlier in this chapter. Of the venous causes, deep vein impairment, unsuitable for simple forms of surgery, is far more likely than superficial vein incompetence.
2. If the oedema extends to knee level or higher. Of the venous conditions, only deep vein problems are likely to cause this.
3. If there is a definite history of deep vein thrombosis, then deep vein impairment must be assumed until proved otherwise.

In the circumstances just outlined, surgery should not be

considered without good quality functional phlebograms which must include the iliac veins and inferior vena cava. The phlebogram may show widely open but valveless deep veins. Here (short of valve reconstruction or auto-transplantation of valves) surgery to enlarged superficial veins will do little harm but will not succeed in relieving oedema. If a normal sized and well-valved long saphenous vein is shown, it cannot be the cause of oedema and should not be removed.

Various deep vein and valve reconstructions are described in Chapter 21 but, again, it must be emphasized that these are procedures only for the specialized expert. Palma's cross-over operation for iliac vein occlusion is perhaps the most promising of these in the relief of oedema if iliac vein occlusion is present.

## Conservative treatment of venous oedema

In summary, when surgery is not appropriate the principles of treatment are:

- Sleeping with the foot of the bed raised 30 cm or more (but check arterial pulses first), and elevation of the feet to a high level whenever possible during the day. The proportion of the day spent in elevation should increase with the severity of the condition.
- Use of elastic support (see Chapters 13 and 18).
- Judicious trial of diuretics.
- Use of intermittent pneumatic pressure devices.
- Massage can be very beneficial when expertly applied.

## The problem case: obscure minor oedema; idiopathic oedema of women

All too often there is the patient who has mild to moderate, but troublesome, oedema which does not fit clearly into any of the categories outlined above. Such cases will not be remedied by a few injections into superficial veins upon which the patient's dissatisfaction has been focused. It is not wise to raise the hopes of the patient, who should be warned that surgery or injection to veins will not change the oedema and that the visible veins are a separate cosmetic issue. This problem is not rare and does require careful individual thought.

There is little doubt that many of these patients have an unidentified inborn predisposition, perhaps tissue structure or hormonal, to dependency oedema. Often they are women aged forty or over and the condition is related to premenstrual or menopausal water retention. There is one easily recognized variety, termed erythro-cyanosis frigida, with blue cold extremities, often subject to chilblains, prone to oedema and giving a rather displeasing and shapeless limb. It is an important condition to recognize as the patient is desperate for any treatment that may provide a remedy but treatment by surgery or injection of veins gives disappointing results. One possible exception to this is when disabling chilblains, occurring each winter, have persisted into adult life and are the main complaint; here a lumbar sympathectomy may bring the patient relief but this is occasionally followed by prolonged distress through post-sympathectomy pain radiating down the thigh. (Post-sympathectomy pain is quite common following sympathectomy by phenol injection or by surgery; it usually comes on about a week after the procedure, that is, after the patient has left hospital, and for this reason it is wise to warn the patient that it may occur but will usually subside after 2 or 3 weeks. It can be most unpleasant but fortunately only a small minority persist.) In all other circumstances sympathectomy must not be carried out, however persuasive the patient may be, as it will not bring benefit and eventually be the cause of profound dissatisfaction; it certainly will not relieve oedema.

Some of the possible explanations for obscure oedema are:

1. A mild degree of lymphatic hypoplasia allowing easy accumulation of tissue fluid (seldom justifies a lymphogram).
2. Hormonal imbalance.
3. Administration of drugs or hormones (see earlier part of this chapter) causing water retention in susceptible patients.
4. Postural causes, such as prolonged standing, or poor habits, such as sleeping at night in a chair (elderly people or alcoholics).
5. It must be remembered that the elderly lose the robustness of their tissues and will be prone to a peripheral oedema more easily provoked than at a younger age. It may be unwise to operate on simple varicose veins in the elderly if a mild oedema is the main complaint as the results can be disappointing.

Many of the patients referred to above fall within the well-recognized category of idiopathic oedema of women; the causation and treatment of this is well discussed by Ledingham (1987).

### Management of the obscure oedema

Cure may not be possible but helpful advice can be given and some suggestions are summarized below:

1. Elevate limbs at night and at every opportunity by day.
2. Use support hose or give trial to elasticated tubular stockinette, 'Tubigrip'. The patients will seldom accept full surgical elastic stockings as these may be less acceptable to them than the oedema itself. They should not be coerced into using them but only used if the patient senses a real benefit. Support hose usually brings equally good control of a mild oedema and is psychologically kinder to the patient.
3. Diuretics used judiciously are often of value. It may

be best for the patient to see a physician for advice upon this and at the same time to have a medical check for possible hormonal inbalance or other general cause for oedema.

4. In more severe cases pneumatic intermittent compression devices used at night may help the patient (see Appendix).

5. Various medications, such as rutosides (Paroven), may bring benefit in the milder cases.

## Oedema of lymphatic origin

Oedema caused by inadequate lymphatic function, lymphoedema, is a major topic, too large to cover fully in this book but, because of its importance in the differential diagnosis of many venous states, a short description of the circumstances causing lymphoedema and how it may be distinguished from other forms of oedema will be given.

### Normal anatomy and function of the lymphatic system in the limbs

The lymphatic vessels possess numerous delicate valves and start as a fine 'capillary' network in the tissue spaces which merges into a series of channels running in broadly defined patterns up the lower limbs. From here they follow the main veins of the pelvis and abdomen, and through the cisterna chyli to the thoracic duct, which in turn runs up the thoracic vertebrae to empty into the left subclavian vein. The lymphatics of the left upper limb similarly join the thoracic duct but the right upper limb drains separately by the right lymph duct into the right subclavian vein. At intervals there are groups of lymph nodes (e.g. popliteal, inguinal, pelvic and aortic) which act as 'filters' and thus offer some resistance (often bypassed by neighbouring channels) to onward movement of fluid within the lymphatics. Like veins, the numerous valves and the general arrangement is dedicated to move lymph in one direction only, towards the thoracic duct. The propulsion of lymph depends on:

1. Periodic contraction of lymph channels so that each segment between valves forms a minute pumping unit responding to distension by contraction and passing fluid from one segment to another, sequentially along the full length of the lymphatic system. This is regarded by many (Hogan and Nicoll, 1979; Johnston, Hayashi and Elias, 1986; Azevedo and Teixeira 1988; McHale, 1988) as the main driving force in the movement of lymph.

2. Intermittent compression of lymph channels when neighbouring muscles contract, by pulsation in arteries and fluctuation in the pressure of veins nearby.

3. External compresssion by body weight and movement. Therapeutically, by massage or pneumatic inter-

mittent external compression devices. Continuous compression by elastic support can scarcely give repeated pumping action but may help to prevent accumulation of interstitial fluid. Gravity is a force to be overcome in the upright position but will favour return of lymph in the elevated limb.

The means by which interstitial fluid is drawn into the lymph capillaries and passed into the lymph channels to become lymph fluid is still debated. It is likely to be a combination of osmotic forces, fluid pressure within the interstitial space and by physical interaction between myoendothelial fibres and anchoring filaments at multiple specialized lymph collecting points in the tissue space to produce a slight suction effect (Reddy, Kronskop and Newell, 1975; Guyton, 1986). Both interstitial and lymph fluids have a similar composition with high protein content.

The normal lymphatics in the lower limbs are arranged in two distinct layers which run separate courses up to join the inguinal glands. One set is in the superficial tissues, outside the deep fascia: the other is beneath the deep fascia, draining the muscles and other deep tissues (Pflug and Calnan 1971). This arrangement explains why it is possible for lymphoedema to be confined to the superficial tissues and not shared by the deep tissues as is usually the case. This is the basis of many attempted cures which seek to establish connection between superficial to deep lymphatic systems.

### The essential role of lymphatics

Normal lymphatics remove about one-tenth of the tissue fluid but their essential role is the removal of all large protein molecules and particulate matter, which otherwise remain trapped in the tissue spaces (Pflug, 1972). If this should happen, the colloid osmotic pressure of the interstitial fluid will rise progressively so that the fluid cannot be reabsorbed by the venous part of the capillary beds and will accumulate (Figure 14.1) to cause lymphoedema.

A further role of the lymphatics is the elimination of invading bacteria which are drawn into the lymph capillaries and driven up the lymphatics to be destroyed in the lymph nodes. This defensive role may be lost in lymphatic obstruction so that the oedematous tissues become prone to infection.

### Lymphoedema

This arises when the essential feature in lymphatic function, its ability to remove large molecule proteins from the tissue spaces, is lost. There is no other route by which these unwanted proteins can be removed and they will accumulate with a corresponding increase in the tissue fluids osmotically attracted to them. The role of the lymphatics in this respect is indispensable; by contrast, their part in removing tissue fluid is only incidental as a necessary accompaniment to removing protein. The venous portion of the capillary bed is fully capable of removing all excess fluid, provided that retained proteins, raising the colloid osmotic pressure, do not prevent this. The various forms of lymphatic disorder leading to oedema will be described presently.

It has already been stated that classical lymphoedema is brawny and does not pit on pressure. The abnormally high protein content, and the reaction of the tissues to this, may determine this characteristic texture of the lymphoedematous limb. In some cases this feature may not be easy to detect, for example, the first appearance of lymphoedema in a young person may well show pitting on pressure and remain like this for some time until the chronicity of the condition accompanied by repeated inflammatory episodes causes diffuse fibrosis with coarse skin and firm non-pitting oedema.

Lymphoedema is a separate entity from venous oedema and in primary lymphoedema (see below) the venous function assessed by plethysmography or by phlebography is normal (Negus, Edwards and Kinmonth, 1969; Struckmann et al., 1986). In some pathologies, for example malignancy, obstruction of lymphatics and thrombosis of a principal vein may share the same cause and occur side by side. Apart from this there seems little relationship between the origin of these two major causes for oedema in the limbs. However, it is possible for the chance development of a venous disorder in the presence of a mild pre-existing lymphatic deficiency, or vice versa, to have a cumulative effect and set up a disproportionate amount of oedema.

The causes of lymphoedema are:

1. Primary lymphoedema:
   (a) Defective development or obliterative disease of unknown cause in the lymphatic system.
2. Secondary lymphoedema:
   (b) Acquired damage by trauma (including surgery), radiation or infection.
   (b) Obstruction to lymphatics by parasitic infestation or malignancy.

**Primary lymphoedema: defective development of lymphatics** Failure of normal development of the lymphatics arises in a variety of patterns (Kinmonth, 1982; Wolfe, 1984) but this may not be evident for many years and it is the first appearance of oedema in a teenager or a young adult that causes the diagnostic problems. The term 'Milroy's disease' is often indiscriminately used and only applies to a distinctive group of patients with congenital oedema and a clear family history of swollen limbs from birth. An hereditary tendency is quite common in primary lymphoedema even in those not evident at birth but here it is not known whether an inborn defect is late in reveal-

ing itself or whether there is an inherited vulnerability to an unidentified obliterative process in an otherwise normal lymphatic system. Some patterns of disorder show predominance of females or an association with particular congenital malformations. Lymphoedema may be classified by age of onset and by lymphangiographic appearances.

Classification by age of onset bears little relationship to the nature of the lymphatic abnormality. Lymphoedema congenita is evident at birth. Lymphoedema praecox may appear at any age before 35 years and is predominately seen in females. Typically it first appears in teenagers or young adults and may cause considerable psychological upset. Lymphoedema tardo is the term given to lymphoedema of late appearance after the age of 35 years. About 66% of lymphoedematous states appear, apparently spontaneously, around puberty, whilst 11% are present at birth; some 5% first appear with pregnancy and others give a history of injury or infection that appear to have precipitated it.

The following patterns of lymphatic abnormality are recognized by lymphangiography (Kinmonth, 1982; Figure 14.3):

*Hypoplasia or aplasia* Over 80% fall in this category. The affected lymphatics are inadequate in number and size; the lymph nodes are fibrotic and there is much evidence that the affected nodes obstruct lymph flow. Wolfe (1984) believes fibrosis in the lymph nodes may appear after birth and causes obliteration of the lymphatics by 'thrombosis' of the high protein fluid within the obstructed vessels; he prefers to use the term 'obliterative disease' rather than hypoplasia. The cause for fibrosis within the affected lymph nodes is not known but does not appear to be related to any identifiable inflammatory disease. The following patterns of hypoplasia are described by Kinmonth: distal hypoplasia; proximal hypoplasia with distal distension of lymphatics; proximal hypoplasia with distal hypoplasia of lymphatics.

In *distal hypoplasia* (Figure 14.3(b)), a scarcity of channels is evident below the inguinal ligament but with normal lymphatics above this level; the lymph nodes in the affected area may show some fibrosis. It causes moderate oedema below the knee, usually bilaterally and symmetrical. One in three patients has a family history of oedema and there is a predominance of young females. Distal hypoplasia is the most likely cause for the distressing development of unsightly swelling in one or both legs of a girl around puberty (lymphoedema praecox) (Figure 14.4).

In *proximal hypoplasia with distal lymphatic distension* (Figure 14.3(c)) there is a failure at pelvic or abdominal level, with fibrotic lymph nodes causing obstruction to lymph vessels below this so that they become dilated and tortuous, giving rise to a severe oedema of the entire limb (Figure 14.5). Males and females are affected equally but only 10% have a family history. It usually occurs

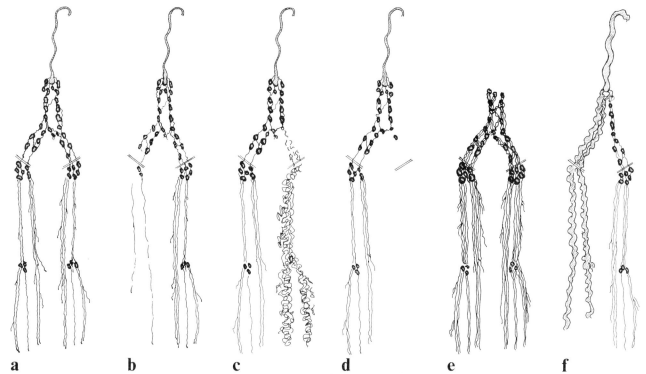

**a**        **b**        **c**        **d**        **e**        **f**

**Figure 14.3** *Diagrammatic representation of the main patterns of abnormality found on lymphography in primary lymphoedema (Kinmonth 1982).*

*(a) Normal arrangement of lymphatics in lower limbs draining via para-aortic glands to the thoracic duct.*

*(b) Distal hypoplasia in the right lower limb.*

*(c) Proximal hypoplasia with distension of distal lymphatics in the left lower limb.*

*(d) Proximal and distal hypoplasia on the left side.*

*(e) Bilateral (numerical) hyperplasia, with failure of the thoracic duct to fill.*

*(f) Megalymphatics in one limb and extending up to involve the thoracic duct; the opposite limb is normal. The lymphatics are grossly enlarged and valveless, resembling varicose veins. Such lymphatics not only fail in upward propulsion but allow reflux downward and this may include chyle*

unilaterally, but often showing latent lymphangiographic changes on the opposite side. The lymph nodes of the affected side show dense fibrosis. This type of proximal obstruction may prove suitable for some form of restorative surgical procedure, such as lymphovenous anastomosis or the enteromesenteric bridge described by Kinmonth.

Various combinations of the distal and proximal varieties occur to give *proximal hypoplasia with distal hypoplasia* and in these the condition may be bilateral but not necessarily symmetrical (Figure 14.3(d)).

A form of hypoplasia usually described separately is Milroy's disease which is the cause of 5–6% of primary lymphoedema. This is a familial condition and is evident at birth (lymphoedema congenita). The term Milroy's disease is not therefore appropriate for oedema appearing at a later age.

Gonad dysgenesis with lymphoedema is a rare (1.4%) condition in which distal hypoplasia is genetically linked with gonadal dysgenesis, usually as Turner's syndrome; other congenital abnormalities may accompany it. Because gonadal dysgenesis may present initially as lym-

phoedema, chromosomal studies should always be carried out in any case of congenital lymphoedema or in females who develop lymphoedema before commencement of menstruation.

*Bilateral hyperplasia* (Figure 14.3(e)) Six to seven per cent of primary lymphoedema patients fall in this distinctive group who develop bilateral and usually symmetrical oedema (Figure 14.6). It has strong genetic linkage. There is often a clear family history and many have other deformities of a set pattern, e.g. double eyelashes. All cases have a defective or absent thoracic duct and the lymphatics widely over the body show evidence of distension, especially marked in the lower limbs. The lymph nodes are enlarged and fibrotic; the lymphatics are broad and hyperplastic in the sense of being more numerous than normal (numerical hyperplasia), but do not show the same degree of obvious distension and tortuosity as those below a proximal hypoplasia. It is thought to be due to early failure in the development of the thoracic duct and consequent obstruction to the lymphatic system.

*Megalymphatics* (Figure 14.3(f)) This is a different form

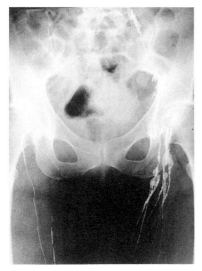

a

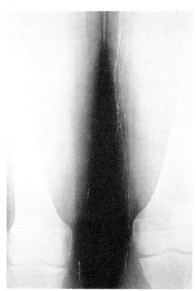

b

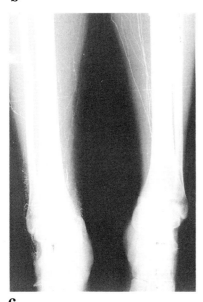

c

**Figure 14.4** *(a)–(c) Lymphograms showing right distal hypoplasia in a young woman. There is a deficiency of lymphatics up the length of the limb and only a few in the groin. On the patient's left side the lymphatics are normal*

of hyperplasia and is found in 3–4% of patients with primary lymphoedema. It is never familial and may be due to an embryonic mishap, perhaps caused by drug or virus, which affects the development of part of the lymphatic system. The lymphatics in the affected area are grossly enlarged and valveless so that it is virtually a lymphatic 'varicosis'. It is always unilateral, affecting only one lower limb, and for this reason is unlikely to be caused by a defective thoracic duct as this would affect both sides; the duct, however, often shares in the abnormal changes. The massive lymph vessels may allow reflux of chyle from the intestinal lymphatics down to the limb and chylous fistulas in the inguinal region or perineum may occur. The lymph nodes in the affected area do not show fibrosis, nor do they appear to be causing obstruction. The accompanying oedema in the limb may be severe. This is not an obstructive phenomenon but the massive lymphatics suggest a failure of the normal upward propulsion of lymph, perhaps due to absence of the valves and lack of contractility in the walls. The component of reflux and fistula formation can be overcome by surgical ligation of the massive lymph channels involved; this should always precede any surgical tissue reduction procedure.

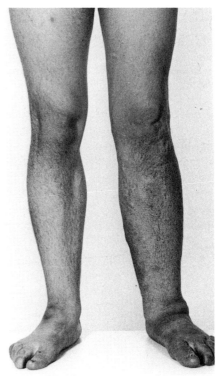

**Figure 14.5** *Clinical picture of proximal hypoplasia with distal distension of the lymphatics in a youth aged 15 years. Fluid vesicles formed intermittently on the front of the thigh and seeped fluid (dermal backflow)*

The proportions (Kinmonth, 1982) in which the primary lymphoedemas arise are as follows:

- Primary hypoplasia 71.3%
- Bilateral hyperplasia 6.7%
- Megalymphatics 3.4%
- Milroy's hereditary lymphoedema 5.7%
- Lymphoedema with gonadal dysgenesis 1.4%

*Surgical excision of a swelling in the groin – a caution*
Surgery to excise an unidentified mass in the groin in the belief that it is a hernia or lipoma is a particular pitfall. It may be due to lymph dysplasia mixed with fibromatous tissue and its removal uncovers an unsuspected lymphatic deficiency with the appearance of severe lymphoedema. Kinmonth (1982) refers to nine such cases, some with family histories of oedema, and advises lymphangiography before any inguinal swelling of uncertain diagnosis is explored or excised. Certainly groin swellings should not be removed from any patient with existing oedema, or a family history of oedema, without being completely certain that lymphatic pathways are not going to be disturbed in any way.

**Primary lymphatic disorders occurring with congenital venous disorders** It is not uncommon to find developmental lymphatic disorders combined in greater or lesser degree with an inborn venous disorder, each aggra-

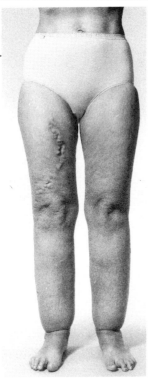

**Figure 14.6** *Patient with bilateral (numerical) hyperplasia. In fact, this troubled her little and her main complaint was of the disfiguring varicosity shown on the upper right thigh. This was due to simple superficial incompetence and a chance development superimposed on the lymphoedema. Surgery to the vein was carried out successfully, with great care not to disturb any lymphatics during saphenous ligation*

vating the tendency of the other to cause swelling in the limb. A lymph disorder on its own is not often associated with overlengthening of the limb and when this is found it should always arouse suspicion of concurrent venous or arterial disorder. The lymphoedematous limb does not ulcerate but when this occurs it is most likely to be due to underlying venous disease and should be investigated along the lines discussed in Chapter 13.

**Secondary lymphoedema: acquired obstruction or loss of lymphatics** Various disease processes may obstruct the lymphatics or the glands progressively, for example, filarial or malignant proliferation within them. The massive and widespread enlargement in filariasis (Dandapat, Mohapatra and Mohanty, 1986), prone to repeated infection from the deep skin crevices, is well known. Malignancy in various forms may cause the rapid development of severe oedema often compounded by compression of the accompanying deep vein by a mass of malignant glands or its actual thrombosis.

Extensive loss or damage to lymphatics will follow surgical block dissection of lymph glands and may give a troublesome oedema. Similarly heavy radiotherapy may cause significant obstruction. The old style radical mastectomy, removing all axillary lymphatic nodes and often combined with radiotherapy, commonly caused an unpleasant oedema of the upper limb. Severe lymphangitis, for example caused by streptococcus, may be followed by lymphatic deficiency and oedema, but here it is possible that there was a pre-existing mild hypoplasia.

*Investigation of lymphoedema* A common problem is to distinguish between a venous and a lymphatic origin for an oedema. Usually there are clear clinical indications but it is often necessary to obtain additional and more positive information. In the identification of a venous origin photoplethysmography is a simple method of particular value because it can give clear identification of defective venous return on exercise; it is, however, less effective in giving full reassurance of normality and, for instance, an occlusion in the iliac veins with undamaged deep veins below the inguinal ligament may show oedema in the limb but give a normal plethysmogram (see Figure 9.6). However, in most cases the plethysmogram will give positive recognition of venous disorder so that a functional phlebogram is appropriate; if the plethysmogram is normal, without history of deep vein thrombosis or clinical evidence of iliac vein occlusion (pubic varicosities or iliac fossa tumour), then a venous cause is so unlikely that phlebography can be omitted and a radioactive colloid uptake test proceeded with as the next step. This test is the simplest way to assess lymphatic function; it requires a single injection of radioactive colloid in the lower part of the limb with the uptake and subsequent distribution of colloid assessed by a gamma camera (see Chapter 23). The results are reliable and it avoids a rather tedious dissection to find and cannulate a lymphatic; moreover it does not cause the widespread, persisting dissemination of radiopaque material through the abdominal, thoracic and pulmonary lymphatic systems, often seen after lymphangiography. Establishing the diagnosis in this way may be all that is needed for appropriate decisions to be made, and lymphangiography is reserved for the more difficult cases where it may be needed to display the pattern of abnormality in greater detail, particularly if some form of surgery is being considered.

**Treatment of the primary lymphoedemas** A specialist work such as Kinmonth (1982) must be referred to for this but a summary is given here.

Mild cases may be controlled by diuretics together with a policy of elastic support with high elevation of the limb(s) whenever possible, certainly overnight. Various mechanical devices giving intermittent pneumatic compression in successive segments up the limb are obtainable and can be very effective in minimizing the oedema; these are used overnight or whenever the oedema is excessive.

If surgery is to be considered a lymphangiogram will be needed to identify the pattern of disorder and whether this will respond to any form of surgery. Massive chylous reflux in megalymphatics can be treated successfully by ligation of these channels. Reconstruction of lymphatics is not possible but transplantation of lymphatics in an enteromesenteric pedicle to the groin can bring benefit to the occasional patient with lymphatic deficiency or obstruction above this level (Kinmonth et al., 1978; Hurst et al., 1985). Likewise relief to obstructive states may be possible by implantation of a bisected lymphatic gland below the obstruction (Nielubowicz and Olszewski 1966, 1968) into a neighbouring major vein, such as the femoral, and can be very successful initially; the benefits, however, are often of limited duration as the newly established lymphatic drainage into the vein eventually seals over. Many operations, such as Thompson's (1967, 1970), have been designed to enable the superficial lymphatics to drain to the oedema-free subfascial layers but the success of these procedures is, at best, very limited. Perhaps the most effective methods are those that do not rely upon establishing new lymphatic routes but aim at surgical reduction of massive oedematous subcutaneous tissue and excess skin. Charles' operation (1912) is the most widely practised and certainly gives a slender limb but with an irregular contour; this is accepted by the patient as preferable to the more unsightly burden of an excessively swollen limb and its attendant complications. None of these surgical procedures should be embarked upon without proper previous experience in this type of surgery.

## Prevention of recurrent cellulitis in lymphoedema

Recurring infection with painfully inflamed areas and general malaise are a common complication of severe lymphoedema and may cause the patient much misery.

This arises from infection in the depths of the stagnant crevices that develop between bulging areas of lymphoedema. The patient finds it difficult to clean these and often a painful fissure has developed in its deepest part. In this environment bacteria flourish, including haemolytic streptococci which will readily invade the adjoining oedematous tissues. The acute attack can be quite serious and must be treated with appropriate antibiotics. Often further attacks follow in quick succession and in these circumstances the patient can be given relief by the prophylactic use of long-term, low dosage antibiotics given orally. Penicillin V (phenoxymethylpenicillin) is particularly effective given at a dosage of 250 mg as a single tablet daily, and forestalls further attacks for prolonged periods.

Severe, recurring cellulitis is, of course, a strong indication for a tissue-reducing procedure such as Charles' operation in order to remove the affected area.

## References

Azevedo, I. and Teixeira, A. A. (1988) Physio-pharmacology of the lymphatics. *Phlebology*, **3**, Suppl. 1, 99–103

Charles, H. (1912) In *A System of Treatment* (eds A. Latham and T. C. English), Churchill, London

Dandapat, M. C., Mohapatro, S. K. and Mohanty, S. S. (1986) Filarial lymphoedema and elephantiasis of the lower limb: a review of 44 cases. *British Journal of Surgery*, **73**, 451–453

Guyton, A. C. (1986) *Textbook of Medical Physiology*, Saunders, Philadelphia

Hogan, R. E. D. and Nicoll, P. A. (1979) Quantitation of convective forces active in lymph formation. *Microvascular Research*, **17**, S145

Hurst, P. A. E., Stewart, G., Kinmonth, J. B. and Browse, N. L. (1985) Long term results of the enteromesenteric bridge operation in the treatment of primary lymphoedema. *British Journal of Surgery*, **72**, 272–274

Johnston, M. G., Hayashi, A. and Elias, R. (1986) Quantitative approaches to the study of lymphatic contractile activity in vitro and in vivo: potential role of this dynamic 'lymph pump' in the re-expansion of the vascular space following haemorrhage. *Lymphology*, **19**, 45

Kinmonth, J. B. (1982) *The Lymphatics: Surgery, Lymphography and Diseases of the Chyle and Lymph Systems*, Arnold, London

Kinmonth, J. B., Hurst, P. A., Edwards, J. M. and Rutt, D. L. (1978) Relief of lymph obstruction by use of a bridge of mesentery and ileum. *British Journal of Surgery*, **65**, 829–833

Ledingham, J. G. G. (1987) Idiopathic oedema of women. In *Oxford Textbook of Medicine* (eds D. J. Weatherall, J. G. G. Ledingham and D. A. Warell), Oxford University Press, Oxford

McHale, N. G. (1988) Neural control of lymphatic pumping. *Phlebology*, **3**, Suppl. 1, 105–108

Negus, D., Edwards, J. M. and Kinmonth, J. B. (1969) The iliac veins in relation to lymphoedema. *British Journal of Surgery*, **56**, 481

Nielubowicz, J. and Olszewski, W. (1966) Experimental lymphovenous anastomosis. *British Journal of Surgery*, **55**, 449

Nielubowicz, J. and Olszewski, W. (1968) Surgical lymphaticovenous shunts in patients with secondary lymphoedema. *British Journal of Surgery*, **55**, 440–442

Pflug, J. J. (1972) The lymphatic system and lymphoedema. *British Journal of Hospital Medicine*, 363–370

Pflug, J. J. and Calnan, J. S. (1971) The normal anatomy of the lymphatic system in the human leg. *British Journal of Surgery*, **58**, 925–930

Reddy, N. P., Kronskop, T. A. and Newell, P. H. (1975) A note on the mechanisms of lymph flow through the terminal lymphatics. *Microvascular Research*, **10**, 214

Struckmann, J., Stranfe-Vognsen, H. H., Andersen, J. and Hauch, O. (1986) Venous muscle pump function in patients with primary lymphoedema: assessment by ambulatory strain gauge plethysmography. *British Journal of Surgery*, **73**, 886–887

Thompson, N. (1970) Buried dermal treatment for chronic lymphoedema of the extremities. *Plastic and Reconstructive Surgery*, **45**, 541–548

Thompson, N. (1976) The surgical treatment of chronic lymphoedema of the extremities. *Surgical Clinics of North America*, **47**, 445

Wolfe, J. N. N. (1984) The prognosis and possible cause of severe primary lymphoedema. *Annals of the Royal College of Surgeons of England*, **66**, 251–257

## Bibliography

Allen, A. J. and Wright, D. I. I., McCollum, C. N. and Tooke, J. E. (1988) Impaired postural vasoconstriction: a contributory cause of oedema in patients with chronic venous insufficiency. *Phlebology*, **3**, 163–168

Gajraj, H., Barker, S. G. E., Burnand, K. G. and Browse, N. L. (1987) Lymphangiosarcoma complicating chronic primary lymphoedema. *British Journal of Surgery*, **74**, 1180

Mardsden, P. D. (1990) Kwashiorkor. *British Medical Journal*, **301**, 1036–1037

Pflug, J. J. and Knox, P. (1987) Interrelationship between veins and lymphatic in chronic venous insufficiency. *Phlebology*, **2**, 93–102

Stringer, M. D., Melcher, D. and Stachan, C. L. J. (1986) The lower limb as a presenting site of malignant lymphoma. *Annals of the Royal College of Surgeons of England*, **68**, 8–11

Weatherall, D., Ledingham, J. G. G. and Warrell, D. A. (eds) (1978) *Oxford Textbook of Medicine*, Oxford University Press, Oxford

# 15

# Venous and other vascular disorders affecting the upper limb

An essential difference between venous problems in the upper and lower limbs is the virtual absence of disorders created by gravitational downflow in the superficial veins of the upper limb. The stresses on the valves, caused by hydrostatic or abdominothoracic pressures, are much less than in the lower limb and, even if the valves of superficial veins should become incompetent, the pressure differences and vigour of consequent retrograde flow within the upper limb are insufficient to create varicose veins (see Chapter 4). This means that for practical purposes varicose veins of the type commonly found in the lower limbs are not seen in the upper limbs. Theoretically, gravitationally induced varicose veins might arise in the greatly enlarged superficial veins of gymnasts or acrobats who repeatedly stand on their hands but even here, in this relatively unnatural position, the pressures generated (dependent upon level below the heart) are considerably less than those prevailing in the lower limb when upright. Thus, the commonest venous disorder of the lower limbs, and the complications arising from it, scarcely ever occur in the upper limb and when tortuous veins are seen only a limited range of causes have to be considered.

## Significance of tortuous veins in the upper limb

As just stated, reversed gravitational downflow causing varicose veins is not found in the upper limb, but when superficial veins are compelled to act as collaterals past an occluded deep vein a forced reversed flow may well occur; collateral veins become enlarged and, where flow is against the natural direction, will also become tortuous just as they do in post-thrombotic syndrome in the lower limbs. Although less common, deep vein occlusion also occurs in the upper limbs and, since simple varicosities are excluded, enlarged tortuous superficial veins may be assumed to signify this. The commonest example of this is axillary and subclavian vein thrombosis which is easily recognizable by a swollen limb with 'varicose veins' on the upper arm, shoulder and upper chest (Figure 15.1).

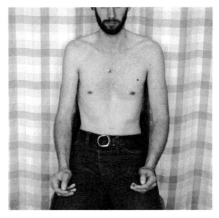

**Figure 15.1** *Clinical photograph of left subclavian thrombosis. This had developed 3 weeks earlier in an enthusiastic oarsman following prolonged use of a new type of training apparatus which required repeated maximal effort. The patient complained of swelling of the limb and increasing discomfort with moderate exertion. In the illustration slight swelling in the left arm is just detectable and a pattern of enlarged veins over the upper left chest is evident. One year later the arm had improved considerably but the patient was still unable to return to rowing. In discussion it was agreed to accept the limitation in full use of the limb rather than attempt any form of restoration to the obstructed venous outlet*

However, the patient may scarcely have noticed the enlarged veins because the predominant symptoms are discomfort and swelling of the limb. These changes must not be confused with the remarkable physiological hypertrophy of normal superficial veins seen in response to strenuous use of the upper limbs in certain manual occupations and a variety of sports, for example, rowing, weightlifting and gymnastics.

Occasionally, another cause for large, tortuous superficial veins, especially peripherally, in the upper limb is arteriovenous fistula, either multiple (congenital) or single (acquired); this is referred to again presently and in Chapters 12 and 17.

## Venous occlusion of the upper limb

Venous occlusion in the upper limb may arise from thrombosis or compression of the main veins. The tendency for thrombosis to occur 'spontaneously' is less than in the lower limb and there is usually an identifiable reason (Figure 15.2). Many cases of thrombosis follow medical interference with the veins of the arm, by intravenous drips, diagnostic catheterization of the veins, central venous cannula or pacemaker lead into subclavian and innominate veins (Figure 15.3) (and see section on digital subtraction angiography, Chapter 22). The thrombosis may be confined to the arm and, with anticoagulant treatment, there may be little long-term after-effect but in more extensive cases it will be followed by prolonged disability. Pulmonary embolus, sometimes fatal, is a recognized occasional occurrence in thrombosis of the upper limb (DeWeese, 1985). The clinical features of swelling, discomfort and prominent veins are similar to those in the lower limb and need not be described further here. With an unexplained thrombosis in the upper limb the possibility of malignancy in axilla, thoracic outlet or upper chest must be considered (Figure 15.4). Apart from this possibility, axillosubclavian thrombosis is a distinctive clinical entity and is discussed below.

## Axillosubclavian vein occlusion

The axillary and subclavian veins form the main outlet for venous blood from the upper limb and a thrombosis here is more severe in its effect than at a lower level. Moreover, these veins pass through complex skeletal anatomy which may compress and damage them so that the deep vein is most vulnerable to thrombosis at the very point where occlusion will cause maximal effect. In some respects it corresponds with the left common iliac vein which is prone to thrombosis causing an obstructed venous outlet syndrome where it is compressed by the overlying right common iliac artery (see Chapter 9).

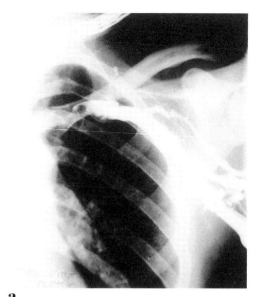

**a**

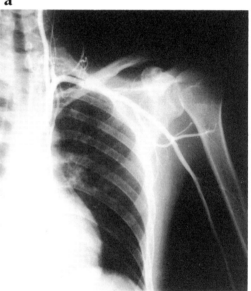

**b1**

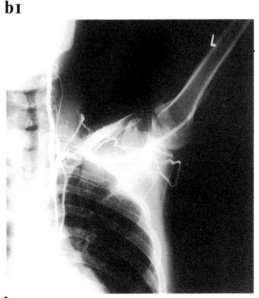

**b2**

**Figure 15.2** *Intermittent vascular occlusion and eventual thrombosis at thoracic outlet due to costoclavicular compression. Investigation was carried out for swelling and discomfort in the left arm.*

*(a) Left subclavian vein thrombosis is shown by phlebography.*

*(b) Subclavian arteriogram in the same patient by aortic catheterization.*
  *1. With the arm to the side, normal outline is shown.*
  *2. With the arm fully raised, severe compression of the subclavian artery is shown where it overlies the first rib and is crossed by the clavicle.*
*It is uncommon for the artery to be affected by costoclavicular compression together with the vein and this does raise the possibility of an accessory ligament or other abnormal anatomy*

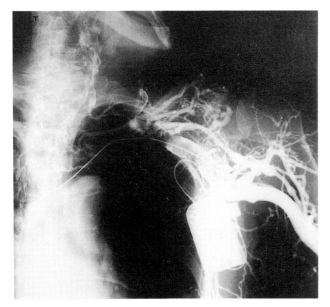

**Figure 15.3** *Axillosubclavian thrombosis in a man aged 76 years and caused by a pacemaker inserted 2 years previously. The subclavian vein is occluded and the axillary vein only thinly outlined due to clot within it. Venous return is by numerous collaterals*

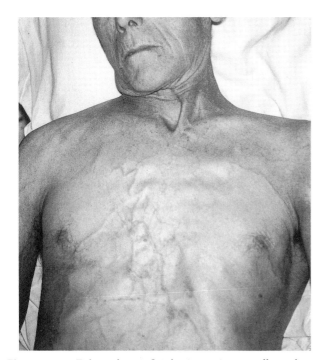

**Figure 15.4** *Enlarged superficial veins acting as collaterals on the right upper chest in a patient with thrombosis and occlusion of the right innominate vein due to mediastinal malignancy*

## The mechanism of subclavian vein compression

The axillary vein crosses the axilla and becomes the subclavian vein at the outer margin of the first rib. Here the vein passes under the costocoracoid ligament (a thickened portion of the clavipectoral fascia) and through a narrow passage bounded by the rib below, the clavicle above and

the robust anterior scalene muscle behind. The potential for damage with such unyielding structures surrounding it is very real if a slight disproportion of the anatomy brings them closer than usual. The vein may be compressed by two different circumstances:

1. Downward and backward movement of the shoulder, as in carrying a heavy weight or strongly bracing back the shoulders. This may pinch the vein between the clavicle, or the costocoracoid ligament, and the first rib.
2. Raising the arm, which causes rotation of the scapula so that the glenoid cavity is directed upwards and the acromioclavicular joint is carried backwards and slightly downwards. This rotates and angulates the clavicle at the sternoclavicular joint to narrow the interval between its medial portion and the first rib in which the vein lies (Figure 15.5). This is probably the more important of the two mechanisms.

Various other mechanisms for compression have been described but are, at best, exceptional causes. These include: compression by anatomical variants of brachial plexus, arteries, ligaments, tendons, or abnormal fibrous bands, possibly extending from a cervical rib; displacement and callous formation in fractures of the clavicle or first rib is an occasional cause. Daskalakis and Bouhoutsos (1980) describe 20 cases, investigated by phlebography and venous pressure measurements, and discuss the likely causes.

### Intermittent costoclavicular compression without thrombosis: thoracic outlet syndrome

There are a number of descriptions of a clinical syndrome of venous congestion of the upper limb occurring with certain movements, such as prolonged elevation of the arm during sleep or attempts to work above head level (DeWeese, 1985). This is thought to be the forerunner to eventual axillosubclavian thrombosis in many cases.

### Cervical rib in relation to arterial and venous compression at the thoracic outlet

There is a corresponding syndrome of ischaemic symptoms by compression of the subclavian artery and brought on by similar movements. In this, the mechanism of compression is between the anterior scalene tendon and the first rib but in the most striking cases a cervical rib is also present (Figure 15.6), often bilaterally. This extra rib, or a ligamentous extension from it, has a sharp upper edge which greatly increases the likelihood of the artery being nipped between it and the scalene tendon (Figure 15.7(c),(h)). The space in which the artery lies is often further reduced by a prominence on the first rib where the cervical rib articulates with it. The venous syndrome is unlikely to occur in a patient with a cervical rib because the subclavian vein lies in front of the anterior

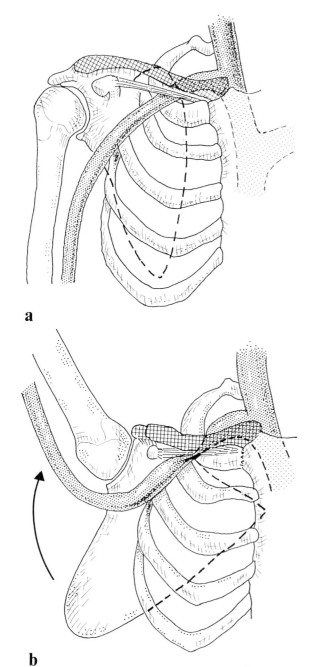

**a**

**b**

**Figure 15.5** *Diagram of the mechanism of costoclavicular compression to the subclavian vein.*

*(a) With the arm to the side, the clavicle and the costocoracoid ligament cross the subclavian vein without compressing it.*

*(b) When the arm is fully raised the curved clavicle rotates backwards together with the scapula so that the subclavian vein is compressed against the first rib. The costocoracoid ligament may also play a part in this*

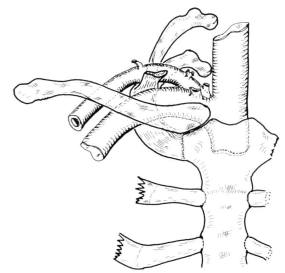

**Figure 15.6** *Diagram of compression of the subclavian artery against a cervical rib. The subclavian artery and vein are shown crossing over the first rib but they are separated by the anterior scalene muscle and its tendon (shown divided here for clarity). A cervical rib is present and the artery crosses over the lower portion of this together with any ligamentous extension from it and its articulation with the first rib. Elevation of the arm, combined with contraction of the muscle, causes compression of the artery against the cervical rib; the subclavian vein, lying in front of the anterior scalene muscle, is unlikely to be involved in this process. Beyond this point the artery may develop a poststenotic dilatation (not illustrated) in which thrombus forms*

scalene muscle and usually well beyond the tip of the cervical rib. The subclavian artery can certainly be damaged by repeated compression between a cervical rib and the firm scalene tendon but seldom, if ever, does the extra rib cause venous compression and thrombosis. The artery immediately distal to the point of compression often develops a poststenotic dilatation (Holman, 1954, who quotes Halsted's earlier description) or aneurysm in which thrombus forms and is shed as microemboli down to the fingers to cause ischaemic attacks or actual gangrene (Figure 15.7). A cervical rib may also affect the lower part of the brachial plexus which crosses over it and cause loss of sensation and paralysis in the hand, usually in the distribution of T1. On clinical examination both arterial and venous syndromes can be reproduced by high elevation of the arm or by bracing the shoulders forcibly backwards. The diagnosis of compression of the subclavian artery is confirmed by arteriography, first with the arm down, and then, when it is raised; in similar fashion compression of the vein can be demonstrated by phlebography with the arm in the two positions. A cervical rib is often easily palpable in the supraclavicular fossa and is, of course, readily displayed on X-ray (Figures 15.7(b)1, 2).

Browse, Burnand and Lea Thomas (1988) illustrate a case of cervical rib with a thrombosed subclavian vein but it is not clear whether the rib was a significant factor in its causation. In 15 personal cases of cervical rib, most bilateral, the author did not see any with evidence of subclavian compression, nor in 10 cases of subclavian vein thrombosis did he find any with cervical rib. Cervical rib occurs in about 1 in 250 people (Eastcott, 1969) so that in the occasional patient with venous compression and thrombosis arising from other reasons it may be

**Figure 15.7** *Ischaemia in the fingers, caused by cervical rib.*

*(a) The fingers of a farm-worker aged 28 years who worked through 2 months of winter believing he had a 'touch of frostbite'. The first and second fingers show mummified gangrene.*

*(b) 1. A cervical rib was palpable and visible in the right supraclavicular fossa.*
*2. X-ray showed bilateral cervical ribs to be present.*

*(c) Arteriogram showing poststenotic dilatation in the distal subclavian artery; debris from this has caused thrombosis in the mid-brachial artery; the digital arteries of affected fingers were also thrombosed (not shown).*

*(d) Photograph taken during surgery showing the subclavian artery drawn aside in a sling to reveal the sharp upper edge of the cervical rib against which it was compressed.*

*(e) Resected poststenotic dilatation in the artery beyond the cervical rib, opened to show thrombus within it. Portions of this periodically break away to cause ischaemic episodes in the fingers. Extensive thrombosis of the main arteries of the upper limb may occur, as in this patient. During surgery on such patients the thrombus in the dilatation is cleared away, the cervical rib resected and, if ischaemia in the hand warrants it, a prestellate sympathectomy carried out. The dilatation need not be resected unless there are unusually severe intimal changes but, if it is removed, direct re-anastomosis of the remaining artery is usually possible without difficulty (see page 314).*

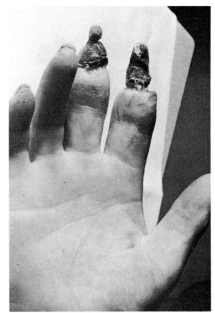

a

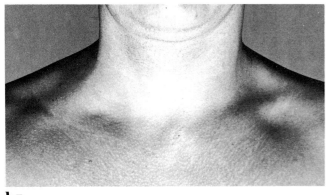

b1

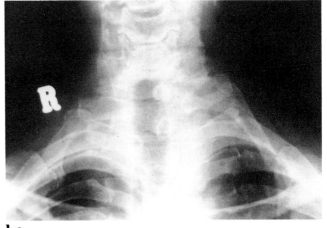

b2

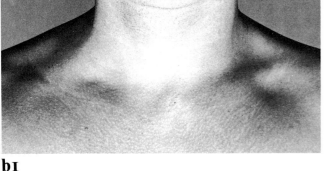

c

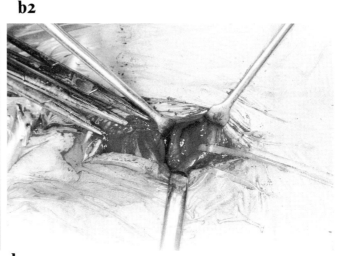

d

**Figure 15.7** *(continued)*

*(f)–(j)  A further patient, a young woman, with recurring attacks of ischaemia in fingers of the right hand.*

*(f)  Ischaemic lesion on forefinger at time of operation.*

*(g)  X-ray shows right cervical rib; a prominent costal process is present on the left transverse process of C7 on the left side and a ligamentous extension from this is likely.*

*(h),(i)Arteriograms to the right subclavian artery with arm to*

*side and arm raised. Severe narrowing of the artery is evident when the arm is raised and a poststenotic dilatation is present beyond this point.*

*(j)  At operation the right subclavian artery has been mobilized and the cervical rib exposed; its tip and articulation with the first rib can be seen just above the artery forceps used as a pointer. The cervical rib was divided close to its neck and removed together with the prominent articulation on the first rib.*

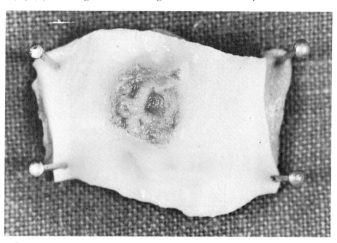

e

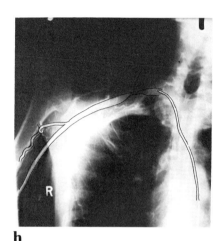

h

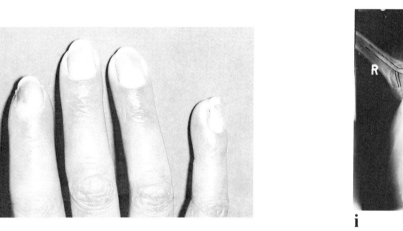

f

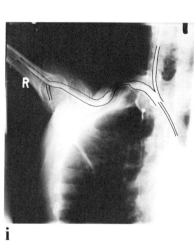

i

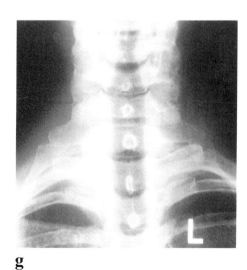

g

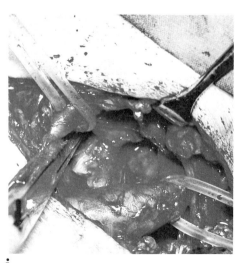

j

**Figure 15.7** *(continued)*
*(k) The dilated portion of the artery opened and a mound of thrombotic debris within exposed. Microembolism from this has been causing the ischaemic attacks in fingers. This was cleaned away and the artery closed; there is no necessity to resect this expanded portion of artery once the provoking factor, the cervical rib, has been removed*

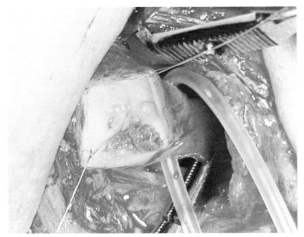

**k**

present by chance and not, in fact, implicated. However, in some cases there is a substantial protrusion where the extra rib articulates with the first rib or fibrous extensions from it and it is conceivable that this might impinge on the vein.

*Conclusion*

Cervical rib is an important cause for arterial (ischaemic) or neurological manifestations but seldom gives rise to venous problems. In any ischaemic phenomenon (i.e. related to arterial supply) in an upper limb, especially if unilateral and affecting fingers, a cervical rib must be the first possibility to exclude. However, this extra rib is a common abnormality, often harmless, and its presence does not necessarily mean it is the actual cause although this is probable. Arteriography with the arm to side and fully raised will clarify its role. Treatment will be by surgical removal of the cervical rib, ligamentous extensions from it and its prominent articulation with the first rib; at the same operation thrombotic debris is cleared from the enlarged portion of the artery, together with any other procedure needed to restore a good arterial supply.

**Treatment of costoclavicular compression of the vein**

This is an uncommon condition and mild forms occur where compression is only partial and sufficient relief is obtained by avoiding the provoking movements. In severe cases phlebography should be carried out and this may show that thrombosis has already occurred. If a vein

which has not thrombosed, or collaterals generated by thrombosis, are clearly compressed on upward movement of the arm then surgery removing the first rib or the inner half of the clavicle may be justifiable (DeWeese, 1985); simple division of anterior scalene muscle, sometimes beneficial when the artery is being intermittently compressed (with or without cervical rib), is not likely to succeed in relieving venous symptoms.

**Axillosubclavian vein thrombosis**

Although this is said to arise 'spontaneously' it is likely that costoclavicular compression, or a similar mechanism damaging the vein, is the underlying cause. Indeed the clinically obvious thrombosis may be the culmination of a number of silent lesser episodes.

**Clinical presentation**

Thrombosis is usually preceded by some prolonged and unusual activity (hence the term 'effort' thrombosis) or positioning of the arm, such as carrying a heavy suitcase over a considerable distance (Figure 15.8), using special training apparatus or falling asleep with the arm over the back of a chair. Within the next 36 hours the patient experiences increasing discomfort or pain in the arm with swelling and limitation of use. On examination the limb is swollen up to the shoulder, with pitting oedema of the back of the hand, the skin has a bluish tint and the veins are prominent. Venous patterning on the upper arm, shoulder and neighbouring chest is more evident and over the coming weeks these veins become larger and more tortuous as they respond to the collateral flow through them (Figure 15.9). Hughes (1948), in a review of 320 cases, termed the condition 'Paget–Schroetter syndrome', after the two surgeons who described it separately over a century ago.

**Investigation**

A Doppler flowmeter over the collateral veins at the shoulder reveals a high flow rate increased by exercising the hand. Simple direct pressure measurement confirms that venous pressure in the forearm is raised and photoplethysmography shows a poor response to exercise. Phlebography gives proof of the diagnosis by showing an obstructed subclavian vein, often with clot extending into the axillary vein, and various side branches taking collateral flow, for example, from the basilic or axillary veins to jugular or intercostal veins (see Figure 1.18). Collateral veins often follow the line of the first rib making their way as a bypass to the jugular vein, and as these collaterals lie in the costoclavicular interval they may be subject to intermittent compression on arm raising (DeWeese, 1985) (Figure 15.9(b)).

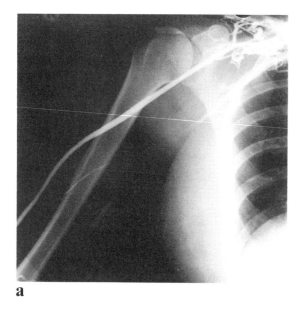

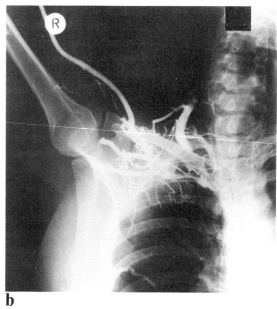

**Figure 15.8**   *Axillosubclavian vein thrombosis due to costoclavicular compression. 'Spontaneous' thrombosis in a woman aged 43 years following carrying a heavy suitcase.*

*(a)   Phlebogram with arm to side. Venous outlet from the right upper limb is almost entirely through the cephalic vein; the basilic vein is extensively occluded by thrombus, the axillary vein is very narrowed and the subclavian vein is occluded. Multiple collaterals run onto the chest wall or follow the subclavian vessels to outline the external jugular vein.*

*(b)   With arm raised, some major collateral vessels under the inner clavicle no longer fill.*

*Resection of the first rib was carried out. (Professor P. Morris' case)*

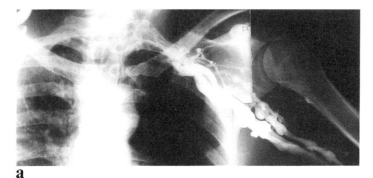

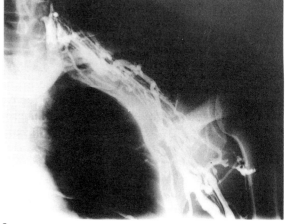

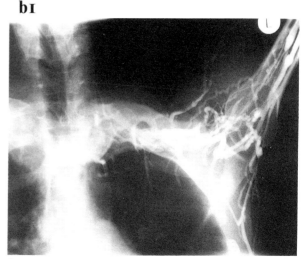

**Figure 15.9**   *Left subclavian vein thrombosis progressing to complete occlusion of the axillary and subclavian veins, in a male patient aged 46 years. He initially presented with swelling and discomfort in the left upper limb which increased in severity over the next 2 months.*

*(a)   Initial phlebogram showing the subclavian vein largely obstructed by thrombus in the portion of vein between first rib and clavicle.*

*(b)   Further phlebogram, 2 months later, showing progression of thrombosis so that the subclavian and axillary veins are now completely occluded.*
    *1. A leash of collateral veins follows the axillary vessels and are shown with the arm down.*
    *2. The arm has been fully raised and many of the collateral veins previously shown now fail to fill, probably because of compression between the clavicle and the first rib. This is an indication for surgical decompression either by removal of the first rib or by resection of the inner portion of the clavicle. In this patient, the first rib was removed through the axillary approach and this brought some improvement. (Professor P. Morris' case)*

These investigations do not however exclude the possibility of causes other than costoclavicular compression and careful thought must always be given to the alternative diagnosis of underlying advanced malignancy with extensive involvement of lymphatic glands in the upper axilla or mediastinum, or direct invasion by pulmonary tumour. As with any major thrombosis in veins, a general screening for any inherent state causing enhancement of thrombosis, such as deficiency of antithrombin III or protein C (see Chapter 16), should be carried out.

### Prognosis and treatment

In most cases of axillosubclavian thrombosis from costoclavicular compression the symptoms will be very troublesome for some months so that only limited use of the limb is possible. After this time there is a slow improvement both in the ability to use the limb and in the swelling. However few limbs will return to complete normality. The improvement is not due to the subclavian vein reopening but to the collateral veins enlarging to become more effective. Eventually an acceptable state may be reached but not full recovery and indeed a significant number are left with quite a severe disability and recurring discomfort with any heavy use of the limb. When seen in the initial stages it must be recognized that this is potentially a cause for moderate to serious disability so that all effort must be made by use of anticoagulants to minimize this. The usual routine is to give intravenous heparin for a week and this to be followed by some 3–6 months of warfarin treatment, both anticoagulants being carefully monitored to ensure an effective dose is being given. Theoretically there is much to support the use of streptokinase but, so far, no convincing evidence based on practical experience has been produced to show that this has a real advantage over heparin and warfarin treatment. The main difficulty is that the basic cause, costoclavicular compression, persists and recanalization of the vein is most unlikely. Here surgery may be able to help either by thrombectomy and freeing the vein from compression in the acute phase, or by a venous bypassing procedure to overcome the obstruction in the subclavian vein later on.

### Thrombectomy in the early stages

Thrombectomy cannot succeed unless the problem of freeing the vein from continuing compression is dealt with at the same time. A number of successes are reported from a procedure resecting the inner half of the clavicle and costocoracoid ligament, together with a thrombectomy so that the bony compression is removed and the vein reopened (Figure 15.10(a)). This gives a very direct approach and is perhaps the procedure to be recommended and there does not seem any significant disability from loss of the inner clavicle. An alternative

method is to remove most of the first rib either by an infraclavicular approach, or via the axillary route, but both of these are likely to require more surgical expertise than going through the bed of a resected clavicle. No series of any great size with any of these methods has been reported so that the consistency of successful outcome is uncertain and caution is advised.

### Axillojugular venous bypass

There is much to commend a policy of treating the initial thrombosis with anticoagulants and then waiting a full year to assess the residual symptoms. If these are tolerable it may be best to accept this but, if severe, then a venous bypass is a possible solution. For this a phlebogram is essential to identify good condition basilic and lower axillary veins to which a venous bypass may be anastomosed. This may be either a free autograft of saphenous vein anastomosed from axillary vein to the internal jugular vein (Figure 15.10(b)1) or, better, by bringing down the divided jugular vein to anastomose end to side with the axillary vein (Figure 15.10(b)2). Again published experience upon this is small and not always encouraging so that in most cases it may be wisest to continue with a conservative policy.

## Other manifestations of venous disorder in the upper limb

As already explained, the venous pressures in the upper limb seldom reach the levels found in the lower limb and venous hypertensive changes, including ulceration, do not ordinarily occur. However, occasionally, hypertension may be caused by arteriovenous fistula, as either congenital or acquired lesions, to give rise to pigmentation and induration progressing on to venous ulceration. The commonest example of the latter is a surgically created arteriovenous fistula for access in repeated renal dialysis (Figure 15.11) and a number of cases of quite severe pigmentation, induration and ulceration in the hand have been reported from this cause (and see Chapter 17 and Figure 12.5(a)).

Other venous manifestions and differential diagnoses are similar to those occurring in the lower limb but some brief comments are given below.

## Congenital venous anomalies, Klippel–Trenaunay syndrome and Parkes-Weber's syndrome of multiple arteriovenous fistulas in the upper limb

Policy and treatment is along the same lines as the lower limb (see Chapter 12), but overlengthening of an upper limb has not the same importance because weight-bearing joints are not involved and there is no long-term likelihood of arthritis in the spine due to malalignment.

**Figure 15.10**   *Treatment of subclavian thrombosis by surgery.*

*(a)  Diagram to illustrate resection of the inner portion of the clavicle to give direct access to the vein so that thrombectomy may be carried out. This simultaneously removes the obstructing thrombus and decompresses the vein. This procedure is perhaps the most suitable for a recent thrombosis where there is some prospect that the vein may remain open.*

*(b)  Surgical bypassing of an occluded subclavian vein.*
  *1.  An autogenous graft of reversed saphenous vein is used to create a bypass between the internal jugular vein and the axillary vein. In order to prevent compression of this new channel the subclavicular tunnel is decompressed by either removing the first rib or resecting the inner half of the clavicle.*
  *2.  An alternative method using the neighbouring internal jugular vein as a bypass. Access is gained by resecting the inner clavicle and the internal jugular vein is divided at high level so that its lower part may be swung down to anastomose with the axillary vein*

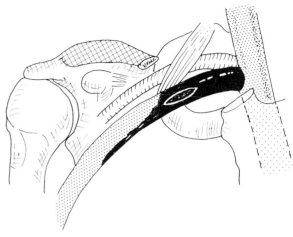

**a**

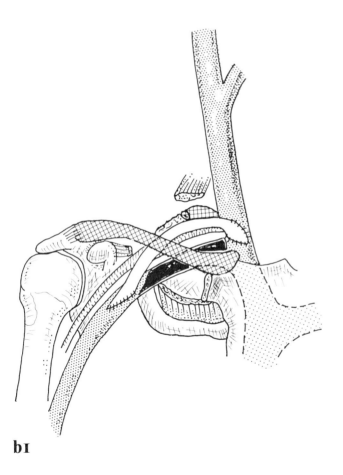

**b1**

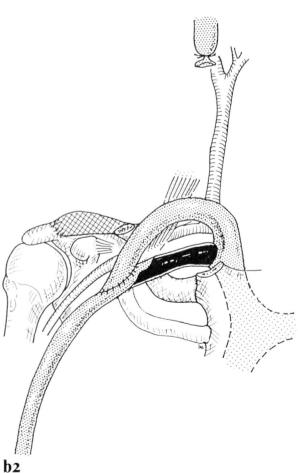

**b2**

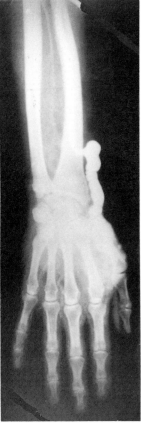
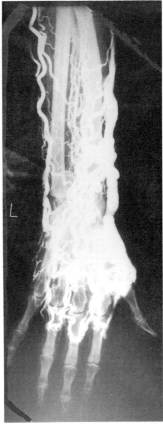

**I**       **2**

**Figure 15.11** *Venotensive ulceration in the hand caused by a surgically created arteriovenous fistula in a patient requiring repeated renal dialysis. After the fistula had been present for 2 years the patient developed brown pigmentation and ulceration on the back of the hand and forefinger. The illustration shows two phases of an arteriogram in this patient:*

*1. Direct flow of opacified blood across the fistula into an enlarged vein near the wrist.*

*2. Rapid and extensive filling of veins on the hand and forearm, giving venous hypertension at a level approaching arterial blood pressure.*

*The ulceration healed and other changes receded soon after the arteriovenous fistula was closed surgically*

The inequality in length may be disregarded and good function expected of the limb.

## Oedema

The range of possible causes for oedema in the upper limb is similar to that in the lower limb (see Chapter 14). However, a generalized oedema from systemic causes, such as heart failure and renal disease, will usually be more conspicuous in the lower limbs and sacrum, because it appears first in those parts furthest below heart level where venous pressure is highest. Causes of oedema unique to the upper limb(s) include:

*Bilateral oedema*

Compression or thrombosis of superior vena cava by tumour or invasive malignancy.

*Unilateral oedema*

1. Primary lymphoedema – relatively uncommon.
2. Secondary (acquired) lymphatic obstruction:
   (a) Malignancy (especially carcinoma of breast or lung).
   (b) Surgery removing axillary lymphatics.
   (c) Radiotherapy.
   (d) Primary skin neoplasm with secondary lymph-nodes in axilla.
3. Venous obstruction by thrombosis or compression:
   (a) Thoracic outlet syndrome.
   (b) Costoclavicular compression and thrombosis.
   (c) Malignancy affecting subclavian or axillary veins.
   (d) Injury or surgery affecting deep veins of upper limb.
4. Arteriovenous fistula – congenital, or acquired by trauma or surgery for easy access in renal dialysis.
5. Hysteria – self-application of constricting band or prolonged immobility of a limb in dependent position.
6. Immobility by paralysis.
7. Venous angiomatosis (congenital).

## Ulceration

This occurs most commonly on the hand. Venous ulceration is a rarity usually only seen with arteriovenous fistula as described above and will be recognized by the accompanying pigmentation and enlarged veins. Apart from this, the range of other causes is very similar to those given in Chapter 13 but some of the more important are summarized below.

1. Ischaemia. This may arise from (and see Chapter 17):
   (a) Embolus, usually from heart disease, fibrillation or recent coronary thrombosis.
   (b) Microembolism from subclavian aneurysm caused by cervical rib.
   (c) Atherosclerosis with thrombosis of main arteries to limb.
   (d) Self-injection of drugs, especially barbiturates.
   (e) Raynaud's syndrome, either the primary disease or secondary to serious systemic disease (see below).
2. Neuropathy (trophic lesions):
   (a) Neurological disease, e.g. syringomyelia.
   (b) Diabetes.
   (c) Nerve injury.
   (d) Leprosy
3. Malignancy:
   (a) Epithelioma.
   (b) Malignant melanoma.
4. Specific infections, including:
   (a) Tropical diseases, e.g. Leishmaniasis or leprosy.

(b) AIDS, syphilis or tuberculosis.
5. Haematological disorder.
6. Self-inflicted injury.

Perhaps the commonest type of ischaemic ulceration in the fingers is seen with Raynaud's phenomenon. Because manifestations of this state are seen most commonly in the hand rather than the feet it may be helpful to include a synopsis of the causes and significance of Raynaud's phenomenon at this point.

## Raynaud's phenomenon: an outline

This is an important syndrome of intermittent pallor, blueness and numbness of the fingers (and possibly the toes). In *primary Raynaud's phenomenon*, a disease in its own right, spasm of the digital arteries in response to cold is the usual precipitating factor and its course is relatively benign. The more severe *secondary states* may be accompanied by vasculitis with extensive closure of the digital arteries giving irreversible damage and persisting ischaemia.

If only *unilateral*, suspect a local arterial cause, e.g. cervical rib or an atherosclerotic lesion in the subclavian artery discharging debris.

If *bilateral*, remember that Raynaud's phenomenon is often the earliest manifestation of a serious generalized disease, such as, lupus erythematosis, widespread collagen disease or systemic sclerosis with scleroderma (Figure 15.12), leukaemia, cryoglobulinaemia or myxoedema. It is therefore imperative at the outset to carry out a complete medical screening which must include a chest X-ray, complete blood picture excluding LE cells and leukaemia, ESR, estimation of cold agglutinins and cryoglobulins, serum T[4], rheumatoid and antinuclear factors. Polycythaemia may present with ischaemic manifestations, especially gangrene, in fingers or toes and be mistaken for Raynaud's phenomenon. Inhaled chemicals (e.g. polyvinyl monomer in the plastics industry) and certain drugs (e.g. ergot) can be causative and must be inquired for.

When a background medical state causing a secondary Raynaud phenomenon has been excluded in this fashion then a diagnosis of *primary Raynaud's disease* is permissible. Even so a number of these patients eventuallly turn out to have a slowly progressive scleroderma (systemic sclerosis). Most patients with Raynaud's disease are women but when it occurs in a man two special states must be considered:

1. Occupational Raynaud's phenomenon due to use of machinery or tools giving rise to high frequency vibrations, e.g. holding a metal part subjected to a grinding process or use of a chain saw. This vibration-induced Raynaud's phenomenon may cause severe ischaemic and neurological changes in the fingers if the cause is not recognized in good time. However,

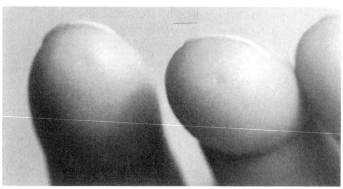

**a**

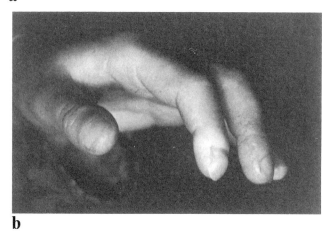

**b**

**Figure 15.12** *Raynaud's phenomenon in scleroderma. In addition to white fingers with numbness or pain, and thickened tissues, other lesions develop.*
*1. Scarring caused by painful, pinhead-sized ulcers (keens) may appear on the fingertips.*
*2. Ischaemia may cause atrophy of the terminal phalanx and overlying pulp of the tip of the index finger. This gives a characteristic curving of the nail with a claw-like appearance. More severe changes with gangrene in one or more fingers may occur. The arterial supply within the hand and finger is severely damaged by thrombosis and, unlike primary Raynaud's disease, will be incapable of vasodilatation even in favourable conditions*

smoking may cause similar changes and at times it is difficult to distinguish between the two conditions.
2. Tobacco-induced arteritis. The first evidence of a 'smoker's arteritis' (Buerger's disease) in a young person may be intermittent pallor of the fingers. The young man with these symptoms must be urged to stop smoking.

### Comment on treatment

Benign primary Raynaud's disease (cold hypersensitivity) seldom gives any useful response to vasodilators or similar agents. At the time of writing a new range of vasoactive materials are being given trial, including nifedipine, GTN paste, enalapril, thymoxamine, ketanserine and stanozolol. The previous generation of vasodilators raised many false hopes and it remains to be seen if the modern variants are any more successful. Upper limb sympathectomy tends to be impermanent and usually gives only temporary relief so that it is employed only as a measure of desperation. It should only be considered if the hands are capable of becoming pink and warm in favourable surroundings, indicating a circulation still able to dilate up.

With secondary Raynaud's phenomenon the cause must be identified and treated if possible. Vasodilators or sympathectomy bring no benefit and when accompanied by arteritis (e.g. lupus erythematosis or systemic sclerosis) it may prove impossible to prevent loss of fingers or even the hands. Although comparatively uncommon these severe states are so damaging, indeed life threatening, that ulcerative lesions of the fingers must always be considered with particular care.

*Note.* Raynaud's phenomenon is well reviewed by Cotton and Khan (1986), and Heidrich (1979).

## References

Browse, N. L., Burnand, K. G. and Lea Thomas, M. (1988) *Diseases of the Veins. Pathology, Diagnosis and Treatment,* Edward Arnold, London, pp. 627–642

Cotton, L. T. and Khan, O. (1986) Raynaud's phenomenon: a review. *International Angiology,* **5**, 215–236

Daskalakis, E. and Bouhoutsos, J. (1980) Subclavian and axillary compression of musculoskeletal origin. *British Journal of Surgery,* **67**, 573–576

DeWeese, J. A. (1985) Management of subclavian venous obstruction. In *Surgery of the Veins* (eds J. J. Bergan and J. S. T. Yao), Grune and Stratton, New York, pp. 365–382

Eascott, H. H. G. (1986) *Arterial Surgery,* Pitman Medical, London, pp. 216–234

Heidrich, H. (ed.) (1979) *Raynaud's Phenomenon,* TM-Verlag, Berlin

Holman, E. (1954) 'On circumscribed dilation of an artery immediately distal to a partially occluding band': post-stenotic dilatation. *Surgery,* **36**, 3–24

Hughes, E. S. (1948) Venous obstruction in the upper extremity (Paget–Schroetter's syndrome): a review of 320 cases. *British Journal of Surgery,* **35**, 155–163

## Bibliography

Boontje, A. H. (1979) Axillary vein entrapment. *British Journal of Surgery,* **66**, 331–332

Browse, N. L. (1987) Lymphoedema of the arm. *British Medical Journal,* **295**, 3–4

Davies, A. H., Walton, J. Stuart, E. and Morris, P. J. (1991) Surgical management of the thoracic outlet compression syndrome. *British Journal of Surgery,* **78**, 1193–1195

Galea, M. H., Berridge, D. C., Gregson, R. H. S., Hopkinson, B. R. and Makin, G. S. (1990) Axillary/subclavian vein thrombosis: a clinical and radiological evaluation of conservative management. *Phlebology,* **5**, 193–199

Gutman, H., Peri, M., Zelikovski, A. *et al.* (1985) Deep venous thrombosis of the upper limbs. *Phlebology,* **39**, 63–68

Hirai, M. and Shionoya, S. (1979) Arterial obstruction of the upper limb in Buerger's disease: its incidence and primary lesion. *British Journal of Surgery,* **66**, 124–128

Hughes, D. G., Dixon, P. M. and Fletcher, E. W. L. (1987) Augmentation of upper limb venography with digital subtraction. *Phlebology,* **2**, 125–127

Jayson, M. T. V. (1983) Systemic sclerosis – a microvascular disorder? *Journal of the Royal Society of Medicine,* **76**, 635–641

Jayson, M. T. V. (1984) Systemic sclerosis: a collagen or micro vascular disease? *British Medical Journal,* **288**, 1855–1856

Kahn, D., Pontin, A. R., Jacobson, J. E., Matley, P., Beningfield, S. and van Zyl-Smit, R. (1990) Arteriovenous fistula in the presence of subclavian vein thrombosis: a serious complication. *British Journal of Surgery,* **77**, 682

Marcus, R. T., Pawade, J. and Vella, E. J. (1990) Painful lymphatic occlusion following axillary lymph node surgery. *British Journal of Surgery,* **77**, 683

Olsen, N., Petring, O. U. and Rossing, N. (1987) Exaggerated postural vasoconstriction reflex in Raynaud's phenomenon. *British Medical Journal,* **294**, 1186–1188

Thompson, N. (1969) The surgical treatment of advanced postmastectomy lymphoedema of the upper limb. *Scandinavian Journal of Plastic and Reconstructive Surgery,* **3**, 54–60

# 16

# Acute and subacute deep vein thrombosis in the lower limb

It is not within the scope of this book to consider acute deep vein thrombosis of the lower limb in great detail because this has become a separate study in its own right. However a surgeon working in venous disorders must know how to minimize this feared complication in his own patients and how to recognize it either as a subacute phenomenon to be distinguished from a chronic venous disorder, or as an acute state, perhaps complicating surgery. Acute venous thrombosis is an all-pervading and dangerous illness appearing unexpectedly in various guises so that no surgeon can escape meeting it sooner or later. Its prompt recognition and treatment can spare the patient progressive and permanent damage to the veins of the lower limb and an increasing danger of pulmonary embolism. The incidence of venous thrombosis and relationship to subsequent post-thrombotic syndrome are discussed in Chapters 8 and 9. A summary of present-day understanding and management of this important condition follows.

## Causation and occurrence of acute venous thrombosis

A wide range of conditions are associated with venous thrombosis and appear to be causative in some way, but it must be said at once that an appreciable number of cases do arise without any other recognizable abnormality and in this respect appear to be spontaneous. The circumstances that may precipitate its onset are summarized below:

1. Surgery or any major illness.
2. Malignancy.
3. During and immediately after pregnancy.
4. Injury to the limb or the body generally. This particularly includes fractures of the lower limbs and the treatment that follows.
5. With any disturbance to the major veins whether from surgery, neighbouring disease or compression from nearby structures.

6. Prolonged immobility, especially accompanied by dependency of the lower limbs.
7. In a wide range of metabolic, hormonal and other disturbances of physiology, such as dehydration, hyperlipidaemia or cardiac failure.
8. Blood dyscrasias and abnormalities of blood coagulation.
9. In hereditary states of enhanced tendency to venous thrombosis (e.g. deficiency of antithrombin III) where any of the circumstances given above may trigger thrombosis with unusual ease.

A most important finding of recent years has been made through the use of the $^{125}$I-fibrinogen test. The reliability of this test in detecting recent thrombus in thigh and leg veins has been confirmed many times by phlebography. A number of independent studies have shown that in about 30% of patients an appreciable amount of clot appears in the veins of the lower limbs within a few days of major surgical operation and has formed either during or soon after surgery. In most cases it resolves harmlessly but in a highly important minority permanent damage to valves or the vein lumen may be caused, or worse, the process may extend to give active deep vein thrombosis with its attendant danger of pulmonary embolism and eventual post-thrombotic syndrome in the limb. Furthermore it has been shown that quite extensive clot may be present with little or no clinical evidence and this implies that a potentially dangerous state is well advanced before it declares itself clinically. The evidence points clearly to the process being initiated either during surgery or soon afterwards so that careful attention has to be given to this danger period.

Virchow, over a century ago, summed up the conditions leading to deep vein thrombosis as increased coagulability, damage to the vein wall and slowing of the venous blood flow. These principles are still accepted but in the interval, extensive research has revealed the complex system of factors that govern or inhibit clotting processes (Figure 16.1) and the key role played by the

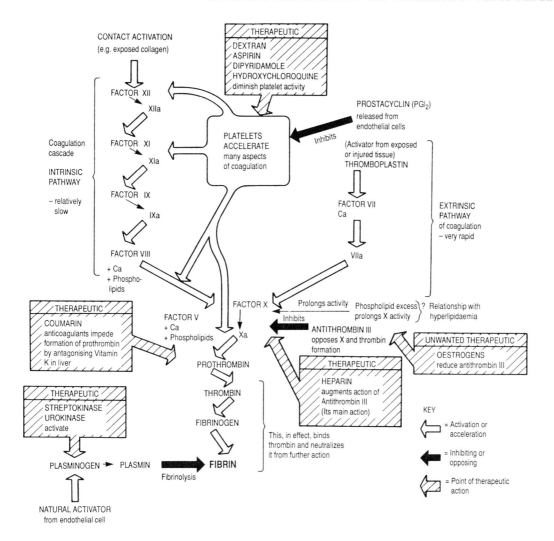

**Figure 16.1** *Diagram of the coagulation cascade. (Adapted from information in Weatherall et al., 1987)*

platelets in initiating thrombosis; lipids or hormonal changes, such as those induced by the contraceptive pill, or bacterial endotoxins can all influence and enhance the tendency for blood to clot. Moreover there is a small group of patients with an hereditary tendency to venous thrombosis who have an identifiable deficiency of such coagulation factors as antithrombin III, proteins C and S, heparin cofactor II, fibrinogen and plasminogen. The balance between fluidity and coagulation of blood is delicate and complex and may be upset by a variety of changes affecting the body generally or locally. Some of the more important aspects of blood coagulation and circumstances leading to an increase in coagulability and a tendency to thrombosis are summarized in Figure 16.1.

## Examples of hypercoaguable states

1. Inherited antithrombin III (heparin cofactor) deficiency, plasminogen deficiency and abnormal fibrinogen. Recurrent and fatal venous thrombosis arises in these states. Heparin is not effective in antithrombin deficiency but oral anticoagulants are.

2. Oestrogens (as in the contraceptive pill) reduce antithrombin III and enhance likelihood of venous thrombosis. Anaesthesia can have a similar effect.

3. Inflammatory states, malignant conditions and trauma, including surgery, may release thromboplastin into the bloodstream.

4. Certain bacterial endotoxins can trigger the coagulation cascade.

5. Thrombocytosis is a well-recognized cause for venous thrombosis, e.g. postsplenectomy and in polycythaemia vera where an additional factor is the increased viscosity of the blood.

**TABLE 16.1** Some basic mechanisms in blood coagulation

| Features preserving normal fluidity | Features promoting coagulation | Features preserving normal fluidity | Features promoting coagulation |
|---|---|---|---|
| Well-maintained flow | Stasis allows build up of clotting factors | Widespread clot may form without a haemostatic plug or incorporation of platelets and without any obvious endothelial damage. Such hypercoaguable states occur in:<br>● congenital antithrombin III deficiency<br>● disseminated intravascular coagulation<br>● experimentally, by infusion of thromboplastins, tryptin, fatty acids and other materials | Interaction of factor X with platelet surface greatly speeds up thrombin formation. Retraction of fibrin strands strengthens thrombus. Platelet membrane accentuates contact activation of coagulation cascade and greatly accelerates formation of thrombin by factor X. Release of antiheparin activity that protects coagulation from inhibitors.<br>Serotonin and other powerful vasoconstrictors are released from platelets and further aggregation potentiated |
| Coagulation mechanism is stable until triggered. Blood in a vein does not coagulate for many hours when trapped between two ligatures | Contact with foreign surface activates coagulation sequence but much quicker response is started by tissue injury factor (thromboplastin); malignant tissue may release this and some bacterial endotoxins have similar action | | |
| Normal endothelium is completely acceptable to blood and works actively to prevent coagulation:<br>● coated with heparin-like substances<br>● synthesizes activators of fibrinolysis<br>● forms enzymes stopping platelet activity<br>● synthesizes prostacyclin (PGI$_2$) which inhibits platelet adhesion and interaction<br>● PGI$_2$ release is increased with thrombin formation thus localizing its effect | Any damage to endothelial cell reduces or destroys its protective role so allowing platelet adhesion and thrombus formation | Inhibitors of coagulation:<br>Antithrombin III (heparin cofactor) is by far the most important (but at least three others including $\alpha_2$-macroglobulin). This inhibits factors XII, XI, IX and X (the most important) and inactivates thrombin. (*Heparin augments antithrombin III*) | |
| Platelets are essential for haemostasis but circulate harmlessly until activated. Their role is the formation of a haemostatic plug to close any breach in the blood vessel and their action is usually localized to vicinity of intimal damage | Any damage to endothelium, especially exposure of collagen, causes rapid adhesion of platelets to that area and to each other; thrombin is concurrently being formed. Granular bodies release adenosine diphosphate (ADP) and thromboxane A$_2$:<br>● this causes aggregation of platelets<br>● increasing mass of platelets stick together to form a haemostatic plug bonded with fibrin; this is reversible by lysis | Fibrinolysis:<br>Plasmin is a potent proteolytic agent derived from circulating plasminogen incorporated in thrombus and is activated by endothelium. Plasmin does not circulate (it would soon destroy all fibrinogen, prothrombin and various coagulation factors) and is instantly deactivated by circulating antiplasmin. Plasmin is only activated in thrombus in close proximity to vein wall where antiplasmin cannot oppose it | |

## Examples of stasis possibly being a factor in venous thrombosis

Shock, congestive heart failure, any state of increased blood viscosity, such as polycythaemia or haemoconcentration, and prolonged immobility. However, immobility on its own is insufficient to cause thrombosis in the presence of a normal intima; some other factor is likely to be present. Prolonged immobility in a sitting position, such as in air flights or sleeping in deck chairs in wartime air raid shelters, may cause deep vein thrombosis in the lower limbs of apparently healthy people. Stasis allows an easy build up of the elements in fibrin formation. Fibrinogen is bound to the surface of red cells which delays its being washed away and also strengthens bonding of thrombus. Stasis probably facilitates, but does not initiate, deep vein thrombosis.

## Risk factors in venous thrombosis

Age, immobilization, bed rest, prior venous thrombosis, congestive heart failure, shock, oestrogens, Gram-negative sepsis, trauma such as injury, surgery and child-birth, malignancy and certain blood groups appear to be susceptible.

## Pharmacological actions in the therapy of venous thrombosis

1. The oral anticoagulants of the coumarin group, such as warfarin, act by antagonizing vitamin K so that the production of prothrombin in the liver is progressively reduced according to dosage. Its effect, and recovery from it, is slow; phytomenadione speeds up regeneration of prothrombin once the drug has been withdrawn.
2. Heparin given intravenously has immediate action and is used to give prompt anticoagulant effect. Its action is to augment the action of the naturally occurring antithrombin III so that formation of thrombin is impeded progressively according to dose. It is also used by subcutaneous injection (or some products orally) in prophylaxis of deep vein thrombosis in doses too low to cause a haemorrhagic state but sufficient to delay thrombin being formed. Protamine sulphate rapidly reverses its action.
3. Dipyridamole amd aspirin inhibit the induction of platelet aggregation; clinical experience has not shown them to be effective in preventing deep vein thrombosis. Some success has been reported with hydroxychloroquine which has a similar effect.
4. Dextran by intravenous infusion is a plasma expander causing haemodilution with lowering of blood viscosity, coating protectively the endothelium and also reducing platelet adhesion and aggregation. It is acknowledged to have a beneficial effect prophylactically.
5. Streptokinase is a bacterial exotoxin and urokinase is extracted from urine. Both are specific activators of plasminogen to form plasmin, a powerful fibrinolytic agent. This can be a valuable, and at times life-saving therapy, but its clinical effect, especially in clot many days old, is unpredictable. It will wreck normal haemostasis for some hours and in no circumstances should it be used if vascular surgery is contemplated because there is no easy way to reverse its action.
6. Ancrod, derived from snake venom, interferes with the conversion of fibrinogen into fibrin so that the end product is structurally different and more susceptible to lysis by plasmin. It does, in effect, bring about a degree of defibrination but with little effect on the overall clotting sequence; nevertheless it is hazardous to use within 48 hours of surgery. Excessively rapid infusion can cause such rapid formation of fibrin, before its lysis, that widespread intravascular clotting may occur. It is as effective as heparin in the treatment of deep vein thrombosis but the greater technical supervision it requires, and the not infrequent reactions to it, outweigh its advantages so that it has not been widely accepted. It remains an intriguing possibility but with little real application in venous surgery.

*Note.* Oestrogen is an agent which is known to enhance any tendency to thrombosis so that its use should be avoided in any patient coming to surgery, especially if there is a history of previous thrombosis. This has particular relevance if oral contraceptives are being used.

## Immediate and long-term consequences of venous thrombosis

### General considerations

Many minor episodes of thrombosis pass unnoticed and resolve spontaneously but others prove progressive. The severity of the condition depends upon its positioning and extent.

1. Localized to calf veins it may give rise to pain on movement and some swelling but, although potentially dangerous, can resolve harmlessly.
2. Positioned in the femoropopliteal portion of deep vein can cause considerable pain and swelling of foot and leg because a major pathway of venous return is obstructed.
3. Thrombosis confined to a common iliac vein may give rise to moderate discomfort and swelling of the limb but if it extends to become iliofemoral its effect will be made much more severe by the increased obstruction to the main venous outlet of the limb.
4. A combination of these will greatly increase the severity and potential for long-term damage. The state may be reached where the limb is entirely dependent upon the superficial veins for its venous return and if the thrombosis spreads to them, as it may, then venous gangrene may develop.

The severe forms give rise to swelling, cyanosis and pain, summed up by the term 'phlegmasia cerulea dolens' (meaning an inflammation – warm and swollen – which is blue and painful) or, if oedema renders the skin colourless, 'phlegmasia alba dolens' (as in white leg of pregnancy). This may occasionally progress on to venous gangrene, varying from small to extensive areas of slate-coloured dead skin in an oedematous limb. In these circumstances the deeper tissues usually survive and the arteries will be shown to be patent on arteriogram or subsequent dissection after amputation or death. Confusion in diagnosis may easily arise, however, because venous thrombosis may develop as a secondary complication to arterial occlusion and is quite commonly found at amputation for ischaemia. It may be difficult to decide which pathology has caused gangrene but it should be remembered that a purely venous gangrene is comparatively rare. In these most severe forms of venous gangrene there is a high mortality rate approaching 50%, probably reflecting the gravity of the causative background state rather than the limb changes. Indeed it is important to realize that the condition is to a large extent reversible until tissue death actually occurs but even here, if the area of skin death is not too large, survival and recovery of a useful limb may still be possible. Amputation should not be resorted to too easily and the highest mortality rate is amongst those coming to amputation; if the arterial supply is thought to be adequate, and not causative, persevering with medical treatment and eventual skin grafting may yield a better outcome.

The rapid accumulation of several litres of oedema fluid in the limb may cause quite marked hypovolaemic shock which can only increase the dangers to life and limb. This must be countered by limb elevation (but only if a good arterial supply has been demonstrated by Doppler flowmeter or by arteriography) to reduce oedema by improved venous return, and when necessary the restoration of blood volume by plasma or dextran (there are additional advantages with the latter by its inhibiting effect on platelet activity).

## Pulmonary embolism

Thromboembolism is, of course, the most common and dangerous complication. This, and the grave illness, such as advanced malignancy, cardiac or pulmonary disease, which may lie behind the original thrombosis account for a high proportion of deaths. In this respect the thrombosis may well be a terminal secondary event rather than the primary illness. Pulmonary embolism, although of paramount importance, will not be discussed further here.

## Long-term effects

Thrombus within a vein in its least damaging form may undergo complete fibrinolysis, but all too often it organizes to leave deformity (Figure 16.2) or lasting fibrotic occlusion of the vein (Scott, 1970) and the valves implicated in this process are irreparably damaged. In this way the essential functions of the deep vein are impaired, often severely, so that the ability for upward pumping against gravity is reduced and widespread incompetence of valves in the deep veins, or in collaterals substituting for occluded deep veins, cause a state of venous hypertension. The clinical manifestations of this late consequence of deep vein thrombosis, the post-thrombotic syndrome, are discussed in detail in Chapters 8 and 9. It is a most important cause for disabling venotensive changes (see Chapter 6 for other causes).

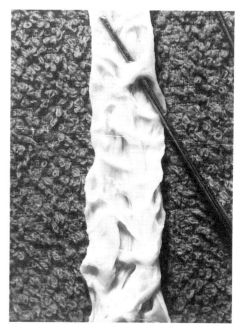

**Figure 16.2** *The interior of a vein which has recanalized following thrombosis. It can be seen that there is irregular fibrous intimal thickening and in two places intimal fibrous septa cross the lumen. This sort of deformity, in varying degree, is the result of organization and recanalization of thrombus within a vein. The delicate valve cusps are buried in the thickened tissue or are severely damaged so that the vein loses the essential attribute of flow permitted in one direction only. Organization of venous thrombus may not succeed in restoring any useful lumen so that in effect the vein remains permanently occluded*

## Clinical aspects of acute deep vein thrombosis

Deep vein thrombosis shows great variation in speed of development, extent and degree of change it may cause in the limb. A fulminating thrombosis may develop apparently within a few hours or the process may build up over some days. The overt clinical manifestations will always have been preceded by quite extensive thrombosis in the deep veins for at least some hours or days but often this silent stage does not prove progressive so that its occurrence may pass unnoticed, overshadowed by other aspects of the patient's illness. Attention may be drawn to the probability of an unnoticed deep vein thrombosis only when a pulmonary embolus occurs; this may vary from a small but painful episode, to a massive and dangerous one, causing breathlessness and cyanosis without pain.

The variability of the condition makes detailed description difficult and here only important generalities will be considered. In a rapidly progressive deep vein thrombosis the main presenting features are discomfort or pain, with prominence of the superficial veins and swelling of the limb (Figure 16.3). The onset of this is typically some 8 days after an operation or commencement of an illness confining the patient to bed (other circumstances are

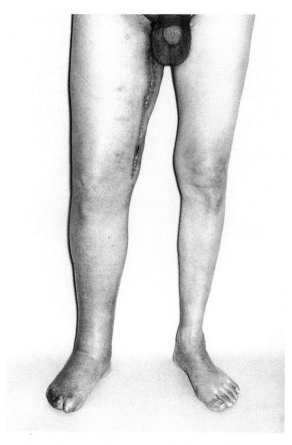

**Figure 16.3** *Gross swelling in lower limb caused by acute deep vein thrombosis following otherwise successful femoropopliteal arterial bypass using reversed saphenous vein. The swelling remained troublesome for about 6 months but suddenly subsided and it was found that the arterial reconstruction had occluded. The limb survived but with severe claudication.*

*In this case a factor in occurrence of deep vein thrombosis was disturbance in the vicinity of the deep veins (see Chapter 17) but, in minor or major form, it is a common complication in many states where there has been no direct interference with the vein (see text)*

given earlier in this chapter). Calf pain often denotes a deep vein thrombosis but not always so, and similarly Homan's sign of pain on stretching of the calf muscles

by dorsiflexion of the foot does not invariably indicate thrombosis in the calf deep veins; nor does absence of these signs exclude an extensive thrombosis especially, for example, if this is in the superficial femoral vein. However, a painful, tender-to-touch set of calf muscles, heavy with oedema and with a positive Homan's sign, in the absence of any other likely cause, such as injury, almost certainly denotes a deep vein thrombosis. It is likely to be accompanied by at least some pyrexia and, if it is extensive, a raised white blood cell count. Venous congestion, that is, distended superficial veins and a cyanotic tinge, is a valuable sign but it may be masked if substantial oedema has accumulated. Even so a Doppler flowmeter may be able to detect strong upward collateral flow in the superficial veins (Figure 16.4). Likewise the Doppler flowmeter may give strongly supportive evidence of obstructive changes in the femoral veins. Clinical and Doppler evidence is not, however, sufficient on its own and should always be backed by phlebography or positive identification by one of the means described below at an early stage if there is any reasonable suspicion that thrombosis has occurred.

## Other specialized diagnostic measures

### Phlebography

The range of techniques, both invasive and non-invasive, capable of diagnosing deep vein thrombosis in the lower limbs has increased steadily. This has been to some extent stimulated by a wish to avoid the invasive technique of phlebography but the introduction of low-osmolar contrast media has improved the safety and comfort of this so much, that there should not be undue hestitation in using it now. Phlebography remains the most accurate diagnostic measure (Figure 16.5) and it is likely that development of computerized digital subtraction techniques will bring considerable further improvement. However, there is an undeniable advantage in having alternative techniques that either give a reliable screening test or allow treatment to proceed without phlebography.

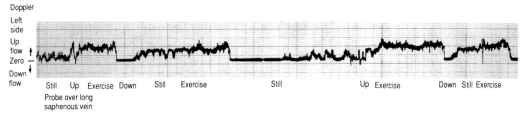

**Figure 16.4** *A Doppler flowmeter tracing in a female patient aged 48 years, with femoropopliteal deep vein thrombosis, 10 days after onset. The left leg and thigh showed about 2 cm of swelling, with shiny and bluish skin. The superficial veins were prominent but without tortuosity. The tracing is from the long saphenous vein in the lower thigh. With the patient standing still there is continuous upflow which is accentuated by exercise and followed by a compensatory pause; flow soon builds up and is again increased by a single movement. This flow pattern indicates that deep vein obstruction (by recent thrombus) is causing the superficial veins to act as collaterals and gives strong circumstantial evidence of the diagnosis*

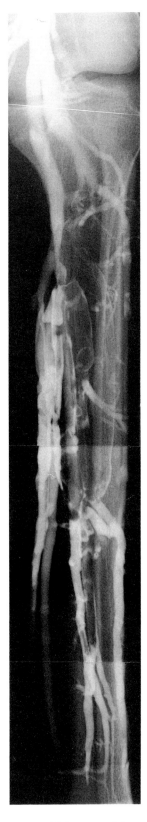

**Figure 16.5** *Composite phlebogram of deep vein thrombosis in the leg. The tibial and peroneal veins in mid-leg show sizeable filling defects, with opacified blood tracking round them to give the characteristic tramline appearance of venous thrombosis. This was accompanied by iliofemoral thrombosis; for further details and the changes evident 3 years later see Figure 8.8(a)*

Some of these techniques are outlined below (and see detailed description in Chapter 23).

### Ultrasound

Use of the continuous wave directional Doppler flowmeter to observe changes in the flow characteristics have already been referred to but real-time B-mode ultrasound is capable of giving good images of deep veins and their valves. Thrombus can be clearly demonstrated by lack of movement of the vein walls and this method is already used in some centres in the assessment of deep vein thrombosis (see Figure 2.12 and the section on ultrasound in Chapter 23). Colour flow imaging is particularly effective in this respect.

### Thermography

A heat camera or, more economically and conveniently, liquid crystal contact thermography can detect the local rise in temperature caused by the collateral flow in superficial veins that accompanies deep vein thrombosis. Most cases can be indentified at an early stage, even before clinical manifestations, by this means and there is little doubt about its potential value as a screening test for thrombosis.

### $^{125}I$-fibrinogen scanning

Although reliable in detecting recent clot and observing progressive extension, this is not a test for everyday use. It has proved a most valuable research technique but it has the disadvantages of a minimal delay of 24 hours before diagnosis, unsuitability in pregnancy or in the young, the possibility of transmission of virus disease by the fibrinogen, and its invalidation if the limb under examination has had any recent injury, operation or inflammatory process.

### Imaging by radioactive isotopes

The gamma camera used after injection of $^{99}Tc^m$ into the veins can give an effective venogram but it is doubtful if this has any advantage over X-ray phlebography using low-osmolar contrast medium which is capable of giving much better definition.

### Scanning by computer-assisted radiography and magnetic nuclear resonance

Computed tomography requires enhancement by contrast medium in order to visualize thrombus and has only limited application. Magnetic resonance imaging identifies flowing blood and this allows good demonstration of thrombus, especially when enhanced by suitable media. It is, however, costly and time consuming and, at present, only used in special circumstances (see Chapter 23).

## Distinguishing acute deep vein thrombosis from acute ischaemia

The severe case with rapid onset will cause considerable pain in the limb accompanied by swelling of the dorsum of the foot, in the ankle region and often upwards to the groin. This makes the arterial ankle pulses difficult to feel and the rapid waterlogging of the tissues with stretching of the skin may cause pallor and conceal the signs of venous congestion. Moreover, vasoconstrictor substances (serotonin) released from the thrombus will shut down the arteries so that the condition is often mistaken for acute arterial ischaemia when first seen. The diagnosis can usually be clarified by giving prolonged firm pressure over the pulses at the ankle in order to squeeze away the overlying oedema fluid and, after a short pause to let the examining fingers recover, to feel again for the pulses. A Doppler flowmeter should be able to resolve all doubts about the vigour of the pulses but even here oedema may make the arteries difficult to locate so that failure to obtain a signal is not sufficient evidence upon which to diagnose ischaemia. Another aid to diagnosis is a photoelectric capillary pulse detector provided by the photoplethysmograph in arterial mode.

Oedema, in itself, is not an early manifestation of acute ischaemia although it may be present incidentally if there is pre-existing cardiac oedema when arterial embolism occurs, or the patient has been sleeping with his leg hanging out of bed in order to relieve ischaemic rest pain. The presence of oedema should always give cause for extra thought before diagnosing acute ischaemia, particularly if the foot has some warmth to it, as it usually will in venous states.

Loss of cutaneous sensation is one of the most important signs of acute ischaemia and good sensation preserved in the toes and foot almost certainly rules out ischaemia of any severity. In deep vein thrombosis appreciation of touch may be blunted by general discomfort and swelling in the limb but the stocking or glove anaesthesia typical of a severe ischaemia soon after onset will not be convincingly present.

It is to be hoped that by these means a correct decision can be made whether to proceed to phlebogram or arteriogram, but in some circumstances both investigations may be needed to ensure that treatment is based upon a complete diagnosis. A limb should never be elevated above the horizontal until the adequacy of arterial supply has been verified. Prolonged elevation of an acutely ischaemic limb is a cardinal error and if there are any doubts the limb must be kept horizontal.

## Other conditions to be distinguished

There are several other conditions which may be mistaken on clinical grounds for deep vein thrombosis (and see Figure 6.13):

1. An actively invading infection, particularly by streptococcus, causing a widespread cellulitis with lymphangitis can have many similarities. Here, the patient will have a raised temperature and a hot, reddened extremity, often with a skin lesion denoting the portal of entry for the infection; this together with tenderness and redness spreading up to enlarged lymph nodes in the groin gives a typical picture. This state may arise in the presence of venous eczema or ulceration, thus enhancing confusion over diagnosis. It may also occur in conjunction with superficial thrombophlebitis to compound diagnostic difficulties further.

2. An extensive superficial thrombophlebitis in widespread varicose veins can give a painful, tensely swollen limb with obvious venous manifestations so that it is erroneously labelled as a deep vein thrombosis. The cords of hard thrombosed veins clarify the diagnosis but these may be concealed in longstanding induration and oedema so that they are not easy to distinguish. It is important to realize, however, that superficial phlebitis is not always localized to one area, perhaps a few inches across, but may involve the entire circumference from foot to knee if this is the underlying pattern of varicose veins. This can be particularly difficult to recognize in the obese patient. Although a deep vein thrombosis may be present simultaneously this seldom arises, but as usual if there is any doubt a phlebogram should be carried out.

3. Rupture of calf muscles or of a synovial cyst in the popliteal fossa (Figure 16.6(a)) will give considerable pain and tenderness in the calf with swelling at the ankle, and on clinical grounds alone may not be easily distinguished from thrombosis. The main clue will be by the abruptness of onset but phlebography may be needed to avoid unnecessary anticoagulation of the patient. Although deep vein thrombosis is the commonest cause for a painful enlarged calf, it must be remembered that other conditions, such as a rapidly growing sarcoma or haemorrhage, do occur (Figure 16.6(b), (c)).

## Establishing the cause of acute deep vein thrombosis

An attempt should always be made to understand why a deep vein thrombosis has occurred. The main triggering events have already been given but if it is apparently spontaneous, and especially in the younger patient, careful thought must be given to any possible background state, either local or general, that may have enhanced coagulation; a full haematological screen should be arranged before any anticoagulant treatment is started.

## Long-term consequences

The limb that 'recovers' will remain swollen and uncomfortable for many months with slow improvement

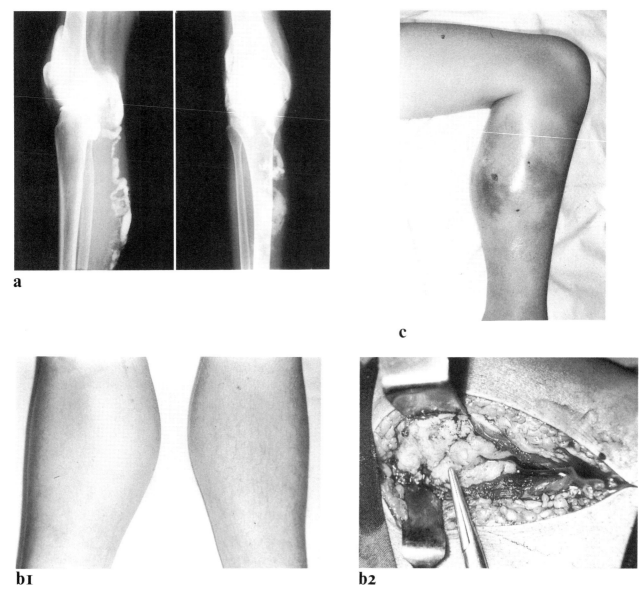

**Figure 16.6**  *Examples of diagnostic pitfalls in patients with a swollen, painful calf.*

*(a)  This patient could easily have been mistaken for a deep vein thrombosis but the abrupt onset and the presence of a large effusion into the knee joint lead to an arthrogram which is illustrated in lateral and anteroposterior views. The knee joint communicates with a popliteal synovial cyst (Morrant–Baker) which has ruptured and its contents are tracking down the calf muscles.*

*(b)  1. Clinical photograph of a women of 32 years who presented with discomfort and firm swelling in the right calf.*
*       2. Exploratory operation revealed a mass of pale, friable tissue deeply placed amongst the calf muscles. Histology confirmed that it was a rhabdomyosarcoma.*

*(c)  Photograph of the calf of a youth with sudden onset of severe pain and swelling in the left calf. Extensive discolouration, shown in the photograph, made it clear that haemorrhage was the cause. There was a family history of haemophilia and this proved to be the diagnosis here*

as the occluded veins are recanalized and collateral vessels enlarge. With many patients there will not be a complete return to normality because the deep veins remain occluded, or are severely deformed with the valves wrecked. These changes are the basis of the post-thrombotic syndrome (see Chapter 8) which may not develop fully, with induration, pigmentation and ulceration, for some years. Even a relatively silent thrombosis which passed almost unnoticed, perhaps following childbirth,

may damage the deep veins sufficiently to lead to this years later. Presumably this is determined by the positioning and extent of the damage. For example, thrombus confined to the common iliac vein may cause mild swelling which may resolve and not cause later problems but a femoropopliteal thrombosis is very likely to cause prolonged disability progressing within 2 or 3 years to a fully developed post-thrombotic syndrome.

# Prevention of deep vein thrombosis in surgical patients

Because deep vein thrombosis has such formidable short- and long-term consequences, a range of methods, based on many years of international research, has been suggested in an effort to use our theoretical knowledge to the advantage of the patient. In this chapter, no more than a review of the more important can be given, but whatever method is favoured it is essential for a surgeon to have a clear policy designed to minimize venous thrombosis amongst his patients. The relative values of the various methods may be debated but the unforgivable sin is to do nothing about the problem and such an attitude amounts to neglect of the patient. The evidence is strong that much can be done to protect the patient but no single method is universally accepted and some of the most effective have decided drawbacks or even dangers. The methods currently used are summarized below.

## Precautions against postoperative deep vein thrombosis

A history of previous deep vein thrombosis below the age of 40 years, or of a family history of such episodes, must give rise to suspicion of an inherited defect in the coagulation inhibitors causing the patient to be especially vulnerable to thrombosis. This may be identified by an expert haematologist who can also advise upon the best way to counteract any such deficiency before surgery is carried out.

## Measures during surgical operation.

The probable ill effects of prolonged immobilization and pressure upon the veins as the patient lies on the operating table are well recognized, and many methods have been suggested to overcome this. Careful positioning upon an even, cushioned surface seems wise but elevation of the heels so that weight is taken off the vulnerable calf muscles is perhaps more debatable. This position will cause the calf muscles to hang with the soleal sinuses gaping and stagnant. Some form of movement to the venous blood would seem a better principle and various systems have been devised to work the musculovenous pump of the calf intermittently by mechanical foot movement, pneumatic compression, or electrical stimulation to the muscles. Certainly an encouraging drop in the incidence of postoperative deep vein thrombosis has been reported in a number of trials.

Employment of such devices will not appeal to all surgeons but it would seem unwise to ignore completely care of the limb veins during an operation. A reasonable policy is one of avoiding stagnation of venous blood in the limb by giving the feet a short series of upward movements at regular intervals, perhaps every half-hour, and at the end of the operation to give brief high elevation to the limbs together with further foot movements and gentle knee bending to ensure a complete change of venous blood.

Needless to say the limbs must be protected from all forms of unnecessary damage. Use of the old type of diathermy pad bandaged to the thigh must certainly be avoided. The use of a tourniquet must be open to strong suspicion and, surprisingly, few studies upon the relationship of tourniquet to deep vein thrombosis have appeared. Certainly the use of a tourniquet for varicose vein surgery cannot be justified when the advantages are so small in comparison to the inherent risks, including deep vein thrombosis.

## Postoperative measures

*Physical means intended to avoid sluggish flow in overdistended veins*
### Active movement and early mobilization of the patient
This is the simplest and most basic requirement, with the intention of preventing stagnant columns of venous blood in lower limbs and pelvis, and also to promote natural fibrinolysins by muscular activity. Whilst in bed, frequent and repeated active movement of the limbs (e.g. foot movements every 5 minutes), accompanied by several deep breaths to move the venous blood centrally, are urged upon the patient. At an early stage the patient is asked to get up and walk about actively (perhaps a minimum of 5 minutes every hour) and in most surgical operations this should be possible the day following operation. Indeed, an operation should be designed to allow this and, for instance, the type of incision and suture material used for an abdominal operation should permit it without any appreciable risk of wound disruption; to immobilize a patient in bed for fear of wound dehiscence is no longer permissible. A distinction must be made between early ambulation and early sitting out of bed. Ambulation will achieve the movement of venous blood and fibrinolysis that is hoped for but a patient sitting upright, perhaps immobile and in discomfort, brings little advantage and possible dangers from overdistended and stagnant veins in the dependent lower limbs. Good flow and avoidance of overdistension in the veins is easier to achieve by active movement on the bed than by sitting in a chair. The term 'bed rest' is one that should be avoided, certainly in surgical patients, because it encourages a state of dangerous inactivity at the very time the effects of illness, injury or surgery are most likely to produce venous thrombosis; 'bed activity' is a much better description if for some reason the patient has to be confined to bed and immediately conveys, perhaps humorously, the attitude that is required.

The specific requirements for venous surgery are given later in this section but there is seldom any reason why the varicose vein patient should not commence hourly walks as soon as he has recovered from anaesthetic and certainly the next day. The patient should be instructed before operation in a system of foot movements every 5 minutes accompanied by several deep breaths and, on the hour, to get up and walk steadily for at least 5 minutes. Fifty-five minutes should be spent on the bed, with foot movements, etc. alternating with 5 minutes' walking; if the walking is interrupted the patient should not stand still but should mark time or 'bob' up and down on the toes. No doubt every surgeon will have his own favourite system along similar lines but failure for the patient to be instructed, and the nurses to understand these requirements, is an error.

**Elevation of the limbs** High elevation of the lower limbs to narrow the veins and speed up the rate of blood flow through them is favoured by many surgeons as a simple protective measure. However, if carried to extreme, it may immobilize the patient and a position of moderate elevation, together with insistence upon frequent movements, would seem a reasonable compromise suitable for venous patients. This will allow the patient to get out of bed easily for hourly walks.

**Elastic support** Thigh-length elastic stockings are often employed as the main protective measure and these are intended to speed flow by reducing the lumen of the veins. The danger is that they may be used to the exclusion of active exercises and if the stockings are less than an ideal fit they may cause undesirable constriction at knee level. If the patient is to be encouraged to sit out of bed, they may have the advantage of preventing overdistension of the veins and thereby increase the rate of flow, but this effect is insignificant compared with the benefits of muscular activity which should always be insisted upon in addition to the use of stockings.

One form of elastic support that is not permissible in the postoperative management is the use of elastic webbing bandages (red or blue line bandages) because these are capable of inflicting damage to the veins. Unskilled application of this type of bandage, using a forceful stretch with each turn and failure to appreciate that any overlapping turn doubles the compression given by the bandage, can cause excessive pressure, or even constricting bands. It is not always easy in a busy ward to guarantee experienced hands will apply the bandage and excessive zeal will not only cause the patient real pain but greatly enhance the possibility of deep vein thrombosis in the limb. These bandages are unsuitable for protection against deep vein thrombosis and caution is needed in their use for chronic venous disorders where they should only be applied either by the patient, who will know the tension that brings comfort to the limb, or a skilled attendant in a special vein clinic. Most certainly they should not be used following venous surgery to the limbs because here every encouragement must be given for easy venous flow without any hint of congestion at any level.

*Pharmaceutical means of reducing tendency to thrombosis*

Another approach upon which most attention had focused over recent years has been the use of anticoagulants and platelet inhibitors. There is no doubt that the judicious use of a variety of these agents can reduce significantly the incidence of postoperative venous thrombosis but, although the methods and materials used have improved in every way, they still represent an additional complexity and cost in treatment to give protection that will not be required by the majority of patients. Moreover any use of anticoagulants is vulnerable to occasional mishap, difficult to guard against in mass application, and this has to be balanced against the undoubted good that it may achieve. In varicose vein surgery many vein ends are left unsecured, after stripping for example, so that the use of anticoagulants would seem undesirable and, in any case, deep vein thrombosis should be a rarity with proper management. However many surgeons in other fields of surgery are persuaded that their use does bring overall benefit to their patients and will either use them on special indication, such as in malignant disease and in major orthopaedic surgery where early mobilization is not easy, or as a routine in all but minor operations. Before reviewing the anticoagulants commonly used, something must be said upon the reverse aspect, that is to say, the withdrawal of any agent that is known to enhance likelihood of venous thrombosis.

**Withdrawal of the contraceptive pill** This does in fact concern patients coming to venous surgery because they tend to belong to the younger age group likely to be on 'the pill'. The evidence that the oestrogen content of current contraceptive pills enhances the likelihood of thrombosis, by diminishing antithrombin III activity, is strong and any patient coming to surgery, including for varicose veins, should cease taking any oestrogen-containing pill 4 weeks before surgery and employ some other form of contraception (Guillebaud, 1985). Progestogen oral contraception does not appear to have the same danger and its continuation or substitution is permissible; oestrogen contraception should not be restarted sooner than 2 weeks postoperatively. The risk of thrombosis occurring in any individual patient who remains on 'the pill' is not numerically high but can take such a severe form that it must be avoided. Protection of the patient is paramount but an additional thought is the surgeon's medicolegal vulnerability if a damaging thrombosis should occur.

Patients under hormonal treatment for carcinoma of the prostate may similarly have an enhanced tendency for deep vein thrombosis and it may be wise to suspend this treatment if major surgery is required.

**Anticoagulants in prophylaxis of thrombosis**
*Heparin* Low dose subcutaneous heparin is perhaps the most widely used of the anticoagulants in prevention of thrombosis. This form of treatment has evolved over

recent years and a typical regimen used currently is to give 5000 iu twice daily by subcutaneous injection, with the first dose being given preoperatively; this is maintained for several days. An appreciable incidence of haematoma found in the early development of this prophylactic use of heparin has been considerably reduced by using smaller doses, given above; it is not necessary to monitor treatment by laboratory tests. Various forms of heparin have been advocated but there is no universal agreement upon the advantages of, say, calcium over sodium heparin. Recently dihydro-ergotamine has been used to increase the speed of venous flow by its constricting effect on veins and combined with a reduced dose of heparin (heparin-DHE). This is thought to diminish further any tendency for haemorrhage whilst under treatment. However in some circumstances excessive vascular spasm involving the arteries may occur, with a possibility of peripheral gangrene, and the contraindications for this regimen must be clearly understood, for example, in the very ill or the shocked patient.

Heparin is a naturally occurring agent and so has considerable appeal in its use. The effort to find improved ways of using it continues; administration by inhalation is under trial and low molecular weight heparin and synthetic heparinoids are being investigated.

*Oral anticoagulants* There is little doubt that the coumarin (vitamin K antagonist) group of anticoagulants is as effective as heparin in the prevention of thrombosis, and warfarin has had extensive use confirming this. However, it does not give immediate effect and cannot be immediately reversed, and it does require careful laboratory control if haematoma is to be avoided. For these reasons it has lost popularity compared with heparin, but its use is still permissible and it is particularly indicated where there are special indications for long-term protection from thrombosis as with many orthopaedic cases or in the prevention of renewed deep vein thrombosis after this has occurred.

*Ancrod (Arvin)* This agent and similar materials are effective in defibrinating the blood and giving good protection from postoperative thrombosis. Four ampoules are injected subcutaneously immediately after surgery and then 1 ampoule daily for at least 4 days. It is used by some centres in hip replacement but it does require availability of laboratory monitoring and can give rise to haemorrhage. An antedote is available should this occur and human fibrinogen may be given. Again it has little advantage over heparin but may be specially indicated in established thromboembolism and given intravenously in a body weight-determined dosage.

### The platelet inhibitors

*Dextran 70* This material is again effective when infused intravenously during and after surgery. It probably interferes with platelet function to change the texture of any thrombus that is formed so that natural lysis occurs more easily. There is some evidence that it is more effective in reducing the incidence of pulmonary embolism than in preventing deep vein thrombosis. It is usually started with induction of anaesthesia and 500 ml given during the operation; a further 500 ml is given soon afterwards and yet again the next day. It has the virtue of simplicity and does not require laboratory control but it is possible to overload the circulation. If more prolonged protection is required then oral anticoagulation can be substituted on the second day. Anaphylatic reactions are possible, although rare, and suitable precautions and treatment should be available.

*Platelet disaggregators* The drugs which inhibit platelet aggregation, such as aspirin and and dipyridamole (Persantin), are used by some centres but the evidence for effective reduction in the incidence of deep vein thrombosis is not so secure as in the other agents described so far. Their effectiveness in certain arterial conditions does not necessarily apply to veins. Certainly they can induce a haemorrhagic state if the patient is abnormally reponsive and cannot be viewed as entirely harmless. In view of this and the uncertainty over their success in the prevention of venous thrombosis, other agents should be preferred if pharmaceutical methods are to be employed.

## Protection from deep vein thrombosis in venous surgery

The importance of ensuring that any patient with a personal or family history of previous deep vein thrombosis is screened to exclude a congenital defect in the natural coagulation inhibitors has already been referred to and, if identified, expert haematological advice will be needed before any surgery is carried out. Oral contraceptives containing oestrogen should be withdrawn 4 weeks before operation and for 2 weeks afterwards; progestogen, or another form of contraception, should be substituted.

### Varicose vein surgery

All of the pharmaceutical methods of reducing the risk of deep vein thrombosis and thromboembolism introduce a small but distinct hazard of their own and their use must be balanced against the advantages they may bring to any individual patient. In the case of varicose vein surgery the risks of thrombosis are small provided that the surgery is performed without unnecessary trauma, a policy of active exercise to the limbs with early, true ambulation is followed and no more than light elastic support is used. The incidence of thrombosis does not justify the use of any of the pharmaceutical means outlined in the previous section apart from withdrawing oestrogen contraceptives. Experience has shown abundantly that a simple surgical procedure, rapid mobilization and return home within a few days is remarkably trouble free. The authors own preference is to admit the patient no more than 3 hours before the operation so that there is not a long overnight wait and, when the veins are marked out before operation, to give instructions upon exercises and walking postoperatively. In this way the patient realizes that the only interruption in activity is during the operation itself. Even here movement should not cease entirely as the surgeon, or theatre nurses, may give the feet a series of passive movements several times during the operation; at the end each limb is elevated in turn, the knee and hip are gently flexed and further foot movements given so that venous stagnation is minimized. Crepe bandages are evenly applied up to the knee, or just above, without undue tension, and tight or constricting bandages are avoided; nothing more than this is required as this form of bandage will give gentle restraint to prevent overdistension of veins when the patient walks a few hours later. Harsh or tight bandaging is highly undesirable and must be avoided. The patient returns to a bed raised at the foot some 18 inches (45 cm).

### Measures in reconstructive surgery to the deep veins

In the case of surgery involving reconstruction to the veins there may be a special need to protect the reconstruction against thrombosis and the surgeon may decide to use anticoagulants postoperatively, but in this case the possibility of resultant haematoma has to be accepted and the surgeon prepared to evacuate this if need be. A temporary arteriovenous shunt is often placed below a venous reconstruction to give high flow through it as protection from thrombosis. For this purpose, a short graft or a side branch of the vein is used to connect it with the neighbouring main artery. A shunt used in this fashion also gives sustained distension to the reconstruction thus preserving maximal calibre, otherwise threatened by compression from surrounding oedema and fibrosis. The shunt is left in place for some weeks until the healing processes are completed and the likelihood of thrombosis or narrowing of the reconstruction after its removal is minimal. It should be designed in a way to make its eventual closure easy. Anticoagulation by warfarin may be given during this time.

### Treatment of acute deep vein thrombosis

Deep vein thrombosis is a serious condition and its treatment will require the use of anticoagulants, which, once started, will require continuing for some months. This treatment in itself is tedious for the patient and has hazards of its own so that it should not be commenced without reliable proof that thrombosis has indeed occurred. Positive identification should always be obtained by phlebography or one of the other methods described earlier in this chapter and careful thought given

to the cause of thrombosis, particularly, in the exclusion of malignancy.

The treatment of acute deep vein thrombus has three aims: to prevent any further extension of thrombosis; to reduce the risk of pulmonary embolism and to minimize the effect of this should it occur; to encourage early resolution of existing thrombus in the hope of minimizing lasting damage to deep vein lumens and valves. There are three main forms of treatment, detailed below.

### Anticoagulation

Anticoagulation is administered by heparin intravenously, to give immediate effect, and after 5–7 days of this changed to an oral anticoagulant, such as warfarin. This will be effective in limiting further thrombosis but does not have any direct lytic action upon thrombus although it does give the natural fibrinolytic processes an opportunity to work. The short-term outcome may appear reasonably satisfactory but many cases develop a typical post-thrombotic limb over the next year or two, or even some years later, and the results cannot be viewed with complacency. This treatment is the most suitable for thrombosis seen a week or more after onset because at this stage other forms of treatment appear no more effective but are more disturbing for the patient.

*Dosages.* Heparin 5000 units is given intravenously as a loading dose, accompanied by commencement of 40 000 units every 24 hours by continuous infusion or 10 000 units every 6 hours by intravenous injection; laboratory control is important to ensure that an effective dose is being given. Warfarin 10 mg daily is given orally for 3 days and then dosage adjusted according to prothrombin time.

### Fibrinolytic therapy

Fibrinolytic therapy is administered by use of streptokinase or urokinase. This is likely to be most effective with recent non-adherent thrombus and in theory should greatly reduce post-thrombotic sclerotic damage within the deep veins. However, its action is often incomplete (Figure 16.7) and long-term follow-up has shown only marginal reduction in the incidence and severity of post-thrombotic limbs. Drawbacks can be pyrexial reactions and dangerous haemorrhage, which are difficult to control, and it is especially contraindicated by recent surgery, trauma, pregnancy or soon after childbirth. However, it is perhaps the treatment of choice when a maximal effort is to be made to protect a young patient, seen soon after onset, from pulmonary embolus and long-term disability. Thrombolytic therapy in surgical practice is well reviewed by Moran, Jewell and Persson (1989).

*Dosage.* Streptokinase 250 000 units by intravenous infusion over 30 minutes and maintained at 100 000 units per hour for 1 week.

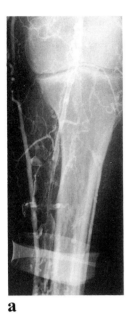 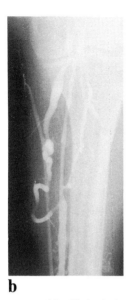

**a**       **b**

**Figure 16.7**  *Deep vein thrombosis treated by fibrinolysis 10 days after onset.*

*(a)  Phlebogram of upper leg before treatment.*

*(b)  Repeat phlebogram after treatment with streptokinase, followed by heparin. The patient's clinical state improved but the phlebogram shows only marginal improvement in the veins, with very little filling of the principal veins. Oral anticoagulant (warfarin) was used for 9 months but moderate disability persisted, with eventual post-thrombotic syndrome. A more complete resolution of the thrombosis might have been achieved if fibrinolytic treatment had been employed at a much earlier stage*

## Surgical thrombectomy and the use of a temporary arteriovenous fistula

Surgical thrombectomy has been given extensive trial over the last few decades (for example, Fogarty *et al.*, 1963; Haller and Abrams, 1963; Mavor and Galloway, 1969; DeWeese, 1978). The procedure removes large quantities of thrombus, particularly from the iliofemoral veins, with immediate relief of venous congestion and oedema in the limb. However, the thrombosis may soon re-establish itself. Nevertheless, the experience at that time showed that it could bring real benefit in terms of preventing pulmonary embolus and possibly reducing the severity of post-thrombotic sequelae, provided it was:

1. Carried out early, before the thrombus had commenced to organize and become adherent to the vein walls; within the first few days it is easily removed and the endothelium has not been sufficiently damaged to cause inevitable, recurrent thrombosis.
2. Directed at the iliofemoral veins which are virtually the sole venous outlet to the limb. The stasis and distension caused by thrombotic occlusion of these veins can only encourage further spread of thrombosis in the veins of the limb below. Freeing venous flow by

opening the iliofemoral veins would seem a fundamental step in combating this.

Undoubtedly, the early exponents showed thrombectomy could be done without undue complications and was capable of giving immediate improvement to the patient. However, on long-term follow-up the incidence of post-thrombotic disability was found to be similar to patients treated by anticoagulation alone. Many surgeons, after giving brief trial to thrombectomy, concluded that the extra effort of this substantial procedure was not worthwhile and swung back to non-surgical treatment with anticoagulation or, more recently, thrombolysis. However, a new factor was introduced in the 1970s with the addition of a temporary arteriovenous fistula to back up venous thrombectomy by giving rapid, sustained flow through the thrombectomized venous outlet until endothelial healing is complete. Evidence has been published that this is a practical procedure, giving good protection from pulmonary embolus, well-maintained patency of iliofemoral veins and a substantial reduction in eventual post-thrombotic syndrome (Zetterquist *et al.*, 1986; Eklof *et al.*, 1987; Gruss, 1988). The same criteria for surgery are required, involvement of the iliofemoral veins and its use only within a few days of onset, before thrombus has become adherent. Preliminary assessment by phlebography to show the extent and state (non-adherent with flow around it or adherent and obstructive) is essential. The procedure is supported by heparin and coumarin anticoagulation which inevitably introduces some hazards but these prove to be within acceptable limits and the complication rate is no greater than with conservative treatment.

Thrombectomy is carried out by opening the common femoral vein and use of balloon thrombectomy catheters; precautions are taken to prevent dislodgement of pulmonary embolus. An arteriovenous fistula is made between the neighbouring saphenous vein, or a major branch of it, and the common femoral artery. It is fashioned in a way to allow easy closure some weeks or months later. This procedure is described in Chapter 21.

At the present time (1992) it does seem that a technique of thrombectomy with temporary arteriovenous fistula has been evolved that gives superior results in a selected, but important, group of patients. The stage has been reached where preliminary assessment of acute deep vein thrombosis by phlebography will allow confirmation of early thrombus suitable for treatment by thrombolysis or by thrombectomy and fistula. Alternatively, a late thrombus is found where the opportunity for thrombectomy has been missed, but it is perhaps still suitable for thrombolysis; failing this, anticoagulation has a most valuable role to play in preventing deterioration and in limiting the damage done. Lesser episodes of thrombosis below the knee should be treated by anticoagulation because at this level the other forms of treatment offer no advantage. The policy of treatment just outlined should give the patient considerable protection from pulmonary embolus and the use of a Greenfield filter device in the infrarenal inferior vena cava is best reserved for pulmonary embolism occurring in spite of such treatment, or when a large floating thrombus in a major vein is recognized and surgery is contraindicated.

Every medical centre should be aware of thrombectomy's new status and decide whether this should be incorporated into their policy of treating acute deep vein thrombosis. This implies diversion of resources and availability of a surgical team skilled in the procedure. The majority of cases will still be best treated by thrombolysis or anticoagulation but those patients likely to benefit by surgical intervention can be rationally selected for this.

## Subacute and recurrent thrombosis of the deep veins

Insidious onset of deep vein thrombosis in an otherwise fit patient does arise from time to time and may catch the physician unawares. It may in fact be the first manifestation of systemic disease or developing hidden malignancy but this is not necessarily so and sometimes a cause may never be identified. However, in every case the possibility of malignancy or other accompanying illness must be given careful thought and any symptoms that might suggest this possibility appropriately investigated; it may be some months before this cause can be eliminated and a policy of vigilance over this time is necessary. Other cases may be provoked by mechanical factors such as prolonged sitting posture, as in air travel, or compression of the vein by anatomical structures, for example, entrapment by gastrocnemius muscle, compression by the left common iliac artery, or, in the upper limb, by costoclavicular compression. When acute or subacute thrombosis arises consideration must always be given to all possible factors, both general or localized to the limb, that may have provoked the attack. In the young patient this should include full haematological screening, with assessment of the coagulation inhibitors, such as antithrombin III. Certainly a phlebogram to the limb is an essential requirement, both to confirm the diagnosis and to look for any abnormality that may have caused it.

Thrombosis may be slowly progressive over some weeks with gradual spread of the thrombus in the vein and a corresponding increase in the patient's discomforts (Figure 16.8). The initial complaint brought to the doctor may be a sense of tightness in the limb which the patient attributes to veins somewhat more distended than the other side and fears he is developing 'varicose veins'. On examination the signs may be minimal, with only a trace of oedema at the ankle and slight tension and tenderness in the calf. The long saphenous vein and its tributaries may be somewhat more prominent than its normal counterpart but, unless previously present, without any true tortuosity of its branches (varicose veins). These signs may be so slight that the doctor is perplexed and may feel it unnecessary to take any immediate action. However examination with a Doppler flowmeter may show undeniable upward flow in superficial veins, accentuated by exercise and indicating a real possibility of blockage in deep veins sufficiently extensive to divert blood up the saphenous system in collateral fashion; similarly liquid crystal contact thermography can detect increased flow in the superficial veins. With such additional evidence, a phlebogram should be obtained and the physician may be chastened by the extent of thrombus revealed in the calf veins or thigh veins. The longer this process is left the more likely it is that permanent damage will be done to the musculovenous pump with eventual emergence of the post-thrombotic syndrome, or that a fulminating deep vein thrombosis will develop with the attendant danger of pulmonary embolism.

Regarding treatment, subacute thrombosis appears to be a process that may simmer on for many weeks unable to resolve itself without the help of anticoagulants. If the condition has been present for some weeks, as is so often the case, then a preliminary course of heparin may be dispensed with and treatment started directly with an oral anticoagulant, such as warfarin. However, there is much to be said in favour of a short spell of hospitalization for heparinization accompanied by elevation and active movement of the limb before long-term oral anticoagulation is started. Use of a fibrinolysin, such as streptokinase, may lead to more complete resolution and minimize the damage to the valves but this has not been proved as yet and may not have any great advantage if much of the thrombus is many weeks old. Oral anticoagulation should be continued for at least 3 months and the patient kept under surveillance for a year or two after this to make sure that there is no recurrence. If caught in time resolution may be virtually complete but often slight calf swelling and mild symptoms on excessive walking may persist. Light to medium weight elastic support up to the knee may be helpful at all stages together with elevation at every opportunity. If phlebography has shown any extrinsic compression to the vein this should be rectified surgically since otherwise the provoking factor will remain and cause recurrent episodes with eventual complete closure of the main vein. This is especially true of the costoclavicular compression syndrome and here warning episodes and positive findings on phlebography indicate thrombectomy with resection of the inner half of the clavicle, or of the first rib. This may prevent permanent occlusion of the subclavian and axillary veins, with the burden of a heavy oedematous limb (see Chapter 15).

**Figure 16.8** *Two examples of subacute deep vein thrombosis presenting as 'varicose veins' in a vein clinic.*

*(a)–(c) A man aged 72 years complaining of 6 week's discomfort, particularly on walking, in the left lower limb. Examination showed moderate swelling in the left calf and lower leg. There was slight prominence of the superficial veins and a Doppler flowmeter detected strong upflow in the long saphenous vein.*

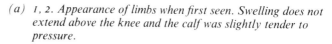

*(a) 1, 2. Appearance of limbs when first seen. Swelling does not extend above the knee and the calf was slightly tender to pressure.*

*(b) Doppler flowmeter tracing showing strong upflow, accentuated by exercise, in the long saphenous vein. Photoplethysmogram showing shallow, but normal, tracing on the right side; on the left side there is little response to exercise, a brief, 6 second recovery period and early appearance of arterial pulsation.*

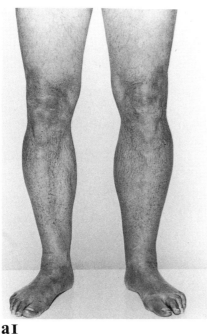

**a1**

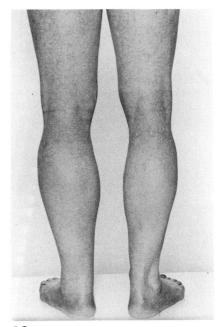

**a2**

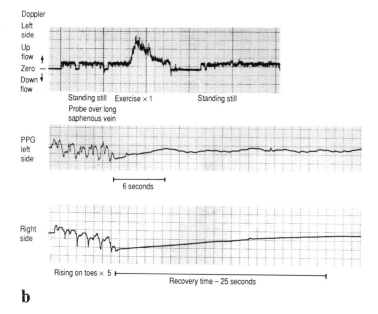

**b**

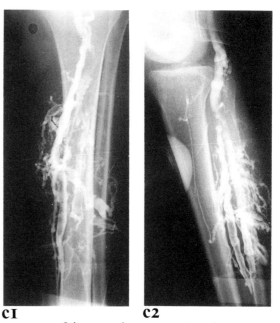

**c1**          **c2**

*(c) 1, 2. Phlebography, with lateral and anteroposterior views of the left leg. The posterior tibial veins and many of the lesser veins, including muscle sinuses, show the 'tramline' sign due to opacified blood flowing thinly around a mass of clot filling the vein. Numerous small vessels are outlined by flow forced into them because there is no other avenue of*

*escape; many of these vessels connect with perforators taking flow to the superficial veins.*

*This patient was treated by intravenous heparin followed by oral warfarin. Symptoms largely disappeared but slight swelling persisted and it is likely that there will always be some deep vein impairment.*

*(d)–(f)  This patient, a business man, aged 51 years, who travelled frequently by air, complained of discomfort in the left leg and increased prominence of the superficial veins. Some varicose veins were present but seemed insufficient to explain his symptoms. Doppler flowmetry to the long saphenous vein showed no more than a minor incompetence. No firm diagnosis was made and the patient returned 1 month later reporting that the discomfort had increased and walking was now difficult. The findings on clinical and Doppler examination were again inconclusive but 4 days later the pain was more severe and swelling had appeared at the ankle. He had also noticed increased prominence in the veins of the foot and lower leg. Measurement showed that there was now 2 cm of swelling not previously present in the calf and Doppler flowmetry to superficial veins now showed continuous upflow accentuated by exercise.*

*(d)  The Doppler flowmeter tracing from the long saphenous vein in the lower thigh with continuous upflow accentuated by exercise. This is characteristic of collateral flow past occluded deep veins and its development coincided with the increased severity of the patient's symptoms and signs.*

*(e)  Phlebogram of the leg at the time of Doppler tracing (d). There is failure of the deep veins to fill, several muscular branches show obvious clot within the veins and many lesser veins are seen taking blood out to the superficial veins. The long saphenous vein in the lower leg, and at higher levels not illustrated here, showed strong upward flow in keeping with a collateral role. The appearances were consistent with extensive thrombotic occlusion of tibial, popliteal and superficial femoral veins.*

*The patient was treated with streptokinase and long-term warfarin. Over the next 2 years the limb improved greatly and the patient became virtually symptom free. Slight calf swelling persisted (1 cm) but the long saphenous vein no longer showed any evidence of collateral function.*

*(f) Doppler tracing 2 years after onset has reverted to a pattern of simple incompetence without the continuous upflow previously present.*

*In spite of extensive investigations no cause for this slowly progressive deep vein thrombosis was found. The patient remains well 4 years later and it is possible that prolonged flying by air was a major factor in the occurrence of an otherwise idiopathic thrombosis. Popliteal entrapment is however possible. The patient, well aware of the potential danger of his orginal condition, refuses to be weaned off warfarin!*

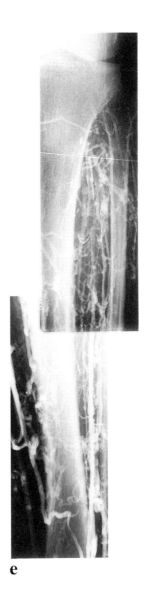

**e**

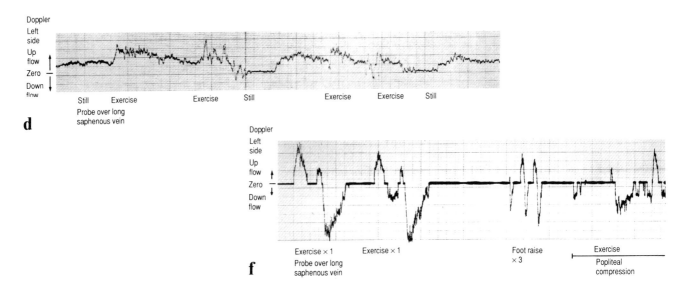

Doppler
Left side
Up flow
Zero
Down flow

Still    Exercise    Exercise    Still    Exercise    Exercise    Still

Probe over long saphenous vein

**d**

Doppler
Left side
Up flow
Zero
Down flow

Exercise × 1    Exercise × 1    Foot raise × 3    Exercise

Probe over long saphenous vein    Popliteal compression

**f**

*Note on authorities consulted in the preparation of Chapter 16.* Over the last few decades, deep vein thrombosis has been the topic of more papers in surgical literature than any other and reflects the immense effort made to banish this scourge. The lists that follow are mainly representative of British publications and the titles of these papers give an idea of the range of activity in this field. Similar prolific work has appeared in America, Europe and, indeed, all nations participating in surgical research.

## References

DeWeese, J. A. (1978) Iliofemoral venous thrombectomy. In *Venous Problems* (eds J. J. Bergan and J. S. T. Yao), Chicago, Year Book Medical, pp. 421–435

Eklof, B. O., Einarsson, E., Endrys, J. *et al.* (1987) Surgical treatment of iliofemoral venous thrombosis. *Phlebology*, **2**, 13–22

Fogarty, T. J., Cranley, J. J., Krause, R. J. *et al.* (1963) Surgical management of phlegmasia cerulea dolens. *Archives of Surgery*, **86**, 256–263

Gruss, J. D. (1988) Venous reconstruction. Part 1. *Phlebology*, **3**, 7–18

Guillebaud, J. (1985) Surgery and the pill. *British Medical Journal*, **291**, 498–499

Haller, J. A. and Abrams, B. L. (1963) Use of thrombectomy in the treatment of acute iliofemoral venous thrombosis in forty-five patients. *Annals of Surgery*, **158**, 561–569

Mavor, G. E. and Galloway, J. M. D. (1969) Iliofemoral venous thrombosis. Pathological considerations and surgical management. *British Journal of Surgery*, **56**, 45–59

Moran, K. T., Jewell, E. R. and Persson, A. V. (1989) The role of thrombolytic therapy in surgical practice. *British Journal of Surgery*, **76**, 298–304

Scott, G. B. D. (1970) Concerning the organization of thrombi. *Annals of the Royal College of Surgeons of England*, **47**, 335–343

Zetterquist, S., Hagglof, R. and Jacobsson, H. (1986) Long-term results of thrombectomy with temporary arteriovenous fistula for iliofemoral venous thrombosis. *Phlebology*, **1**, 113–117

## Bibliography

Ackerman, F. R. and Estes, E. (1951) Prognosis in idiopathic thrombophlebitis. *Annals of Internal Medicine*, **34**, 902–910

Adamson, A. S., Littlewood, T. J., Poston, G. J., Hows, J. M. and Wolfe, J. N. (1988) Malignancy presenting as peripheral venous gangrene. *Journal of the Royal Society of Medicine*, **81**, 609–610

Berquist, D. and Hallbrook, T. (1978) Thermography in screening postoperative deep vein thrombosis: a comparison with the [125]I-fibrinogen test. *British Journal of Surgery*, **65**, 443–445

Bonnar, J. and Walsh, J. (1972) Prevention of thrombosis after pelvic surgery by British Dextran 70. *Lancet*, **i**, 614

Browse, N. L. (1988) Prevention of postoperative deep vein thrombosis. *British Journal of Surgery*, **75**, 835–836

Browse, N. L., Gray, L. and Morland, M. (1977) Changes in the blood fibrinolytic activity after surgery (the effect of deep vein thrombosis and malignant disease). *British Journal of Surgery*, **64**, 23–27

Browse, N. L., Burnand, K. G. and Lea Thomas, M. (1988) *Diseases of the Veins*, Edward Arnold, London

Brozovic, M. (1979) Mechanisms of deep vein thrombosis: a review. *Journal of the Royal Society of Medicine*, **72**, 602–605

Cantwell, B. M. J., Carmichael, J., Ghani, S. E. and Harris, A. L. (1988) Thromboses and thromboemboli in patients with lymphoma during cytotoxic chemotherapy. *British Medical Journal*, **297**, 179–180

Carter, A. E. and Eban, R. The prevention of postoperative deep venous thrombosis with Dextran 70. *British Journal of Surgery*, **60**, 681–683

Charig, M. J. and Fletcher, E. W. L. (1987) Emergency phlebography service: is it worth while? *British Medical Journal*, **295**, 474

Coleridge Smith, P. D., Hasty, J. H. and Scurr, J. H. (1990) Venous stasis and vein lumen changes during surgery. *British Journal of Surgery*, **77**, 1055–1059

Coleridge Smith, P. D., Hasty, J. H. and Scurr, J. H. (1991) Deep vein thrombosis: effect of graduated compression stockings on distension of the deep veins of the calf. *British Journal of Surgery*, **78**, 724–726

de Cossart, L. and Marcuson, R. W. (1983) Vascular plasminogen activator and deep vein thrombosis. *British Journal of Surgery*, **70**, 369–370

Cunningham, M., de Torrente, A., Ekoe, J. M. *et al.* (1984) Vascular spasm and gangrene during heparin-dihydro-ergotamine prophylaxis. *British Journal of Surgery*, **71**, 829–831

Dalen, J., Hull, R. D. and Nicolaides, A. N. (1986) Deep vein thrombosis and pulmonary embolism: developing a protocol for effective prophylaxis. *Phlebology*, **1**, 75–96

Davies, J. A. and Tuddenham, E. G. D. (1987) Haemostasis and thrombosis. In *Oxford Textbook of Medicine* (eds D. J. Weatherall, J. G. G. Ledingham and D. A. Warell), Oxford University Press, Oxford

Dejode, L. R., Khurshid, M. and Walther, W. W. (1973) The influence of electrical stimulation of the leg during surgical operations on the subsequent development of deep-vein thrombosis. *British Journal of Surgery*, **60**, 31–32

Dodd, H. and Cockett, F. B. (1976) *The Pathology and Surgery of the Vein of the Lower Limb*, Churchill Livingstone, Edinburgh

Doran, F. S. A. (1971) Prevention of deep vein thrombosis. *British Journal of Hospital Medicine*, 773–779

Dormandy, J. A. and Edelman, J. B. (1973) High blood viscosity: an aetiological factor in venous thrombosis. *British Journal of Surgery*, **60**, 187–190

Duruble, M. and Ouvry, P. (1991) Haemodilution in venous disease. *Phlebology*, **6**, 31–36

Eriksson, B. I., Zachrisson, B. E., Teger-Nilsson, A. C. and Risberg, B. (1988) Thrombosis prophylaxis with low molecular weight heparin in total hip replacement. *British Journal of Surgery*, **75**, 1053–1057

European Fraxiparin Study (EFS) Group (1988) Comparison of low molecular weight heparin and unfractionated heparin for prevention of deep vein thrombosis in patients undergoing abdominal surgery. *British Journal of Surgery*, **75**, 1058–1063

Evans, D. S. and Negus, S. (1971) Diagnosis of deep vein thrombosis. *British Journal of Hospital Medicine*, 729–740

Fennerty, A., Campbell, I. A. and Routledge, P. A. (1988) Anticoagulants in venous thromboembolism. *British Medical Journal*, **297**, 1285–1287

Field, E., Nicolaides, A. N., Kakkar, V. V. and Crellin, R. Q. (1972) Deep-vein thrombosis in patients with fractures of the femoral neck. *British Journal of Surgery*, **59**, 377–379

Fredin, H. O., Rosberg, B., Arborelius, M. and Nylander, G. (1984) On thrombo-embolism after total hip replacement in epidural analgesia: a controlled study of dextran 70 and low-dose heparin combined with dihydroergotamine. *British Journal of Surgery*, **71**, 58–60

Gordon-Smith, I. C., Hickman, J. A. and Le Quesne, L. P. (1974) Postoperative fibrinolytic activity and deep vein thrombosis. *British Journal of Surgery*, **61**, 213–218

Harvey Kemble, J. V. (1971) Incidence of deep vein thrombosis. *British Journal of Hospital Medicine*, 721–726

Hughes, G. R. and Pridie, R. B. Acute synovial rupture of the knee – a differential diagnosis from deep vein thrombosis. *Proceedings of the Royal Society of Medicine*, **63**, 587–590

Hurlow, R. A. and Strachan, C. J. L. (1978) The clinical scope and potential of isotope angiology. *British Journal of Surgery*, **65**, 688–691

Irvine, A. T. and Lea Thomas, M. (1991) Colour-coded duplex sonography in the diagnosis of deep vein thrombosis: a comparison with phlebography. *Phlebography*, **6**, 103–109

Kakkar, V. V. (1971) Medical treatment of deep vein thrombosis. *British Journal of Hospital Medicine*, 741–750

Kakkar, V. V. (1987) Venous thrombosis and pulmonary embolism. *Surgery (Oxford)*, **1**, 948–957

Kakkar, V. V. and Jouhar, A. J. (1972) *Thromboembolism: Diagnosis and Treatment*, Churchill Livingstone, Edinburgh

Kakkar, V. V., Flanc, C., Howe, C. T. *et al.* (1969) Treatment of deep vein thrombosis. A trial of heparin, streptokinase and arvin. *British Medical Journal*, **1**, 806–810

Kakkar, V. V., Howe, C. T., Laws, J. W. and Flanc, C. (1969) Late results of treatment of deep vein thrombosis. *British Medical Journal*, **1**, 810–811

Kohn, H., Mostbeck, A., Lofferer, O. *et al.* (1986) Non-invasive screening for deep vein thrombosis: comparison between $^{99m}$Tc-labelled compounds, thermography, $^{131}$I-fibrinogen uptake test and X-ray phlebography. *Phlebology*, **1**, 65–72

Lassen, M. R., Borris, L. C., Christiansen, H. M. *et al.* (1988) Heparin/dihydroergotamine for venous thrombosis prophylaxis: comparison of low-dose heparin and low molecular weight heparin in hip surgery. *British Journal of Surgery*, **75**, 686–689

Laverick, M. D., McGivern, R. C., Crone, M. D. and Mollan, R. A. B. (1990) A comparison of the effects of electrical calf muscle stimulation and the venous foot pump on venous blood flow in the lower leg. *Phlebology*, **5**, 285–290

Lawrence, J. C., Xabregas, A., Gray, L. and Ham, J. M. (1977) Seasonal variation in the incidence of deep vein thrombosis. *British Journal of Surgery*, **64**, 777–780

Lea Thomas, M. (1982) *Phlebography of the Lower Limb*, Churchill Livingstone, Edinburgh

Levin, H. O. and Al-Hassan, H. (1990) Ultrasonic diagnosis of iliofemoral venous thrombosis: merits and disadvantages. *Phlebology*, **5**, 107–112

Leyvraz, P. F., Bachmann, F., Hoek, J., Buller, H. R., Postel, M., Samama, M. and Vandenbroek, M. D. (1991) Prevention of deep vein thrombosis after hip replacement: randomised comparison between unfractionated heparin and low molecular weight heparin. *British Medical Journal*, **303**, 543–548

Loew, S. (1977) Aspirin in the prophylaxis of venous and arterial disease. *Proceedings of the Royal Society of Medicine*, **70**, 28–31

Mansfield, A. O. (1972) Alteration in fibrinolysis associated with surgery and venous thrombosis. *British Journal of Surgery*, **59**, 754–757

Mavor, G. E. (1971) Surgery of deep vein thrombosis. *British Journal of Hospital Medicine*, 755–764

Mavor, G. E., Dhall, D. P., Dawson, A. A. *et al.* (1973) Streptokinase therapy in deep vein thrombosis. *British Journal of Surgery*, **60**, 468–474

Michiels, J. J., Stibbe, J., Bertina, R. and Broekmans, A. (1987) Effectiveness of long term oral anticoagulation treatment in preventing venous thrombosis in hereditary protein S deficiency. *British Medical Journal*, **295**, 641–643

Mitchell, D. C., Grasty, M. S., Stebbings, W. S. L., Nockler, I. B., Lewars, M. D., Levison, R. A. and Wood, R. F. M. (1991) Comparison of duplex ultrasonography and venography in the diagnosis of deep venous thrombosis. *British Journal of Surgery*, **78**, 611–613

Moloney, G. E., Morrel, M. T. and Fell, R. H. (1972) The effect of electrical stimulation of the legs on postoperative thrombosis. *British Journal of Surgery*, **59**, 65–68

Mudge, M. and Hughes, L. E. (1978) The long term sequelae of deep vein thrombosis. *British Journal of Surgery*, **65**, 692–694

Negus, D. (1985) Prevention and treatment of venous ulceration. *Annals of the Royal College of Surgeons of England*, **67**, 142–148

Nicolaides, A. N. (ed.) (1975) *Thromboembolism*, MTP, Lancaster

Nicolaides, A. N. and Gordon-Smith, I. (1972) The prevention of deep venous thrombosis. In *The Treatment of Venous Disorders* (ed. J. Hobbs), MTP, Lancaster

Nicolaides, A. N. and Lewis, J. D. (1972) The management of deep venous thrombosis. In *The Treatment of Venous Disorders* (ed. J. Hobbs), MTP, Lancaster

Nicolaides, A. N., Kakkar, V. V., Field, E. S. and Fish, P. (1972) Venous stasis and deep-vein thrombosis. *British Journal of Surgery*, **59**, 713–716

Nicolaides, A. N., Clark, C. T., Thomas, R. D. and Lewis, J. D. (1976) Fibrinolytic activator in the endothelium of the veins of the lower limb. *British Journal of Surgery*, **63**, 881–884

Parker-Williams, J. and Vickers, R. (1991) Major orthopaedic surgery on the leg and thromboembolism. *British Medical Journal*, **303**, 531–532

Rickles, F. R. and Edwards, R. L. (1983) Activation of blood coagulation in cancer: Trousseau's syndrome revisited. *Blood*, **62**, 14–31

Roberts, V. C., Sabri, S., Petroni, M. C. *et al.* (1971) Passive flexion and femoral vein flow: a study using a motorized foot mover. *British Medical Journal*, **3**, 78–81

Sabri, S., Roberts, V. C. and Cotton, L. T. (1971) Prevention of early postoperative deep vein thrombosis by passover exercise of leg during surgery. *British Medical Journal*, **3**, 82–83

Sandler, D. A. and Martin, J. F. (1989) Autopsy proven pulmonary embolism in hospital patients: are we detecting enough deep vein thrombosis. *Journal of the Royal Society of Medicine*, **82**, 203–205

Sandor, T., Laszlo, E., Magyary, F. *et al.* (1986) Prophylaxis of postoperative thromboembolism with heparin-dihydroergotamine combination. *Phlebology*, **1**, 57–64

Sagar, S., Stamatakis, J. D., Thomas, D. P. and Kakkar, V. V. (1976) Oral contraceptives, anti-thrombin III activity, and post-operative deep-vein thrombosis. *Lancet*, **i**, 509–511

Schindler, J. M., Kaiser, M., Gerber, A., Vuilliomenet, A., Popovic, A. and Bertel, O. (1990) Colour coded duplex sonography in suspected deep vein thrombosis of the leg. *British Medical Journal*, **301**, 1369–1370

Scurr, J. H., Ibrahim, S. Z., Faber, R. G. and Le Quesne, L. P. (1977) The efficacy of graduated compression stockings in the prevention of deep vein thrombosis. *British Journal of Surgery*, **64**, 371–373

Sevitt, S. and Gallagher, N. G. (1959) Prevention of venous thrombosis and pulmonary embolism in injured patients. *Lancet*, **ii**, 981

Sigel, B., Edelstein, A. L., Felix, W. R. and Memhardt, C. R. (1973) Compression of the deep venous system of the lower leg during inactive recumbency. *Archives of Surgery*, **106**, 38–43

Stamatakis, J. D., Kakkar, V. V., Lawrence, D. and Bentley, P. G. (1978) The origin of thrombi in the deep veins of the lower limb: a venographic study. *British Journal of Surgery*, **65**, 449–451

Sue-Ling, H. M., Johnston, D., Verheijen, J. H. *et al.* (1987) Indicators of depressed fibrinolytic activity in pre-operative prediction of deep venous thrombosis. *British Journal of Surgery*, **74**, 275–278

Sutton, G., Hosking, S. and Johnson, C. D. (1991) We still still have insufficient evidence to support perioperative heparin prophylaxis against venous thromboembolism. *Annals of the Royal College of Surgeons of England*, **73**, 111–115

Swedenborg, J., Hagglof, R., Jacobsson, H. *et al.* (1986) Results of surgical treatment for iliofemoral venous thrombosis. *British Journal of Surgery*, **73**, 871–874

Thomas, P. R. S., Butler, C. M., Bowman, J., Grieve, N. W. T., Bennett, C. E., Taylor, R. S. and Thomas, M. H. (1991) Light reflection rheography: an effective non-invasive technique for screening patients with suspected deep venous thrombosis. *British Journal of Surgery*, **78**, 207–209

Tibbutt, D. A., Williams, E. W., Walker, M. W. *et al.* (1974) Controlled trial of ancrod and streptokinase in the treatment of deep vein thrombosis of lower limb. *British Journal of Haematology*, **27**, 407–414

Various authors (1978) In *Venous Problems* (eds J. J. Bergan and J. S. T. Yao), Year Book Medical, Chicago

Various authors (1979) In *Surgery of the Veins of the Leg and Pelvis* (ed. R. May), W. B. Saunders, Philadelphia; Georg Thieme, Stuttgart

Various authors (1985) In *Surgery of the Veins* (eds J. J. Bergan and J. S. T. Yao), Grune and Stratton, New York

Various authors (1986) In *Phlebology '85* (eds D. Negus and G. Jantet), John Libbey, London, pp. 375–511

Vessey, M. P., Doo, R. and Fairbairn, A. S. (1970) Post-operative thromboembolism and the use of oral contraceptives. *British Medical Journal*, **3**, 123–126

Virchow, R. (1846) Thrombosis and embolization. *Beitr Exp Path Physiol*, **2**, 227–380. (This is reprinted in Sudhoff (1910) *Klassiker der Medizin*, Bd. 7–8, Leipzig, and included in: Virchow, R. L. K. (1856) *Gesammelte Abhandlungen zur wissenschaftlichen Medicin*, Meidinger, Sohn u. Co., Frankfurt, pp. 219–732)

von Kaulla, E., Droegemueller, W., Aoki, N. and von Kaulla, K. N. (1971) Anti-thrombin III depression and thrombin generation acceleration in women taking oral contraceptives. *American Journal of Obstetrics and Gynecology*, **109**, 123–126

Walker, M. G. (1972) The natural history of venous thromboembolism. *British Journal of Surgery*, **59**, 753–754

Walker, M. G., Shaw, J. W., Thomson, G. J. L. *et al.* (1987) Subcutaneous calcium heparin versus intravenous sodium heparin in treatment of established acute deep vein thrombosis of the legs: a multicentre prospective randomised trial. *British Medical Journal*, **294**, 1189–1192

Watts, R. A. and Bretland, P. M. (1990) Necrotizing fasciitis mimicking a ruptured popliteal cyst. *Journal of the Royal Society of Medicine*, **83**, 52–53

Weatherall, D. J., Ledingham, J. G. G. and Warell, D. A. (eds) (1987) *Oxford Textbook of Medicine*, Oxford, Oxford University Press

Whitehouse, G. (1987) Radiological diagnosis of deep vein thrombosis. *British Medical Journal*, **295**, 801–802

# 17

# Interrelationship of venous disorders with ischaemia and other conditions

Most arterial and venous disorders are quite distinct from each other. Widmer *et al.* (1981) in the comprehensive Basle study of venous and arterial conditions did not report any direct relationship beween them beyond occurrence in similar age groups and both being common causes for complaint in the lower limbs. However, in certain states, especially ulceration, there are sufficient superficial similarities for misdiagnosis to be possible. This may lead to the serious error of an arterial lesion being given treatment in direct conflict with its requirements. The important matter of distinguishing between arterial and venous lesions will be considered in the first part of this chapter; also discussed is the recognition of those states where both arterial and venous disorders are present simultaneously in the same limb.

## Distinguishing arterial and diabetic ulcers from venous ulcers

The term ischaemia, in connection with an ulcer, can be used in two ways. It may refer to a local ischaemia caused by microangiopathy in the fibrotic tissue surrounding a longstanding venous ulcer (Haselbach *et al*, 1986), a diabetic or rheumatoid ulcer, but more usually it is used to describe the overall reduction in the arterial supply to the distal part of a limb, commonly caused by arterial disease, especially atherosclerosis. It is in this last sense that the term will be used in this chapter.

There are three categories of ulceration of vascular origin, around the ankle and foot, that are of particular importance to the venous specialist

1. Ischaemic ulcer purely due to arterial insufficiency. To misdiagnose this as a venous ulcer can bring unnecessary misery to the patient and may eventually cause loss of the limb. In the description of this given below, the diabetic ulcer has been added even though it is usually more neuropathic than ischaemic; this is included because it has some similarities with an ischaemic ulcer and is often accompanied by arterial disease so that its diabetic origin may be overlooked; no description of an ischaemic ulcer is complete without the warning of this possibility.

2. Venous ulcer purely due to venous hypertension. This may result from massive superficial vein incompetence combined with a weak pumping mechanism (see Chapter 6), or severe impairment of the pumping mechanism due to post-thrombotic damage (see Chapter 8) or congenital absence of valves (see Chapter 7), or, occasionally, from arteriovenous fistula (see Chapter 12 and later in this chapter). Venous disorder is by far the commonest cause for ulceration in the leg and it will respond to measures counteracting venous hypertension. Venous ulcer is discussed at length in Chapter 13 in addition to the chapters given above.

3. A state of venous hypertension combined with arterial disease. Whether an ulcer is predominantly arterial or venous may be difficult to decide but, however viewed, it is an unhappy combination. Treating only one component may not succeed in healing an ulcer and every effort must be made to find ways to improve both aspects. The difficulty here is that conservative treatment suitable for the venous component conflicts with the requirements of the arterial side and vice versa. Moreover, there is the possibility that a limb-threatening arterial insufficiency may be overlooked because of the obvious evidence of venous disorder.

## The ischaemic ulcer

Because an ischaemic ulcer caused by arterial disease (atherosclerosis) occurs in the same age group, is near the ankle and causes pain, there is a tendency for this to be misdiagnosed as a venous ulcer; moreover, an ischaemic ulcer may even be accompanied by oedema for reasons given presently. Beyond these features in common, there is little similarity and the distinction is crucial because the treatment of an ischaemic ulcer by venous principles can only do harm.

### The effect of elevation and elastic compression in an ischaemic limb

An ischaemic ulcer is due to an arterial insufficiency that reduces the arterial pressure in the distal part of the limb (Figure 17.1). An arterial ulcer does not develop unless the horizontal perfusion pressure is reduced below 60 mmHg and at this level the pressure is inadequate to compete with any elevation of the foot. Every 1.3 cm of elevation reduces the arterial perfusing pressure by 1 mmHg (specific gravity of mercury is 13.55 and that of blood 1.06; thus, mercury is 13 times heavier than blood); 13 cm of elevation brings the arterial pressure down by 10 mmHg and at 52 cm it is reduced by 40 mmHg so that at this height a horizontal perfusion pressure of 60 mmHg is reduced to 20 mmHg, that is, insufficient to maintain tissue viability, let alone healing of an ulcer. Similarly elastic compression of, say, 30 mmHg in a horizontal limb will compress the vessels and threaten to reduce the precarious blood suppply to a critical level; if the limb is elevated at the same time the circulation may cease completely in the most distal parts, the toes and forefoot.

When a patient is upright, arterial pressure is hydrostatically increased and allows a slow build up to a higher level, possibly able to withstand external compression, but as soon as there is any exercise, blood is diverted through the muscle beds and the pressure falls away, often to become irrecordable. Collateral arteries, compensating for an occluded main artery, only provide a meagre rate of delivery and cannot meet the extra requirements of muscular exercise. This is often made apparent by the pallor and sensory numbness developed in a critically ischaemic foot on walking. When upright, hydrostatic and arterial pressure may reach a level able to withstand 30–40 mmHg compression but on exercise will immediately reduce to a critical point at which elastic compression seriously threatens the circulation.

### Oedema in a critically ischaemic limb

If the limb is kept down without exercise, there is only passive venous return and a very slow turnover of circulation, with high venous pressure and accumulation of oedema. A patient with a critically ischaemic limb will often sleep with the leg hanging out of bed in order to relieve the ischaemic rest pain (Figure 17.2(a)). The oedema caused by this (Figure 17.2(b)) may appear to confirm a venous condition that requires elevation but nothing could be further from the truth. Oedema is commonly seen in patients with rest pain from critical ischaemia. In these circumstances, *treatment by elevation or elastic compression is potentially disastrous and must be avoided.*

On a number of occasions in years gone by, the author has seen arterial ulceration that has been mistakenly treated by application of heavy elastic webbing bandage and the leg put into high elevation. The significance of the white, numb forefoot and the great misery of the patient from ischaemic rest pain has not been appreciated, with the result that irreversible tissue changes have left no alternative but amputation to bring the patient relief. Many of these limbs could have been saved quite easily by arterial surgery if the true state had been recognized at the outset and such damaging mistreatment avoided. One of the battles fought by arterial surgeons 30 years ago was to bring enlightenment on this. Surely, there can be no excuse nowadays for this grave error, but like all fundamental principles, the lesson cannot be repeated too emphatically or too often. *No limb should be subjected to elevation and/or compression without a careful arterial assessment, and no ulcer can be assumed to be venous just because it is near the ankle.* Comparative youth is not sufficient reason to neglect this precaution as young people do occasionally suffer severe arterial disease (Figure 17.3), but the likelihood of ischaemia is much greater in the elderly. There must always be conscious

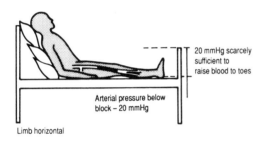

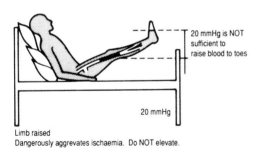

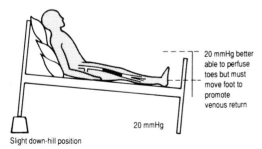

**Figure 17.1** *Diagram to show the effect on the foot of raising an ischaemic limb above the horizontal. If an ischaemic ulcer is present the arterial perfusion pressure is likely to be severely reduced in the distal part of the limb and may not be sufficient to lift flow to the forefoot and toes in elevation*

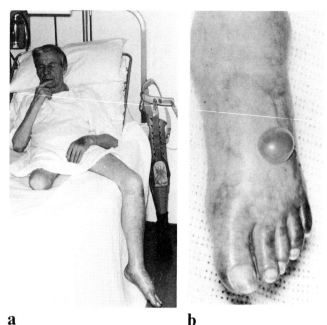

**a**        **b**

**Figure 17.2** *Oedema may accompany severe ischaemic rest pain.*

*(a) This patient has severe ischaemia and seeks relief by hanging the leg out of bed throughout the night. The oedema is a postural phenomenon; on its own the reduced perfusion pressure in the capillary beds of an ischaemic limb is not sufficient to form oedema but this certainly becomes possible with the congestion and raised pressure caused by prolonged dependency. It is an important diagnostic trap and the presence of oedema must never be used as a reason for excluding the diagnosis of ischaemia as the underlying cause. In a venous state the patient would seldom choose to sleep with the leg hanging down in this fashion, although some may greatly aggravate their problems by sleeping in a chair. In this illustration, the patient has already lost the other limb and arterial reconstruction did not prove feasible to the remaining side so that amputation was the only way of relieving the patient's pain.*

*(b) A closer view of the foot. Bullous oedema is present; this is unusual but emphasizes the severity of the oedema that may occur. If ulceration were present this would allow easy bacterial invasion but, because of inadequate blood supply, the resulting cellulitis would show scarcely any inflammatory response so that the gravity of the situation may be underrated. Antibiotics could improve matters but the patient's pain can only be truly relieved either by arterial reconstruction or by amputation*

exclusion of the ischaemic ulcer and this is a skill that is essential to all venous specialists.

Table 17.1 summarizes the features distinguishing between arterial and venous ulceration.

*Some guiding rules in recognizing an ischaemic ulcer*

Although the features distinguishing between purely arterial and purely venous ulceration are summarized in Table 17.1, some of the key features are repeated below:

1. The ischaemic limb will usually have a clear history of intermittent claudication and/or nocturnal rest

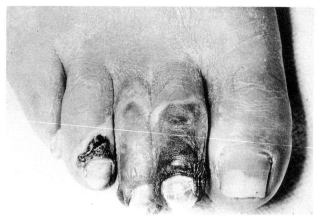

**Figure 17.3** *Ischaemia and gangrene of the toes due to Buerger's disease (thromboangiitis obliterans) in a young man aged 19 years. Smoking is a key factor in this and the disease may cease to progress if smoking is stopped completely. This is an essential requirement and if it is strictly observed, a lumbar sympathectomy may bring considerable additional improvement*

pain; however this can be misinterpreted as a painful venous ulcer, so beware.

2. A dry, painful ulcer with poor or absent granulation tissue is likely to be arterial.

3. An ulcer without evidence of accompanying venous stasis (pigmentation, induration, etc.) is most unlikely to be venous and may well be ischaemic; there are, of course, many other alternative diagnoses to be considered (see Chapter 13).

4. Venous ulceration never occurs on the underside of the foot and only occasionally on the upper aspect and toes.

5. Ulceration over a bony prominence is likely to be due to arterial disease or to sensory loss from diabetic neuropathy.

6. Ischaemic ulceration may occur with faint but detectable pulses throughout the limb if the arterial occlusion is at a high level in, say, aorta or iliac arteries, and this may give false reassurance.

7. Oedema does not automatically signify a venous origin because a critically ischaemic patient may find relief by sleeping with the leg hanging out of bed.

8. Failure to feel pulses at the ankle may be due to induration and oedema. Examination with Doppler flowmeter should resolve this but, for the same reasons, the pulses may not be easy to locate. A pressure index (ratio of ankle to brachial Doppler measured pressures) below 0.5 strongly suggests an ischaemic cause; above this level it is increasingly less likely.

9. No venous condition should be treated by elevation or the use of elastic compression unless a good arterial supply has been confirmed with adequate ankle pulses identified either by palpation or by Doppler flowmetry.

10. If a patient responds to elevation, or elastic

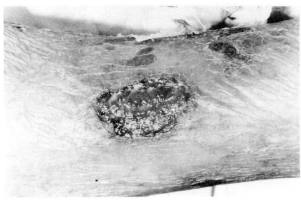

a

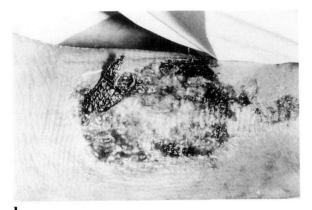

b

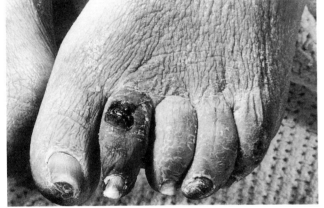

cI

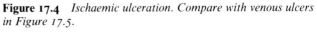

**Figure 17.4**  *Ischaemic ulceration. Compare with venous ulcers in Figure 17.5.*

(*a*)  *Ischaemic ulcer on the shin in a patient with claudication and rest pain. There is no surrounding pigmentation or induration, and the ulcer is 'dry' with only poor granulation tissue. The wrinkled skin is due to recent subsidence of oedema caused by the patient hanging the leg out of the bed. This ulcer healed following arterial reconstruction.*

(*b*)  *A similar ischaemic ulcer on the shin.*

(*c*)  *1.  Ulceration over, and into, the proximal joint of the second toe, which is black and shrunken (mummified) in its distal part. The patient had severe rest pain and had been hanging his foot out of bed. The wrinkling of skin on the foot is due to recent subsidence of dependency oedema and cellulitis in response to treatment by analgesia, avoidance of dependent positioning and use of antibiotics.*
*2.  Photoplethysmograms in arterial mode from the great toes of the patient in (c)1.* Upper: *left side, very diminished arterial pulsation with only occasional extrasystoles coming through, in keeping with marked ischaemia.* Lower: *right side, showing good pulsation interrupted by extrasystoles, in keeping with good arterial supply. This method of assessment is quick and easy to apply. It is valuable when ankle pulses cannot be detected and will indicate the adequacy of a diminished arterial supply when the limb is elevated.*

(*d*)  *A massive ischaemic ulcer with extensive necrosis of superficial layers and deep fascia with exposure of underlying tendons. An ulcer due to venous hypertension alone does not expose the deeper structures in this fashion but ischaemia commonly does; a deeply invading neoplasm may do so but is recognizable by its proliferating malignant tissue (Figure 13.7(a)). Note the absence of venous pigmentation which is always present around a venous ulcer*

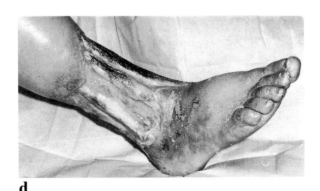

d

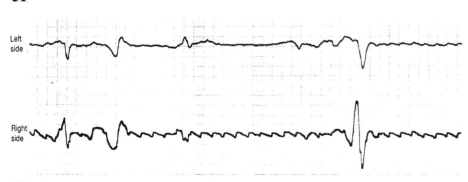

Left side

Right side

c2

**TABLE 17.1** Main features of ulcers of arterial origin compared with those of venous origin

| Features | Arterial ulcer | Venous ulcer |
|---|---|---|
| Age group | Usually over 55 years but occasionally in young patients (Figure 17.3) | Occurs over a wide age group but mostly over 50 years |
| History and presentation | Claudication and possibly numbness on walking; nocturnal rest pain | Longstanding vein problems, with or without previous deep vein thrombosis |
| Site of ulcer | Toes, foot and leg, especially the shin; often over bony prominences of joints of toes, metatarsal heads, heel and malleoli (beware diabetes) where skin is vulnerable to pressure | Most common in 'gaiter' area but may occur at higher level, on the foot or even the toes but never on the underside of the foot. Behind ankle and outside of leg not uncommon |
| Appearance of ulcer | 'Dry' ulcer, may be necrosis and blackening, possibly exposing tendons and ligaments<br><br>Little or no pus, poor or absent granulation tissue (Figure 17.4) | Moist ulceration with exudate and often pus. Strong, often prolific granulation tissue but may have superficial slough. Never exposes deeper structures |
| Surrounding skin | Comparatively normal colour or possibly bluish. Possibly black gangrenous skin or cynanosed devitalized skin | Brown pigmentation and often oedematous changes, may show scarring from previous ulcers and atrophie blanche (Figure 17.5) |
| Comment | Ischaemia prevents usual inflammatory reaction to infection, either absent or muted; if pus forms, ischaemia is minimal and ulcer is capable of healing | Reacts to infection with pus formation and surrounding cellulitis |
| Oedema | No oedema, unless patient hanging leg out of bed due to rest pain (Figures 17.2, 17.7) | Some oedema usual, although may be partially concealed by other changes |
| Surrounding induration | Not present | Extensive induration due to liposclerosis usual |
| Bacteriology | May grow pathogens, especially *Staph. aureus*, and tissue death caused by this is without inflammatory response; cynanotic devitalized surrounding skin characteristic of this | Mixed flora usual but may include specific pathogens, especially *Staph. aureus*, and often the cause of much pain |
| Edges of ulcers | Ragged and flat with no epithelial ingrowth, unless ischaemia is minimal and ulcer is healing | Variable: when deteriorating, edges are sharply cut; when healing, shelving with grey epithelial ingrowth |
| Accompanying features | Absent or very diminished ankle pulses, often popliteal and sometimes femoral pulses absent | Ankle pulses present but may be concealed by oedema and induration |
| | Doppler pulses diminished and damped, or absent | Normal Doppler pulses may be more difficult to find because of oedema |
| | Probably pallor of forefoot on elevation (Figure 17.6) | Good colour maintained in forefoot on elevation |
| | Possibly reduced sensation (beware diabetes) | Normal sensation, unless nerve injury from a previous operation! |
| | After elevation, very slow recovery of colour and filling of venous gutters on returning to horizontal | Normal colour and quick refilling of venous gutters on returning to horizontal after elevation |
| | Marked rubor on dependent position of limb | Marked venous congestion on dependency; may be difficult to distinguish from ischaemic rubor but is blue from outset unlike ischaemic dependency rubor |
| | Coincidental varicose veins always possible but without gross evidence of venous stasis unless both conditions are present | Visible evidence of venous disturbance, venous flares at ankle, pigmentation, eczema, induration, oedema, etc., enlarged veins giving deep venous gutters when elevated |
| | May have areas of skin gangrene on toes, foot, heel, lower leg or shin | Black areas may be part of ulcer but if so beware ischaemia and/or diabetes |
| Posture adopted by patient | Characteristic ischaemic posture, sitting up on bed, in knee up-position or hanging leg over side of bed, in order to relieve pain (Figures 17.2, 17.7). Oedema from this likely | No characteristic posture but will often elevate limb because, unlike the ischaemic state, patient has learnt that dependent position causes pain and deterioration of ulcer |

*Note.* Dependency favours the ischaemic state (at least temporarily) but aggravates the venous state
    Elevation aggravates (often severely) the ischaemic state but eases the venous state

**TABLE 17.1** *(continued)*

| Features | Arterial ulcer | Venous ulcer |
|---|---|---|
| Response to treatment by elevation and/or compression bandage | Causes pain, which may be severe, and deterioration in ulcer | May cause pain if ulcer infected with pathogen but more usually relief of discomfort. Ulcer commences to heal |
| *Special investigations* Doppler flowmeter | Over peripheral arteries: Diminished pulsatility and damped waveform, or absent signal. If absent, is probe located properly – compare with other side | Over superficial veins, on exercise in upright position: May confirm massive incompetence with downflow in varicose veins; shows preferential flow up saphenous if there is deep vein impairment |
| Photoplethysmography | Arterial mode: Feeble or absent pulsation. Very reduced or absent on elevation Venous mode: May show normal or excessive response to exercise | Venous mode: poor response to exercise with very short recovery time (under 7 seconds). If simple incompetence, blocking of saphenous vein or varicosities may restore recovery time to near normal Arterial mode: full pulsation |
| Arteriography | Irregular narrowing or occlusion of arteries | Normal arteries or minimal changes consistent with age |
| Functional phlebography | No significant change | Obvious venous abnormality (detailed elsewhere) |

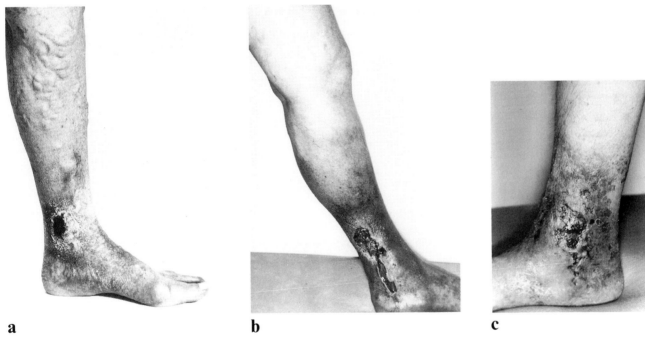

**a**                    **b**                    **c**

**Figure 17.5**   *Venous ulcers, each of different causation, but all showing the hallmarks of venous disorder, particularly surrounding pigmentation.*

*(a) Encrusted ulcer, caused by massive incompetence in superficial veins. The varicosities arising from the long saphenous vein, the multiple enlarged venules on the foot and the pigmentation around the ulcer give immediate recognition of a venous ulcer. Atrophie blanche is evident on the skin anterior to the ulcer.*

*(b) Chronic ulceration due to post-thrombotic syndrome. There is swelling up the knee, superficial veins acting as collaterals show prominence but not varicosity, and the ulcer is surrounded by heavily pigmented skin overlying thickened, indurated subcutaneous tissue. Atrophie blanche is present below and in front of the ulcer, and distended venules are visible on the foot.*

*(c) Chronic ulceration in a patient with severe incompetence in the deep veins but with no history or other evidence of deep vein thrombosis (valveless syndrome). The skin in the vicinity of the ulcer is pigmented and eczematous, with induration and thickening of the underlying tissue. The superficial veins show no undue enlargement*

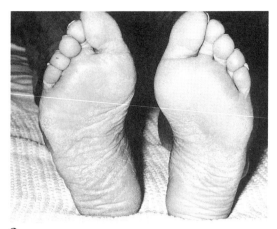
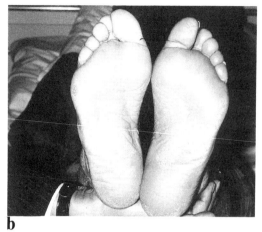

a
b

**Figure 17.6** *Diagnosis of ischaemia by colour changes in the forefoot and toes in response to elevation (see also Colour Plates 10 and 11).*

*(a) Good colour is present in both feet in the horizontal position.*

*(b) Pallor in the ischaemic right foot persists after being blanched by gentle hand pressure whilst in elevation at 0.5 m above horizontal. This is a valuable clinical test which confirms the diagnosis and shows that the foot will be damaged by prolonged elevation; it also gives warning that after local surgery, for example, amputation of a toe, healing will not be satisfactory. Similarly this foot will not be able to show an inflammatory response to warn of infection*

compression, with increased pain or distress the limb should be returned to horizontal and the arterial state checked again. If there is still doubt the limb must not be elevated until a good arterial supply has been identified with certainty (Figure 17.8). Elevation or compression do great harm to the ischaemic limb but the horizontal position, combined with movement, is safe and suits a venous problem quite well. In any event the patient should be encouraged to move the feet frequently and have a short walk each hour.

### Useful additional clinical tests

*Colour changes in response to elevation*

*Part 1.* Foot is elevated to 0.5 m (20 inches) and the forefoot and toes gently compressed with the hand to empty dermal capillary beds and cause blanching. The limb is maintained in elevation for at least 1 minute to see if colour is regained (Figure 17.6). With normal arterial supply colour returns immediately or within a few seconds; any delay above 20 seconds indicates a significant impairment in arterial perfusion pressure; increasing severity is indicated by a longer time before recovery of colour, with persistent pallor in severe ischaemia.

*Part 2.* The foot is now returned to the horizontal and watched to observe the speed of recovery in colour and in filling of the venous gutters caused by elevation. If pallor and guttering persist for more than 30 seconds this indicates a very restricted arterial inflow and a severe ischaemia. Sensory numbness may be caused by severe ischaemia, diabetes, or, of course, a separate neurological state.

*Response to dependency* The patient is asked to sit with the legs over the side of the examination couch. A steady

development of a strong rubor within 30 seconds is in keeping with moderate to severe ischaemia; this will gradually take on a cyanotic tint. If there is also a venous disorder venous congestion will occur quickly and confuse interpretation so that this test has little value in the presence of venous problems.

### Special investigations

*Photoplethysmography in arterial mode* If this shows pulsation on foot or great toe it may be used to measure the arterial pressure at the level of a pneumatic cuff placed on the lower or upper calf. If a suitable cuff is available the same method can be used to measure perfusion pressure in a digit. In an ischaemic limb, pulsation may disappear with elevation.

*Arteriography* If the tests just given confirm an impaired arterial supply, arteriography should only be carried out if circumstances indicate that arterial reconstruction should be considered, either to relieve disabling claudication or to relieve rest pain and avert the need for amputation. Arteriogram should not be used as a diagnostic adjunct but only as a preliminary to arterial reconstruction.

Exclude diabetes by routine check of urine in all patients or by blood sugar estimation. Remember an ulcer on the foot or leg may not be vascular in origin (see Chapter 13); an arterial or venous ulcer will always have strongly positive clinical evidence, backed by the special investigations, of the causative vascular disturbance. If this is not present then another diagnosis must be considered.

*Bacteriology in an ischaemic ulcer*

An ischaemic ulcer cannot respond to infection by

**Figure 17.7**  *Examples of typical postures adopted by patients with ischaemic rest pain (see also Colour Plate 12).*

*(a)  Knee-up position on the bed. The downward slant of the leg below the knee gives a small improvement of perfusion to the foot by gravitational downflow from the relatively good circulation at knee level. The patient will often seek relief in this position. Note the tobacco-stained fingers of this patient; it is most unusual for a non-smoker to reach this predicament.*

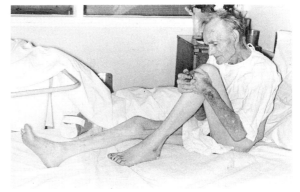

a

*(b)  The various positions adopted by an elderly woman who refused to come into hospital for 3 months, in spite of severe rest pain. She either sat with her feet hanging over the side of the bed (1) or in the knee-up position (2). As a result, hip, knee and spine stiffened in flexion, with widespread weakening of muscle, so that the patient was unable to stand without aid and then only in a bent position (3). This patient also had severe ulceration (shown in Figure 17.4(d)) and, although arterial reconstruction was feasible, amputation immediately above the knee had to be resorted to. Prolonged physiotherapy greatly improved movement in the hip joint and straightening of the spine. She eventually walked quite well with an artificial limb and 9 months later had a good result from arterial reconstruction to the left side which threatened to follow the same course as the right side*

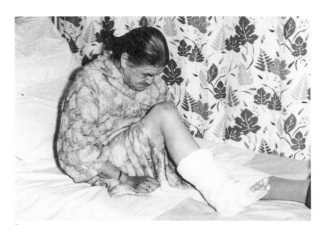

b2

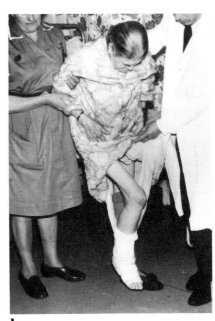

b1

b3

developing an inflammatory response or pus because the blood supply is insufficient for this. If a damaging pathogen, such as *Staphylococcus aureus*, is present it may cause a steady deterioration in the skin around the ulcer which becomes cyanosed, devitalized and eventually gangrenous. The significance of this change is often not appreciated because of the lack of inflammation so that it is regarded as just part of the ischaemic process. This is far from so and if nothing is done the area of damage will extend so that amputation may become inevitable even if the blood supply can be improved by arterial reconstruction. Recognition of this change, readiness to

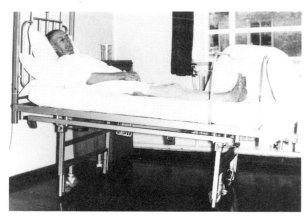

**Figure 17.8** *Care of the critically ischaemic foot. When a decision upon the feasibility of arterial reconstruction awaits urgent arteriography the patient should be nursed as shown here; the bed is placed in a slight foot-down position because this gives marginal assistance to the arterial supply and it also indicates to everyone that, in no circumstances, should the limb be elevated. A cage is used to protect the toes and forefoot from the slightest weight of bedclothes. The patient is asked to give the feet frequent movements in order to promote venous return, and every hour to get up and walk about for a few minutes. In this way joints and the antigravity muscles can be kept in good condition. The patient should not be allowed to hang the leg out of bed and adequate analgesia must be given. The room temperature should be warm enough to release sympathetic vasoconstrictor tone and the foot allowed to assume room temperature*

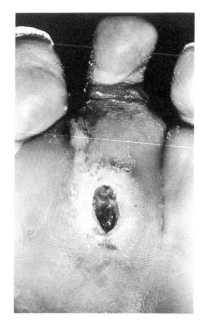

**a**

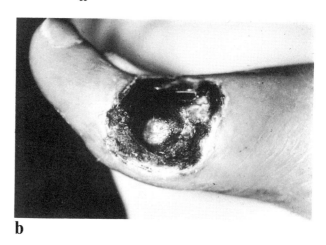

**b**

**Figure 17.9** *Diabetic ulceration and neuropathy.*

*(a) A perforating ulcer on the sole of the foot under a metatarsal head is one of the commonest diabetic lesions in the foot, due to neuropathy (see also Colour Plate 8). Although painless, it is an unstable condition which will eventually allow entry of infection which causes a slowly spreading diabetic cellulitis that will eventually destroy a large part of the foot, with the patient scarcely aware that anything is amiss. This may be forestalled by excision of the head of the metatarsal, together with the corresponding toe, to allow redistribution of the weight to other bony prominences, and it may be some years before they too are involved in a similar process*

*(b) The arterial circulation is quite good but loss of the protective reflexes due to diabetic neuropathy has caused pressure necrosis and skin gangrene over the head of the first metatarsal bone. In diabetic neuropathy, the skin over any bony prominence in the affected area is vulnerable to pressure.*

culture and the use of an appropriate antibiotic can stop this process and give the foot its best opportunity if arterial reconstruction proves feasible.

Similarly, in the ischaemic foot, a streptococcal cellulitis spreading widely from an ulcer may prove very deceptive because of the muted response. It will be accompanied by pain, a diffuse dull redness, and slight swelling. If the patient is hanging the leg out of bed the swelling will be more marked and in elevation the colour in the forefoot will change to pallor. Crisis can often be delayed by an antibiotic which will give time for the feasibility of arterial reconstruction to be assessed.

Bacteriology of the venous ulcer is also important although there is a tendency for some authorities to be dismissive over this. In the author's experience the presence of a pathogen, especially *Staphylococcus aureus*, can be the cause of considerable pain in an ulcer and failure to respond to treatment. Certainly a range of harmless organisms is usual in the venous ulcer but, unless it is looking in a 'healthy' and settled state, culture is advised, with treatment by an appropriate antibiotic if a known pathogen is identified.

Similar considerations apply to a diabetic lesion.

## Diabetic lesions

Certain aspects of diabetes can affect both arterial and venous lesions, and, of course, diabetes may produce its own characteristic ulceration. A diabetic ulcer is caused by three factors:

1. The presence of a diabetic neuropathy with diminished appreciation of pain so that there is loss of the

protective reflexes and trophic ulceration develops. This occurs over bony prominences, such as the head of a metatarsal bone, where the skin may be crushed by prolonged pressure between hard bone and the ground. Because there is no pain, this does not provoke a protective change of position to transfer the weight elsewhere and in this way an ulcer is created. This ulcer is a sensory phenomenon and is often seen in the presence of a good arterial supply. The usual sites are under a metatarsal head or heel, or over a toe joint or malleolus (Figure 17.9) because these areas are particularly vulnerable to pressure, but for the same reason a purely ischaemic ulcer is also likely to occur at these sites. Occurrence of an ulcer at one or more of these places is almost certain to be due to sensory loss (as in tabes or diabetes), or ischaemic, or a combination of the two.

2. Nevertheless, ischaemia in varying degree is common in diabetes and may either combine with sensory loss to produce an ulcer or be the sole cause of skin gangrene and ulceration.

3. Diabetic tissue is prone to infection and unless the diabetes is well controlled any open ulcer is likely to allow infection into the surrounding tissue. A characteristic form of this is a slowly invasive cellulitis (Figure 17.10(a), (b)) causing necrosis of all deeper tissues, including ligaments and tendons, and invasion of joints. In the presence of diabetic neuropathy this very destructive process will cause no pain and will not be noticed by the patient. The area of tissue involved becomes oedematous but may show little true inflammation and no tenderness. The overlying skin

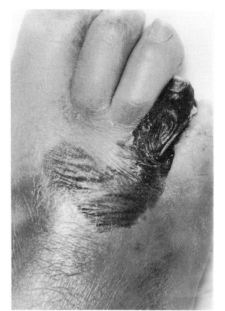

**a**

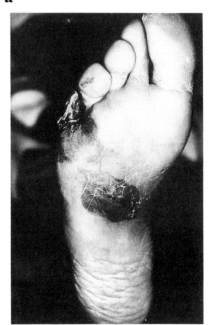

**b**

**Figure 17.10**  *'Silent' destruction of a foot by infection in diabetes.*

*(a)  Diabetic cellulitis (tunnelling gangrene) spreading from a gangrenous toe. There was no pain in this foot which showed only moderate oedema, little inflammatory response and no tenderness to pressure. In fact most of the tendons on the underside of the foot were necrotic and infection too deeply entrenched for the foot to be saved so that below-knee amputation was necessary. This 'silent', low-grade cellulitis, smouldering through the foot over many weeks, is very destructive and typical of diabetes.*

*(b)  Similar extensive damage within the foot in another diabetic patient, spreading from a gangrenous little toe. This process was painless but lead to loss of the foot. Any break in the skin of a diabetic is a potentially dangerous portal of entry for infection (see also Colour Plate 9).*

*(c)  The ultimate stage of a neuropathic diabetic foot. After many years with surgery at intervals, removing various bony prominences, diabetic cellulitis has escaped and inflicted severe damage through the foot and into the lower leg. A below-knee amputation was necessary here but earlier recognition of the diabetic cellulitis with a forefoot amputation might possibly have given this foot further use, but the ulceration underneath indicates that the neuropathic changes are too extensive and the limit of usefulness has been reached*

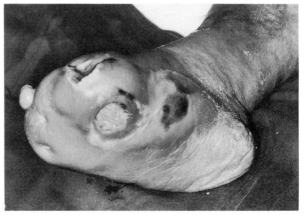

**c**

is intact but yet there is extensive destruction of underlying tissues. At this stage the cure can only be by removing all the necrotic tissue which usually means excision of, at least, the metatarsal head with associated ligaments and tendons, or if more extensive, a forefoot amputation; in many cases the process is so extensive and involving the lower leg that amputation below the knee may be necessary (Figure 17.10(c)). All too often this process has passed from a recoverable state to an irrecoverable one whilst under medical observation. An excellent account of surgical conservation of the neuropathic foot is given by Warren (1989).

Such a patient may, of course, also have an incidental venous disorder which may be blamed for a small ulcer under a metatarsal head, or over a malleolus, with oedema extending from it. Delay in effective action may lead to loss of the foot and it is therefore essential that the venous specialist should be alert to the possibility of a primary diabetic lesion or of diabetes concurrent with venous or arterial problems. The only defence against this insidious diagnostic pitfall is conscious awareness of this possibility and routine checking of the urine for sugar or by estimation of the blood sugar level.

## Venous ulceration with unsuspected concurrent arterial disease

It has already been pointed out that a venous disorder in the middle aged or elderly patient may well be accompanied by at least some arterial disease and ischaemia. Symptoms of arterial origin, such as intermittent claudication or rest pain, may all too easily be attributed to the clearly visible venous state and this may have a number of undesirable consequences, similar to those considered with ischaemic ulcer above:

1. There will not be any satisfactory response to treatment, pain will continue and the ulcer will fail to thrive.
2. Elevation or use of elastic compression may do harm and increase the patient's discomfort and cause an ulcer to deteriorate.
3. A possibly treatable condition, occlusion of main arteries, may remain untreated and eventually cause loss of the limb.
4. If occlusion in the main arteries is not recognized the best means for arterial reconstruction, the saphenous vein, may be needlessly discarded by an operation removing it to treat less serious venous manifestations. An operation removing the long saphenous vein and using it, reversed, as an arterial bypass may be a brilliant success by dealing with the arterial and the venous problems at the same time; this is an opportunity that must not be wasted (Figures 17.11, 17.12). The same considerations apply (see below) to the

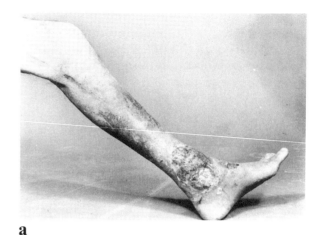

**a**

**b**

**Figure 17.11** *(a), (b) Extensive ulceration on both aspects of the leg due to combined atherosclerotic femoropopliteal arterial occlusion and massive incompetence in the long saphenous vein. Both the limbs showed similar changes and, on one side, removal of the saphenous vein, reversing it, and using it for femoropopliteal arterial bypass, gave an excellent result with complete healing of the ulceration. However, the same procedure carried out on the opposite side gave only temporary benefit to the ulcers which eventually reappeared (shown here) even though the arterial reconstruction continued to work well and allowed a below-knee amputation to heal well when this became necessary. If the cause of venous stasis is saphenous incompetence, the opportunity must not be missed to use this vein for arterial reconstruction*

patient who has coronary heart disease and may be suitable for aorta to coronary bypassing.

## Relationship of arterial insufficiency (ischaemia) to venous disorder

Although various studies have shown that the incidence and severity of venous disorders and arterial disease increase with age, there is no evidence of a direct relationship in the development of the two conditions; they happen to share rather similar age groups. However, arterial disease may well have direct influence on the ability of a limb to tolerate the ill effects of venous

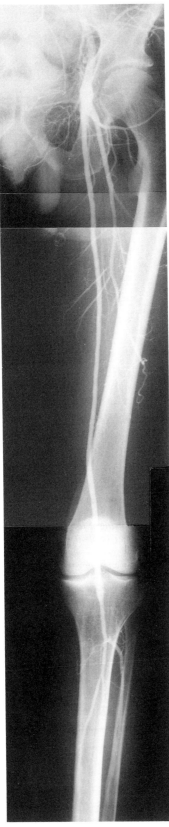

**Figure 17.12** *An example of the good result that can be obtained by arterial reconstruction, using an autogenous graft of reversed long saphenous vein running from common femoral to lower popliteal artery (patient's left side). This arteriogram was obtained during assessment of the opposite side 6 years later*

hypertension, particularly on the skin, leading to ulceration. Cornwall, Dore and Lewis (1986), in a study of 117 lower limbs with ulceration, found that 90% had evidence of a venous defect and 31% of these had significant ischaemia, shown by Doppler flowmeter assessment of the blood pressure in the leg. It was concluded that reduced arterial supply is a factor in delayed response to treatment of venous ulceration. Although in a venotensive limb, with a certain amount of oedema and liposclerosis, there may be some doubt about the accuracy of Doppler-based assessment, it is certainly possible that moderately severe ischaemia aggravates any tendency to venous ulceration and in older patients may account for a significant number of cases where a venous ulcer fails to respond to treatment. Nevertheless, many cases of venous ulceration occur in young patients without any hint of arterial disease and, conversely, many quite severely ischaemic limbs with coexisting venous disorders do not develop ulceration. Whilst it must be acknowledged that ischaemia can be a significant factor in the elderly patient, there is no evidence that this is an essential requirement for venous ulceration to occur in all patients.

The dire consequences of misdiagnosing and treating a purely ischaemic ulcer as a venous ulcer have been considered at length earlier in this chapter, but the hazard of treating venous ulceration when there is unrecognized accompanying arterial disease can be just as serious. In a very comprehensive study of 600 patients with chronic venous ulcers (827 legs), Callam *et al.* (1987a) assessed the arterial supply by Doppler measurement of the ankle/brachial pressure index and found this to be at or below 0.9 in 21%, and below 0.7 in 10%; in 11% the pedal pulses could not be felt, 136 patients had an associated history of cerebrovascular or coronary heart disease and 31 patients had intermittent claudication, all with a low Doppler pressure index in the ulcerated limb. In patients under the age of 40 years, venous ulcers showed no evidence of associated arterial disease but the incidence rose steadily with increasing age to reach 50% over the age of 80 years. In a separate control group, 176 legs were indentified with reduced arterial supply and of these 52% had definite evidence of venous insufficiency. It is clear from this that arterial disease and venous disorder with ulceration share an increasing prevalence with age and if one is present there is a real likelihood that the other is also present in greater or lesser degree. These authors, quite rightly, stress the danger that arterial disease may be overlooked in patients with chronic venous ulceration and urge that arterial assessment should be carried out in all patients before any treatment by compression bandage is employed. They give as factors pointing to the presence of a significant ischaemia, increasing likelihood with the age of the patient, evidence of arterial disease elsewhere, and an ulcer positioned on the foot. The most damaging error arises when a patient with severe ischaemia has obvious, but incidental, venous changes so that the condition is wrongly attributed to these. The same authors quote eight cases in their own experience where application of compression bandage actually precipitated the need for amputation and a survey amongst surgeons in their area indicated that many had encountered the same mistake in the management of patients with ulceration.

The findings in the study referred to above have been given at some length because they are in full accord with our own experience, given earlier in this chapter, when ischaemic ulceration is mistaken for a venous ulcer. With such mistreatment the limb may have little chance of survival, but fortunately there is now much wider recognition of this danger. Equally important is to recognize when a limb with typical venous ulceration also has an ischaemic component and may not tolerate strong elastic compression or high elevation. Elevation was not specifically mentioned in the study by Callam *et al.*, but it must be stressed that this can be even more damaging than elastic compression. In the limb with ischaemic ulceration the arterial supply may be so reduced that elevation of the foot by 0.5 m above the horizontal renders the forefoot and toes totally bloodless with tissue death within a few hours.

## Checklist of additional questions and examinations when arterial disease is possible

If the patient has moderate to severe venous stasis with all the usual manifestations, including threatened or actual ulceration, especially if middle aged or older, or the ulcer is not a typical exudative venous ulcer with surrounding pigmentation, then additional information must be obtained upon:

1. Any history suggesting intermittent claudication or sleep disturbed by rest pain (but beware of confusion with nocturnal cramps which are commonplace).
2. The femoral, popliteal, posterior tibial and dorsalis pedis (normally absent in 10%) pulses must be checked by palpation.
3. If there is any uncertainty about pulses, check with Doppler flowmeter for pulsatility and waveform of ankle pulses; estimate ankle/brachial Doppler pressure index. Below 0.8 this is becoming a significant reduction but is only truly meaningful when it is 0.7 or below; 0.5 or below indicates a severe ischaemia sufficient to account for ulceration and rest pain; at this level certainly preserve the saphenous vein for reconstructive surgery. Other appropriate clinical tests and special investigations have been given earlier in this chapter in the section on ischaemic ulcer, including the need to exclude diabetes.

## Policy decisions; preservation of the saphenous vein

If the various tests above indicate significant arterial disease is present, the saphenous vein should not be sacrificed in an attempt to improve the venous state without most careful evaluation and this will now be considered.

*Factors to be considered if venous ulceration is present together with ischaemia due to arterial occlusion*

When obvious venous stasis with ulceration is present together with arterial occlusion some complex considerations may arise. The long saphenous vein is a most valuable 'spare part' in arterial reconstruction in the lower limbs (Figure 17.12) and coronary arteries, and, especially if arterial disease is present, must never be sacrificed for purely venous reasons without careful thought upon the patient's possible essential need for this vein in arterial reconstruction.

If the ischaemia is severe and arterial reconstruction is known to be feasible, and is regarded as essential, then these facts must be born in mind:

1. Balloon angioplasty may be a simple way out but the arterial lesion may not be suitable for this or it has been tried and failed. In this case, reconstruction using the long saphenous vein as a bypass should give the best long-term result in comparison with alternatives such as the use of a synthetic arterial prosthesis.
2. If the long saphenous vein is massively incompetent it is likely to be grossly enlarged, with saccules beneath leaking valves, and not suitable for use as a bypass arterial substitute.
3. If the venous hypertension causing the ulcer is due to deep vein impairment, as in a post-thrombotic limb, then the long saphenous may be acting as an important collateral. If this vein is removed and used to restore the arterial supply, there will be two adverse effects: (a) The venous state may be aggravated. (b) A successful arterial reconstruction in the presence of venous obstruction may considerably increase oedema in the limb. This makes it undesirable in many cases of post-thrombotic limb to use its long saphenous vein for arterial reconstruction.

The key to the situation is the role being played by the saphenous vein. Is it the cause of the venous ulcer or is it playing a compensatory role, as in the post-thrombotic limb? Appropriate action in these two cases is now considered further.

*Case report 1.* The saphenous vein is causative as evidenced by: unequivocal control given by a Trendelenburg test (carried out as described in Chapter 2); photoplethysmography shows a very short recovery period after exercise which is restored to normal when the long saphenous vein is temporarily blocked; additional confirmation, if it is needed, is given by a functional phlebogram showing spillover down the saphenous vein and a widely patent deep vein throughout. In these circumstances the following options are available:

1. The saphenous vein is removed, reversed so that valves do not oppose flow, and used as best as can be as an arterial bypass. Large saccules beneath leaking saphenous valves must be excised and the vein resutured, otherwise rupture of a saccule under arterial pressure may occur. Massive oversize in the saphenous vein, together with repairs of this sort do, of course, reduce the chance of success. However, this would seem preferable to raiding the opposite limb for its saphenous vein; experience shows that this may be needed in its turn to save that limb. The technique of 'in situ' bypass with the saphenous vein is an alternative but if saccules are present these may be ruptured during instrumental division of valve cusps. The author's preference would be to remove the vein, inspect it and carry out any necessary repairs to make sure that the best possible use is made of an otherwise unsatisfactory vein. This procedure, although with a reduced chance of success, stands a reasonable chance of restoring the arterial supply to near normal and at the same time removing the principal cause for the venous problem. In these respects it is ideal.

2. Raiding the opposite limb is an option but it may be regretted later on if that too needs rescuing, as is often the case. Instead, use the best alternative technique for arterial reconstruction, such as balloon angioplasty, use of a synthetic arterial prosthesis or endarterectomy. This will allow the saphenous vein to be left undisturbed as a final reserve, admittedly unsatisfactory, for possible future reconstruction to a limb or coronary artery; when the arterial supply has been successfully restored the venous state can be treated by the usual conservative means, elevation and external support. Alternatively, with a good arterial circulation established there is no real contraindication to removing the saphenous vein if it is badly at fault and regarded as worthless for any future reconstruction.

*Case report 2.* The long saphenous vein is not at fault and is not causing the ulcer but is acting as an important collateral in a post-thrombotic limb. Removing this may do harm and certainly, with arterial reconstruction, will increase oedema. Therefore, reconstruct the artery if possible by using another vein, for example, a cephalic vein, or by one of the other techniques given in the last paragraph but, as stated there, try not to raid the opposite limb for its vein. Once arterial supply is restored the venous problems in the post-thrombotic limb may be treated by the usual principles (see Chapter 8).

*Note on the use of allograft (homograft) veins for arterial reconstruction.* Using the saphenous vein from another patient, abundantly available from varicose vein surgery, is a tempting proposition but most certainly will not give

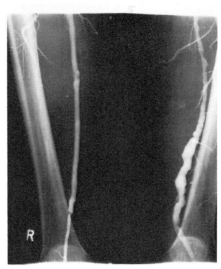

**Figure 17.13** *Allograft or homograft vein, taken from another patient, should not be used for arterial reconstruction. In this patient an incompetent long saphenous vein, removed from another patient, was used as an arterial bypass in order to avoid amputation. This arteriogram, 2 years later, shows irregular aneurysmal change through the graft; soon after this it thrombosed and ceased to work. Homograft arteries, used extensively in the 1950s, showed similar changes after a year or two and usually gave benefit of rather short duration. By contrast, use of the patient's own living tissue, an autogenous vein graft, for arterial reconstruction, is capable of giving prolonged good long-term results. For this reason, and for its possible use in coronary artery bypass, the long saphenous vein should never be sacrificed without good reason, particularly when the patient already has evidence of arterial disease. Although an oversized, incompetent long saphenous vein is less than ideal for this purpose it may offer the best prospect of a successful result*

the same good results as an autogenous graft of the patient's own vein; indeed, like the homograft arteries used in the 1950s (Eastcott, 1969; Sawyer and Kaplitt, 1978), the inevitable degenerative changes in an allograft might eventually create a dangerous aneurysmal state in the graft (Figure 17.13) or at best lead to its early occlusion. Moreover, there are serious medical and legal implications from the possibility of conveying viral infections, such as hepatitis B or HIV, if fresh tissue is used. Without a most careful screening and subsequent processing, use of an allograft vein as a 'one off' procedure is not permissible.

*Policy if arterial surgery is not carried out but may be needed in the future so that it is desirable to preserve the long saphenous vein*

If arterial reconstruction is not considered essential and is not carried out, but it is recognized that the saphenous vein should be preserved in case the limb deteriorates further, or possibly because it may be required for a coronary bypass procedure, what can be done to improve the venous state without damaging the saphenous vein?

If the venous problem is post-thrombotic the question is scarcely relevant because, in all probability, this vein should not be removed because of its valuable collateral role. Not only will its removal fail to bring benefit to the venous state but it may aggravate it; cautious conservative treatment of the venous condition (see below) is all that is available and there is no conflict of interest.

If, however, the problem is of massive incompetence in the saphenous system causing ulceration, then one of the following options can be considered:

- If the long saphenous vein is so abnormal as to be totally worthless for any form of arterial reconstruction it may be permissible to remove it.
- Inject the varicosities only, in the hope that this will bring improvement without damage to the saphenous vein itself.
- Remove the varicosities surgically but leaving the saphenous vein itself intact.
- Treat the venous problem with a cautious, modified, conservative programme of elevation and external support.

These possibilities are now discussed further.

**Removing saphenous veins** The long saphenous vein may be so enlarged and with multiple saccules that it is clearly going to be far less satisfactory for use in arterial reconstruction than alternative techniques, say, balloon angioplasty or using a synthetic graft. After weighing up all the factors involved, and, if necessary, discussion with an arterial surgeon, it may be permissible to remove the saphenous vein. This should only be done if the venous tests give strong indication of real benefit in doing this and if the ischaemia is not too severe. Even so the improvement in the ulcer may be less than expected.

**Injection of varicosities only** Sclerotherapy by injection to varicose branches of the saphenous vein is probably not wise. The firm compression bandage necessary to achieve sclerosis with minimal thrombus formation may cause harm or even danger to the limb if the ischaemia is moderately severe. Moreover, if the varicosities are not compressed to prevent filling, then excessive thrombus may form and extend into the saphenous vein itself. The likelihood of damaging this vein so that it is no longer suitable as an arterial bypass graft must be appreciable and in this case surgery to the vein would have been more effective and less troublesome for the patient. A severe ischaemia, indicated by pallor of the forefoot on elevation, is a direct contraindication to sclerotherapy. This limb is in a highly precarious state, easily pushed into severe rest pain or gangrene requiring amputation, and in any case treatment should be directed to improving the arterial state rather than treating the lesser venous problem.

**Surgery to varicosities only** Surgical removal of the varicosities, with preservation of the long saphenous vein, is a permissible option and may well be beneficial if clinical tests are favourable, especially if there is good control of the varicosities by localized finger pressure to their upper end. A cautious approach is desirable and the surgeon must ensure that there is an adequate arterial supply for satisfactory healing in the vicinity of the proposed operation. Surgical dissection should be minimized and whilst tunnelling is permissible, undermining a large area of skin is not. This procedure is again contraindicated in limbs with pallor of the forefoot or toes on elevation; once more, the main priority here should be to restore blood supply by arterial reconstruction if possible.

**Conservative treatment** The well-tried venous measures of elevation and external support may be given cautious trial if the ischaemia is not too severe (pressure index above 0.8). A large proportion of the day can be spent with the leg horizontal, but not raised above this unless ischaemia is minimal and colour well maintained on elevation. The horizontal position is safe and, from the venous standpoint, greatly to be preferred to prolonged periods of dependency. Regarding elastic support this may be used with a low compression of 20 mmHg, provided the ischaemia is minimal. This can be given trial and a useful check would be to confirm by a photoplethysmograph that it continues to show arterial pulsation in the forefoot or toes with the stocking on and the limb horizontal. Far better is to use external support without compression, that is, by inelastic support, the paste bandage. This must be applied snugly but without any compressive force, with the leg in a horizontal position and the forefoot circulation checked a few hours later; the patient should be instructed to return immediately if there is any undue discomfort.

## Notes in brief on other venous to arterial relationships

### Does venous disorder encourage arterial disease?

The presence of obvious venous disorder may mislead the examiner so that a more significant arterial state is ignored and this has been considered in some detail earlier in this chapter. On the separate question, whether venous disorder encourages arterial disease, there is no evidence of this but the consequence of arterial disease, ischaemia, may well be accentuated by a background of venous hypertension. Ischaemic ulceration may occur more readily in skin already damaged by venous stasis and prove more intractable. However, this observation is of little help in the practical management; it is the recognition that ischaemic and venous damage are interacting that is important and this has been considered at length previously.

*Venous thrombosis in relation to arterial disease or injury, and small vessel disorders*

1. Buerger's disease (Eastcott, 1969), an occluding arteritis in young adults who smoke (Figure 17.3), is well recognized to give localized, or sometimes extensive, venous thrombosis (phlebitis migrans) and no doubt there are other rare forms of arterial disease that may do the same. Here artery and vein seem to be victims of the same thrombotic process.

2. There is little evidence that atherosclerosis in older patients directly encourages venous thrombosis. However, extensive venous thrombosis in leg veins, superficial and deep, not infrequently complicates a severe ischaemia of the limb and finally determines its loss. This may be accompanied by a moderate to extensive oedema, perhaps even a moist gangrene (Figure 17.14) (other causes for moist gangrene include sudden ischaemia in a previously oedematous limb, as in arterial embolism complicating heart failure, or gangrene occurring as a complication of diabetes). In these circumstances thrombosis is encouraged by severe ischaemia, together with prolonged immobility and dependency resulting from this, rather than the arterial disease per se. It is a consequence of ischaemia rather than part of the intrinsic arterial pathology.

3. As part of widespread intravascular thrombosis due to increased coagulability, for example, in polycythaemia, thrombocythaemia or some types of leukaemia.

4. Following amputation. In the author's experience, mid-thigh amputation is more prone to massive iliofemoral thrombosis than below-knee or Gritti–Stokes' amputations. An important factor in this may be the near-complete stasis in the remaining large capacity veins now deprived of virtually all source of flow. To this must be added factors related to all the circumstances leading up to the amputation. Prolonged immobility by sitting, especially with the stump hanging down, must be undesirable here.

5. When artery and vein are injured simultaneously it is necessary to clear the ends of the divided vein of clot and thrombus before repairing the vein (see section upon injury and repair of veins, Chapter 21).

6. Prolonged oedema following arterial reconstruction. This may be due to unmasking of a pre-existing tendency for oedema due to impaired deep veins, usually post-thrombotic, or lymphatic insufficiency. This may be unavoidable and indeed predictable beforehand. With the renewed arterial supply, control of the oedema by elevation and elastic support may be used more freely.

   An acute deep vein thrombosis may have preceded or may follow arterial surgery (Figure 16.3). This will require the usual treatment, but beware of fibrinolytic therapy within 10 days, or heparin treatment within 5 days, of surgery. Oedema may be very persistent from this cause and, as a point of interest, the sudden disappearance of this oedema signifies that the arterial reconstruction has closed off.

   The oedema may have lymphatic origin due to disturbance of lymphatics in the track of a bypass procedure or, more likely, to damage of lymphatics and glands in the groin. Dissection in this region must not disregard these structures. They are not difficult to recognize and can often be displaced rather than divided.

7. Venous thrombosis after using a tourniquet. Outmoded methods, indiscriminately using tight bands as tourniquets around a limb, certainly produced unacceptable complications, including venous thrombosis. With well-regulated present methods, using a pneumatic cuff at a controlled pressure, few cases are reported but there appears to be insufficient studies of possible complications following their use during surgical operations. Even if the present complication rate is low there must be some degree of increased risk in using a tourniquet so that it should never be employed without good reason. For instance, its use to avoid a small blood loss in varicose vein surgery (Corbett and Jayakumar, 1989) would not seem justifiable, although it must be admitted that statistical evidence to support this view is not available. One does however see the occasional case where a tourniquet appears to have precipitated venous thrombosis and caused a post-thrombotic limb, but other factors beside the tourniquet will have been present at the same time and no valid conclusion can be drawn. An attitude of considerable respect for the potential danger inherent in a tourniquet is advisable (Klenerman, 1982; Fletcher and Healy, 1983).

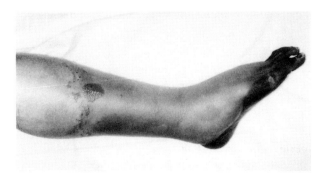

**Figure 17.14** *Extensive gangrene with oedema, caused by deep vein thrombosis superimposed on severe ischaemia. A 'moist gangrene' of this sort is prone to infection which can spread to the surviving upper part of the limb and into the bloodstream. This form of gangrene may require an amputation as a matter of urgency. In the example shown there was no break in the skin and infection had not supervened; the black shrunken toes, mummified by drying of the tissues, show that the onset of gangrene was at least 2 weeks previously*

*Relationship of venous to small vessel disorders and vasospastic conditions*

Raynaud's phenomenon (Heidrich, 1979; Cotton and Khan, 1986) and acrocyanosis with chilblains are two quite common conditions in this category. Venous thrombosis may occur in secondary Raynaud's phenomenon but caused by the process that is responsible for the phenomenon, for example, in leukaemia. Apart from this no definite relationship has been established between venous problems and these very distinctive vascular disorders in small blood vessels. However, an important association arises because the patient so often blames any varicosities that may be visible. Treating these may improve the strictly venous aspects but will not relieve the manifestations of Raynaud's or acrocyanosis and patients should be clearly warned of this. They often have high expectations that it will do so. The veins they complain of may be trivial and their real distress is over the spasms of numbness and pallor or the blue discolouration and chilblains in winter. It is wise to avoid sclerotherapy or surgery to veins in these circumstances unless they are undoubtedly defective, and the limited benefit to be expected is clearly understood by the patient.

Raynaud's phenomenon is, of course, a vasoconstrictive state caused by a wide range of conditions and only in the primary variety is it, perhaps, a disease in its own right. It may have serious significance and should have expert evaluation, supported by the appropriate laboratory tests.

Some of the causes of Raynaud's phenomenon and other ischaemic manifestations in the upper limb are detailed below:

1. Unilateral and asymmetrical:
   (a) Arterial disease in main artery, especially atherosclerosis.
   (b) Cervical rib or thoracic outlet syndrome (see Chapter 15).
   (c) Injection of thrombogenic material into an artery, e.g. barbiturates or a venous sclerosant. This may arise from a medical procedure (Figure 17.15) or from self-injection in drug addiction* (Figure 17.16).
2. Bilateral and symmetrical:
   (a) Primary Raynaud's disease, that is, where no cause can be demonstrated (cold sensitivity).
   (b) Secondary Raynaud's phenomenon: attacks of pallor in response to an endogenous disease process or due to external influences.

*This form of arterial injury is not likely to occur more than once and, for this reason, is not really in the category of Raynaud's phenomenon, which is a recurring state rather than an isolated episode. However, intra-arterial injection of thrombogenic agents is a disaster against which every precaution must be taken during the injection of varicose veins. Because of its importance to the venous specialist a section on this is included below and also see Chapter 19 on Sclerotherapy.

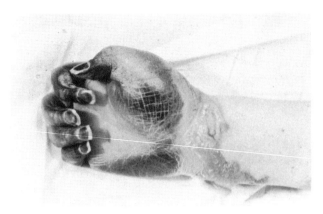

**Figure 17.15** *Many commonly used drugs, especially barbiturates, injected intra-arterially, cause severe damage to the intima, soon followed by thrombosis in the peripheral arteries. In the early days of pentothal (thiopentone) intravenous anaesthesia a number of cases were reported due to injection into the brachial artery in the cubital fossa. One such case is illustrated, a child in whom the entire hand was lost. The list of drugs capable of doing this is long and includes all agents used to sclerose varicose veins. Never give an intravenous injection in the vicinity of an artery, particularly in attempts to sclerose a perforatoring vein near the ankle*

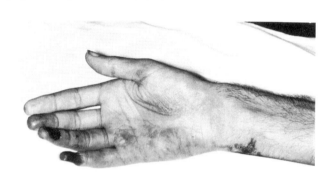

**Figure 17.16** *The hand of a drug addict who injected himself with barbiturates by self-insertion of a needle into the cubital fossa. The brachial artery was entered and there has been substantial loss of the fourth and fifth digits with ischaemic damage to the third digit, the ulnar portion of the hand and wrist. Accidental injection of a venous sclerosant into an artery near the ankle will cause corresponding damage to the foot and might well be even more extensive*

3. Examples of secondary Raynaud's phenomenon:
   1(a) Endogenous causes:
      (i)   Autoimmune diseases, rheumatoid arthritis, scleroderma and other collagen disorders.
      (ii)  Lupus erythematosis.
      (iii) Blood disorders, leukaemia, thrombocytosis, polycythaemia vera.
      (iv)  Circulating abnormal proteins, cryoglobulins, cold agglutinins, macroglobulinaemia, hyperfibrinogenaemia.
   (b) External influences:
      (i)   Inhaled or ingested chemical or drugs; e.g.

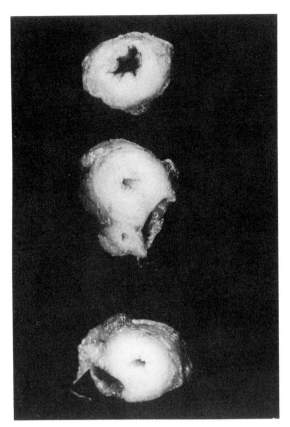

**Figure 17.17** *Ergot poisoning due to indiscriminate use of rectal suppositories containing ergotamine tartrate to relieve migraine is not particularly rare. The portions of artery shown here come from a young women who had not understood the importance of limiting her use of ergot and developed extensive bilateral gangrene in the lower limbs and eventually died. The sections are through a popliteal artery and show the contracted, thickened walls of the artery and narrowing of the lumen characteristic of severe ergotism. All patients on this therapy must understand the great danger of overdosage and that the warning given by pale, cold extremities, epecially with numbness or areas of gangrene on the digits, must be heeded if disaster is to be averted*

polyvinyl chloride (industrial), ergotamine (Figure 17.17).

(ii)  High frequency vibration, usually industrial, e.g. chain-saw, pneumatic riveter, a grinding process.

(iii)  Related to smoking, especially in early Buerger's disease (thromboangiitis obliterans) (Figure 17.3).

(iv)  Contraceptive pill or oestrogen therapy.

## Intra-arterial injection of thrombogenic agents

If injected into an artery, a wide range of otherwise well-accepted therapeutic agents cause intense damage to the endothelium distally, soon followed by heavy deposition and aggregation of platelets, with thrombosis of the affected vessels. There is immediate onset of severe pain and rapidly increasing ischaemia in the parts supplied by the artery, and widespread tissue death occurs within a few hours. Once initiated there is no reliable way of averting this sequence of events. The same agents injected into a vein may cause no more than a local thrombosis because the thrombogenic effect is quickly diminished by dilution as the stream enters ever larger veins as it travels centrally; with arteries, the stream of material travels distally in unreduced concentration through ever smaller vessels upon which the tissues are dependent for their blood supply.

The materials that may cause this certainly include a number that are commonly used intravenously. Many disciplines in medicine have had to learn the bitter lesson of a familiar drug, that can be injected safely into a vein, causing extensive gangrene, with loss of an extremity, when accidently injected into the neighbouring artery. Barbiturates are in this category and the introduction of pentothal (thiopentone) in the 1940s brought a crop of disasters (Figure 17.15). This arose because of the proximity of the brachial artery to the cubital vein, at that time commonly used for introducing intravenous anaesthetic agents. Since then the anaesthetists have insisted upon an exemplary set of precautions to prevent this happening, mainly by total avoidance of any vein near an artery and a system of pausing before the main injection is put in; usually a small vein on the back of the hand is used.

*Avoidance of intra-arterial injection during sclerotherapy*

The materials used in sclerotherapy, by their very nature, are particularly damaging to arteries. Cockett (1986) refers to 18 cases, known to medical defence societies, or that have been published by various surgeons over the last 10 years, of injection of a sclerosing agent into or around an artery during sclerotherapy for varicose veins. The resulting gangrene led to below-knee amputation in two patients and transmetatarsal amputation in a further twelve, with persisting disability in the other four. Undoubtedly other cases, not published, have occurred. The consequences in terms of distress and disability to the patient, and the medicolegal and professional implications for the medical attendant do not need emphasis. Cockett in his analysis makes these points:

1.  All of the sclerosants in common use are equally capable of causing arterial damage and none can be considered to be safe in this respect. The only safe course is to avoid any possibility of entering an artery, even a small one (Figure 17.18).

2.  All the cases referred to arose from attempts to inject a perforating vein just above the ankle on the inner aspect of the leg, where the posterior tibial artery is near to the surface and easily entered by a needle. Injection into this area must be avoided. Although Cockett does not refer to the front of the ankle, the anterior tibial artery must be vulnerable here and this is another area for special care or avoiding completely.

In addition to the areas just described, injection at any

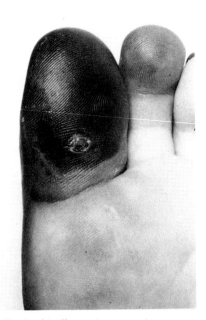

**Figure 17.18** *In this illustration extensive gangrene of the great toe has been caused by the injection of sodium tetradecyl sulphate into a plantar wart of a boy aged 12 years; only 0.1 ml of 3% solution was used but it must have entered the artery of supply to the wart and was sufficient to cause loss of the great toe*

level may strike a small artery and cause local skin gangrene. To minimize these risks, the point of the needle must never be plunged deeply out of sight or touch; it must be seen to enter a varicose vein and must not probe for the invisible or inpalpable vein. Blood should be withdrawn before injecting and if this is bright red, or certainly if it is pulsatile, the needle should be withdrawn without any injection. (Blood from veins can be unexpectedly bright red at times but it is better to heed the warning and reinsert the needle elsewhere rather than ignore any hint of danger.) Having withdrawn a little blood satisfactorily, a small amount of sclerosant is injected, followed by a pause before putting in the full amount (0.5 ml as maximum), so that any adverse effect may be judged; if the patient experiences pain then nothing further should be injected at that site and possibly, depending on the severity of pain, the procedure should be abandoned altogether.

The venous specialist must ensure that his junior staff fully understand the danger and are well trained in good techniques of injection before permitting them to carry out sclerotherapy unaided.

Drug addicts, injecting themselves in the cubital fossa, where the vein they seek overlies the brachial artery, not infrequently enter the artery and cause severe ischaemic damage to digits, hand and often the forearm. The author has seen three such cases due to injection of barbiturates (Figure 17.16).

## Treatment

Prevention here is infinitely preferable to attempted cure. At best, treatment promptly given can do little more than reduce the extent of damage. Probably nothing can avert the rapidly progressive changes in the main area affected, and only the fringe areas can be protected. The usual advice is to give heparin (500 units) into the artery immediately, through the same needle if it is still in place, and maintain full heparin anticoagulation for some days afterwards by intravenous means. There is a danger that the anxious medical attendant may increase the damage by excessive treatment unlikely to improve matters. In this category, sustained administration of heparin or other materials by cannula into the artery may inflict further trauma upon it, and should only be used for a short period if it is essential to deliver the therapeutic agent locally, for example, when prostacylins are employed. An attempt to combine sympathectomy, by surgery or by injection of phenol, with anticoagulant therapy may produce yet further severe difficulties; experience has shown that the high incidence of haemorrhage and other complications this may cause is not justified by the benefits. However, a 'physiological sympathectomy', by keeping the patient's body well warmed, is recommended because it gives the desired effect and is safe.

Other agents that, theoretically, may prove helpful include dextran, cortisone and defibrinogenation with ancrod (Arvin). However, such polypharmacy is not free from problems and may complicate further an irredeemable situation. Use of fibrinolysis by streptokinase or platelet disaggregation with prostacyclins, given by direct infusion into the affected artery, is again of theoretical value but as yet unproven and should only be attempted by those fully conversant with this form of treatment.

## Permissible intra-arterial injections

A number of medical procedures involve deliberate injection into an artery, for example during arteriography, but here the medium used is carefully selected and is known to be suitable for intra-arterial use. No material should be injected intra-arterially without being certain it is safe; if there is any uncertainty, it must be assumed that it is not suitable until 'proved otherwise'. Arteries are far too vulnerable to chemical injury to take any chance upon this. Low-osmolar opaque medium, introduced comparatively recently, has proved a considerable advance upon previous media by having much lower thrombogenicity and causing virtually no discomfort on intravascular injection. It is a most satisfactory medium for venography and it is rare to see any reaction in the vein used for its injection.

## Venous thrombosis mimicking acute ischaemia; 'pseudo-ischaemia'

It is well recognized that the first onset of a deep vein thrombosis in the lower limb may be mistaken for the acute ischaemia of a sudden occlusion or interruption of a main artery, as in arterial embolism or by trauma. The limb is in great discomfort and the patient often describes it as a numbness of the leg (as might occur in acute ischaemia) and on examination this seems to be so; with this there is quite marked pallor without any venous congestion or prominence of the superficial veins; oedema is present but appears slight, and perhaps most deceptive, the ankle pulses cannot be felt but are easily located on the normal side. Within a few hours, or the next day, the situation clarifies and the usual appearances of deep vein thrombosis are fully evident. A possible factor in this 'pseudo-ischaemia' is that rapid, extensive formation of thrombus causes the release of considerable serotonin (5-hydroxytryptamine) which produces an element of arterial spasm. Added to this is a rapid accumulation of oedema giving discomfort and remoteness of sensation, together with a pallid appearance. Although it is building up quite quickly and creating these disturbances, the oedema is not at first so very obvious to the observer but it is sufficient to cause these changes and to make ankle pulses difficult to detect. Similarly the Doppler flowmeter may find the arteries difficult to locate because their relationship to the surface is altered by oedema in all layers.

It is a good rule that a 'spot' diagnosis should always be followed by a logical evaluation to justify the instinctive one. Any suspected ischaemia of acute onset must include in its differential diagnosis the possibility that this is a pseudo-ischaemia due to early venous thrombosis. The presence of slight oedema and warmth in the foot and leg should heighten suspicion that this is so. The pulses may well be identified if the oedema fluid is squeezed away by prolonged firm pressure followed by careful palpation. A Doppler flowmeter should pick up the pulses and the search to locate an artery must not be given up too easily. In a true acute ischaemia a cause, such as heart disease (embolism) or trauma, is always apparent (Figure 17.19(a)), the limb will soon loose temperature and should not have any oedema (unless it was there beforehand) when compared with the other side. If there are continuing doubts an arteriogram can be used to confirm a normal arterial system but this should seldom be necessary. The clinical diagnosis of venous thrombosis should usually be sufficiently certain to proceed to venogram as a prelimary to anticoagulant or fibrinolytic therapy.

## Summary of main physical signs in a limb with acute ischaemia

The march of events in a limb with extensive, acute loss of arterial supply, and the accompanying physical signs, will be:

Within the first few hours:

- Pain, swiftly turning to numbness, with loss of sensation.
- Pallor and coldness to the touch in the extremity, with a cyanotic zone above this.
- Loss of arterial pulses by palpation or Doppler flowmetry.
- Cutaneous anaesthesia and, depending on extent and severity, loss of power of movement (due to loss of nerve function).

After 6 hours (in severe cases):

- Ischaemic contracture of muscle (exactly analogous to rigor mortis).

After 24 hours (in severe cases):

- Fixed staining of skin, giving a slate-blue colour which does not blanche on pressure (due to death of skin) (Figure 17.19(b)).

After many days:

- Drying of dead surface tissues with darkening colour through brown to black; skin becomes hard and shrunken (mummified). This is manifest gangrene (Figure 17.19(c)).

Figure 17.19 illustrates some of the features given above. In extreme cases there may be only 6 hours before massive irreversible death of tissue (muscle) occurs but often cessation of arterial supply is not absolute and the changes occur more slowly and are less extensive. Nevertheless, it is essential to recognize the acute ischaemia which may cause irretrievable damage and loss of the limb within 6 hours. A policy of 'wait and see' is not justifiable and in case of doubt an expert arterial opinion must be obtained immediately. In ischaemia resulting from trauma, reduced blood volume (haemorrhagic shock) may prevent assessment of the circulatory state of the limb and this will have to wait until the general state of the patient has been improved. In trauma, sensory loss from nerve injury may be confused with that caused by ischaemia.

## Ischaemic episodes due to microembolism of atheromatous debris

This is a very different form of ischaemia to that caused by abrupt blockage of main arteries as described above. Its onset is sudden in an older patient, with one, or sometimes both, feet becoming very painful and swollen

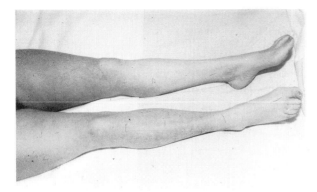

a

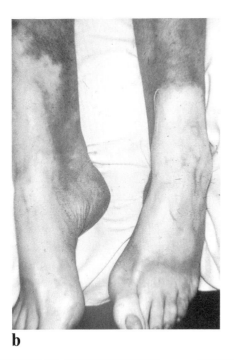

b

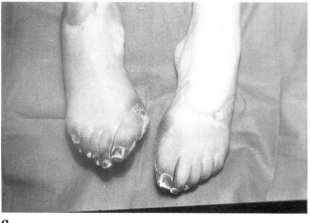

c

**Figure 17.19** *Acute ischaemia and its consequences.*
*(a) Acute ischaemia, bilaterally, caused by a 'saddle embolus' in a young women with mitral stenosis and auricular fibrillation. At onset there was acute pain which soon receded to numbness in the feet and legs. The illustration shows pallor extending almost to the knees with a cyanotic zone above this and normal colour in the thighs. The extremities were cold to the touch, with*

*complete loss of sensation; the femoral and all pulses below this were absent, and the patient was unable to move the feet or toes. Ischaemic calf muscle contracture had not yet occurred so that viability of the tissues was assumed and embolectomy to the aortic bifurcation was carried out successfully. Ischaemic contracture may occur within 8 hours of onset and is due to massive death of muscle so that amputation of the limb may be the only way of saving the patient. Fixed staining of the skin is another indication of tissue death and together with muscle contracture denotes irreversible changes which, if extensive, mean that the limb has been irretrievably lost. Ischaemia sufficient to cause anaesthesia should never be 'observed' overnight without effective treatment.*

*(b) This patient, similar to that above, was seen too late to save her limbs or her life. Medical advice was not sought until 48 hours after onset and this photograph was taken on admission to hospital. Both limbs were cold and without arterial pulses; below the knees there was no sensation and the skin showed fixed staining, that is, a slate-blue colour not blanched by pressure and denoting death of the skin; the white areas over the feet, shown in the photograph, are where her well-intentioned husband had placed a hot-water bottle to 'warm' her numb feet. Also seen in the photograph, are down-drawn feet caused by extensive ischaemic contracture of the calf muscles; this represents a massive death of tissue, analogous to rigor mortis, and gives warning that attempts to restore circulation to the limbs will put the patient's life in danger from highly toxic products of devitalized muscle entering the general bloodstream.*

*(c) This patient had similar but less severe ischaemia than the preceding one and her feet are shown 3 weeks after onset. All the features of late manifest gangrene in both feet are present. A demarcation line between living and dead tissue is shown and beyond this there is widespread fixed staining in keeping with skin death; the toes are blackened and wrinkled, typical of 'mummification' due to drying out of moisture, and this change confirms that it is several weeks since tissue death occurred. Some ischaemic contracture is present. This patient was very frail and succumbed soon after admission*

(Figure 17.20). On examination the foot and toes have a blotchy blue discolouration and are tender, but warm, to the touch; the ankle pulses may be present although the swelling may make their detection difficult without a Doppler flowmeter. Over the next few days small patches of gangrene develop on the toes. These changes can gradually recede with recovery of the foot. The likely explanation is microembolism of atheromatous debris, usually from the aorta, and causing diffuse blockage in capillary beds of the skin. It is unlikely to be confused with a venous thrombosis which is rarely confined to the foot.

## Some other circumstances affecting veins

### Venous obstruction by extrinsic pressure

This is seen in its most severe form when malignant glands surround the veins (Figure 9.11). Other firm swellings that may obstruct the deep veins are: malignant tumour, aneurysm, cysts near popliteal or hip joint. Entrapment

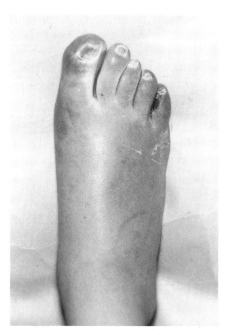

**Figure 17.20** *Ischaemia due to microembolism of atheromatous debris from the aorta. This elderly patient had sudden onset of a painful and slightly swollen right foot, seen here 4 days after onset. The foot was warm and the toes slightly blue with small patches of gangrene on them. Good ankle pulses were present but it was clear that the foot had sustained diffuse vascular damage. This recovered slowly over the next 2 months*

by muscle and tendons in the popliteal fossa (Connell, 1978; Iwai *et al.*, 1987), at the thoracic outlet (DeWeese, 1985) or axilla (Boontje, 1979), may cause intermittent obstruction and finally thrombosis in the vein. Obstruction of the left common iliac vein by the overlying right common iliac artery is described in Chapter 9.

## Venous thrombosis

This is not infrequently seen as a form of phlebitis migrans or an extensive deep vein thrombosis as an expression of hidden malignancy elsewhere in the body, particularly in carcinoma of the pancreas or bronchus. The contraceptive pill may precipitate venous or arterial thrombosis in a very small number of women, and in men hormonal treatment of prostatic carcinoma may have the same effect.

## Venous dilatation in large and small vessels with apparent weakening of the walls

This may be seen in widely differing circumstances and taking different forms:

1. In pregnancy the enlarged and, often, varicose veins are largely due to hormonal changes, principally oestrogen, but also in part caused by haemodynamic stresses, including raised venous pressure in pelvic veins resulting from the large return of blood from the placenta.

2. Hormones used therapeutically or circulating due to endocrine gland disturbance, such as Cushing's disease, may have a strong effect on all tissues including the veins; corticosteroids are particularly active in this respect.

3. Excessive consumption of alcohol, either as a direct effect on the veins or because of secondary effects by liver damage, appears to affect the veins in at least some people. An undue proportion of truly massive varicose veins that appear to have a structural weakness, are seen in publicans or other people who stand a great deal and drink excessively.

4. In prolonged dependency, particularly in neurological disorders, for example, in the paralysed lower limb after poliomyelitis, the foot and leg may have a deep puce colour with some oedema. It is also seen following injury to a limb, or in amputation stumps where physiotherapy to promote active exercise is not being carried out. Hysterical paralysis, especially if a self-applied constricting band is being used (oedeme bleu), has the same effect. In all the examples given above it is the capillary beds and venules that are affected to give the colour, in effect, a form of venous congestion. In neurological disorders, there may be an accompanying loss of vasomotor control. The patients are sometimes referred to the venous specialist but it is most unlikely that any treatment to the superficial veins, even if varicosed, will improve this state. Sympathectomy in this state is not helpful.

5. In heart failure distended venules and veins, with a generally congested appearance in the foot and lower leg, are commonly seen.

6. In old age, perhaps accentuated by heart failure, the thinned tissues and changed hormonal pattern, a bluish congested tint is often seen in the capillary beds of hands and feet, especially in dependency. This may give rise to unnecessary concern to doctor and patient.

## Acquired arteriovenous fistula in the limbs

Arteriovenous fistula or shunt (Branham, 1890; Holman, 1923, 1924, 1937; Allen, Barker and Hines, 1947; Eastcott, 1969; Gomes and Bernatz, 1970; Sako and Varco, 1970) is the term given to a communication between artery and vein without any intervening capillary bed so that blood at arterial pressure flows without resistance into low pressure veins. This may be a congenital condition, usually with multiple communications, and is described in Chapter 12. The acquired arteriovenous fistula is usually the result of some form of injury which opens up artery and vein simultaneously but occasionally arises spontaneously due to arterial disease. The acquired fistula is usually a single aperture, the size of which varies according to the circumstances.

*Note on pulsating varicose veins.* If pronounced pulsation, in time with the heart beat, is clearly visible, or found by Doppler flowmeter, in the varicose veins of a supine patient, it will inevitably suggest an arterial fistula and if it is accompanied by a typical machinery murmur then this is likely to be true. However, the pulsation may be similar to that seen in the jugular vein and caused by tricuspid valve regurgitation in a patient with heart disease. This can allow the pressure wave of right ventricular contraction to be transmitted down to an incompetent saphenous vein and its varicose branches (Blackett and Heard, 1988; Dayantus *et al.*, 1990). In this case a machinery murmur would not be present in the limb and this should alert the examiner to the probability of diagnosis other than arteriovenous fistula.

In similar fashion, thoracic pressure may by transmitted down to varicose veins and cause variation in their size from one moment to another. The obvious example is a cough impulse but any prolonged expiratory effort may cause a visible change, for example, the author recalls a lady musician with large varicose veins who was fascinated by their undulation in size as she played the French horn.

A photoplethysmograph will quite often detect a weak pulsation in flow in the capillary bed of a patient who has been standing for 30 seconds or more but this is not necessarily abnormal and, indeed, is a well-accepted method of recording pulse beats or arterial inflow into a limb. It indicates that the bed is well filled and responding to arterial inflow. The possible role of arteriovenous shunts in the formation of varicose veins and in venous disease generally is discussed in Chapter 23 under 'Diagnosis by ultrasound' in the section on pulsatile flow, and under 'Radionuclide scintigraphy' in the section on haemodynamic appraisal of pathogenesis in varicose veins.

## Arteriovenous fistula from injury: iatrogenic causes

Any form of injury which breaches artery and vein in close proximity may cause this condition (Figures 17.21, 17.22). The range of injuries is very wide but knife wounds, missiles and high velocity fragments are the commonest causes. The patient will therefore have a clear history of penetration through the skin but a closed injury can occasionally cause the condition by trauma from fractured bone ends. The condition may be seen in war injuries, knife fights or industrial injuries but less frequently in car accidents. It may also be caused, accidentally or deliberately, by surgical and medical procedures. There are many possible iatrogenic causes of this sort:

### As a planned procedure

1. To create large veins to facilitate repeated renal dialysis (Figure 17.23).

2. Following venous thrombectomy or reconstruction in order to maintain high flow of blood and distension of the vein for some weeks until vascular healing is complete with an endothelialized surface. The fistula may then be closed off by a further procedure.

3. In support of an arterial bypass procedure involving anastomosis to small distal arteries, such as the tibial vessels, especially when using synthetic or allogenic (e.g. umbilical) artery grafts. Again the object is to maintain high flow to the immediate vicinity of the restricted outlet into the distal artery. The advantages of this are debatable.

### As an accepted or incidental complication

1. Fistula may follow arterial bypassing when a long saphenous vein is used *in situ*. In this, the vein is left in place with its valve cusps divided by an instrument so that retrograde flow can occur. Any branches with defective valves may become, in effect, arteriovenous fistulas but these are usually detected during operation and ligated. Some may escape detection and require a separate procedure later on.

2. In attempts to save an ischaemic foot by arterializing the distal saphenous vein to create a circulation in reverse direction at full pressure into the capillary beds of the foot. This has not proved successful and is not recommended.

### Surgical accidents

1. During arterial bypass operations a recognized mistake is to insert the saphenous vein graft into the popliteal vein below the knee instead of into the artery. The vein here is robust, overlies the artery and contracts down so that it is quite easily mistaken for the artery. All arterial surgeons are aware of this trap and consciously identify both artery and vein. A number of cases are reported and in most the error was recognized within 48 hours and corrected without undue difficulty.

2. Various surgical procedures can simultaneously damage artery and vein and perhaps the best known example arises during lumbar intervertebral disc surgery where a cutting instrument penetrates anteriorly into aortic bifurcation and iliac vein (Eastcott, 1969).

3. Various orthopaedic nailing and pinning procedures can damage neighbouring artery and vein.

4. A surgical ligature around both artery and vein can necrose away to allow an arteriovenous fistula to form. Many surgeons ligate artery and vein separately to avoid this possible complication.

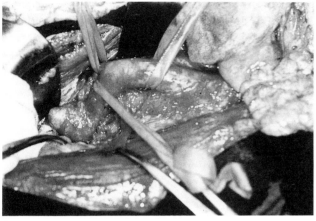

**a**

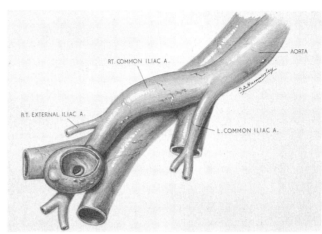

**b**

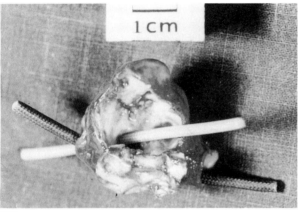

**c1**

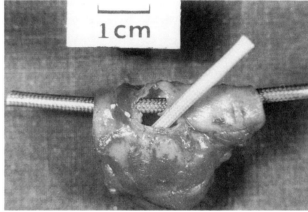

**c2**

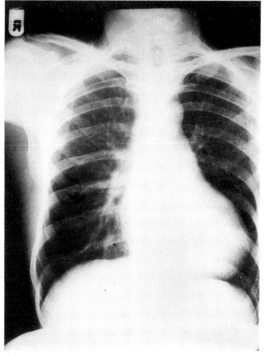

**d**

**Figure 17.21**   *Arteriovenous fistula with aneurysmal varix. This patient presented as a pyrexia of unknown origin and Streptococcus viridans was found on blood culture. A loud 'machinery' bruit was present in the lower abdomen which led to identification of an arteriovenous fistula between the right internal iliac artery and vein. The patient gave a history of falling off a haystack, 8 years previously, onto a pitchfork which penetrated the lower abdomen; on arrival at hospital he was at first thought to be dead but eventually recovered without any abdominal exploration. He returned to farm work over the following 8 years until he was disabled by bouts of fever. This unusual presentation of an arteriovenous fistula was due to infection on the endothelium of the fistulous aperture, comparable to a bacterial endocarditis.*

*(a)   A general view of the findings at operation. The aneurysmal varix can be seen to the left of the picture. The right common and internal iliac arteries, supported by tapes and greatly enlarged, are prominent in the centre.*

*(b)   An artist's depiction of the vascular changes. An aneurysmal varix forming a communication between the right internal iliac artery and vein is present. The common and internal iliac arteries leading down to the fistula have hypertrophied to the same size as the aorta itself, whilst the left iliac arteries remain unchanged.*

*(c)   1, 2. Interior views of the aneurysmal varix and the site of bacterial endothelial infection.*

*(d)   X-ray showing considerable cardiac hypertrophy caused by the arteriovenous shunt. The heart was otherwise healthy and was not the origin of the bacteraemia which arose from the arteriovenous fistula*

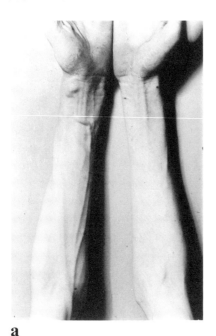

**a**

**Figure 17.22**  *An arteriovenous fistula at the wrist following penetration by a splinter of glass in a youth.*

*(a)  In this picture, the small bulge on the left wrist indicates an aneurysmal varix communicating between the radial artery and vein. This has caused widespread increase in venous pressure which is clearly indicated by the prominence of the superficial veins throughout the left forearm. A Doppler flowmeter showed a continuous rapid flow through the veins towards the heart.*

*(b)  A directional Doppler flowmeter tracing from superficial veins leading away from the fistula at the wrist. Continuous fast flow towards the heart is shown but arterial pulsation is obscured by turbulence until the artery is temporarily occluded above the fistula; flow is then maintained by side branches at a reduced rate and its pulsatile pattern is more evident. High velocity pulsatile flow of this nature is not ever found in normal circumstances in the limbs and is characteristic of arteriovenous fistula. A weak pulsatile action may be found in fully distended superficial veins in the lower limb of a patient who has been standing still for 30 seconds or more but the accompanying flow is sluggish and it is more of a transmitted arterial 'bounce' than true arterial pulsatile flow*

Flow towards heart

Zero

**b**

Unimpeded flow  ‖ Vein ‖ Unimpeded ‖ compressed  flow  Compression of artery above fistula  ‖ Unimpeded flow

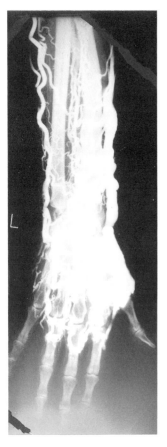

**Figure 17.23**  *Angiogram of an iatrogenic arteriovenous fistula in the forearm, created to facilitate access for renal dialysis. This one had to be dismantled after 2 years because it had given rise to the typical venous hypertensive changes of pigmentation and ulceration on the hand*

### Spontaneously acquired arteriovenous fistula

Aneurysmal degenerative arterial disease may involve the adjoining vein and eventually give rise to a fistula between the two. The best example of this is in the abdominal aortic aneurysm which erodes into vertebral bodies and into the neighbouring inferior vena cava or an iliac aneurysm into iliac vein (Figure 17.24). A similar process may be seen when either primary or secondary neoplasms involve the vessels; mycotic aneurysm from infective endocarditis may have the same effect if the infection destroys both artery and vein walls as the initiating process. This must be distinguished from the occasional arteriovenous fistula which falls prey to secondary infection by *Streptococcus viridans* giving infective vegetations at the aperture; this is secondary to the presence of the vascular abnormality and not the initiating process (Figure 17.21(c)).

### Mechanism of formation

It is not too difficult to imagine a penetrating injury that lacerates adjoining artery and vein, or even punches a hole in both structures. The fistula may be established immediately or not be apparent at first because the potential communication is filled with blood clot which eventually yields or is absorbed so that the communication opens up fully. Organization of clot and repair of the

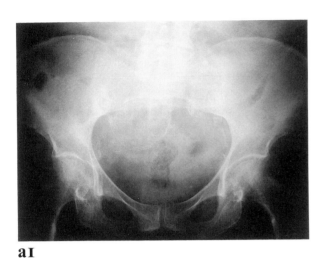

**a1**

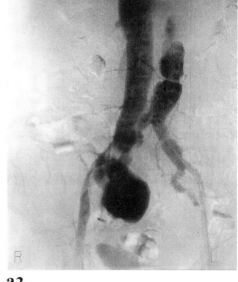

**a2**

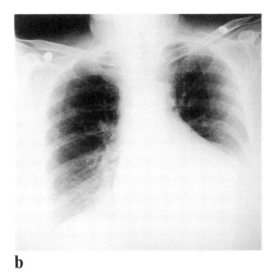

**b**

**Figure 17.24** *Spontaneous arteriovenous fistula between iliac vessels. This patient had presented with acute swelling and discomfort in the right lower limb which was, at first, diagnosed as a deep vein thrombosis but the presence of a loud bruit suggested an arteriovenous fistula.*

*(a)  1. Abdominal X-ray showing a rim of calcium outlining an iliac aneurysm.*
*2. An angiogram showing an irregular aorta leading down to a right iliac aneurysm which communicates with the neighbouring iliac vein. Surgical repair and reconstruction with a bifurcated aortofemoral Dacron graft was successful.*

*(b)  Chest X-ray of this patient showing considerable cardiac enlargement caused by the arteriovenous fistula. (By permission of W. B. Campbell)*

injured vessel walls is completed by an endothelial lining laid down upon it and this prevents any tendency for thrombus to build up and effect a natural cure. Here nature's own protective mechanism of endothelializing diseased or injured vessels actually smoothes over and makes permanent this unwanted communication (Figure 17.25). The aperture may be quite small, perhaps only a few millimetres, or massive so that major vessels, such as iliac artery and vein, are in full communication through an aperture 1 cm across (Figure 17.21(b), (c)). Clearly there is a size of aperture above which the heart is unable to support the massive shunting of blood from arterial to venous systems and is inconsistent with continued life.

*The aneurysmal varix*

This is a variant of the process just described and arises

when the injury causes a large haematoma to lie between the damaged artery and vein. The artery establishes an endothelial-lined hollow within this which extends to give full communication with the vein. The intervening aneurysm is, in fact, a false aneurysm with its walls formed from organized clot and not from expanded vessel wall. It is an unstable state which is likely to enlarge progressively.

**The consequences of arteriovenous fistula**

*In the limb*

The veins running from the fistula back towards the heart will become enlarged as a result of the increased pressure and rate of flow within them. Veins below this level will also be affected by the raised venous pressure and become

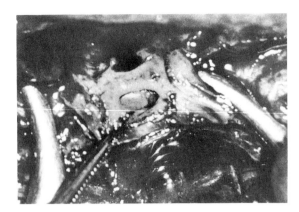

**Figure 17.25** *The aperture formed between a brachial artery and a large false aneurysm resulting from laceration by a high velocity fragment of metal. This has been present for 4 weeks and the aperture has become lined with a smooth new intima covered with endothelium to give an entirely congenial surface free from any tendency to thrombosis. This exemplifies the natural process of repair within a blood vessel; at first the injured portion is irregular and highly thrombogenic but, provided flow does not cease, this is soon endothelialized to give a non-thrombogenic surface. In the case of a false aneurysm or an arteriovenous fistula it is this process that forms an aperture perfectly fashioned to maintain flow indefinitely. Thus, the defensive mechanism to maintain flow may have undesirable consequences at times, but nevertheless is often greatly to be preferred to a cessation of flow in the vessels concerned. At least it gives time and opportunity for surgical reconstruction*

enlarged, but the manifestations vary considerably and, for example, if the main vein has been occluded by the injury, massive tortuous collateral vessels, with rapid pulsatile flow, may proliferate in the area. If a major artery and vein are involved, the raised pressure within the vein will cause oedema, possibly extending up to a high level. The artery leading down to the fistula will become enlarged due to the collapsing nature of the pulse caused by loss of peripheral resistance (just as in the development of collateral arteries connecting a major artery above a block to the low pressure area below it; it seems that the wide excursion of the pulse in these vessels is the stimulus to their hypertrophy).

### Infective endophlebitis

As previously mentioned, *Streptococcus viridans* may eventually colonize on the aperture, just as in cardiac valvular disease, to cause constantly proliferating vegetations giving rise to fever, bacteraemia and micro-embolism. This is however a rare complication (Figure 17.21).

### General circulatory and cardiac effects

A substantial shunt between artery and vein will cause venous return to be greatly increased and, because of the large defect in arterial resistance, it may be difficult for the heart to maintain normal arterial pressure. Thus a vicious cycle is set up with the cardiac output being increased to maintain pressure but this in its turn increases venous return to the heart which strives all the harder to deal effectively with this. The collapsing nature of pulsation in the arteries leading down to the fistula creates a constant tendency for these vessels to enlarge and for the aperture of the fistula itself to increase. Thus the process may steadily augment with increasing cardiac hypertrophy and, finally, dilatation of the heart which can no longer support the demands made on it so that cardiac failure occurs. Smaller fistulas will not be sufficient to affect the heart in this way but nevertheless will show the same tendency to increase steadily with time.

### Physical signs

The condition will cause local swelling with enlarged, possibly tortuous, veins radiating from it. If it is sufficiently large to give widespread effects, the raised venous pressure causes the characteristic changes of venous hypertension in the distal part of the limb, that is, oedema, pigmentation of the skin, induration, eczematous changes and ulceration (lipodermatosclerosis). In this way the venous specialist may be confronted with features associated with commonly occurring venous conditions, namely enlarged veins, oedema, pigmentation and other skin changes in the lower part of the limb giving a typical picture of a venous disorder. It is indeed true that the patient has the characteristic features of venous hypertension but the list of causes for this state does, of course, include congenital and acquired arteriovenous fistulas. The author has seen several cases where surgical attempts to remedy enlarged veins have been made without realizing their true cause was an underlying arteriovenous fistula (Figure 17.26) (Braithwaite and Tibbs, 1955).

The patient is likely to complain of discomfort, which may be considerable, in the vicinity of the fistula where swelling is maximal. A careful history will usually give a clear story of an injury, but this may have been some years before, now almost forgotten and the scar perhaps insignificant, or, because it was due to medical intervention the patient is not aware of its possible relevance.

There is usually visible and palpable pulsation in and around the lesion but the most distinctive feature is a loud bruit heard on auscultation, set up by the turbulent jet of blood passing through the fistulous communication. The rhythmical pumping quality of this is often described by such terms as a 'machinery' or 'to and fro' bruit. This is widely conducted by all vessels in the limb, both arteries and veins, but in the enlarged main artery leading down to the fistula a somewhat different bruit, due to high speed flow within it, may be recognized as a continuous thrumming note. A Doppler flowmeter applied to the

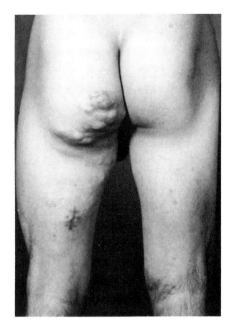

**Figure 17.26** *These varicose veins in a young man aged 19 years were due to arteriovenous fistulas between the internal pudendal artery and vein beneath the gluteus maximus muscle. It is uncertain whether these were congenital in origin or due to an injection into the buttock 2 years previously. The scar on the back of the thigh is due to a previous surgical attempt to remove varicosities emerging there a year previously*

veins leading away from the fistula will show continuous fast flow with added peaks at each arterial pulse (Figure 17.22(b)). This is far greater than the pulsation which may be found in other venous disorders when the subject has been standing motionless for 30 seconds or more so that the venous system in the lower limb is completely filled and transmitting arterial input; this is very weak and easily abolished by a short spell of exercise or putting the limb horizontal. It is not to be compared with the intensity and persistence shown in the presence of an arteriovenous shunt. Photoplethysmography will confirm very strong arterial pulsation but otherwise is non-specific and will give the reduced response to exercise and shortened recovery period found in various forms of venous hypertension.

These changes and the bruit described above will be abolished if the main artery is temporarily occluded by finger pressure above the fistula. If the fistula is of sufficient size to put a load upon cardiac output there will be a marked tachycardia and based on this a valuable physical sign may be elicited.

### Branham's sign

This was described by Branham in 1890 who noticed that the tachycardia in an "aneurismal varix of the femoral artery and vein following gunshot wound" was temporarily abolished when the main artery leading down to it was compressed. Clearly this only applies to a fistula

of sufficient haemodynamic importance to cause tachycardia. When the sign is present it is a clear indication of the load upon the heart and the need to close the arteriovenous shunt.

### Arteriogram

The most informative investigation will be by serial arteriography with injection of the opaque medium into the artery leading down to the fistula. The features shown will be, rapid transit of medium down the artery and appearing almost immediately in the corresponding vein as an upward stream starting at the fistula. In the acquired fistula with the usual single opening, the communication can usually be accurately indentified. Other confirmatory evidence will be an obvious, often massive hypertrophy of the artery leading down the fistula and enlargement of the outgoing veins, often with tortuosity in the neighbouring lesser branches.

*Treatment* The main purpose in this chapter is to describe the features of arteriovenous fistula to help the venous specialist in its recognition, and treatment will only be outlined here.

This is a condition which will become more formidable to operate upon with time. Ideally the diagnosis is made early and surgery carried out without delay before the whole area becomes matted with dense fibrosis.

Clearly the objective is the reliable closure of the fistula but this must be accomplished without any significant interference to the arterial supply, or venous return, to and from the limb. This means that if major vessels are involved their continuity must be maintained or restored as an essential feature of the operation, since otherwise considerable disability may follow or even loss of the limb.

A small fistula, in some circumstances, can be shut off by plugging it with a suitable device introduced by arterial catheter (iatrogenic or therapeutic embolization). More usually, however, surgery will be necessary and for this the following steps will be required:

1. The main artery leading to the fistula must be temporarily shut off by surgical exposure and clamping, or by balloon catheter introduced into the artery to occlude it at an approriate level, or if the lesion is low down in the limb by use of a pneumatic tourniquet.
2. If a major artery and vein, such as the femoral, are involved these structures must be preserved and restored to full function.
3. Dissection is started a short distance above and below the fistula where the tissues are not too matted. The main vessels and branches in the vicinity are all exposed and clamped off. Dissection is continued towards the fistula from above and below and along the artery. This may allow it to be separated from the vein, so that both structures may be trimmed and repaired. However, the densely fibrotic tissue in the

immediate vicinity of the fistula may make this very difficult and in this case the artery and/or vein may be opened into by longitudinal incision so that the fistulous opening is clearly identified from within. This will allow a fingertip to be placed in the opening and by sharp dissection round this to separate the vessels completely, each with a side aperture at the site of the fistula.

4. The vessels are now repaired. With a comparatively recent fistula it may be possible to excise each opening and repair it by suturing. Alternatively it may be more satisfactory to resect perhaps a centimetre of the entire vessel including the fistulous opening, followed by joining the vessels together by end-to-end anastomosis. In the case of the vein this is best done by multiple interrupted sutures (see Chapter 21). Restoration of continuity may only be possible by some form of graft and this is preferable to dragging the vessel ends together with excessive tension. A portion of saphenous vein, reversed and used end to end, should be ideal for the artery. The same vein can be used to fashion a tube suitable to match the diameter of the vein in maximal distension and sutured into place with multiple interrupted sutures.

If the vessels involved in the fistula are of no great consequence, for example, in the internal iliac artery and vein shown in Figure 17.21, it is permissible to ligate both vessels above and below the fistula which is then resected without restoration of continuity in the vessels. Alternatively quadruple ligation can be carried out, leaving the fistula in position, but this does run the risk of leaving in major branches which can maintain an active fistula.

## Injury to artery and vein: brief notes

Major trauma quite frequently divides a major artery and vein simultaneously in the limbs, for example in popliteal or superficial femoral vessels. This will cause a critical ischaemia and urgent repair of the vessels must be carried out. The venous injury may only be discovered at the time of operation and with any arterial injury the state of the neighbouring main vein should be checked upon. It is an essential principle that both artery and vein should be restored. This is often surprisingly easy and avoids the highly unsatisfactory result of an arterial supply restored without any adequate venous outlet; this will give a swollen congested limb that may fail to survive. If the vein alone is repaired this will be prejudiced because without an accompanying arterial repair the venous flow will be meagre and may lead to early thrombosis.

### Order of proceeding

Stabilize any major fracture in collaboration with an orthopaedic surgeon; clean and debride the wound if necessary, expose the injured vessels, trim the ends, extract thrombus and clot, and flush the vessels with heparin solution. Arterial 'spasm', a narrowed segment of artery (Figure 17.27) with no pulsation below it, usually

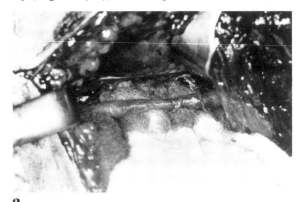

a

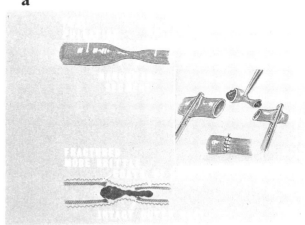

b

**Figure 17.27** *The term 'arterial spasm' in connection with arterial injury is misleading and gives rise to the misconception that this state is likely to be recoverable.*

*(a) This shows a portion of superficial femoral artery that has just been unhooked from the jagged end of a fractured femur during exploration for critical ischaemia of the foot observed a few hours after the injury. A narrowed portion of artery is clearly visible; the artery leading down to this showed strong pulsation, but below, it was easily compressible and without pulsation. The narrowed artery 'in spasm' was opened and the presence of fractured intima, with complete occlusion by thrombus, confirmed. Surgical repair by excision of the damaged artery and reanastomosis was successful. Spontaneous reopening of an injured artery showing narrowing due to fractured intima will not occur and a policy of waiting for 'vascular spasm' to resolve may cause loss of the limb.*

*(b) Diagram illustrating the mechanism of intimal fracture giving rise to apparent 'arterial spasm'. The intimal layer of an artery is brittle compared with the outer elastic layers so that any form of crush, or impact by passage of a missile nearby, may disrupt the intima but leave the outer coats intact. The ruptured intima, with exposed deeper layers, is highly thrombogenic and occlusion is completed by local thrombosis. The diagnosis at operation can be confirmed by arteriotomy and surgical repair carried out by excision of the damaged portion of artery followed by, either, direct reanastomosis, or, if this causes too much tension, by bridging the gap with a graft of reversed autogenous long saphenous vein*

means that the intimal layer has been disrupted or fractured by crushing (Hardy and Tibbs, 1960; Tibbs, 1962). This should be confirmed by arteriotomy and the segment excised (Figure 17.28). If the vein has also been injured

it should be repaired first, by end-to-end anastomosis using multiple interrupted sutures. In this way the vein is ready to accept full venous return as soon as the artery is repaired and opened without troublesome venous congestion and bleeding (Figure 17.29 and see Chapter 21).

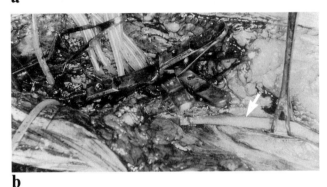

a

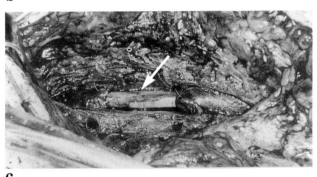

b

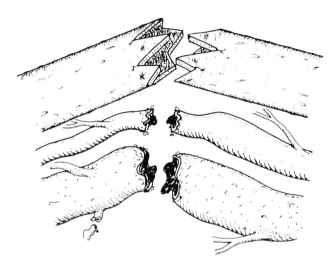

c

**Figure 17.28** *Traumatic thrombosis, with fractured intima, in a common femoral artery. A reciprocating machine had struck the patient forcibly in the left groin. Soon after this the limb became cold, numb and pulseless. It was clear that localized injury to the common femoral artery had caused its thrombosis and immediate surgical exploration was carried out.*

*(a) At operation the common femoral artery was found to be contused and pulseless. This photograph was taken immediately after arteriotomy and shows the shattered intima within. Such gross disruption of the intima cannot resolve spontaneously and excision, with replacement by a graft of autogenous saphenous vein, was decided upon.*

*(b) The neighbouring upper end of the long saphenous vein was mobilized and removed.*

*(c) The damaged portion of the artery has been excised and clot removed from the adjoining ends. The gap has then been bridged by end-to-end anastomosis with a graft of saphenous vein, shown in this photograph; the vein was reversed in case a valve was present*

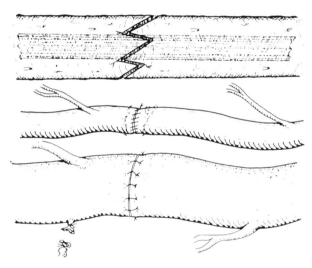

**Figure 17.29** *Diagrams to show repair necessary when both the main artery and vein are divided by an injury. If the neighbouring long bone is fractured this is stabilized, by pinning, as a first step. The opportunity to repair the vein must not be missed, since otherwise, survival of the limb will be jeopardized or, at best, considerable disability from inadequate venous return will persist. Venous engorgement during the operation is avoided by restoring the vein before the artery.*

*The vein is repaired first, by cleaning away clot, trimming the ends and then reanastomosing it. Interrupted sutures are used to prevent separation and collapse of the vein ends. The artery is then cleaned, trimmed and anastomosed end to end. The vein anastomosis is checked to ensure that it distends with flow once the arterial supply has started again. If there is a deficiency of artery or vein this may need to be bridged, preferably by autogenous graft from saphenous vein; for vein replacement, this will need to be fashioned to give an adequate lumen (see Chapter 21)*

If a deficiency in one or both vessels has been created and there is a gap between the ends too great to permit anastomosis, then this must be bridged by a graft. For the artery a graft of reversed saphenous vein is very suitable. For the vein it will be necessary to fashion a tubular graft of matching size from saphenous vein as described in Chapter 21.

With more extensive injuries and accompanying tissue damage, it becomes much more difficult but the same process of repairing both artery and vein is more important than ever if the limb is to be saved; the surgeon must work hard to achieve this because blood supply is the ultimate determinant in limb survival. In the tibial region vessels may be too small for repair to be feasible except by microsurgery, but fortunately the multiplicity of neighbouring vessels is likely to provide adequate collateral arteries and veins so that loss of an individual tibial artery and accompanying veins is not critical. The most difficult level is where there is a single main line of vascular supply breaking into several lesser vessels, that is, at the division of the popliteal artery and vein into tibial and peroneal branches. This complex arrangement of the main vessels is close to the upper shaft of the tibia and liable to be torn across in fractures here to give a critical ischaemia; local repair of the arteries and veins is not really possible and much will depend on the collateral circulation around the knee. In extremis, if the foot remains severely ischaemic after the fracture has been reduced and the patient resuscitated, then an arterial bypass from upper popliteal to mid posterior tibial artery may be justifiable; venous return would depend largely on the saphenous veins so that any vein graft used in the bypass should be taken from the opposite limb. Above this level, where surgery is more straightforward, it is essential that popliteal, superficial and common femoral vessels should be repaired, particularly if there is extensive accompanying damage and fractures. Again it must be stressed that the main vein must be repaired as well as the artery if the limb is to be given its best chance. This may only take an additional 10 minutes and bring benefit far in excess of the small extra time and trouble required to do this.

# References

Allen, E. V., Barker, N. W. and Hines, E. A. (1947) *Peripheral Vascular Diseases*, Saunders, Philadelphia

Blackett, R. L. and Heard, G. E. (1988) Pulsatile varicose veins. *British Journal of Surgery*, **75**, 866–868

Boontje, A. E. (1979) Axillary vein entrapment. *British Journal of Surgery*, **66**, 331–332

Braithwaite, F. and Tibbs, D. (1955) A case of localised arteriovenous fistulae. *British Journal of Surgery*, **42**, 442–443

Branham, H. H. (1890) Aneurismal varix of the femoral artery and vein following gunshot wound. *International Journal of Surgery*, **3**, 250–251

Callum, M. J., Harper, D. R., Dale, J. J. and Ruckley, C. V. (1987a) Arterial disease in chronic leg ulceration: an under-estimated hazard? Lothian and Forth Valley leg ulcer study. *British Medical Journal*, **294**, 929–931

Callum, M. J., Ruckley, C. V., Dale, J. J. and Harper, D. R. (1987b) Hazards of compression treatment of the leg from Scottish surgeons. *British Medical Journal*, **295**, 1382

Cockett, F. B. (1986) Arterial complications in treatment of varicose veins. *Phlebology*, **1**, 3–6

Connell, J. (1978) Popliteal vein entrapment. *British Journal of Surgery*, **65**, 351

Corbett, R. and Jayakumar, K. (1989) Clean up varicose vein surgery – use a tourniquet. *Annals of the Royal College of Surgeons of England*, **71**, 57–58

Cornwall, J. V., Dore, C. J. and Lewis, J. D. (1986) Leg ulcers: epidemiology and aetiology. *British Journal of Surgery*, **73**, 693–696

Cotton, L. T. and Khan, O. (1986) Raynaud's phenomenon: a review. *International Angiology*, **5**, 215–236

Dayantus, J., Liatus, A. C. and Lazarides, N. (1990) Pulsatile varicose veins caused by tricuspid valve regurgitation. *Phlebology*, **5**, 189–191

DeWeese, J. (1985) Management of subclavian venous obstruction. In *Surgery of the Veins* (eds J. J. Bergan and J. S. T. Yao), Grune and Stratton, New York, pp. 365–382

Eastcott, H. H. G. (1969) *Arterial Surgery*, Pitman Medical, London

Fletcher, I. R. and Healy, T. E. (1983) The arterial tourniquet. *Annals of the Royal College of Surgeons of England*, **65**, 409–417

Gomes, M. M. R. and Bernatz, P. E. (1970) Arteriovenous fistulas: a review and ten-year experience at the Mayo Clinic. *Mayo Clinic Proceedings*, **45**, 81–102

Hardy, E. G. and Tibbs, D. J. (1960) Acute ischaemia in limb injuries. *British Medical Journal*, **1**, 1001–1005

Haselbach, P., Vollenweider, U., Moneta, G. and Bollinger, M. A. (1986) Microangiography in severe chronic venous insufficiency evaluated by fluorescence video-microscopy. *Phlebology*, **1**, 159–169

Heidrich, H. (ed.) (1979) *Raynaud's Phenomenon*, TM-Verlag, Zum Ostersiek

Holman, E. (1923) The physiology of an arteriovenous fistula. *Archives of Surgery*, **7**, 64–82

Holman, E. (1924) Arteriovenous aneurism. *Annals of Surgery*, December, 801–816

Holman, E. (1937) *Arteriovenous Aneurysm*. Macmillan, New York

Iwai, T., Sato, S., Yamada, T. et al. (1987) Popliteal vein entrapment caused by the third head of gastrocnemius muscle. *British Journal of Surgery*, **74**, 1006–1008

Klenerman, L. (1982) The tourniquet in operations on the knee: a review. *Journal of the Royal Society of Medicine*, **75**, 31–32

Sako, Y. and Varco, R. I. (1970) Arteriovenous fistula: results of management of congenital and acquired forms, blood flow measurements, and observations on proximal arterial degeneration. *Surgery*, **67**, 40–61

Sawyer, P. N. and Kaplitt, M. J. (1978) *Vascular Grafts*, Appleton-Century-Crofts, New York

Tibbs, D. J. (1962) Acute ischaemia of the limbs. *Proceedings of the Royal Society of Medicine*, 593–596

Warren, A. G. (1989) The surgical conservation of the neuropathic foot. *Annals of the Royal College of Surgeons*, **71**, 236–242

Widmer, L. K., Stahelin, H. B., Nissen, C. and da Silva, A. (1981) *Venen-Arterien-Krankheiten, koronare Herzkrankheit bei Berufstatigen*, Huber, Bern

# Bibliography

Browse, N. L., Burnand, K. G. and Lea Thomas M. (1988) Cystic degeneration of the vein wall. In *Diseases of the Veins* (ed. N. L. Browse), Edward Arnold, London, pp. 661–663

Flanigan, D. P., Burnham, S. J. Goodreau, J. J. and Bergan, J. J. (1979) Summary of cases of adventitial cystic disease of the popliteal artery. *Annals of Surgery*, **189**, 165–175

Gillespie, G. (1973) Peripheral gangrene as the presentation of myeloproliferative disorders. *British Journal of Surgery*, **60**, 377–380

Macfarlane, R., Livesey, S. A., Pollard, S. and Dunn, D. C. (1987) Cystic adventitial arterial disease. *British Journal of Surgery*, **74**, 89–90

Mestres, C. A., Ninot, S., Guerola, M., Morales, M. A. and Mulet, J. (1987) Spontaneous iliacocaval arteriovenous fistula: the case for differential diagnosis. *British Journal of Surgery*, **74**, 1178–1179

Scott, H. J., Cheatle, R. R., McMullin, G. M., Coleridge Smith, P. D. and Scurr, J. H. (1990) Reappraisal of the oxygenation of blood in varicose veins. *British Journal of Surgery*, **77**, 934–936

Welch, G. H., Reid, D. B. and Pollock, J. G. (1990) Infected false aneurysms in the groin of intravenous drug abusers. *British Journal of Surgery*, **77**, 330–333

# 18

# Treatment of varicose veins and other manifestations of superficial vein incompetence. 1. Conservative management; varicose veins in pregnancy

This chapter is concerned with principles in the treatment of varicose veins and other manifestations of simple incompetence of the superficial veins. Much of it will be presented in summary form because it has been discussed in other chapters but certain aspects, such as conservative treatment and the management of varicose veins in pregnancy, will be given in more detail.

## Treatment available for superficial vein incompetence

There are three levels of treatment available to be used either alone or combined:

1. *Reassurance*. This is undoubtedly valuable in an appreciable number of patients who are unduly worried by: large but normal veins, insignificant varicose veins, a family history of massive varicose veins and ulceration, or when sclerotherapy or surgery is not considered desirable (e.g. in old age) for relatively harmless varicosities.
2. *Conservative treatment*. This entails measures that do not involve any physical obliteration or removal of veins. It may be used on its own or to back up active treatment. The basis is elevation of the limb(s) and use of external support in some form.
3. *Active intervention*. This is usually to obliterate the pathway of incompetence and its varicose veins (see Chapters 3 and 4) by surgical removal or by sclerotherapy.

## Are the veins at fault?

Because varicosities are so apparent, they are often blamed for symptoms which in fact have other causes. The first essential is to review the evidence that the veins are at fault and that they are going to respond favourably to the treatment proposed.

Discomfort caused by superficial incompetence is nearly always accompanied by evidence of venous abnormality in that general vicinity. The absence of any detectable abnormality should cause serious doubt whether there is a venous cause, however convinced the patient may be that varicose veins must be the cause for her discomforts, even though none are visible. Nevertheless, certain patterns of superficial incompetence may be 'concealed' to some extent and will require careful examination to uncover proof of their existence. Discomfort well away from varicosities must be viewed with suspicion, for example, groin pain is unlikely be related to calf varicosities if the groin is free from abnormal veins. Sometimes patients will blame discomforts onto varicose veins in the opposite limb, and although a relationship is possible in cross-over incompetence, it should not be accepted without good evidence of venous changes in the limb complained of. Conversely, symptoms in the area of varicose veins are not necessarily related to them, so that it must not be assumed too readily that removing the veins will give relief. In cases of uncertainty for any of these reasons the trial use of elastic support (elastic tubular bandage is suitable), to see if this brings relief, may be helpful in resolving doubts. The approach to any patient must be analytical and not an automatic response to the sight of varicose veins; the association between symptoms and the varicosities must always appear reasonable and be backed by satisfactory clinical tests if disappointing results are to be avoided.

Venous eczema and ulceration will always have clear evidence of an accompanying venous disorder and hypertension, usually pigmentation and induration in surrounding skin; without this, other causes for the ulcer must be considered (see Chapter 13).

The presenting manifestations of superficial vein incompetence are summarized below:

1. Aching discomfort especially towards the end of a day's standing, and most marked just before menstruation. Intradermal venules and small veins immediately under the skin may cause stinging discomfort premenstrually.
2. Disfiguring varicose veins. However, with the 'straight-through' variety of saphenous incompetence (see Chapter 4), there may be no intervening varicosities and the evidence of an unnaturally enlarged saphenous vein may be concealed from sight in subcutaneous fat.
3. Evidence of venous hypertension, such as venous flares on foot and ankle, pigmentation, oedema, fibrosis, eczema or ulceration. *Note.* Oedema on its own, without accompanying venotensive changes, must not be attributed to varicosities too readily; other possible causes must be given careful thought.
4. Complications of varicose veins, such as superficial thrombophlebitis or haemorrhage (see Chapter 6).

## Reasons for treatment

An appreciable number of patients are unnecessarily perturbed by minor varicosities and will require no more than reassurance. Fear that their veins may deteriorate to the state suffered by one or other parent is a common motive for seeking advice. Clearly there is an ill-defined border between changes so minimal that no treatment is needed and those where it has become desirable either for cosmetic or medical reasons. Each doctor will have his own level of response and this will depend upon his willingness to treat minor blemishes and ability to detect the relatively concealed states of incompetence. In cases of uncertainty the question of treatment must be decided by the self-question: 'How much real benefit can I bring this patient, psychologically or physically?'

There should always be a clear reason for active intervention. Varicose veins should never be removed just because 'they are there'. Reasons for intervening might be:

- To relieve discomfort and anxiety ('I do not want to have veins like my mother').
- To improve appearance and therefore self-confidence.
- To prevent progressive deterioration and possible eventual ulceration, particularly when venotensive changes are already present.
- To cure eczema or ulceration.
- To prevent recurrence of complications such as haemorrhage or superficial thrombophlebitis.

Most varicose veins are only slowly progressive and relatively harmless. The reason for treating them is that they are bringing, or threaten to bring, a disadvantage to the patient and this may range from distress over appearance or discomfort, through to skin changes that are likely to prove increasingly troublesome. The middle-aged man who is merely curious about some harmless veins on his calf may require nothing doing, but the 40-year-old woman whose children have grown up, and is now free to consider herself, may gain considerable self-confidence in having her unsightly veins banished and a longstanding discomfort relieved. If there are accompanying venotensive skin changes, it may be justifiable firmly to advise surgery to forestall eventual ulceration, but without such evidence there is insufficient reason to justify pressing a reluctant patient to have surgery at this stage, and treatment should be offered rather than advised.

## Diagnostic evidence necessary before active treatment is advised

Active treatment involves the obliteration of superficial veins either by surgery or sclerotherapy. This should not be done without positive recognition of incompetence in these veins, that is, retrograde flow with exercise in the upright patient, and demonstration that removal of the veins will be effective in controlling this. This evidence will be provided by:

1. A clearly identified pathway of incompetence and a 'selective occlusion' (Trendelenburg) test applied to this giving good control to enlarged veins; similarly Perthes' test, selectively applied, showing a partial collapse of varicosities (see Chapters 2 and 4).
2. Doppler directional flowmeter applied to pathway of incompetence showing characteristic downflow after exercise (see Chapters 4 and 24).
3. When venotensive skin changes are present, proof that they are caused by superficial incompetence, as distinct from deep vein impairment or valvular deficiency. This may be provided by plethysmography, volumetry or direct venous pressure measurement which show a shortened recovery time after exercise but restored to near normal by temporary occlusion of the pathway of incompetence (see Chapters 6 and 24).
4. Functional phlebography, if necessary, demonstrating that flow in abnormal superficial veins is predominantly downwards and into the deep veins at lower level. It should also confirm that the deep veins are widely open throughout the limb and pelvic region, are undeformed and have adequate valves. This should only be required in cases of unusual complexity or when there is a history of possible thrombosis so that deep vein impairment (post-thrombotic limb) has to be excluded (see Chapters 8, 9 and 13).

## Choosing a policy of treatment

In the treatment of venous disorders in the lower limbs there is a broad range of conditions which can be cured or greatly improved by active intervention but there is also a large sector that cannot be improved and the patient can only be offered advice upon useful measures to ameliorate the condition. A surgeon's duty is to pick out the curable problems, and to recognize those that are not, so that useless and possibly damaging interference may be avoided.

The method of treatment decided upon varies considerably from surgeon to surgeon and often there are several alternatives of equal merit (Eklof, 1988) so that it would be wrong to be too dogmatic but at the same time it is our purpose to give guidance upon this. Table 18.1 summarizes the author's approach and gives lines of treatment that would seem reasonable for the circumstances.

## Conservative treatment

Whether it is used as a holding measure whilst awaiting surgery, or as a considered policy because surgery or sclerotherapy is inappropriate or refused by the patient, conservative treatment has a valuable role. In essence, the patients are taught simple measures to compensate for the defects in the veins. Old habits may have to be changed and, depending on the severity of the condition, some self-discipline may be required, but usually the advantage of increased comfort is obvious to the patient. The condition is controlled but not cured. Pharmaceutical adjuncts to treatment are discussed in Chapter 13, Part 1.

## The principles

When the patient is standing upright, downflow in incompetent superficial veins, unguarded by effective valves, causes a rapid return of full venous pressure in the lower part of the limb. Small movements of the musculovenous pump are insufficient to relieve this, so that the veins are subjected to long periods of sustained maximal tension. During walking, the musculovenous pumps repeatedly strive to relieve the pressure, but any slackening of the deep veins leads to increased superficial downflow and counteracts the benefits; moreover the downflow in the superficial veins is turbulent, giving considerable sideways thrust, again overstretching the veins and, in the longer term, causing tortuosity. In this way the efforts of the deep vein pumping mechanism are defeated and indeed, by enhancing retrograde flow, aggravate the stresses on the vein walls. The effects of this are compounded if, as is often the case, the patient has inherently weak walls to the veins so that they allow overdistension of the valve rings, separation of the cusps and increased leakage of the valves. Moreover, the foot veins may dilate to form a massive venous 'pool' so that at each step blood drains rapidly to the foot as it is raised, only to surge back again when it returns to the ground. If, in addition, the deep vein pump is poorly valved or has been damaged by previous thrombosis then a further disadvantage appears because the pump is easily overwhelmed by the

abnormal superficial downflow and only reduces the venous pressure very briefly or not at all. The resulting sustained, unrelieved venous hypertension causes its characteristic changes and eventual ulceration. This is a formidable catalogue of harmful events, most of which can be mitigated by two simple measures, elevation and external support, and are the basis of conservative treatment of superficial vein incompetence.

### Elevation

When the limbs are elevated above the horizontal there is perfect venous drainage without the need for a pumping mechanism and unhampered by gravitational 'downflow' in the incompetent veins. This gives an opportunity for recovery from the damage done by venous hypertension and the greater the time spent in elevation the less the limb will be affected by venotensive change. However, in practical terms, only limited periods are possible and, indeed, long periods of immobility are deleterious to other aspects of bodily health, so that exercise sessions will be needed to counteract this. Nevertheless, it does give the patient an important means of controlling the worst manifestations of venous hypertension.

### External support by bandage or by elastic stocking

The object of this is twofold: to reduce, if not completely prevent, the unwanted downflow in the superficial veins and to protect the veins from overdistension. External support in the treatment of superficial incompetence is usually by elastic stocking, to upper calf or thigh, or as tights. A variety of elastic materials is used, for example, one-way or two-way stretch and in varying strengths to give graduated compression diminishing up the length of the limb so that there is no tendency to constrict venous return. Inelastic support, by paste bandage, is seldom required for superficial vein incompetence, although even here it might have an advantage with severe ulceration from this cause; its main use is in ulceration due to deep vein impairment (post-thrombotic and valveless syndromes). Elastic support in superficial incompetence is highly effective in giving relief from symptoms and in healing an ulcer, but much less so in deep vein impairment. This is principally because elastic support can eliminate the most damaging component in the former, retrograde flow in the superficial veins, and in this way restore effective musculovenous pumping; in deep vein impairment the pumping mechanism itself is defective and external support can only make a small contribution by combating overdistension and reducing the amount of pooled venous blood in the leg and foot that surges back and forth with exercise. A well-fitted stocking should resist the moderate pressures of downflow in the superficial veins but should not impede deep vein return which is pumped upwards at considerably greater pressure than

**TABLE 18.1** Summary of policy for treatment

| Venous lesion | Reason for treatment | Proof required | Suitable treatment |
|---|---|---|---|
| Minimal or no venous lesion | Patient unnecessarily anxious | Insignificant or no venous abnormality | Reassurance |
| Minor vascular blemish | Appearance | Self-evident | Sclerotherapy or laser |
| Small to moderate sized varicose veins, origin uncertain | Appearance and/or discomfort | Self-evident and absence of a leading vein | Sclerotherapy |
| Small to moderate sized varicose veins. Origin from a well-defined, straight-walled branch of saphenous vein | Appearance and/or discomfort | Control by pressure over a leading (or stem) vein or saphenous vein | If first treatment, by injection into stem vein and varicose veins. If previous sclerotherapy but veins have recurred, then ? surgery |
| Moderate sized varicose veins with obvious enlargement and downflow in saphenous vein | Appearance and/or discomfort, threatened or actual complication | Control by finger over the stem vein or saphenous vein. Doppler downflow after exercise | Surgery preferable but injection to stem vein and varicose veins is permissible if patient prefers this, or as 'first aid' for haemorrhage or ulcer |
| Large varicose veins with saphenous or other clearly defined origin | Appearance and/or discomfort, threatened or actual complications | Control by finger over the saphenous vein or other evident pathway of incompetence. Doppler downflow after exercise | Surgery is best; occasionally sclerotherapy as 'first aid' for haemorrhage or ulcer |
| Venous stasis, threatened or actual ulcer with clearly defined superficial incompetence | Appearance, discomfort and skin changes; cure or prevention of ulcer | Control by finger over the saphenous vein or other pathway of incompetence. Doppler downflow after exercise. Plethysmography with restoration of recovery time when 'controlled'. If in doubt, phlebography showing good deep veins with spillover and downflow in saphenous vein (see text) | Surgery must be first choice. If surgery is not permissible sclerotherapy may be justifiable and can give prolonged benefit |
| Superficial thrombophlebitis with simple varicose veins | Discomfort and possible extension of condition | Tender swelling in presence of varicose veins; control of unaffected varicose veins as described above. Doppler downflow, and this may be found in phlebitic vein | Conservative treatment by firm bandaging and elevation whenever possible. Surgery to saphenous system to remove incompetent veins when sure that phlebitis has no systemic cause |
| Haemorrhage | Likely to recur soon | Control of superficial veins leading down to bleeding point and Doppler downflow | Immediate firm bandage. Early surgery to incompetent veins with excision of vein that has bled. Sclerotherapy as 'first aid' or in the infirm patient |
| Recurrent varicose veins | Any of reasons above | Convincing demonstration of the origin, that is the point of spillover from deep to surface veins. This often possible by clinical tests, otherwise phlebography essential before surgery | If origin demonstrated clearly, then surgery best. If origin uncertain sclerotherapy may give good results but is likely to require repeating at intervals |
| Post-thrombotic limb | Venotensive change, ulcer, etc. | Control of enlarged superficial veins not possible and they show upflow with Doppler. Plethysmography shows short recovery period which cannot be improved by attempted control. Phlebography shows preferential upflow in long saphenous vein and deformed deep veins | Avoid surgery or sclerotherapy. This case requires most careful evaluation and it is likely that conservative treatment will be in the patient's best interests (see text) |
| Valveless syndrome | Any of reasons above including severe ulceration | Control not possible. Doppler shows surge. Plethysmography gives shortened recovery period which cannot be improved. Phlebography shows widely open and valveless deep veins | Sclerotherapy will not be effective. Surgery to superficial veins likely to be disappointing but probably will do little harm. Conservative treatment can give real benefit (see text) |

that exerted by the stocking. External support is also discussed in Chapters 8 and 13.

Thus, the disagreeable features of superficial venous incompetence, the bulging veins, the discomfort and skin changes, are caused by *unwanted superficial vein downflow, overstretching of the vein walls and inadequate relief of venous pressure*. These key components are maximal when the patient is standing but disappear completely as the limb is raised above the horizontal. Herein lies the essence of conservative treatment:

*Minimize standing, elevate the limbs whenever possible and give the veins external support to shut off superficial downflow and protect from overdistension.*

*Note.* Elevation and elastic compression must never be employed without checking that a good arterial supply is present. If the limb is ischaemic, these measures are totally inappropriate, and may endanger the limb (see Chapter 17).

## Conservative treatment in practice

The account just given, of the physical processes causing venous stress within a limb, has described a severe sequence of events, but in practice all gradations of severity are encountered and to give better perspective examples are given below in order of ascending severity. Advice given to the patient is made much more effective by a pamphlet illustrating practical ways of counteracting the ill effects of 'varicose veins' (Figure 18.1).

1. The young housewife, who prefers to avoid active treatment but seeks improved appearance and comfort, will be helped by:
   (a) Support hose, as stockings or tights (light, Class I, 14–17 mmHg compression at ankle).
   (b) A policy of sitting rather than standing for household tasks, making time for several breaks to elevate the limbs well above the horizontal during the day, and certainly in the evening. Veins tire and overdistend so that they benefit from recovery periods.
   (c) Control of obesity.
2. The same housewife, 10 years later, with varicose veins considerably larger and with increasing pruritis and pigmentation of the skin. She still wishes to avoid surgical treatment in spite of being reminded that her limb is deteriorating and may eventually ulcerate. The following will be required:
   (a) A stronger elastic support to limit downflow and prevent overdistension of veins. Medium-weight, two-way-stretch elastic stocking (Class II, 18–24 mmHg compression at ankle), thigh length, is likely to be the most suitable and give the best appearance. It will require a suspender and may prove uncomfortable behind the knee or unpleasant in hot weather. An alternative is a stocking up to the knee, but the down-pull of a two-way-stretch stocking at this level may cause it to slip down if the calf is narrow; in this case a one-way-stretch stocking up to the knee, which has no down-pull, may serve well but has a slightly coarser appearance.
   (b) A rigorous policy of giving the veins recovery periods by high elevation several times a day, with a prolonged session in the evening.
   (c) Diet to reduce overweight.
3. The same patient has not heeded advice and has now developed an ulcer. Although told that her state is still curable by surgery she refuses to have this. The ulcer must be healed by conservative means and this may be achieved by:
   *Either*, use of a strong elastic stocking or an inelastic paste bandage up to the knee (see Chapter 13), combined with a policy of giving a large proportion of the day to putting the leg(s) in high elevation and restricting time spent up and about to essential tasks and short walks to maintain general fitness.
   *Or*, if the ulcer does not respond to mobile treatment in non-elastic paste bandage, several weeks of near-continuous elevation will be required. This must not be viewed as 'bed rest' because it is essential that the patient's muscles and joints should not be allowed to deteriorate through inactivity.

*Healing an ulcer; elevation with activity*

The patient is instructed to lie on a bed or couch with the limbs in a position of high elevation (see Figure 13.21) and is shown an exercise routine to be followed repeatedly whilst in elevation. In addition, each hour the patient should get up for a 5-minute spell of active walking (to use the antigravity muscles) and to perform any essential tasks, such as visits to the bathroom; there should be no standing still or sitting and if necessary the patient should mark time or rise on toes whilst doing a standing task. The walking periods must not exceed the brief period specified. Care of the ulcer by dressings is described in Chapter 13; firm bandaging with crepe, reapplied twice daily, is sufficient support for the brief periods of walking; when the patient increases the duration of walks, stronger elastic support or an inelastic paste bandage must be substituted. This regimen of 'elevation with activity' will require considerable support from the family if the patient is not to be forced back to full household duties.

When the ulcer has healed then a progressive return to more normal life is permitted but the patient must understand that any relaxation of care for the limb will lead to return of the ulcer. The bed need not be raised more than, say, 30 cm, but a considerable proportion of the day should still be given to elevation of the limb and proper elastic support must always be worn before getting up (at least medium support stocking, Class II, 18–24 mmHg, or strong support stocking, Class III, 25–35 mmHg compression at ankle).

Surgical treatment to remove the cause of the ulceration – superficial vein incompetence – should be, once again, discussed with the patient!

## Obesity

Obesity is a factor which appears to aggravate superficial vein incompetence although the precise mechanics of this are uncertain. Undoubtedly some of the worst sets of varicose veins are seen in obese people and these often show a massive cough impulse. It is possible that an accumulation of fat within the abdominal cavity hydraulically transmits intra-abdominal pressure to veins more effectively than in patients of normal build. Also, the weight of fat may compress the iliac veins and the inferior vena cava to cause prolonged distension of all the veins in the lower limbs with consequent valve failure, particularly in superficial veins. Whatever the cause, it is generally agreed that obesity is an undesirable factor. Moreover, it may delay diagnosis because varicose veins concealed in subcutaneous fat are not easily visible to the patient or the medical attendant, who may underrate their extent until ulceration appears.

Obesity brings a number of medical disadvantages and its correction is always desirable. However, its significance must be considered before dietary measures are urged on the patient. Causes other than overeating should be excluded, including endocrine or metabolic disturbance and alcoholism. If necessary the advice of a specialist physician should be obtained. Weight loss on its own is unlikely to cure the patient's venous condition but will certainly make the management of this easier. Many obese patients will respond well to a simple diet, but in other cases, such as the obese alcoholic, with a complex background of psychological and metabolic problems, a satisfactory result may be difficult to obtain.

## Treatment of superficial thrombophlebitis

This has been considered in Chapter 6 but since the treatment is often conservative it will be referred to briefly here. This is usually a straightforward complication of varicose veins but thought should always be given to the possibility of the phlebitis being the early manifestation of a systemic, and often serious, disorder. If this is not the case then treatment will usually be conservative but there is a place for early surgery in many of these patients. The basis of conservative treatment is to prevent blood from entering the affected vein, either by use of a firm supporting bandage or by elevation of the limb. If blood is allowed into the vein it will generate yet more thrombus with further painful distension and spread of the process. Anticoagulants are usually not necessary but may be used if the condition is very extensive or is failing to repond to the compression treatment. Non-steroidal anti-inflammatory agents, such as indomethacin, can be

helpful in alleviating the discomfort but antibiotics are unlikely to bring any benefit. Extrusion of the clot through a stab incision or excision of the affected vein, combined with surgery to cure superficial vein incompetence, is often to be preferred.

## Treatment of haemorrhage from a varicosity

This has been described in Chapter 6 and is only briefly considered here. Initial treatment to stop the haemorrhage is by elevation of the limb and application of a pressure pad by firm bandage over the bleeding point. Continued treatment by compression will eventually allow the open varicosity to seal but this is often unsatisfactory with no more than a plug of dried clot which eventually breaks away with renewal of bleeding. Far more satisfactory is full surgical treatment of the underlying superficial incompetence together with excision of the ruptured vein and the thinned skin over it; this may be carried out at the first convenient opportunity. However, in the elderly and infirm, in whom operation is to be avoided, sclerotherapy to the vein above and below the point of haemorrhage will ensure that further bleeding does not take place.

## Varicose veins in pregnancy

Varicose veins often appear for the first time, or become much worse, during pregnancy. However, after childbirth, the abnormally enlarged veins will usually regress considerably so that many patients return to apparent normality, but in others there is only partial improvement and the veins persist as an ongoing problem. Most mothers with varicose veins will say that their veins first appeared in pregnancy and deteriorated progressively over the years since then. It is clearly a major factor in the development of superficial vein incompetence in women and probably the main reason they are more commonly afflicted than men. The patterns of

---

**Figure 18.1** *These diagrams have served well for many years, as a means of informing patients in the author's vein clinic.*

*(a) Raise the foot of the bed to obtain maximal benefit with overnight rest.*

*(b) Put on the elastic stocking before getting up in the morning.*

*(c) Avoid standing like this.*

*(d) Sit whenever you can.*

*(e) Make several opportunities in the day (and especially in the evening) to sit with the legs raised high so that the blood is running back effectively. This gives the veins and tissues recovery periods and reduces the ill-effects of unrelieved distension due to standing. Move the feet often.*

*(f) A reclining chair that elevates the feet above the horizontal is a good investment*

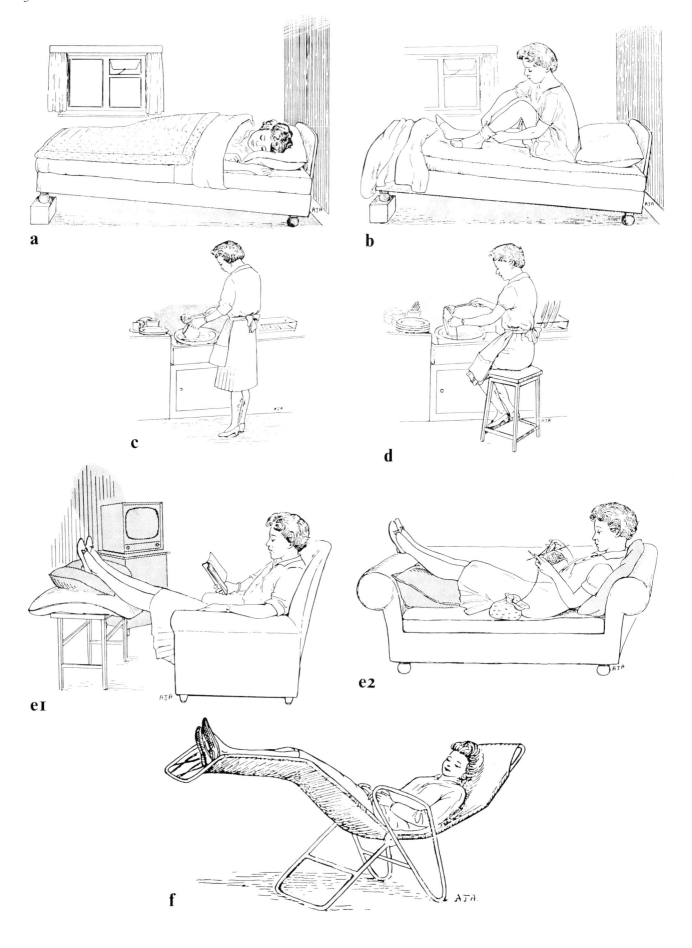

incompetence in pregnancy are more florid but essentially the same as those already described in Chapters 4 and 5, and often with varicosities in the vulva becoming a dominant problem. Vulval varicosities will be considered separately later in this chapter.

## Aetiology of varicosities in pregnancy

The development of varicosities in pregnancy is accompanied by all the usual signs of valve failure in the superficial veins, with retrograde flow down a saphenous vein and the varicosities. At an early stage the superficial veins become more prolific and enlarged; this relaxation of vein walls is shared by the valve rings supporting the cusps, so that they tend to separate and leakage occurs. After pregnancy the vein walls contract down again and the cusps usually regain their former competence but may fail to do so. Outside pregnancy this process is often seen in miniature during the premenstrual stage of the monthly hormonal cycle which, in fact, is the earliest preparation for possible pregnancy. At this time a patient with incipient or actual varicose veins will find they are noticeably more prominent and troublesome. If pregnancy occurs this influence is not withdrawn and will prove progressive. In the first few months the main cause for these changes is hormonal but later the physical and vascular changes in the pelvis will tend to enhance any weakness in the veins caused by hormones.

### The hormonal influence

The veins are in fact sharing in the widespread changes of pregnancy which cause tissues to soften and yield throughout the body. These changes are caused by oestrogen-related hormones, which relax the pelvic ligaments in preparation for childbirth. Involvement of other structures such as veins and ureters seem to be incidental rather than serving any useful purpose. The response to this varies from patient to patient and, indeed, may differ in the same patient in succeeding pregnancies. Little can be done to prevent this influence without endangering the pregnancy.

### The physical and vascular influences

Two obvious influences that may also affect the veins of the lower limbs are the physical weight and bulk of the developing uterus, and the massive vascular changes associated with the increasing size of the placenta. The changes in the veins, however, are well established before these factors have become significant so that they are aggravating factors rather than causative. The gravid uterus may compress and partially obstruct iliac veins with further distension of the already oversized valve rings in the lower limbs. Similarly the placenta forms a virtual arteriovenous fistula tending to raise pressure

within the pelvic veins. The changes of pregnancy are so complex and widespread that it is difficult to pinpoint the key factors, but little can be done to change them and usually the only ways for the patient to ease her discomforts are by elevating her limbs as much as possible and by use of well-fitted elastic support.

## The management of varicose veins in pregnancy

The obvious question is 'why not treat the veins by surgery or sclerotherapy?', and certainly there have been advocates of this (Dodd and Payling Wright, 1959; Fegan, 1960; Fegan, Beesley and Fitzgerald, 1964; Fegan, 1967; Abramowitz, 1973). Sigg (1977) reports successful results with sclerotherapy in over 3000 pregnant women and quotes Fegan, and Tournay and Wallois in support of his opinion that this is justifiable in pregnancy in order to bring relief from severe complaints, but cautions that the first 3 months and the last month must be avoided to minimize risk to the fetus. However, the advocates of active intervention in pregnancy are significantly few and there are several strong arguments for avoiding active intervention during pregnancy:

1. Nothing should be done that might bring harm to mother or fetus; their protection is paramount.
2. The varicose veins usually recede quickly after pregnancy so that treatment may not ever be needed.
3. Varicose veins (superficial incompetence), including vulval varicosities, seldom cause great harm or danger to the patient either during pregnancy or at childbirth. The discomforts are bearable in the knowledge that they will have to be accepted for only a few months and that, if treatment is eventually required, this can be more safely and effectively carried out after pregnancy. Unnecessary treatment is avoided and, at worst, it is no more than a postponement of treatment until a more suitable time.
4. Surgery during pregnancy may present difficulties in a 'hypervascular' pregnant patient and this need not arise if another time is chosen. The florid varicose veins seen in pregnancy are altogether different from the usual well-defined varicose veins seen outside pregnancy. Instead of the single source and pathway of incompetence, so satisfactory to treat, there appears to be a general enlargement of all superficial veins with large varicosities and tortuous venules sprouting from them and apparently filling from multiple sources. A convincing demonstration of the benefits that should follow surgery is not possible. The picture is almost one of a general weakening and stretching of vein walls with superimposed patterns of incompetence. To the surgeon contemplating surgery it seems likely that many veins capable of recovery after childbirth are going to be removed without achieving any significant advantage.

Most surgeons are convinced by the wisdom of these arguments and it will be exceptional for them to carry out active treatment at any stage during pregnancy (Dodd and Cockett, 1976; May, 1979). Moreover, there is universal agreement that active treatment should be avoided during the first 2 months of pregnancy because of the unknown risk to the fetus. A minority of authorities advocate surgery or sclerotherapy after this time but only for quite strong indications.

Undoubtedly the safest policy is to manage the problem of varicose veins in pregnancy conservatively and to reassess the veins some 3 or 4 months after childbirth. This reassessment should not be delayed too long because sometimes a further pregnancy forestalls the surgeon! If the veins have not receded then appropriate surgery should be carried out without delay, particularly if there is any question of further pregnancy. The patient should be encouraged to have this follow-up inspection and follow the advice given, since otherwise the veins may be given low priority and continue enlarging insidiously over the years.

### Should treatment be postponed until the family is completed?

This question is often asked in the belief that the good results of treatment will soon be lost in another pregnancy. There is some truth in this if the treatment has been by sclerotherapy alone but, even if further varicose veins do temporarily appear, further pregnancy is unlikely to have lost the advantages gained by surgery when the patient is assessed a few months after childbirth. The probability of having further children is in fact a good reason for a surgical 'tidy up' at the first opportunity.

In summary the advice given to the patient should be:

1. Varicose veins are a temporary nuisance and pregnancy is not the time to treat them. If they do not subside after pregnancy then the veins can be surgically tidied up (or, if minimal, by sclerotherapy) and the possibility of further pregnancies need not prevent this. Motherhood does not mean that the patient need endure varicose veins for years to come.
2. During pregnancy the veins should be given good support by elastic stockings which will improve comfort and help prevent their excessive enlargement, so that regression is more likely after childbirth. During the day, time must be found to have a number of breaks with the legs raised above the horizontal, for example, on a settee banked with cushions. In this way the veins have recovery periods and are not subjected to unremitting distension. This will also prevent a build up of discomfort and will help minimize the severity of the condition.
3. If oedema is troublesome this must be discussed with the obstetrician who may wish to check upon its sig-

nificance and possibly to prescribe diuretics or other treatment.

### Comment

The worst varicose veins the author has seen is when the patient has had a succession of pregnancies with only a few weeks' interval between them. The large varicosities of the earlier pregnancies have scarcely begun to recede before the veins are burdened yet again and the mother with a family of young children has to work all day without respite. In these circumstances the veins may become alarmingly large in mid-pregnancy and so widespread, with multiple points of filling, that only a very prolonged (and therefore most undesirable in pregnancy) surgical procedure could bring benefit. Such a patient is very difficult to help; suggestions for tubal ligation are rejected and often the husband shows little inclination to allow an interval for the much needed operation to be carried out, or to consider vasectomy. Nevertheless, medium-weight elastic stockings, tubular elastic bandage (see below) or even light-weight stockings can be invaluable to this patient; strong stockings may be too uncomfortable and lose her cooperation.

### Elastic support in pregnancy

It is all too easy to prescribe heavy elastic stockings that make the patient so miserably uncomfortable that she abandons any attempt to use them. The usual mistake is to provide excessively strong thigh-length stockings that crease behind the knee and are uncomfortably hot in warm weather. This can add considerably to the inevitable discomforts of pregnancy. Given below are some suggestions for prescribing stockings in pregnancy:

1. For minimal to moderate varicosities support tights or light-weight elastic stockings or tights are comfortable and will provide sufficient support with improved appearance. Most maternity centres can give advice upon this and there are also independent organizations specializing in mother care who will provide tights suitable for the changing girth of pregnancy.
2. If varicosities are large in terms of size and extent, and mainly below the knee, then medium-weight two-way-stretch stockings (18–24 mmHg compression at ankle), up to the knee (calf length), should prove comfortable for the patient and avoid the difficulties that may arise with elastic stockings crossing the knee joint. Thigh varicosities do not necessarily require support unless they are excessively large; the main requirement is to give support below the knee. Worn bilaterally the appearance is neat and well accepted by most patients. However, when the upper calf is not well rounded there may be problems because the uppermost part of the stocking has insufficient purchase to resist the

downward pull of a two-way-stretch stocking. The solution here is to extend the stocking up to full thigh length, or, perhaps better, use a below-knee one-way-stretch stocking which will not tend to pull down. Tights in these weights of elastic material will be cumbersome, uncomfortable and hot so that they should only be prescribed in special circumstances. Below-knee one-way-stretch stockings are usually very effective and satisfactory but, although somewhat thicker and coarser than the two-way stretch, most women will accept this for a temporary need. Another good alternative is to use a tubular elastic bandage, such as Tubigrip; this may be worn in a single or a double layer and used up to the knee (size D is suitable for most patients) is, in effect, a one-way-stretch stocking without any downward pull. The same material can, of course, be worn as a full thigh-length stocking and in this case it is best to obtain the shaped variety (SSB-shaped support bandage, sizes D–F, long). This usually requires support with suspenders but is comfortable to wear, neat in appearance and well ventilated so that it is not unduly hot. The material will require renewal about every 4 weeks but it is strongly recommended when other types of elastic support prove unsuitable. Indeed many clinics make it their first choice for use in pregnancy.

3. In the severe case, where there is much discomfort, with swelling and purple congested areas near the ankle, perhaps the threat of ulceration, and accompanied by massive varicosities, it may be essential to use the strong support provided by one-way-stretch stockings (25–35 mmHg compression at the ankle) but again keeping this below the knee unless there are unusually large thigh varicosities. If these are present, thigh-length medium-weight or strong one-way-stretch stockings may be used, but the alternative is, again, to use shaped tubular bandage, as a double layer up to the top of the thigh. Yet another alternative is to use a one-way-stretch stocking up to the knee combined with tubular elastic bandage to support the thigh.

4. If the patient has a post-thrombotic limb so that there are pre-existing venous problems then probably she is already well adapted to elastic stockings and should continue with these. It must be remembered, however, that in this condition increasing the strength of the stockings does not necessarily bring increased benefits and may indeed impede collateral venous return. Good quality stockings giving graduated compression, maximal near the ankle, but lessening up the limb so that collateral veins are not unduly compressed, will be required and these will need expert fitting by a specialist in elastic garments. The criterion of success is that they should bring comfort to the patient, and if this is not so, they are probably giving little or no benefit and may indeed be harmful. Usually

one-way-stretch up to the knee, fitted individually for that patient, will provide the best answer.

When severe vulval varicosities are present these will require specially made garments and this will be referred to in the following section.

## Varicosities of the vulva in pregnancy

Vulval varicosities developing during pregnancy can be a source of considerable discomfort and may become quite alarming in size. Characteristically the varicosities, which may occur on either side and occasionally bilaterally, bulge downwards from the labium major and from here further varicosities may radiate through the perineum and down the neighbouring thigh. They become maximal in mid-pregnancy and are more likely to occur in multiparous women than in the first pregnancy. They are commonly seen with associated development of varicose veins in the lower limb, and perhaps one patient in four having both conditions. Overall about 2% of pregnant women will develop significant vulval varicosities (Dodd and Payling Wright, 1959).

The discomforts arise from protruberance, with a sense of weight and heat, in the vulval region. When fully developed the overlying skin becomes chaffed with walking, causing additional discomfort to the patient.

In spite of the considerable size the varicosities may reach, they seldom seem to cause any real harm. There appears to be little reliable information upon complications arising from vulval varicosities but personal discussion with the Department of Obstetrics, John Radcliffe Hospital, Oxford, revealed that no cases of thrombosis or haemorrhage from these varicosities, either before or during childbirth, could be recalled. This Department regards them as a great nuisance for the patient but one in which active treatment is best avoided and conservative measures, using devices giving support, should be used to see the patient through pregnancy. After pregnancy the varicosities usually subside rapidly into insignificance and do not necessarily recur at subsequent pregnancies. However, a certain number do continue as moderate-sized varicosities in the vulva or upper thigh but are often symptomless. These surviving varicosities will be referred to again presently.

### The source of vulval varicosities

The massive increase in vascularity, in both arteries and veins, within the pelvis scarcely needs emphasizing here and it is not surprising that veins communicating with the exterior veins should become grossly enlarged and allow free communication, in either direction. When this occurs, not only are intra-abdominal pressures immediately transmitted to the exterior, as shown by the massive cough impulse in a vulval varicosity, but, when the patient is standing, considerable gravitational downflow will occur through these varicosities to link with an incompetent saphenous system or its own system of varices running down the thigh posteromedially.

The main communications on each side between pelvic and exterior veins that may enlarge in this fashion are:

1. The obturator vein, which arises from the internal iliac vein and has communication with both uterine and ovarian veins through the venous plexus in the broad ligament.
2. The internal pudendal and inferior gluteal veins, also branches of the internal iliac vein and communicating freely with the uterine and ovarian veins.
3. Less frequently, by veins accompanying the round ligament. These veins communicate with the external iliac and ovarian veins, and with the obturator veins by pubic branches.
4. All these veins communicate with the opposite side within the pelvis by venous plexuses in the broad ligament, internal iliac branches and presacral veins, and by vaginal, vulval and pubic exterior veins.
5. Any of these veins emerging from the pelvis may connect with the common femoral and long saphenous veins via their deep and superficial external pudendal branches.

A venogram, through vulval varicosities persisting after pregnancy, will quite often show communications by all these routes but usually one or two components predominate and offer a possible means for controlling the varicosities. However, in active treatment during pregnancy, when the veins are so large and freely communicating, the technical problems are daunting although there are some reports of successful procedures (Dodd and Payling Wright, 1959); needless to say, phlebography during pregnancy should be avoided, but without this surgery would be blindly directed and limited in its prospect of success. Stein (1977) states that vulval varicosities can be injected in pregnancy but advises that it is best left for those that persist after childbirth; we agree with this and regard pregnancy as a strong contraindication, with possible dangers, and real doubt whether any effective response would be obtained in this hypervascular state.

## Management of vulval varicosities in pregnancy

For surgical control to be successful, a preliminary venogram will be required to identify the main communications which are to be removed. Reluctance to do this during pregnancy and the wish to avoid any surgical procedure weigh heavily in the usual decision to manage the veins conservatively. The basis of this is to give mechanical support to the varicosities by specially made elastic garments. Most maternity centres will know of a specialist (orthotist) who will fit the patient individually and

this garment can be combined with appropriate elastic support for varicosities in the lower limbs which are so often present as well. A garment such as this is a tedious burden for the patient who, nevertheless, may well prefer it to the miseries and soreness that otherwise occur. As with varicosities in the lower limb, the vulval varicosities may become slightly less troublesome in the later stages of pregnancy.

## Persisting vulval varicosities after pregnancy

At least 3 months should elapse before making any critical assessment of persisting varicosities in the vulva or upper thigh. Usually these are symptomless and appear harmless, so that active treatment should only be considered if they are causing the patient some form of discomfort, or, because a further pregnancy is likely and it is hoped to prevent the previous problems. If this is so, the first step must be an evaluation of the source of the varicosities and their downward communications. If this appears comparatively localized without an associated long saphenous incompetence then trial of sclerotherapy is justifiable. If there is obvious incompetence in the long saphenous system, with communication to vulva varices through external pudendal veins, then it will be reasonable to advise surgery to correct this, combined with removal of pudendal branches by following them to the labial varicosities. If this is planned, it is advisable to obtain an upward trace venogram, either a short while before the operation or as a preliminary preoperative measure. In the occasional case where pelvic congestion syndrome (see Chapter 5) is suspected, phlebography by selective catheterization of the ovarian veins will be necessary. The post-thrombotic state of internal and exterior varices crossing the pelvis as collaterals to common iliac occlusion must be clearly distinguished from the purely incompetent states referred to above and if there is any uncertainty phlebography should be used to clarify this beyond doubt.

### Sclerotherapy

It has already been suggested that when there is gross incompetence in the long saphenous system then surgical treatment of this and the vulval veins may be best. However, in other circumstances sclerotherapy can be satisfactory (Stein, 1977), although there is not universal agreement over this. The injection needle is usually inserted into a varicosity in the uppermost thigh or perineum adjacent to the vulval varicosity. It can, however, be inserted into the labium majus itself if necessary. The total amount of sclerosant should be limited to 0.5 ml of 3% sodium tetradecyl sulphate and the veins immediately compressed with the fingers for 2 minutes. It is usually not really practicable to maintain compression for long in this region but often a small pad supported by an elastic adhesive strip can be kept in place for 24 hours. A satisfactory response with thrombotic occlusion of the vein is usually obtained and this causes little discomfort to the patient. The author believes that the long term success is reasonably good but there is little to substantiate this specific point in any published work. However, in view of the ease and apparent success of this procedure, there is much to be said for giving it a trial before considering surgery and it need not be preceded by venography.

### Phlebography for persisting vulval varicosities

With the patient lying horizontally, low osmolar contrast medium is introduced, either by needle, or at operation by actual cannulation into any convenient varicosity close to the vulva. 30 ml of contrast medium should be injected quite quickly to ensure a representative distribution through all the branches, and a static film is taken (Figure 18.2). It may be repeated if necessary. This simple form of varicography is usually sufficient but when it is suspected that the vulval veins arise from the pelvic varicosis of ovarian vein incompetence (pelvic congestion syndrome – Chapter 5) the more sophisticated examination of descending phlebography by bilateral selective catheterization of the ovarian veins will be required.

### Surgical treatment of persisting vulval and pudendal varicosities

There are few comprehensive reviews upon surgical treatment and the techniques are still developing (see Chapter 5). However, the following procedures will bring a good yield of success:

1. As described above, long saphenous incompetence should be corrected by ligation flush with the common femoral vein together with all its uppermost branches, stripping of at least its thigh component and surgical removal of the major varicosities in the thigh. The deep external pudendal branch arising from the common femoral vein is looked for and divided, and the superficial pudendal vein traced, if possible, to the labial varicosity. A small incision may be made on the outer aspect of the labium majus to dissect away the varicosity itself but the surgeon must be warned that these varicosities have the thinnest of walls and seem to disappear at a touch. Nevertheless, a direct assault on a vulval varicosity in this fashion usually succeeds in obliterating it.

2. If a venogram has identified an impressive communication with obturator, internal pudendal, inferior gluteal or round ligament veins then surgery may be directed to one or more of these sources. The round ligament and accompanying varicosities can be removed from within the inguinal canal down to the labium. The varicose labial branches of pudendal

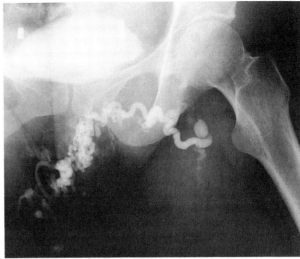

a

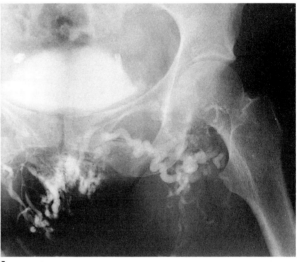

b

**Figure 18.2** *Phlebograms showing interconnection between the external pudendal vein on the left side (persisting after saphenofemoral ligation without stripping) and vulval varicosities. These provide a cross-over circulation to the opposite side. Two phases of filling are shown*

and gluteal veins can be located where they cross the perineum and traced from here but these flimsy veins are not easy to handle satisfactorily.

3. In the unusual case where the vulval varices are part of a system of incompetence through ovarian and pelvic veins, and onwards down the limb, proven by appropriate varicography, then a very different form of surgery is required. This will entail ligation and part removal of the ovarian veins and pelvic varices through an abdominal retroperitoneal approach (Lechter, Alvarez and Lopez, 1987; Hobbs, 1990 – and see Chapter 5).

# Support stockings and bandages

## Elastic support

### Characteristics, design and types of elastic stocking: graduated compression

An elastic stocking, used to control venous disorders, is intended to provide even compression and support, maximal on the foot and ankle, but reducing up the limb in similar fashion to hydrostatic venous pressure in a standing patient. Without such graduation, compression, suitable to counteract ankle venous pressure when standing, would be excessive in the thigh and would restrict venous return from the limb. Graduated compression, avoiding this, is considered a necessary feature and is incorporated in virtually all present-day elastic stockings (Cornwall, Dore and Lewis, 1987; Drug Tariff (National Health Service England and Wales), 1989).

Patients' limbs vary considerably in the strength of compression required, for example, support hose or light support stockings to control and conceal minor varicose veins may only need to exert 14 mmHg compression at the ankle, and are made of thin, attractive-looking material. At the other extreme, a patient with massive varicosities and recurring ulceration may require a strong support stocking, giving compression of 35 mmHg at the ankle, with an easily discernible fabric, but greatly preferable in appearance to the varicose veins it covers. There is an upper limit above which increased compression ceases to give benefit to venous conditions and may become harmful. This maximum is probably about 40 mmHg at ankle level (Fentem, Goddard and Gooden, 1976; Jones et al., 1980; Chant, Magnussen and Kershaw, 1985; Burnand and Layer, 1986; Struckman et al., 1986). Few conditions will benefit from a stocking giving stronger compression than this but it may be necessary in some, for example, widespread congenital arteriovenous fistulas.

### Some terms used in designation of support stockings

**Support hose (or hosiery)** This is the lightest form of support, virtually indistinguishable from ordinary nylon, and obtainable, either as stockings or tights for women, from any 'high street store'. Self-supporting knee-length stockings, designed for men, and substituting for ordinary socks, are also available. Used to enhance appearance and relieve discomforts, for minor blemishes or small varicosities and aching legs, this class of support is freely available without needing medical advice.

**Elastic or 'surgical' hose as stockings or tights** This includes the range of elastic support from light to strong, usually only obtainable from special centres on medical recommendation. They are regarded as a form of medical treatment and, in the wrong circumstances, could be

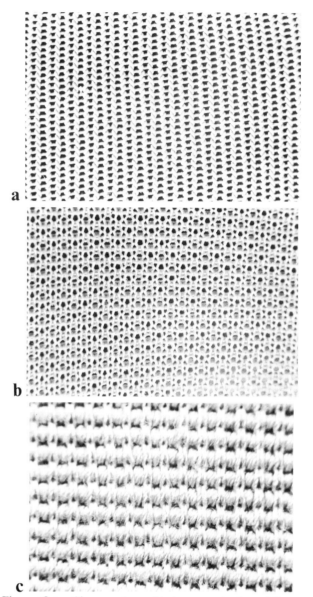

**Figure 18.3** *Close-up views of knit pattern in three different elastic stockings; all are at the same magnification.*

*(a) A uniform knit of elastane giving two-way elasticity. When pulled onto the limb this stocking will conform well and give the desired compression but will give quite strong downpull. It will require firm support by suspender and thus may cause the stocking to be pulled up uncomfortably against the toes.*

*(b) A complex interweaving of horizontally running thread of elastodiene (natural rubber) and vertically running knit of elastane (synthetic) thread. Although it is two-way stretch it will give good circumferential compression with only light longitudinal elasticity; this enables it to conform well without unduly strong downpull.*

*(c) A one-way-stretch stocking designed to give strong compression without downpull and, hence, very suitable for use below the knee. The thick horizontal fibres, running circumferentially, are of natural rubber with cotton wound over it and provide the compression; the vertically running knit is of inelastic cotton strand so that there is no longitudinal elasticity. This type of stocking requires individual manufacture and is regarded by some as outdated. Nevertheless, it is often the most satisfactory type for post-thrombotic syndrome*

harmful, hence the need for prescription. In the past they were mostly prescribed by surgeons and the designation 'surgical' presumably arises from this.

**Stretch characteristics** Endless ingenuity and effort have gone into the design of the stockings now available, with each manufacturer incorporating his own special features and arrangement of strands in the attempt to approach the ideal (Figure 18.3). The most commonly used principle is a two-way-stretch material, which when stretched up the length of the limb conforms well to the contours in the majority of limbs. There are many variants of this fabric which is highly adaptable and allows easy fitting within a limited range of sizes, so that most patients can be supplied from stock 'off the shelf'. A small penalty for this great convenience is that the stocking has a tendency to pull down the limb. This is easy enough to combat by a suspender with thigh-length stockings in women, but may be a nuisance in below-knee stockings. Modern two-way-stretch stockings are seamless and give an excellent appearance without banding or wrinkling. The component of downward pull has of recent years been minimized and the term 'two-way-stretch' is often omitted so that the stocking is simply referred to by strength of support, for example, graduated compression stocking, medium support (Class III), will be generally understood to be of this sort.

The other category is one-way-stretch material, which is elastic circumferentially but not longitudinally, so that a stocking does not suffer from any tendency to pull downwards. The strongest support stockings are often made in this material.

The pros and cons of these two basic materials are considered further presently, but first it may be helpful to describe something of the structure of the fabrics and the technical terms that are used.

**The types of thread and knit** The principle strands will, of course, be elastic and this may be of natural rubber (elastodiene), or a synthetic elastic thread of polyurethane-based fibre (elastane) with special varieties carrying their tradenames, for example, Lycra (DuPont) or Spanzelle (Courtaulds). There is much debate whether synthetic elastic (elastane) is better than natural rubber (elastodiene) in terms of elastic properties and ability to withstand wear, skin moisture and ointments, and detergents. Synthetic fibre is now widely used in light and medium support hosiery but many manufacturers still prefer natural rubber for all grades. The fibre content is usually clearly stated on each pack, together with size and compression class.

The thickness of a strand or yarn is gauged in denier or decitex and indicates the weight in grams of 9000 metres or 10 000 metres respectively; thus a slender strand will have a low denier of, say, 40, but a thick one, used in a strong elastic material, might be 350 denier. These elastic yarns are wrapped in one or more layers of cotton or nylon strand, partly to protect the underlying elastic

core but also to improve the appearance; in addition it may reduce the likelihood of skin sensitivity reactions to the elastic filaments. Interwoven with these threads are other strands, usually nylon, which help to distribute the elastic forces evenly. The exact disposition and method of using these strands varies from one manufacturer to another and in large part give the stocking its particular characteristics. In the preparation of the fabric there are two main types, detailed below.

*Circular knitted* Here the elastic yarn is knitted in a circular pattern of interlocking stitches to give a continuous seamless tube, amongst which are interwoven other strands designed to distribute the elasticity evenly. Graduation of compression is achieved by an increased density of the knitted elastic strands in the lower part of the stocking. Until it is put on the limb the stocking is about half the length of the limb to which it is to be applied and has a rather shapeless outline. However, when it is stretched to full length its component strands conform closely to the limb contours and give graduated compression up its length, without any undesirable banding, for example, behind the knee. This knit is the most widely used in the manufacture of typical (two-way-stretch) elastic stockings in common use today.

*Flatbed* This is knitted on a flat frame which allows variation in width. It can be used to produce a seamless stocking or a fabric that can be sewn into shape with a seam. Here the essential elastic thread runs in a shallow spiral around the circumference of the stocking for its entire length. A pattern of interweaving strands closely enmesh the elastic spiral to complete the fabric of the stocking. Graduated compression is obtained by varying the circumference of the elastic course along the length of the stocking, so that this is least at the ankle but increases up its length. This gives the stocking a shaped appearance when it is off, but in this contracted state it is appreciably shorter than the limb and does require some stretching onto it. This technique of knitting is used to produce stockings made to measure and where a special shape is required for an unusual limb, it may produce a seamed or seamless stocking and has the advantage of giving comparatively little downward pull. Again, the appearance is good with excellent conformity to contour and even lie on the limb.

There are many variants, according to the manufacturer, of these two basic knits with different patterns of interweaving strands, or combinations of elastic yarn. This variation explains why some makes suit one patient more than another, or why there is a difference in cost. Many properties such as durability, and withstanding washing without loss of its resilience, will vary, but even the best will require careful washing and this is described later.

It is usual for all these stockings to have a closed heel and the lighter varieties also have a 'closed toe'. The stronger versions are often supplied with an 'open toe' and this is desirable so that the toes are not crowded.

Because of the appreciable variation between the makes of stocking, the patients may have to experiment to find out which brand suits them best. Tights as light support hose are very popular and are no more than strengthened, lightly elasticated, nylon stockings. They are easily available in ordinary hosiery departments without the need for specialist fitters. A common difficulty with these is the purchase of an inadequate length so that the tights are overstretched and, being fixed by the pelvic portion, give an upward pull, transmitted uncomfortably to the toes. Most brands supply tights specially designed for the longer limb. The patient must be advised of this and should try several makes before concluding that support tights are 'too uncomfortable' to use; they are not all identical and there is nearly always one that will prove suitable. With 'surgical' elastic stockings a good starting point is to have the stocking fitted and supplied by a specialist centre where an expert orthotist is available for the unusual fit.

*Selection of the most suitable elastic support*

The term 'two-way-stretch' indicates that the stocking is elastic both circumferentially (predominantly) and longitudinally. This term is not used so commonly as it used to be because manufacturers feel that they have now eliminated most of the undesirable downward pull associated with the older types of two-way-stretch material. Nevertheless, some downpull remains with any stocking that is stretched by 30% or more of its resting length in order to cover the limb. Graduated compression, achieved by increased density of the knit in the lower part, is easily recognizable by comparing closely the texture in upper and lower parts.

**Two-way-stretch elastic stockings** It has already been pointed out that two-way stretch has the great advantage of considerable adaptability so that, say, three standard sizes can conform to 80% of limbs. Thus very little skill in fitting is required and the stocking can be taken 'off the shelf' and not specially made to measure. However, to attain this means that the stocking has to be stretched onto the limb and held in this stretched position, that is to say, appreciable downpull has to be resisted by suspender belt, a slip-resistant garter or by taking advantage of the limb contour. The inverted-cone shape of the thigh, particularly in heavily built people, causes an elastic stocking to slip easily or to roll down to form a constricting band and certainly will require support by a suspender. Only a minority of thighs are slender enough and sufficiently uniform in width to permit wearing light elastic support without this. The lower thigh, just above the expansion of the knee joint, may prove a suitable level for a self-maintaining stocking in some people.

With elastic support as tights, taken above the pelvic and gluteal bulge, the body shape holds them in good position. The amount of downpull by a 'surgical' stocking varies with the type of knit and arrangement of additional interwoven strands employed, so that some makes give less downpull than others. Other variants are, of course, the length, circumference and contour of the limb and the patient may have to experiment to find the make that suits her best. Another disadvantage of longitudinal pull is that it may extend to the foot, so that the toes are uncomfortably forced against the closed end of the stocking, especially in the longer limb of a tall person. The solution here is to ensure that a brand of stocking manufactured for the longer limb is used, or an open-ended stocking.

If a below-knee stocking is to be used, the shape of the calf is important. Its upper part is slightly narrower just below the knee and this usually gives the stocking sufficient purchase to resist slight elastic downpull, but in a sizeable minority of patients, with a less rounded calf, repeated creeping down can be a problem. One answer to this is to use a thigh-length stocking and suspender belt, but, for a man, a better solution is to use a one-way-stretch stocking, or shaped elastic tubular bandage (Tubigrip – see below), below the knee.

*Measurements required when ordering* All manufacturers supply diagrams to assist in the ordering of stockings and making clear the key measurements and other information required for selecting the correct size and category of stocking for the patient. The patient should not be measured in an oedematous state; this should be reduced by elevation overnight, or longer if there is considerable oedema, and seen early in the day before it reaccumulates.

**One-way-stretch elastic stocking** In this material the stretch is only circumferential (horizontal) and there is no downward pull so that they have the great advantage of providing robust support below the knee without pulling down. The principal elastic course runs spirally around the circumference of the stocking and the diameter of this varies according to the graduated compression required. Its heavier weight gives it a somewhat coarse appearance, acceptable in men, trousered women or when a severe venous disorder is present. These stockings are unnecessarily strong for lesser varicosities but if massive simple varicosities are present, and surgical treatment is not possible, they can prove an excellent answer as below-knee stockings.

These stockings are made in 'fine thread' and 'stout thread', both seamless, but the latter having a somewhat coarser appearance. Both are a robust material which is best limited to below the knee. Thigh-length stockings made in this material are too strong and uncomfortable for most circumstances but may be the only means of controlling severe congenital venous disorders or severe multiple congenital arteriovenous fistulas. The stocking is usually supplied with an open heel which can cause discomfort, but upon request the supplier will insert a heel and this should be ordered. In common with most stronger stockings it has an 'open toe' and this is to be preferred. This fabric is well ventilated and conforms well below the knee to give a neat appearance. It gives strong support (Class III) and is therefore only required for the more severe varicose vein problems or in deep vein impairment. In spite of its heavy appearance many patients prefer this material because of its effectiveness and comfort without any downward creep when used below the knee. It does however require more skilful fitting.

*Measurement and fitting of one-way-stretch stockings* Measurements should be taken with the the leg elevated so that the veins are not distended. Ideally, when on, with the leg elevated, the stocking should be a snug fit with only slight elastic compression; when the patient stands and the veins try to fill, the strong elastic support resists distension of the veins but pressure within the stocking rises only to the venous hydrostatic pressure. Its potentially strong elastic compression should not be used to give heavy continuous compression but rather to resist overfilling of the veins, thus employing the 'containment' principle (see Chapter 13) so important with the inelastic paste bandage and described presently. A one-way-stretch stocking requires experienced fitting and the usual mistake is for it to be supplied gripping the leg far too tightly even when the leg is elevated. The ideal would be an inelastic stocking but this would not allow it to be pulled on and off over the heel; the one-way-stretch stocking, allowing this, is the nearest approach to one able to use the containment principle rather than giving powerful elastic compression even when all the veins are empty in elevation.

Another variety of one-way-stretch stocking comes in the form of an elastic tubular bandage (Tubigrip), which is described below.

*An alternative one-way-stretch elastic support* An excellent one-way-stretch material of moderate strength is provided as a tubular bandage (Tubigrip) supplied in various sizes. This may be obtained in rolls of uniform width from which appropriate lengths are cut, or, as shaped lengths (shaped support bandage or SSB), narrow in the lower part and wide above to accommodate either calf or thigh; it is supplied in various sizes and lengths, intended for use up to the knee or up to the top of the thigh. This shaping gives good graduated compression and, due to the absence of downpull, stays in place well on the calf, but in the thigh may require a suspender to stop downward rolling forming a constricting band. It is available in white or flesh colour and, when covered with an ordinary nylon stocking, gives a reasonably good appearance. It is well ventilated and comfortable to wear so that it is particularly suitable for an elderly patient; if extra compression is required, two layers, worn one on top of the other, may be used. The cut edge of this material has a frayed appearance but the patient must resist the temptation to double or roll this over to make it neater because this creates a constricting band. These stockings only last for about 6 weeks but this is offset by their comparatively low cost; they may be washed and dried overnight, using lukewarm water and good quality soap.

**Stockings made to special measure** Perhaps 10% of patients depart so far from the average limb that it is not possible to fit them with any of the standard sizes available. Most manufacturers make special provision for this and will make a stocking to special measurement and requirements. This is done either by adjusting the knit to give the size and shape required, or by shaping the material which is then sewn together by a seam at the back. The manufacturer's order forms give diagrams of the measurements they require.

*Effects of elastic compression upon abnormal venous physiology*

An elastic stocking may alter favourably the abnormal physiology of venous disorders in a number of possible ways, given below. This has been investigated clinically and scientifically by numerous authors but the value of many of these publications has been diminished by failure to distinguish between superficial venous incompetence, where the main failure is excessive downflow in superficial veins, and deep vein impairment, especially the post-thrombotic syndrome, in which the pumping mechanism is damaged, the deep veins are deformed or obstructed, and enlarged superficial veins act as collaterals. These collateral superficial veins are important for venous return and therefore must not be impeded by external compression. However, their enlargement has often caused their valves to become grossly incompetent and to treat this aspect by elastic compression may conflict severely with their collateral function.

In superficial vein incompetence, elastic compression simply prevents or limits downflow and this can only be beneficial, as experience has abundantly shown. In contrast, elastic compression in deep vein impairment can, at best, only give moderate benefit and, if misjudged, may easily cause adverse effects. It is wrong to put superficial incompetence and deep vein impairment into the same category of 'chronic venous insufficiency'; both may share similar venotensive changes but the causation and treatment of each is very different. Fortunately, most authors today do recognize the difference and in their studies only compare like with like, making it clear that only superficial vein incompetence is being considered, or, say, only post-thrombotic syndrome is included. There are, of course, 'grey' areas between these two states, for example, complex patterns with the features of both valveless and weak vein syndromes, certain varieties of perforator incompetence, and congenital venous abnormalities, but these are being increasingly recognized and separated off in comparative studies.

Some possible ways in which elastic support or compression, by stocking or bandage, may favourably affect venous disorder are listed below:

1. *In superficial incompetence:*
   (a) Reduces or prevents downflow in the incompetent veins.

(b) Restores valvular functions by giving support to expanded valve rings.

(c) Reduces surge to and from venous pool of foot and by this improves effectiveness of foot pump and musculovenous pumps of leg.

(d) Reduces perforator outflow, if this is present.

(e) Supports capillaries and, by reducing their over-

**TABLE 18.2** Comparison of elastic support in superficial vein incompetence and in deep vein impairment

| *Superficial vein incompetence* <br> *(simple varicose veins and complications)* | *Deep vein impairment* <br> *(post-thrombotic and valveless syndromes, and some types of perforator incompetence)* |
|---|---|
| 1. Reason for using: <br> To improve appearance <br>    Usually very successful in flattening bulging <br>    veins and smoothing out limb contour | Protuberant veins not necessarily a problem; if present, will flatten to give smoother surface but a strong stocking detracts from appearance. General enlargement of the limb, so often present, is unchanged |
| 2. Reason for using: <br> To support and compress superficial veins, maximally at ankle with graduated reduction in compression up the limb <br>    *Is very successful in limiting or preventing* <br>    *downflow in incompetent superficial veins,* <br>    *including varicosities.* If a component of <br>    perforator outflow is present, it will limit this. <br>    Prevents overdistension and pooling of venous <br>    blood in foot and leg. Effectiveness of <br>    musculovenous pumps greatly improved <br>    because no longer burdened by superficial <br>    downflow or surge from pooled blood. <br>    Summary: *very effective in controlling the basic* <br>    *defect in superficial vein incompetence* | Compression to control incompetent downflow conflicts with need to encourage collateral upflow. However, it does reduce or prevent overdistension and pooling in superficial veins of foot and leg; this nullifies surge so that priming of pumps is more effective and blood mainly directed upward instead of into an unwanted venous pool. This is the main benefit given by medium to strong elastic support and may bring moderate improvement by some reduction in venous hypertension. Undue compression to upper leg, and above, can constrict collateral superficial veins and cause harmful venous congestion. <br> Summary: *cannot control basic defect of impaired deep veins. Can only limit one secondary effect, venous pooling, and in this way give modest improvement in musculovenous pumping* |
| 3. Reason for using: <br> To reduce oedema <br>    May help in reducing a mild oedema by: <br>      Control of the venous disorder <br>      External support resists the accumulation of <br>      extracellular fluid and prevents <br>      overdistension of capillary bed so that <br>      transudation is limited | May help to reduce oedema but overall swelling in limb usually persists. Excessively strong compression to control oedema may restrict collateral flow and be counter-productive; elevation is a more effective way to reduce oedema |
| 4. Ease of obtaining a satisfactory fit <br>    Since limitation or prevention of superficial <br>    downflow is a key requirement, graduation is <br>    not a critical matter. With light and medium <br>    weight (Classes I and II) it is usually easy to <br>    obtain a satisfactory fit 'off the shelf' | *It is very important not to compress superficial veins acting as collaterals; therefore proper graduation of compression up the limb is critical.* A poor fit or unsuitable stocking may cause congestion and discomfort which the patient cannot endure. It is usually much more satisfactory to use stocking up to knee only; here one-way stretch stays in position well but two-way stretch may creep down |

*Notes:*

1. Although most patients fall decisively into the category of either superficial vein incompetence or of deep vein impairment, there is a sizeable minority who have the features of both conditions (see Chapter 10 – Complex patterns). In these patients, compression of superficial veins may be beneficial to one aspect but adverse to the other. Where a complex pattern of this sort is suspected it is safest to limit the length of stocking to below knee so that any component of collateral function in superficial veins above knee is not interfered with.

2. The considerations above do not include the use of elastic support in the prevention of postoperative deep vein thrombosis and pulmonary embolism (thromboembolic disease). This is referred to in Chapter 16.

3. Some patients with deep vein impairment find they fare better without any elastic support and they control swelling or ulceration by regulating the time given to elevation. There is no virtue in an elastic stocking unless the patient finds it brings real benefit in terms of comfort, control of ulceration and reduction of swelling. Many of these patients learn by experiment how to manage their leg(s) and may only put on the stocking when they visit the doctor! The doctor's duty is to advise the patient on the various factors that may be beneficial, so that the patient may try the merit of these; it would not be right for the doctor to insist that a stocking should be worn if the patient finds it causes miserable discomfort.

distension, decreases excessive transudation and formation of oedema.

(f) Compresses extracellular spaces so that capillary transudation is resisted and oedema is lessened.

2. *In deep vein impairment – especially post-thrombotic syndrome:*

(a) Reduces venous pool in overdistended veins of lower leg and foot. This reduces surge back and forth on exercise and directs blood more effectively into remaining musculovenous pumps.

(b) May improve component of incompetence in collateral superficial veins by supporting valve cusps but this may be offset by interference with collateral upflow.

(c) Supports capillaries and, by reducing their overdistension, decreases excessive transudation and formation of oedema.

(d) Compresses extracellular spaces so that capillary transudate is resisted and oedema is reduced.

(e) In complex patterns it may reduce undesirable component of incompetence but this may conflict with collateral requirements.

(f) Perforator outflow is an inherent part of collateral flow in the post-thrombotic syndrome and restricting this can be undesirable. At ankle or foot level, firm support is unlikely to cause harm in this respect and, for reasons given above, may be beneficial.

3. *In other venous disorders:*

Any of the factors listed above may prove helpful or harmful, according to the circumstances. The effect of elastic support is difficult to predict but always worth trial as below-knee support if venous hypertensive changes are present. If large varicosities are present in the thigh, elastic support can be extended to this level provided Doppler flowmetry has shown that these veins are not acting as collaterals.

**Scientific investigation of elastic compression** It is not proposed to attempt to review the scientific evidence upon benefits of elastic support here, but the papers of Struckman (1986), Brakkee and Kuiper (1988) and others listed in the references for this chapter are instructive in themselves and give a comprehensive bibliography of the work in this field.

A comparison between the use of elastic stocking support in superficial incompetence and in deep vein impairment is summarized in Table 18.2.

*Selection of stocking strength*

**Superficial vein incompetence** According to the severity of their varicosities most patients with superficial vein incompetence will be suited by support hose, light-weight elastic stockings (Class I) or medium-weight elastic stockings (Class II), either thigh length or below the knee. One-way-stretch shaped tubular elastic support (Tubigrip SSB) up to the knee, is particularly suitable for the elderly.

Stockings of strong, one-way-stretch material (Class III) are only suitable for unusually massive varicosities or when there is recurrent ulceration.

**Deep vein impairment (post-thrombotic syndrome, valveless syndrome and certain types of perforator incompetence)** These patients will usually require at least medium-weight (Class II) graduated compression up to the knee. If calf shape does not allow the stocking to stay in place at this level then use either a one-way-stretch stocking or a double layer of Tubigrip, or a thigh-length medium-weight stocking. Unusually severe cases, e.g. congenital vascular abnormalities, may require strong elastic support (Class III) either one-way or two-way stretch.

A guide to selection of stocking strength in the various venous conditions is given in Table 18.3; lymphoedema has not been included.

**TABLE 18.3** Guide to strength (class) of stocking to be used (Classes given are those in the Drug Tariff of National Health Service, England and Wales)

| Reason for use | Support recommended |
|---|---|
| *In superficial vein incompetence* | |
| 1. Appearance | Support tights, light-weight elastic stocking or tights, Class I, compression at ankle 14–17 mmHg |
| 2. Moderate varicosities with some discomfort | As above |
| 3. Substantial varicosities and venotensive changes; concealed incompetence with early venotensive changes; varicosities in pregnancy | Medium support, Class II, compression at ankle 18–24 mmHg |
| 4. Massive varicosities or concealed incompetence with marked or progressive venotensive change or ulceration | Medium support, Class II, may be sufficient, otherwise strong support, Class III, compression at ankle 25–35 mmHg. Often best as one-way stretch below knee |
| 5. Severe varicosis in pregnancy, including vulva | Class II or III, maternity version, with expandable or adjustable 'panty top' |
| *In deep vein impairment* (post-thrombotic limb, valveless syndrome and some types of incompetent perforators) | Medium to strong support (Classes II and III) is usually required. Often below knee is preferable – one-way stretch may be best |

*Contact sensitivity to elastic materials*

All elastic stockings contain materials, notably rubber (elastodiene), synthetic elastic (elastane) or other synthetic fibres (nylon, polyamide or polyurethane polymers) and these are potential allergens to which the patient may become sensitive, causing mild to severe skin reaction.

The medical attendant must be constantly aware of this possibility with patients using elastic support. A patient who has a venous eczema will be particularly likely to react in this way to the materials in elastic stockings. Complete change of the elastic materials used may be successful in avoiding the allergen but the advice of an expert dermatologist should be obtained. As a last resort, uncoloured cotton crepe bandage, reapplied several times a day, may prove sufficient support without causing skin reactions.

### Care of elastic stockings

**Durability** Elastic stockings do require to be handled with reasonable care, both as regards putting on and taking off, and in regular washing. The slender fibres easily catch on any sharp edges, such as badly cut fingernails or metal objects worn on the hands, for example, mounted rings or wrist watches. When putting on a stocking it must not be forcibly dragged on, as this can be very damaging; it should be turned inside out and eased on, foot first, by gentle pull and stretch; likewise it should be peeled off, rather than rolled off or tugged off by a strong pull from its lower part.

**Washing** A stocking should be hand washed several times a week, using lukewarm water and good quality soap or soap flakes; detergents should not be used as these are likely to degrade the elastic fibres quite soon. Do not use a washing machine. Rinse thoroughly and remove excess moisture by folding in a towel; do not wring out or twist the material. Allow to dry at room temperature and not by any heat source; drying in strong sunlight (ultraviolet light) will damage the fabric. Having two stockings, or two pairs, ensures that there should be clean dry ones always ready.

At first, the precautions given above may seem tedious but soon become a routine and the effort is amply rewarded by the stocking being kept in an effective state for many months.

### Elastic and inelastic support bandages

#### Elastic webbing bandage

This is a strong elastic bandage, usually 7.5 cm wide. The compression it exerts is entirely dependent upon the tension used when it is applied and for this reason it should never be applied by an unskilled person. The usual error is to believe that there is virtue in applying it under strong tension and not understanding that turns of the bandage laid on top of each other give cumulative pressure; this may be far in excess of what is desirable or safe. Nevertheless, in experienced hands it can be of value and, in fact, with training, the patient can become very adept at self-application at a safe but effective tension. Its range

of usefulness in the main venous disorders is summarized below.

**Superficial vein incompetence** Here, elastic webbing bandage is unsightly and seldom necessary. An elastic stocking is usually equally effective and of better appearance. Elastic webbing (red or blue line) is easily misused by unduly tight application to cause great discomfort and harm. It seldom brings any special advantage in superficial vein incompetence but a few obese or elderly patients do prefer to use it and should be allowed to continue; they may find it easier to put on than a stocking and they can adjust it to give most comfort.

**Deep vein impairment** Elastic webbing bandage skilfully applied below the knee can give effective external support for those patients who accept its poor appearance because they appreciate the benefits it brings. However, unskilled application using excess pressure can cause great discomfort and harm. It is best applied with the limb in elevation and only laid on, not forcibly stretched on; in this way, when the patient stands, venous overfilling of the leg and foot is resisted and excessive compression, restricting circulation, does not occur. Careful training of the patient in self-application, or a member of family, or community nurse, can be well worthwhile. It may help to have a loop for the foot at one end to facilitate the awkward first turn.

#### Elastic webbing bandage:

- Must not be used in an ischaemic limb – overtight application too easily occurs.
- Must not be used if it causes pain – it is either being applied badly or is inappropriate for the circumstances, or the limb is ischaemic.
- Can be used in the presence of an ulcer if discharge is not too great and the ulcer is not too tender; it allows daily renewal and cleansing of ulcer.

#### Light to moderate strength elastic bandages

There is a great variety of these.

**Adhesive elastic bandage** This class has been widely used for many years and can be applied directly to the skin, but skin sensitivity reactions to the adhesive, or the elastic material, are quite common so that their use in this fashion in venous conditions is not recommended. However, they are very valuable for applying over an inert cotton bandage to form a flexible encasement in sclerotherapy or the treatment of ulcers. The interposition of the cotton bandage (usually crepe) largely prevents skin reaction to the adhesive.

**Self-adherent bandage** Other light elastic bandages are designed to cling or interlock to themselves (cohesive bandage) but do not adhere to the skin, for example, Coban. These are very useful in venous work and skin reaction does not commonly occur. However, the fact that the material binds strongly to itself can bring the disadvantage that any crease tends to form a tough band of rolled up bandage which cuts into the underlying skin. For this reason it should be used with care, or avoided, in the vicinity of a joint, or on the upper thigh where down-rolling may occur.

**Cotton crepe bandage** There is a wide range of non-adhesive, non-interlocking bandages made variously of cotton or synthetic material and some containing elastic strands. These are of value in the dressing of ulcers or skin reactions but care must be taken to use one that does not contain allergens. A good quality crepe bandage should not be spurned as a means of giving support to varicose disorders, especially varicose veins in the elderly. For a few hours after application it can give significant support to the veins and comfort to the patient; because it slackens quite quickly, it may be necessary for the patient to reapply it once or twice a day.

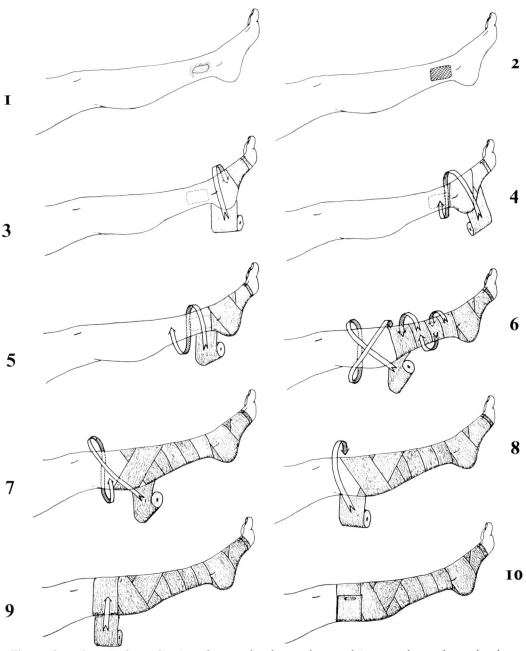

**Figure 18.4** *Steps in the application of a paste bandage and an overlying outer layer of crepe bandage. Care is taken to envelop the heel and ankle. This forms an inelastic encasement up to the knee and by using the containment principle is the most effective way of improving venous return in the post-thrombotic syndrome and valuable in the ambulatory treatment and healing of ulcers. It lacks the convenience of a pull on-off stocking and for this reason tends to be used only during a phase of active treatment under medical supervision rather than for long-term maintenance*

*Inelastic support*

**Inelastic paste (occlusive) bandage** The undoubted benefits of the paste bandage in healing a venous ulcer are due to inelastic 'containment' or 'encasement' of the leg and the term 'occlusive' is not really suitable because this is not their main virtue. Applied without any tension, closely laid onto the foot and leg whilst the limb is in elevation, the material sets into a firm inelastic support (Figure 18.4); when the patient stands, venous filling is limited by the 'container' but the pressure within this never rises above venous hydrostatic pressure for that part of the limb (see Chapter 13). This is an excellent and effective principle in many patients with ulcer. It does require experienced application and renewal every week or two, but a near relative can be trained in this. It is only suitable for application up to the knee. Comparison between its use in superficial vein incompetence and deep vein impairment is summarized in Table 18.4.

**TABLE 18.4.** Inelastic paste bandage: comparison of use in superficial vein incompetence and in deep vein impairment

| *Superficial vein incompetence (simple varicose veins and complications)* | *Deep vein impairment (post-thrombotic and valveless syndromes and some types of perforator incompetence)* |
|---|---|
| Not necessary unless ulcer is present. If ulcer does not respond to mobile treatment in elastic support by stocking, check that the diagnosis of superficial incompetence is correct – if so, a paste bandage is permissible until the ulcer is healed | Inelastic paste bandage is excellent principle for mobile treatment of ulcer. The remaining function in damaged or defective musculovenous pumps is assisted by the minimized venous pooling, so that useless venous surge to and from foot on exercise is largely eliminated; by supporting extracellular space, capillary transudate is reduced; because bandage is resisting expansion rather than compressing tissue it will not impede collateral flow in superficial vessels |

*Choice of length*

**Below-knee stocking (Figure 18.5(a))**
- In men – as men's support hose, one-way stretch or Tubigrip SSB; or as two-way stretch if preferred, according to severity and other circumstances.
- In women who can accept knee-length stocking and have a full shaped calf that will give good purchase above its main circumference. Two-way stretch gives best appearance but, if there are massive varicosities, a one-way stretch may be better.
- Below knee is often the most effective in deep vein problems.

**Thigh-length stocking**
*To lower thigh (Figure 18.5(b))* Seldom used, but in a slim person, a two-way-stretch stocking pulled up to the lower thigh can be successful in staying in place just above the knee expansion but a lot depends on characteristics of manufacture. A young patient may prefer this length but it is not advisable to prescribe it as a routine.

*To upper-mid thigh (Figure 18.5(c))* This is the usual length of thigh stocking, prescribed as 'thigh length' without other qualification. It is by far the most commonly used length for women with varicose veins, in all strengths of stocking. It will require some form of suspender. In slim limbs, a light support stocking with anti-slip gartertop may stay in place. Usually has closed toe and the stocking length must be appropriate for the limb, otherwise toes may be 'crumpled' by excessive upward pull; or use open toe (less popular).

*High thigh and waist length* Popular as tights in support hose, or light-weight elastic support (Figure 18.5(d)). Do not prescribe tights for medium or strong support unless patient wishes it or there is a special reason; they can be uncomfortably hot in summer and a thigh stocking with suspender is kinder.

- High thigh and waist length, as medium or strong support, will be required for unusual venous problems involving the upper thigh and pelvis, for example, congenital vascular disorder (Figure 18.5(e)).
- If high thigh support is necessary bilaterally, a stronger alternative to support hose tights is waist-length panty stockings, obtainable in all strengths and suitable for men and women (Figure 18.5(f)).
- Maternity elastic support with expandable panty top is available for pregnancy varicosis (Figure 18.5(g)).

**Points to remember in prescribing elastic support**

1. Always exclude arterial insufficiency (ischaemia); elastic compression can cause harm and, in severe ischaemia, lead to loss of the limb.
2. Thorough clinical and instrumental examination is necessary to ensure that the diagnosis is correct between superficial vein incompetence and deep vein impairment. If the diagnosis is superficial vein incompetence, then surgery or sclerotherapy is usually the best treatment; elastic support can control but not cure.
3. Elastic support is justifiable in superficial vein incompetence:
   (a) As a temporary measure, whilst the patient is awaiting surgery and there is likely to be a long delay before this.
   (b) In the elderly, or when surgery is not advisable for other reasons.
   (c) When the patient is reluctant to have either surgery or sclerotherapy.

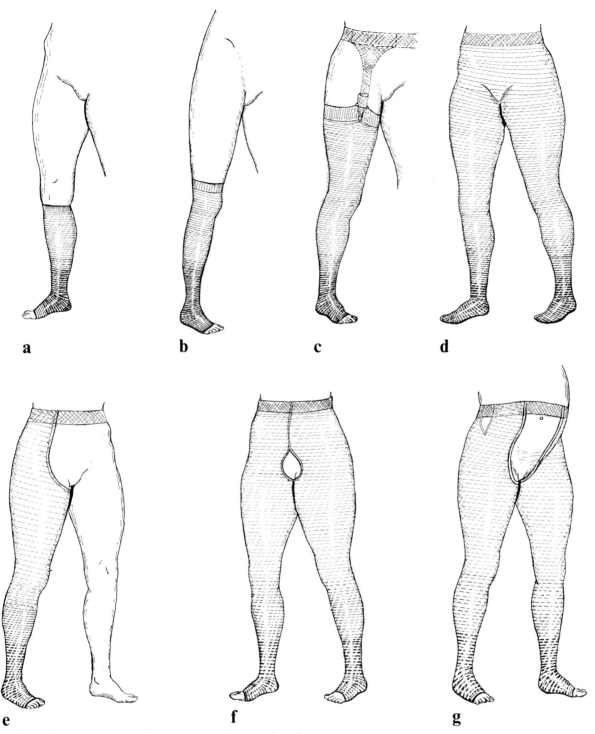

**Figure 18.5**   *The main levels to which elastic stocking may be taken.*

*(a)   Below knee; this should be self supporting but requires a well-rounded calf if two-way stretch is used.*

*(b)   Above knee (lower thigh). Only suitable for a slender thigh; seldom used.*

*(c)   Thigh length (half or mid-thigh), usually supported by suspender.*

*(d)   As tights but only suitable in the lighter weights in ordinary use.*

*(e)   Thigh length with a waist attachment for support. This is specially useful for extensive congenital vascular malformation.*

*(f)   Waist length panty stockings, used for special problems.*

*(g)   Maternity stockings either as support tights (often helpful with vulval varicosities), or more substantially, as waist length panty stockings with adjustable top*

(d) Where there is uncertainty about the diagnosis and the success of active treatment is in doubt.

(e) As a diagnostic measure attempting to clarify whether symptoms are related to varicose veins.

4. In superficial vein incompetence, support tights or an elastic stocking is nearly always to be preferred to other forms of elastic support by bandage.

5. A bandage support may be necessary:

(a) When sensitivity to elastic materials is a problem and, here, a cotton (crepe) bandage may be used.

(b) When obesity and shape of patient prevents successful fitting of stocking.

(c) Because it is the patient's preference.

(d) As an inelastic paste bandage to give mobile treatment in unusually stubborn venous ulcers (but check diagnosis is correct).

The effectiveness is not necessarily related to the strength of compression; choose the lightest compression likely to bring benefit. If the stocking is unduly heavy and ill fitting it may be hot and uncomfortable to wear, with banding behind the knee and the appearance may be unnecessarily dowdy, so that the patient despairs and neglects the veins. Never insist that the patient continues wearing a stocking that causes great discomfort; it is either an unsuitable weight and fit, or is being fitted prematurely over an active, infected ulcer which should be healed first, or the limb is ischaemic.

# References

Abramowitz, I. (1973) The treatment of varicose veins in pregnancy by empty vein compression sclerotherapy. *South African Medical Journal*, **47**, 607–610

Brakkee, A. J. and Kuiper, J. P. (1988) The influence of compressive stockings on the haemodynamics of the lower extremities. *Phlebology*, **3**, 147–153

Burnand, K. G. and Layer, G. T. (1986) Graduated elastic stockings. *British Medical Journal*, **293**, 224–225

Chant, A. D. B., Magnussen, P. and Kershaw, C. (1985) Support hose and varicose veins. *British Medical Journal*, **290**, 204

Cornwall, J., Dore, C. J. and Lewis, J. D. (1987) Graduated compression and its relationship to venous refilling time. *British Medical Journal*, **295**, 1087–1090

Dodd, H. and Cockett, F. B. (1976) *The Pathology and Surgery of the Veins of the Lower Limb*, Livingstone, Edinburgh

Dodd, H. and Payling Wright, H. (1959) Vulval varicose veins in pregnancy. *British Medical Journal*, **1**, 831–832

Drug Tariff (National Health Service England and Wales) (1989) Graduated Compression Hosiery. HMSO, London, (Jan.), 79–83a

Eklof, B. (1988) Modern treatment of varicose veins. *British Journal of Surgery*, **75**, 297–298

Fegan, W. G. (1960) Continuous uninterrupted compression technique of injecting varicose veins. *Proceedings of the Royal Society of Medicine*, **53**, 837–840

Fegan, W. G. (1967) *Varicose Veins*, William Heinemann, London

Fegan, W. G., Beesley, W. H. and Fitzgerald, D. E. (1964) Prophylaxis of superficial and deep venous thrombosis in the lower limbs. *Journal of the Irish Medical Association*, **LIV**, 110–113

Fentem, P. H., Goddard, M. and Gooden, B. A. (1976) Support for varicose veins. *British Medical Journal*, **1**, 254–256

Hobbs, J. (1990) The pelvic congestion syndrome. *British Journal of Hospital Medicine*, **43**, 200–206

Jones, N. A. G., Webb, P. J., Rees, R. I. and Kakkar, V. V. (1980) A physiological study of elastic compression stockings in venous disorders of the leg. *British Journal of Surgery*, **67**, 569–572

Lechter, A., Alvarez, A. and Lopez, G. (1987) Pelvic varices and gonadal veins. *Phlebology*, **2**, 181–188

May, R. (1979) *Surgery of the Veins of the Leg and Pelvis*, W. B. Saunders, Philadelphia, Georg Thieme, Stuttgart

Sigg, K. (1977) Treatment of varicose veins by injection-sclerotherapy: a method practised in Switzerland. In *The Treatment of Venous Disorders* (ed. J. Hobbs), MTP Press, Lancaster, pp. 113–137

Stein, D. (1977) The management of varicose veins: a method practised in South Africa. In *The Treatment of Venous Disorders*, MTP Press, Lancaster, pp. 184–194

Struckman, J. (1986) Compression stockings and their effect on the venous pump – a comparative study. *Phlebology*, **1**, 37–45

Struckman, J., Christensen, S. J., Lendorf, A. and Mathieson, F. (1986) Venous muscle pump improvement by low compression elastic stockings. *Phlebology*, **1**, 97–103

# Bibliography

Anderson, J. H., Geraghty, J. G., Wilson, Y. T., Murray, G. D., McArdle, C. S. and Anderson, J. R. (1990) Paroven and graduated compression hosiery for superficial venous insufficiency. *Phlebology*, **5**, 271–276

Cheatle, T. R., Scurr, J. H. and Coleridge Smith, P. D. (1991) Drug treatment of chronic venous insufficiency and venous ulceration: a review. *Journal of the Royal Society of Medicine*, **84**, 354–358

Christopoulos, D. and Nicolaides, A. N. (1991) The long-term effect of elastic compression on the venous haemodynamics of the leg. *Phlebology*, **6**, 85–93

Christopoulos, D. G., Nicolaides, A. N., Szendro, G. *et al.* (1987) Air-plethysmography and the effect of elastic compression on venous hemodynamics of the leg. *Journal of Vascular Surgery*, **5**, 148–159

Horner, J., Lowth, L. C. and Nicolaides, A. N. (1980) A pressure profile for elastic stockings. *British Medical Journal*, **1**, 818–820

Large, J. (1990) The treatment of varicose veins: a personal review. *Phlebology*, **5**, 141–146

Stemmer, R. (1969) Ambulatory elasto-compressive treatment of the lower extremities particularly with elastic stockings. *Der Kassenarzt*, **9**, 1–8

# 19

# Treatment of varicose veins and other manifestations of superficial vein incompetence. 2. Sclerotherapy and compression bandaging

The history of treating varicose veins by injection goes back for over 100 years, perhaps starting with the use of ferric chloride by Chassaignac in 1853 (Hobbs, 1978). Since then a great range of materials and methods have been advocated and, according to the vogue of the time, the popularity of treatment by injection has swung back and forth. It has always had its critics and supporters. Many of its misfortunes in the past can be attributed to the injection materials used and the variety of these gives some idea of the constant search for something better, for example, carbolic acid, iodine solution, mercuric chloride, sodium salicylate, hypertonic saline, dextrose solutions, quinine, urethane and many others, have all been tried. Undesirable features were related to their systemic effects, such as renal damage, or locally, to severe necrosis and ulceration at the site of any misplaced injection. Ethanolamine had a long run of popularity until recently and proved reasonably satisfactory, but over the last 25 years it has been largely superseded by other agents, notably sodium tetradecyl sulphate (proprietary names: S.T.D. in UK, Sotradecol in USA, Trombovar in France) and hydroxypolyethoxidodecaine or polidocanol (not on official drug lists in UK but widely used on Continent and USA as Sclerovein and Aethoxyskerol). These have proved effective in sealing the vein and relatively harmless both as regards general reaction or local damage from material injected outside the vein. Although these agents have a broad limit of tolerance, dangers can arise through misuse or sensitivity reactions and these important aspects will be considered later. The fact remains that injection techniques have evolved over the years so that they are now widely accepted and used. In competent hands they have a good safety record and the main debate is centred upon their effectiveness as compared with surgery.

Much credit must go to Fegan for emphasizing the need for a careful technique (1960, 1967) and renewing interest in a method that was in danger of falling into disrepute through haphazard application. His publications were followed by a substantial swing over to treating varicose veins by injection using his principles, in the hope that this would prove to be an effective and economical answer to the problem of dealing with the large number of patients requiring treatment. Perhaps because of dramatic advances being made in other aspects of surgery, many surgeons at that time viewed varicose veins as a tedious chore and were glad to turn to an outpatient method that freed them for more 'interesting' operations. Certainly in the British Isles the 'Fegan technique' of empty-vein compression sclerotherapy was used on a massive scale for 10 years before it was realized that many patients, after an initial response, returned a few years later, perhaps worse than ever, so that the treatment had merely shelved the problem (Hobbs, 1974, 1978; Jakobsen, 1979). Its popularity declined and disillusionment was for a while carried too far, but now it is possible, backed by accumulated experience, to form a balanced opinion upon the proper role of sclerotherapy today. In many countries, France for example, sclerotherapy is widely favoured and many specialists treat varicose veins exclusively by this method with great success. However, surgeons are quick to point out that clinics specializing in sclerotherapy usually advise their patients to return each year to see if further injections are required, whereas with surgical treatment there is not the same need for long-term surveillance. Each method has its merits and undoubtedly there are many circumstances in which sclerotherapy is not only an alternative form of treatment but actually to be preferred. It is necessary for the venous surgeon to be skilled both in surgical and injection methods (Eklof, 1988) so that he can advise whichever is appropriate for any individual patient.

In the account that follows an attempt is made to give a balanced opinion based on the accumulated experience of the last 30 years.

## Some basic considerations

1. The treatment of simple (primary) varicose veins caused by superficial vein incompetence is always by the removal or obliteration of the pathway of superficial vein incompetence; the more completely this is done the more effective and lasting the treatment will be. Injection sclerotherapy sets out to cause a chemically induced reaction which will eventually obliterate the pathway of incompetence.

2. Injection of a sclerosing agent, such as sodium tetradecyl sulphate, damages the intima and will be followed by a repair process which can, in favourable circumstances, seal the interior of the vein with fibrous tissue binding the luminal surfaces together and effectively destroying the lumen. Thus the vein is converted to a fibrous cord after a few weeks (Figure 19.1).

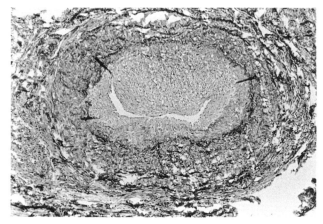

**Figure 19.1** *Histology of a varicose vein, 9 months after compression sclerotherapy. The lumen has been largely obliterated by fibrous tissue but a small endothelialized slit remains that could expand to cause recurrence*

However the process is seldom as complete as this because any trapped clot can and does recanalize so that the unwanted venous pathway is eventually reopened. It is inevitable that clot will form at the site of damaged intima unless the vein is flattened by firm compression which will prevent any entry of blood and hold the walls together to allow fibrous union. This will have to be maintained for at least several weeks and is not easy to acheive in the obese limb.

3. Sclerotherapy will exert maximal effect at the site of injection but there is always considerable spread of the effect which may be very desirable if this is confined to the pathway of incompetence. This is usually the case, but if it should involve other veins, especially the deep veins, the consequences are highly undesirable. This possibility is combated by a careful technique with strict limitation upon the dosage of injection used and by insisting that the patient exercises by repeated walking for several weeks, so as to avoid any stagnation that might encourage thrombosis in the deep

veins. There is much misunderstanding upon the role of exercise and its real purpose is to limit unwanted thrombosis. For similar reasons the patients are asked to elevate the limbs, with frequent foot movements, whenever they are sitting for any length of time.

4. The method is imprecise in its degree and extent, but the experienced user will usually obtain the results he requires. Tortuous veins respond well but with large varicosities it is more difficult to avoid accumulation of substantial quantities of clot in the injected vein with consequent lumpiness, tenderness and a tendency to eventual recanalization. The least predictable long-term results are obtained by injection into the saphenous vein itself, which may fail to seal completely and then will soon recanalize. In a recanalized saphenous vein the valves will have been severely damaged with total loss of their former function, which although imperfect, was still capable of limiting the force and rapidity of downflow.

## Advantages and disadvantages of compression sclerotherapy compared with surgery

### Advantages

It is a 20-minute outpatient procedure with minimal disturbance to the normal pattern of life and immediate free mobility is encouraged. Surgical operation, with probable admission to hospital and general anaesthesia, is avoided (surgery is possible as an outpatient under local anaesthesia but this may limit its scope and the completeness of the result). There are no incisional scars (however most surgeons have developed methods which usually give inconspicuous scars that fade within a few months). It appears to be the most economical method of treating varicose veins (but see comment later).

### Disadvantages

**Compression bandaging** Although the initial treatment is quick, the compression bandage worn for some weeks afterwards becomes very wearisome for the patient and it must be borne in mind that several spells of this will be required if both sides have extensive varicosities; this may require repeating every few years. Most patients endure the compression bandage but certainly would much prefer to be without it both from the point of view of appearance and the constraints it puts upon ablutions. Surgery requires, at most, only a short spell of lightweight elastic support that has neat appearance and may be removed at night and for bathing.

**Discomfort** Most patients experience very little discomfort with either method but in an appreciable proportion there is marked discomfort in the first few days following injection and this appears to be greater than in those patients with corresponding postsurgical discomfort. Perhaps it is fair to say that neither method has a clear advantage here and it would not be right to use the argument of 'less pain' to persuade a patient to have treatment by injection; indeed many patients who have had both methods, state that they have found surgery easier with less discomfort.

**Cosmetic considerations** Sclerotherapy is commonly followed by pigmentation overlying the knotty cord of occluded vein and this takes many months to clear. For this reason, sclerotherapy is often slow to give good cosmetic results and it is wise to caution the patient upon this ('I am going on holiday next month, doctor!'). Surgery is better in this respect with no pigmentation and only a brief period of discolouration from extravasated blood but, of course, both methods may have their misfortunes. Sclerotherapy, in the least favourable circumstances, can give extensive discolouration over visibly lumpy veins, tense with clot and accompanied by considerable tenderness. Much can be done to improve this by releasing the pent up clot but it is still disappointing for the patient. Occasionally surgical incisions give problems but the cosmetic result at 2 months is more likely to be satisfactory than with sclerotherapy; however some patient's scars retain a vivid colour for many months, become keloid or spread, no matter how careful the surgeon has been. Neither method can guarantee to avoid such imperfections.

**Permanence of a good initial result** Neither method is free from recurrence and much will depend upon the quality of the patient's veins. The patient with veins that distend with great ease and whose valves are poor is inherently prone to recurrence with either method. However in patients with a substantial incompetence in the long saphenous system there is little doubt that a conscientiously performed operation gives the best chance of lasting benefit (poorly planned and inadequately performed surgery will give a correspondingly low score of success). In similar circumstances sclerotherapy will produce a number of recurrences within a few years and, as has already been pointed out, this is so well recognized that a policy of regular attendance for possible further injections is often advised. The valves in a recanalized saphenous vein will have been severely damaged and will have lost any previous protective value so that the recurrence that follows is likely to be severe and best treated surgically.

**Morbidity and mortality** Fortunately the mortality rate is exceedingly low with either method. Pulmonary embolism can very occasionally follow either surgery or injection (Hadfield, 1971), but anaphylactic reaction to a sclerosing agent is an alarming and potentially dangerous complication occurring perhaps in 1 : 5000 patients. It is essential that any medical attendant is fully prepared to meet this emergency and always has the appropriate counter measures at hand (injections of adrenaline, hydrocortisone and antihistamine; laryngoscope, endo-

tracheal tube and suction) and in this way the dangers can be greatly reduced. Four deaths, attributed to anaphylactoid reaction to sodium tetradecyl sulphate, were reported to the Committee on Safety of Medicines for the United Kingdom between 1963 and 1988, and about 22 non-fatal, allergic reactions, such as urticaria, were also noted over the same time interval; these figures are likely to be a considerable understatement of the true incidence. The author has experience of one case only, out of several thousand patients receiving sclerotherapy with sodium tetradecyl sulphate, in whom extreme anaphylaxis occurred and the patient probably survived only because the correct therapeutic agents were at hand; this occurred in a fit man without any history to arouse suspicion of allergy and it is the totally unexpected way in which this arises, after hundred of patients without incident, that makes it so dangerous. Polidocanol carries a similar small, but highly significant, incidence of sensitivity reactions. Known allergy to a sclerosant is, of course, an absolute contraindication to sclerotherapy.

Simple fainting may occur after insertion of a needle but before any material has been injected. For this reason injection in the standing position is unwise and if the patient is in a sitting or lying posture no undue problems arise.

Deep vein thrombosis should be rare with either technique but the principles of avoidance should always be scrupulously followed.

Intra-arterial injection will almost certainly cause severe peripheral tissue damage and even put the limb at risk. The dorsalis pedis and posterior tibial arteries are particularly vulnerable near the ankle and even a small injection of sclerosant will cause gangrene of the toes (Mac Gowan et al., 1972, Fegan and Pegum, 1974; Cockett, 1986; Oesch, Mahler and Stirnemann, 1986). There is no really effective way of reversing the effect of an intra-arterial injection and this feared complication must be avoided by constant awareness of its possibility, by a careful technique of inserting the needle and by checking the character of flowback of blood into the syringe. Unskilled employment of sclerotherapy (and of course surgery) can be ineffective and dangerous.

**Economic considerations** With a substantial set of varicose veins, surgery aims at achieving a successful long-term result with a mimimum of follow-up. In this way the relatively high cost of an operation is offset by the absence of additional costs. In similar veins, sclerotherapy, although initially inexpensive, may require many visits and treatments over the years so that the eventual cost may actually be greater than surgery. Experience in the British National Health Service has not shown that sclerotherapy is a cheap and fully acceptable alternative to surgery except in lesser varicose veins. This is difficult to evaluate because so much depends on skill in selection and application of method, but any system has to be judged by what is attainable in average hands.

Medical insurance societies and politicians concerned with cost would be unwise to assume that sclerotherapy is a low cost solution to the problem of dealing with a large number of varicose veins. It has a valuable role to play in a selected range of patients, just as surgery is preferable in other circumstances, and our next task is to try to define this more clearly.

## Indications for compression sclerotherapy

Compression sclerotherapy is much more effective in obliterating peripheral varicosities than in giving lasting occlusion to the principal superficial veins from which these usually arise, the saphenous veins. Thus, the source vein may remain open, continually seeking to establish renewed connections with the low pressure areas below the musculovenous pumps. The elimination of the visible outlying varicosities for at least several years may be all that is required and this is the basis of widespread successful use of the injection method; eradication of the origin is on far less secure ground. With this overall view in mind a list of more specific indications follow; the recommendations apply only to veins which show undoubted simple incompetence, that is, downflow demonstrated by a selective Trendelenburg test or Doppler flowmeter.

Indications:

1. *For comparatively small varicosities where the corresponding saphenous vein is not easily detectable* or shows little downflow with a Doppler flowmeter (Figure 19.2). However, in assessing this it must be

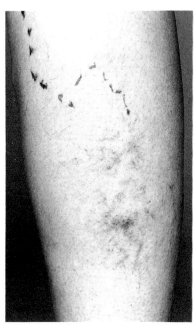

**Figure 19.2** *The ink marks trace a single 'feeding' vein which could be felt running to the area of venous mottling without other evidence of saphenous incompetence. A good result was obtained with local compression sclerotherapy*

remembered that the superficial veins are structures that are very variable from hour to hour. If a patient is seen on a cold day when the veins, especially the saphenous veins, are in a contracted state then the scale of the problem may be greatly undervalued. On a warm day, after a hot bath or during menstruation the veins may be quite large and the involvement of the saphenous system clearly evident. This phenomenon is commonly seen when a patient is attending for a second time and the veins originally noted are scarcely discernible; the patient will often express annoyance that 'my veins are not showing today'. Veins assessed as small early varicosities are very likely to arise from a variably leaking saphenous system and any injection should be strictly limited because excess sclerosant entering the saphenous vein, as it will if the limb is horizontal or elevated, may irreparably damage its valves without occluding it. Even these leaking valves have protective value and their loss can only make severe recurrence more likely.

2. *Larger varicose veins without obvious evidence of saphenous vein incompetence* can well be treated by injection if this is the first time of treatment (Figure 19.3). If they recur it is likely that the saphenous system is at fault and this aspect should be reassessed. Varicose veins meandering down the front and outer aspect of the thigh usually arise from one of the uppermost branches of the long saphenous vein which otherwise may be fully competent (see Figures 5.4 and

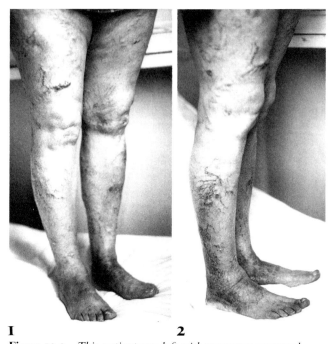

**I**            **2**

**Figure 19.3** *This patient was left with numerous scattered varicose veins and intradermal venules following pregnancy 5 years earlier; two views are shown. No single source could be identified but several sessions of sclerotherapy, first to the larger varicosities, and then to the venules, gave a good result. Surgery to the venules would not have been a practical form of treatment*

19.5(a)). These veins can respond well to injection with properly applied compression, but recurrence by reopening of the same vein is not uncommon. However, it is reasonable to give sclerotherapy one trial if the patient prefers this form of treatment. Injecting varicose veins on the thigh is fully permissible provided the typical downflow of simple incompetence is clearly demonstrated by selective Trendelenburg test or by Doppler flowmeter, and the injection dose is strictly limited in order to minimize its entry into the femoral vein. Varicosities in the groin region may be part of a collateral mechanism due to occlusion of the femoral or iliac veins on the same or the opposite side and for this reason require particularly careful assessment before deciding to inject them.

3. *As an immediate measure for a vein that has actually bled or threatens to bleed* because the covering skin is so thin (Figure 6.14). This arises most often in the elderly and injecting it is a simple alternative to an operation but, apart from this, surgery excising the vein and eliminating the associated superficial incompetence is usually to be preferred.

4. *As an adjunct to surgical treatment.* Surgery may be used as the mainstay of treatment, taking out a saphenous vein for example, but, without completing the operation by removal of the more obvious outlying varicosities (Figure 5.20). If these remain clearly visible, as is often the case, then sclerotherapy can be used to tidy them up subsequently. This may be a deliberate policy in an overloaded clinic to speed up the throughput of surgical patients, because outpatient time is easier to find than theatre time, and it is regarded as the best way to use limited surgical resources. This is a legitimate policy but perhaps not producing the best results and rather hard on the patient; moreover it may result in a large ongoing sclerotherapy clinic which is in itself a significant demand upon resources.

Another reason for leaving unsightly varicosities after dealing with the source surgically, is because they are so near the surface or so thin walled and fragile that they cannot be removed satisfactorily by surgery. In this case it may be wiser to abandon the attempt in the knowledge that sclerotherapy can eliminate them effectively later on.

The question may be asked whether outlying veins may be injected at the time of surgery. A single small injection will produce the usual response and may be permissible but most authorities are worried about the delay before movement starts and the possibility of precipitating a deep vein thrombosis. Medicolegally the surgeon could be in a weak position if this arose after he had acted counter to current opinion. However, a combination of high ligation and stripping of the long saphenous vein, with injection of the vari-

cosities, as one procedure under anaesthesia in 150 patients, without any undue complications, has been reported by Conrad (1975); Goren (1988, 1989) advocates a slightly different combination of sclerotherapy and surgery under local anaesthetic without any reported incidence of deep vein thrombosis. Until there is more published evidence to support the safety of such methods, simultaneous surgery and sclerotherapy should, perhaps, be avoided. (In fact, since writing the papers referred to above Goren has written a further paper (1991) expressing disappointment with the high rate of recurrence found on reviewing the results of sclerotherapy and now advocates 'ambulatory stab evulsion phlebectomy' under local anaesthesia (see Chapter 20).)

5. *As a first aid measure for an active venous ulcer* in the presence of undoubted superficial vein incompetence and when a large vein, showing retrograde flow, can be easily identified running under the ulcer. The best treatment is by surgery, but in the elderly patient, or if early admission is not possible, sclerotherapy can prove to be a very effective answer giving a cure for a prolonged time (Figures 4.8(a), 13.12(b)). It must be emphasized that this is for expert hands only and there must be a positive identification of massive superficial incompetence, by Trendelenburg's test, by Doppler flowmeter and with plethysmography showing reversion to near normal when the veins to be injected are temporarily occluded. Needless to say, good arterial pulses must be present at the ankle to exclude ischaemia. If ischaemia is present it may be appropriate to remove the long saphenous vein surgically and use it for an arterial reconstruction thus curing both conditions; this opportunity must not be lost by an inexpert attack upon the saphenous vein (see Chapter 17). Moreover, compression sclerotherapy in the ischaemic limb may well have disasterous consequences (see 'Contraindications', below).

6. *Recurrent varicose veins after surgery* often give a confused pattern of incompetence in which it is difficult to identify the source of the incompetence by clinical examination. However, this can usually be demonstrated by functional phlebography and varicography, and then surgical treatment is best. If a clearly defined origin cannot be demonstrated then compression sclerotherapy is advisable and can give good results. The treatment may require repeating every few years but the patient is usually satisfied to have the veins controlled in this way. The technique of injection must be good, using only small injections at intervals, to a high level in the thigh and backed by an effective compression bandage for some weeks. This does come as a reminder that the best opportunity to cure varicose veins is by the first operation because the superficial venous system becomes fragmented by surgery and progressively more difficult to treat. The

first operation must not be wasted by inadequate surgery, but when this does arise then it can be one of the most satisfying uses for sclerotherapy.

7. *Small vascular blemishes*, such as isolated venous flares (spider veins) or telangiectasis on the thigh or leg (Figure 19.8), usually respond well but care must be taken to avoid intradermal injection which produces a small area of blackened necrotic skin. When the needle is outside the target venule and into the dermis there is definite resistance to injection which should be a warning of its likelihood; if the injection is intradermal a visible wheal is raised progressively and is an indication to cease injecting immediately. Subdermal injection of dilute sodium tetradecyl sulphate or hydroxypolyethoxidodecaine (polidocanol) outside the vein in small amounts is relatively harmless but best avoided; it can spread rapidly without resistance and it is always best to see the venules clearing as an initial injection of fluid passes through them before proceeding further (and see section on 'Sclerotherapy for spider veins' later in this chapter for more detailed discussion on this topic).

## Contraindications and precautions with compression sclerotherapy

1. *History of allergy or anaphylaxis*, particularly towards the sclerosant that is to be used.

2. *Present or recent acute deep vein thrombosis or active superficial thrombophlebitis.*

3. *If the contraceptive pill is being used.* Although the risk is small, the consequences of arterial or deep vein thrombosis are so formidable that it is not advisable to carry out sclerotherapy if the patient is on an oestrogen-containing contraceptive pill (see Chapter 16 under 'Prevention of deep vein thrombosis in surgical patients', the section on 'Withdrawal of the contraceptive pill'). However, the inconveniences of a compression bandage after injection are not sufficient to prevent an unwanted pregnancy so alternative means of contraception must be arranged!

4. *Uncertainty in the diagnosis.* Enlarged and tortuous veins should not be attacked without confirming that they are part of a pathway of simple incompetence and that their obliteration will do no harm. If they cannot be controlled by a selective Trendelenburg test or, certainly, if a Doppler flowmeter shows continuous upward flow, then they may be part of a collateral system indicating impaired deep veins and more information is required before obliterating these veins. This is especially true in the groin.

5. *When substantial or massive incompetence in a saphenous vein is present.* The benefit here may only be temporary and surgery gives a more satisfactory result. Injection into the long or short saphenous vein seldom gives lasting closure and when it reopens all remaining valve function will have been lost. The rare case of pulmonary embolus comes from this group where sclerotherapy may be followed by massive clot formation in the long saphenous vein with protrusion into the femoral vein and it is not easy to prevent this in an unusually large vein. Injection into massive varicosities tends to give an untidy lumpy response with considerable discomfort which takes a long time to resolve and all too often opens up again quite soon. It is not suitable as a cosmetic procedure which is much better performed by surgery. However, accepting these disadvantages is permissible, for example, in order to control an ulcer or a bleeding varicosity when surgical treatment of the incompetent veins is undesirable or not possible (see 'Indications' above):

6. *Pregnancy.* Here sclerotherapy is often inadequate and carries unknown dangers. It is far wiser to control the veins with elastic support and tidy up the veins, if necessary, some months after childbirth (see Chapter 18).

7. *In the immobile patient.* Active mobility is regarded as the best safeguard against deep vein thrombosis and if this is not possible sclerotherapy is best avoided.

8. *In the obese patient.* A complete understanding of the venous problem is often not possible in the truly obese patient, positioning of an injection needle may be uncertain and the size of the underlying varicose veins unknown. Effective compression bandaging cannot be achieved in the obese limb and there is a belief that these patients are at appreciable risk from deep vein thrombosis and embolus. All effort must be made to encourage the patient to lose weight before a policy of treatment is decided upon.

9. *In the elderly patient.* The older patient may become worried by varicose veins which are, in fact, comparatively harmless and here treatment should not be carried out too readily for purely cosmetic reasons. When treatment is necessary, as in venous ulceration or bleeding from varicosities, the risks of carefully used sclerotherapy are not so great as to preclude it, particularly if the alternative is surgery. As compression bandaging will have to be employed it is essential that the presence of a good arterial supply is confirmed by normal arterial ankle pulses and the absence of any history of claudication. Discomfort in the lower limbs is often attributed to the visible defect of varicose veins when in fact the real cause is an ischaemia that might not tolerate compression sclerotherapy and could even develop gangrene as a result. Elderly veins are noticeably fragile and easily extravasate blood when punctured and compression bandaging is just as necessary as in younger patients in preventing an uncontrolled phlebitic response to injection of sclerosant (see below). Another

drawback is that the patient's willingness and ability to exercise may be uncertain.

10. *If the patient is in a state of poor health* sclerotherapy is unwise and should be postponed or avoided altogether. There are really no indications of overriding urgency for injecting veins; appropriate support bandaging or stocking will control most problems until a more suitable time.

## The principles of compression sclerotherapy

An essential principle in the treatment of simple varicose veins is to remove or obliterate the pathway of superficial vein incompetence that is causing the veins. Sclerotherapy aims to achieve this by converting it into a fibrous cord. However, merely injecting a sclerosant without further precautions will lead to the vein becoming packed with clotted blood to form, what is in fact, an induced superficial thrombophlebitis which will be painful for the patient, slow to settle and may soon reopen again. To prevent this undesirable sequence of events the sclerosant is put into the vein *whilst it is empty and is then kept empty by use of a compression bandage*; this will also ensure that the sclerosant has maximum, undiluted effect on the intima.

The basic steps to accomplish this are as follows:

1. With the patient standing the veins forming the 'pathway of incompetence' are indentified and appropriate sites for injection marked in.
2. The patient is then repositioned in a sitting-up posture so that the veins are keep sufficiently filled to allow easy insertion of injection needles, with syringes containing sclerosant attached, into the chosen veins. Up to six needles and syringes may be used and each is secured in place by semi-transparent adhesive tape.
3. The patient then lies flat on the couch and the limb to be injected is elevated some 18 in (45 cm) so that the veins are emptied but with the needle points still within their lumina.
4. The sclerosant in the syringe(s) is now injected into the empty veins, no more than 0.5 ml at any one site.
5. With the patient still lying flat with the limb elevated, a compression bandage is applied.
6. The patient is then asked to get up and walk for the next 20 minutes in order to disperse any unfixed sclerosant from the limb.
7. The patient returns to normal activities, but is asked to follow a simple programme of exercise by walking at intervals during the day and to elevate the limb when sitting for any length of time. The compression bandage is maintained for several weeks.

The details of applying these principles will vary from one vein specialist to another but the following illustrated passage sets out the method found most satisfactory by the author.

## A technique of compression sclerotherapy

### Materials required

- Examination couch and a support on which limb may be elevated. Skin marking pen. Skin sterilizing swabs.
- 2 ml plastic syringes. (Some clinics prefer all glass syringes because of the smooth easy movement of the plunger, others accept the stiffer piston of the disposable plastic syringe because it is lighter, used once only and there is certainty that blood-born disease cannot be transmitted by it.)
- 25 gauge $\times \frac{5}{8}$ in needles (27 gauge $\times \frac{1}{2}$ in or 30 gauge $\times \frac{1}{2}$ in for fine veins).
- Sclerosant: sodium tetradecyl sulphate 3% (STD) (or hydroxypolyethoxydodecane (polidocanol) 0.5–3%).
- $\frac{1}{4}$ in rayon (Micropore) adhesive tape.
- Compression pads (cotton dental rolls, folded lint, rubber or synthetic foam).
- 4 in (7.5 cm) Elastocrepe bandages. 4 in (7.5 cm) Elastoplast adhesive elastic bandages. Tubigrip, tubular elastic bandaging, straight (size D and E) and shaped, long SSB (size D/F).
- *To counter anaphylactic reaction*: adrenaline 1 : 1000 (1 ml amps with adrenaline 1 mg/ml) for intramuscular injection; hydrocortisone (vials or amps of 100 mg) for slow intravenous injection; antihistamine (chlorpheniramine maleate 10 mg/ml in 1 ml amps) for slow intravenous injection; laryngoscope, endotracheal tube and suction apparatus.

### Selection of injection sites (written and illustrated for right-handed operator)

Selection of injection sites should be done with the patient standing, preferably on a strengthened examination couch or a special platform (Figure 19.4(a)). It is best to confine injections to one limb and avoid bilateral procedures unless these are to be very small; the intention is to treat the limb as completely as possible.

The pathway of incompetence must be traced throughout its length (for example, from groin, down thigh portion of long saphenous vein and via varicosities to lower leg). The saphenous vein itself, or sacculations on it, will not usually be selected for injection, but branch veins with parallel walls feeding tortuous veins below them are key veins that will give a high yield of success and should be indentified and marked for injection whenever possible. In the varicosities themselves, sites for injection should be chosen and marked every few inches down the thigh and leg (up to six sites); the choice is dictated by ease of access and at points where branch varicosities are given off; avoid veins where the overlying skin is paper thin but use a site just above or below this. Do not inject through areas of unhealthy skin but move to the nearest healthy area.

**Figure 19.4** *Serial diagrams illustrating a method of compression sclerotherapy.*

*(a) Patient standing on couch with veins being mapped out and suitable injection sites being chosen.*

*(b) Patient sitting upright with one limb down (1) or with limbs horizontally on couch (2).*

*(c) Patient sitting up with limb down and surgeon inserting needle and syringe. Tape on back of left hand is ready to secure syringe to skin.*

*(d) Inserting the needle with a slight lifting action; the skin is steadied by a finger of the left hand.*

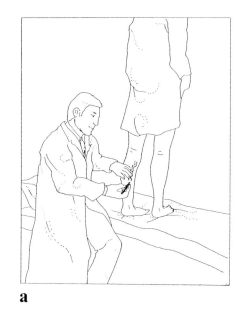

a

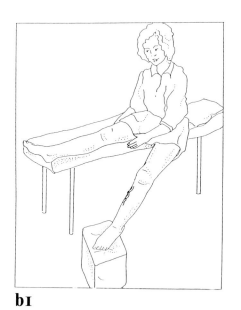

b1

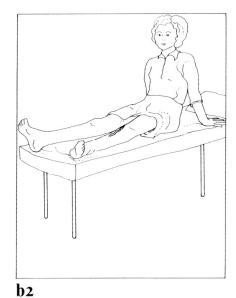

b2

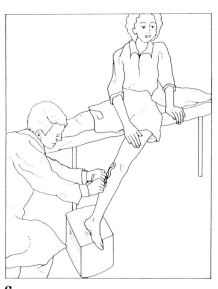

c

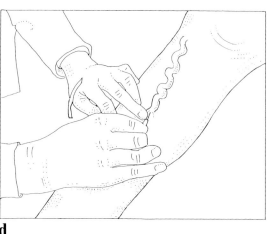

d

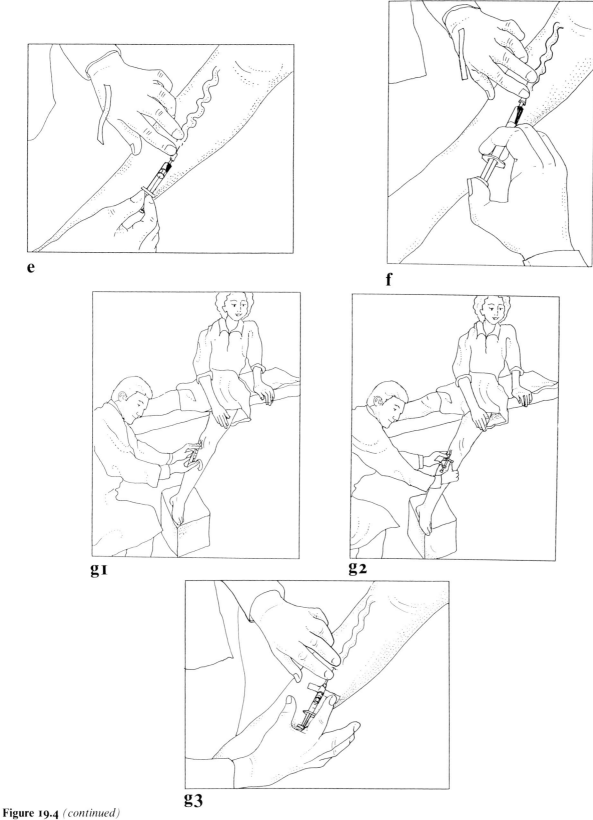

e

f

g1

g2

g3

**Figure 19.4** *(continued)*

*(e) Syringe and needle fixed by left index finger over the needle hub, whilst checking that the needle point is in the lumen by sucking back venous blood.*

*(f) Clearing the needle of blood by injecting a small amount of sclerosant.*

*(g) 1–3. Fixing syringe and needle in place with tape from the back of the left hand. Further tape can be placed gently over the point of needle entry through skin as a safeguard against inward or outward movement, if required.*

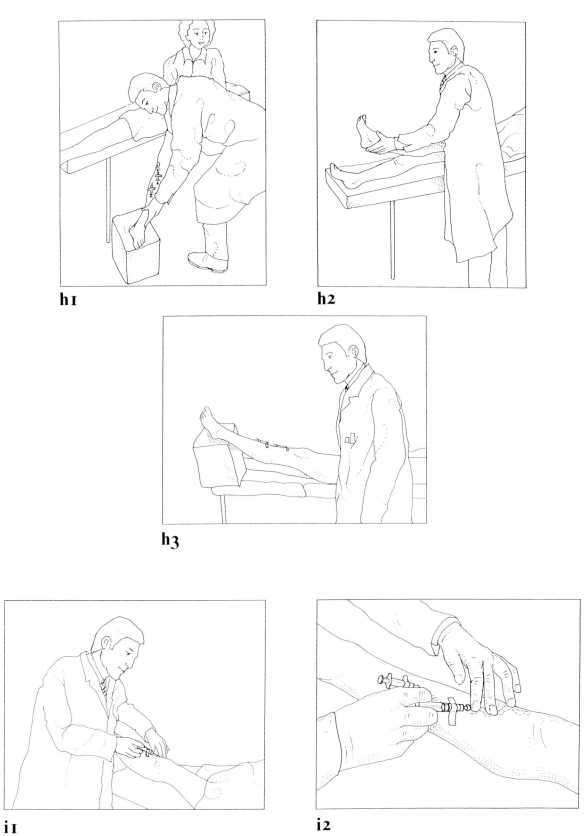

**Figure 19.4** *(continued)*

*(h)* *1–3. The limb is swung into elevated position for main injection of sclerosant.*

*(i)* *1, 2. Use of fingers during injection; left index finger steadies syringe, middle finger is over point of needle to detect any bulge, and the ring finger is used to delay spread of sclerosant 'up' the vein.*

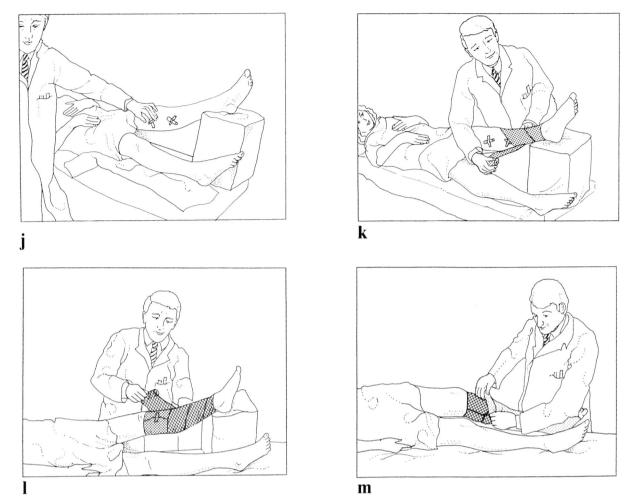

**Figure 19.4** *(continued)*

*(j)  Cotton pads are taped over the injection sites.*

*(k)  A crepe bandage is applied from ankle to above the uppermost injection site.*

*(l)  Application of the second layer – elastic adhesive bandage.*

*(m)  Application of the third layer – elastic tubular support*

When the pathway of incompetence runs to the underside of the foot pump it is often desirable to inject veins crossing the ankle and foot. This is certainly permissible but *beware of selecting sites overlying anterior tibial, dorsalis pedis or posterior tibial arteries because intra-arterial injection is a disaster and will lead to gangrene of the toes or foot* (see Chapter 17 and Figures 17.15, 17.16, 17.18). Great care must be exercised here and even the most experienced worker must be vigilant (see further comments below).

Mark in reserve sites so that if there is any difficulty an alternative site is available nearby.

*Insertion of injection needles*

Do not insert the needles with the patient standing because fainting (syncope due to vasovagal attack) is not uncommon even before any sclerosant has been injected. Always reposition the patient to sit upright on the couch (Figure 19.4(b)) or, if fainting has occurred before, to a lying position so that fainting is less likely and if it does occur causes minimal disturbance to the procedure and no harm to the patient. Another disadvantage of injection to a standing patient is that the full venous pressure may cause a large perivenous haematoma to form before the needle is properly placed and further attempts to enter the vein are prevented. An alternative, preferred by some surgeons, is routinely to have the patient lying and to use the transfixion technique (see below) to enter the vein.

At each chosen site, a needle, with syringe attached and containing no more than 0.5 ml of sclerosant, is inserted into the vein (Figure 19.4(c), (d)) and taped to the skin with 0.25 in Micropore.

The left index finger steadies the skin; the needle is inserted with a scooping action so that the skin is raised as the needle passes through it and in this way does not flatten and close the vein lumen as it is approached. There is a characteristic loss of resistance as soon as the point has passed through the skin and the needle should not be advanced beyond here as it is likely that the point is already in the lumen. There is usually no sense of resistance as the needle enters a varicose vein unless it is a more deeply placed stem vein.

Immediately after the needle point has passed through the skin there should be a pause to give cautious suction with the syringe to check for reflux of blood (Figure 19.4(e)). Care must be taken to avoid dislodging the needle in doing this either by withdrawal or advancement; the left index finger gently clamps the hub of the syringe whilst the right index finger and thumb are rolled against the crossbar of the syringe and the plunger to give suction (do not pull at the plunger as this may displace syringe and needle). If blood comes spontaneously in arterial spurts, or is bright red, withdraw the needle and chose another site; no individual site is worth the slightest risk of intra-arterial injection (venous blood can be surprisingly bright red at times but do not risk it, go elsewhere).

Alternative techniques for entering a vein:

1. The skin is punctured alongside the vein which is then approached from the side without any flattening by skin pressed inwards as the needle traverses it.
2. The transfixion technique is useful when the patient is lying and the veins are only partially filled. The needle is passed directly through skin and vein to emerge on the far side and then slowly withdrawn, with slight suction on the syringe, so that it is immediately apparent when the needle point is in the lumen. In fact, the lumen can usually be entered reliably without transfixion but is a useful reserve method if the initial insertion has overshot the mark.

*Minimizing the risk of entering an artery.* The danger of an injection misplaced into an artery causing extensive gangrene has already been emphasized above and the point made that injections should never be attempted in the vicinity of a known artery that lies close to the surface, such as those near the ankle. Arterial blood spurting back, or even bright red blood sucked back, into the syringe is an obvious and urgent warning to abort the injection and many specialists prefer to use an open-ended butterfly needle because it is likely to show arterial flowback more easily than a needle with syringe attached. Nevertheless, it is better to avoid entering an artery in the first place and it is a good rule never to plunge the needle deeply, probing blindly for a vein, but to keep its point always 'in sight'; this is easier when the veins are moderately distended by the patient being in a sitting position, and by manipulating the needle to enter the lumen without transfixion.

Suck back no more than a trace of blood and, having obtained this confirmation, clear the needle of blood that might block it with clot (Figure 19.4(f)). The fingers of the right hand are adjusted to inject about 0.1 ml of sclerosant; whilst doing this the middle finger of the left hand is placed lightly over the needle point to check that a bulge is not caused by fluid going outside the vein; there should be no sense of resistance and no bulge. Injection of a small quantity of sclerosant at this stage can do little harm (unless an artery has been entered) and not only checks satisfactory positioning of the needle point but also ensures some result even if the needle is displaced before the main injection. If no blood is withdrawn the needle point is gently moved to locate the lumen and test suction repeated; the most usual error is to have passed right through the vein and out the other side. If there is obvious resistance to injection the needle point is probably still in the dermis and forceful injection will cause skin necrosis; the needle should be repositioned. If the test injection causes a bulge, felt by the finger over the needle point, it is usually best to assume this is outside the vein and to reposition the needle; this is distinct from the ripple sometimes felt as injection fluid enters the vein.

*Fixing needle and syringe*

Having confirmed that all is well the syringe is now fixed in place with the tape from the back of the left hand across the lower part of its barrel (Figure 19.4(g)). At certain sites where skin shift may occur, such as near the knee joint, or where sudden contraction of quadriceps muscles may flick the syringe out of position, an additional tape can be placed across the needle where it enters the skin.

Insertion of further needles and syringes proceeds in a similar fashion but should not exceed a total potential dosage of more than 3 ml spread through the limb.

*Pain – its significance*

A well-placed injection of sclerosant into a vein should not cause any immediate pain but may be followed a minute or so later by a slight stinging sensation. If the vein is well compressed and not allowed to distend with clot there will be very little, if any, discomfort over the following hours; if compression is inadequate then, in effect, an uncontrolled superficial thrombophlebitis is set up and will cause marked discomfort some hours after the injection. Real pain should not be a feature at any stage and if it occurs is a clear warning that something is amiss.

*Intra-arterial injection of sclerosant* Severe scalding pain, distal to the injection site, occurring during either the initial test injection or the main injection, is an absolute indication to cease immediately, because the most likely cause is intra-arterial injection of sclerosant; this will be confirmed by blanching or cyanosis in the affected area. If this arises, the syringe should be detached without disturbing the needle so that free bleeding back through the needle may occur. If this confirms that the needle is in an artery then it is used to inject 500 units of heparin before it is withdrawn. If there is no bleeding back, or the needle has been removed with the syringe, there should not be any attempt to re-enter the artery because this may damage it further and it is better to rely on immediate intravenous general heparinization (10 000 units).

An intra-arterial injection is a major emergency requiring admission to a vascular unit for an attempt to minimize the damage. It is probable that little can be done to reverse an inevitable thrombosis of the artery and the possible measures that can be taken are discussed in Chapter 17, pages 359–360.

Less severe pain, during or soon after injection, will be caused if this is outside the vein and especially if it is forced intradermally. At a later stage uncontrolled extension of thrombosis beyond the vicinity of injection, for instance, up the full length of the long saphenous vein, is the most common cause and is usually relieved by active walking rather than by rest. If there is severe and persistent pain the compression bandage should be removed to inspect the limb and reapplied firmly if the arterial supply appears satisfactory and no more than a sharp thrombophlebitic reaction is found. A badly applied bandage, cutting into the skin, can, of course, be the cause of considerable discomfort.

## Note upon syncope and anaphylaxis

The patient who is about to faint always gives warning of this by becoming restless, sighing, breaking out in a sweat or becoming pale. This usually occurs whilst needles are being inserted and before any significant injection of sclerosant. With any of these manifestations the patient should be laid flat upon the couch before complete collapse occurs, which could possibly hurt the patient and is certainly likely to displace syringes. The radial pulse should be checked and if this found to be characteristically slow the injections may be proceeded with after a short wait.

Distress occurring at a later stage, soon after the injections have been given, is likely to be due to a sensitivity response or anaphylaxis. Unlike the harmless faint this is potentially dangerous and the procedure of injecting must be abandoned at once and all care given to the patient. The features of anaphylaxis may include dyspnoea, bronchospasm, cyanosis, shivering or rigors, oedema of the face and eventually laryngeal oedema, nausea and vomiting, rapid pulse and low blood pressure. **Treatment of anaphylaxis** This is summarized at this stage because no one should inject sclerosant without being aware of the small but definite risk of anaphylaxis and be fully prepared to meet this emergency.

If the patient is showing definite distress as described above, the following steps should be taken:

1. Adrenaline, 1 ml of 1 : 1000 solution should be injected intramuscularly.
2. Hydrocortisone, 100 mg is injected over 5 minutes by intravenous injection.
3. Chlorpheniramine maleate, 10 mg in 1 ml fluid, or similar antihistamine, is given by slow intravenous injection.

This is usually sufficient to control the reaction but because it may return or prove progressive the patient should be admitted to hospital overnight so that help is immediately at hand if the condition does deteriorate or laryngeal obstruction develops. It is important to have the skills of endotracheal intubation nearby until there has been no sign of reaction for some hours. Needless to say the causative agent must not be used again and indeed sclerotherapy by any other material is best avoided in the future.

## Injecting the sclerosant

Before the actual injection of sclerosant the patient is repositioned to lie on the couch with the foot elevated 18 in (45 cm) upon a plastic foam support (Figure 19.4(h)). This empties the veins of blood so that the sclerosant can have maximal effect on the intima and formation of clot is minimized.

The sclerosant is injected from the various syringes in an unhurried and methodical fashion. As this is done the left index finger steadies the nozzle of the syringe, the middle finger is positioned lightly over the needle point to detect any bulge caused by extravasation and the ring finger compresses the vein beyond the needle (Figure 19.4(i)) to delay spread of sclerosant 'up' the vein (this placing of the fingers is perhaps a policy of perfection and can be omitted without appreciable disadvantage). The order in which injections are carried out is probably immaterial but it is perhaps best to dispose first of those with easily displaced needle points, for example near the ankle or knee joints, or those that are awkwardly placed, perhaps overlapping another syringe; otherwise move 'up' the limb systematically from the lower leg. It is usually convenient to leave needle and syringe in place until all have been used.

The needles should be withdrawn with care to avoid leaving a track of sclerosant oozing through the skin puncture. The syringe is clamped with the left index finger and the tape peeled off; pressure is then applied with a cotton wool ball over the needle whilst it is withdrawn still attached to the syringe. Whilst the limb is elevated leakage of fluid or blood is unlikely so that prolonged pressure is not needed and a compression bandage will be applied before the patient stands.

In order to protect all concerned from possible blood-borne virus disease, it is important to handle needles carefully and to make adequate provision for safe

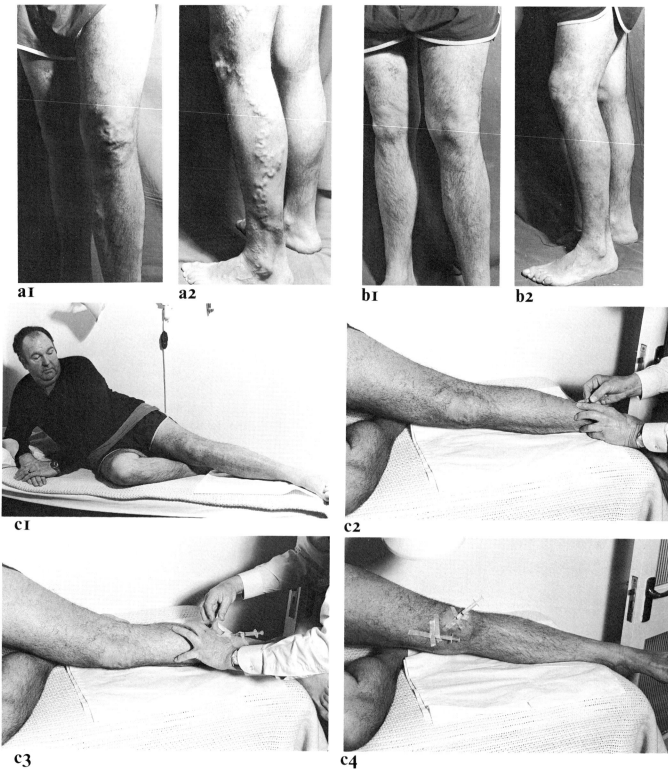

**Figure 19.5**   *Photographic record of injection procedure and compression bandaging in a male patient aged 45 years.*

*(a)   Before sclerotherapy. Front (1) and outer (2) aspects of left leg showing extensive varicose veins running down to the ankle and foot; the origin appears to be from an incompetent anterolateral branch of the uppermost saphenous vein. An extremely tortuous vein, directly under the skin, such as this, should respond well to compression sclerotherapy.*

*(b)   1, 2. Two months after sclerotherapy. A slightly discoloured, knotty cord shows that the varicose vein has been well sealed. This gradually disappeared over the following months without any residual varicosities. Seen again two years later this good result was confirmed, with no sign of recurrence.*

*(c)   The same patient, showing sclerotherapy being carried out.*
*1. The vein has been marked out whilst standing and the patient is now in a semirecumbent position on the couch; this maintains slight filling of the veins.*
*2. Insertion of needle with syringe containing 0.5 ml of STD sclerosant into varicosity on outer leg.*

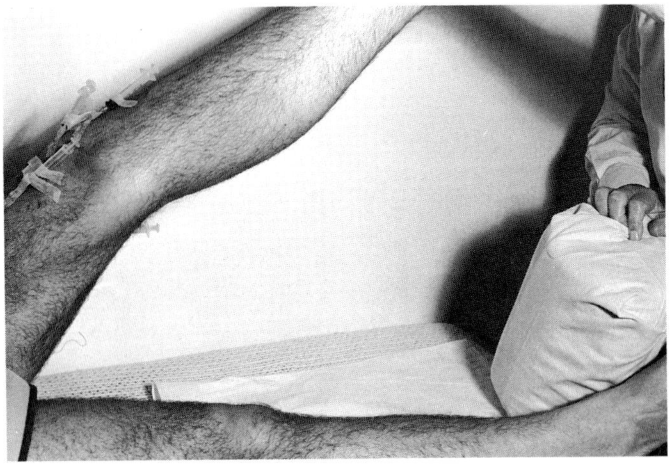

c5

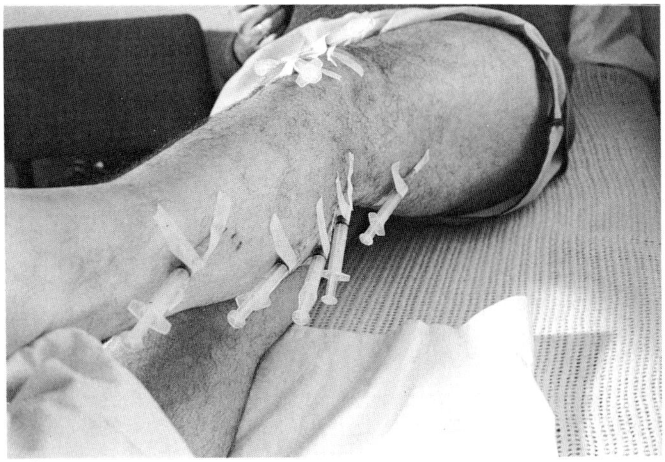

c6

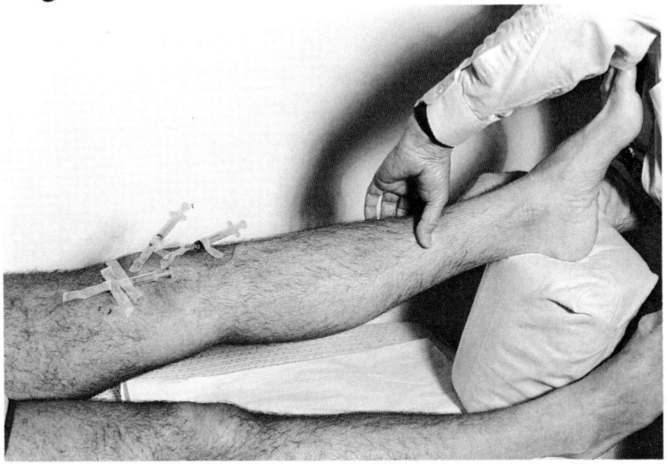

c7

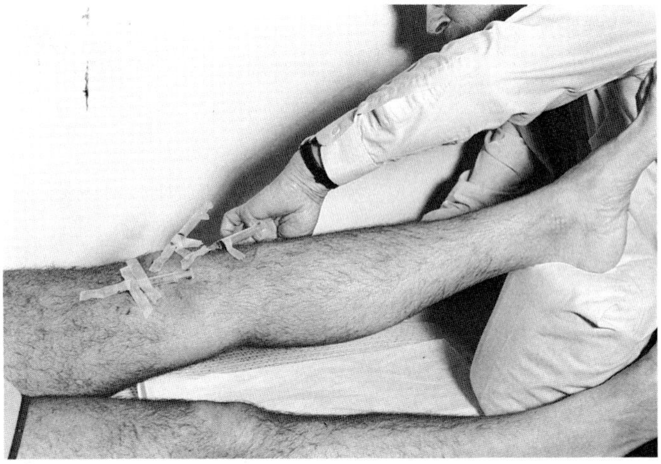

c8

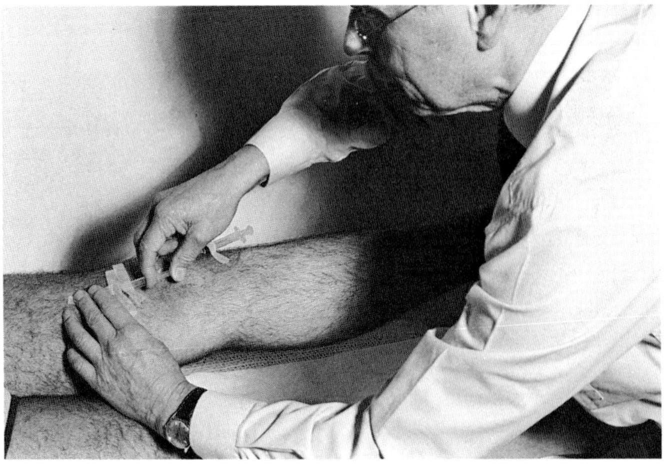

c9

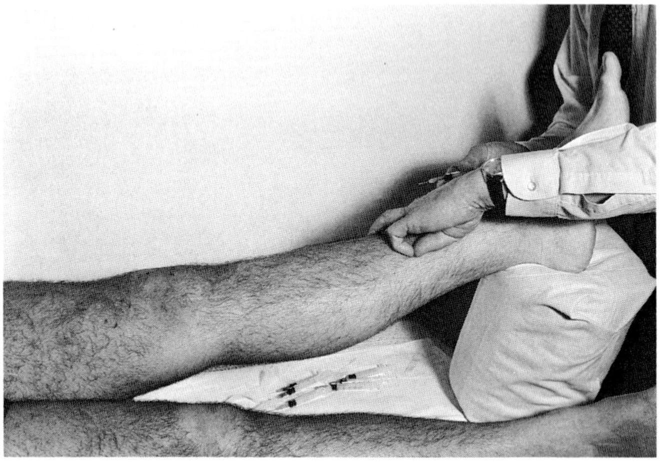

c10

**Figure 19.5** *(continued)*
*3. Five needles and syringes are inserted at intervals along this vein. All are fixed to the skin with Micropore adhesive tape.*
*4. The limb is rotated slightly to insert further syringes into the varicose vein on front of the knee. The double tape on the syringe barrel, with a further tape over the needle point, is used in case the patient contracts the quadriceps.*
*5. The limb is briefly put into high elevation to empty the veins and then placed in moderate elevation on a firm bolster 23 cm (9 in) high.*
*6. View of multiple syringes taped to outerside of leg and ready for injection of sclerosant.*
*7, 8. Sclerosant is injected in sequence up the outer leg.*
*9. Injection into varicose veins over knee.*
*10. Syringes and needles are systematically removed. Care is taken by the operator to avoid needle pricks.*

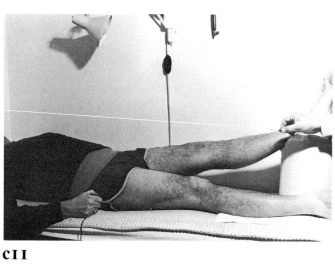

**c11**

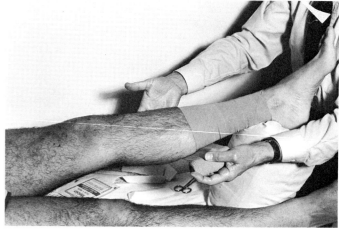

**c12**

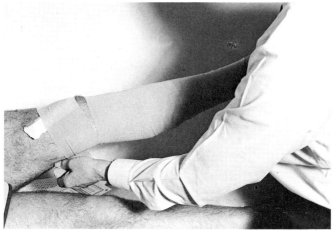

**c13**

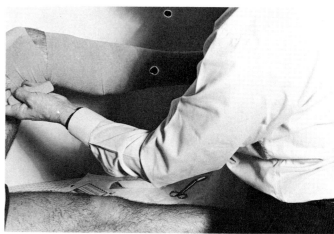

**c14**

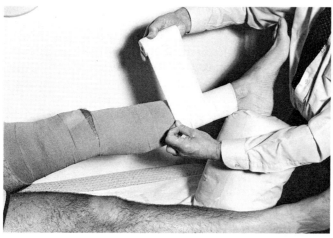

**c15**

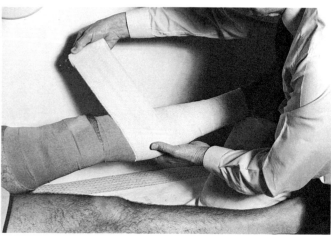

**c16**

**Figure 19.5** *(continued)*

*11. The limb is maintained in elevation ready for bandaging.*

*12. Cotton pads have been laid over injected veins (not visible) and crepe bandage is firmly applied from the ankle upwards.*

*13, 14. Bandaging is continued over the knee where a single large cotton pad is laid over the vein. A gap is left to permit flexing of the knee.*

*15–17. The next layer of bandage is adhesive elastic bandage. This locks the underlying crepe bandage and forms an inelastic*

**Figure 19.5** *(continued)*

*directly to the skin for fear of sensitivity reaction to adhesive, except in the upper thigh, where it is needed to prevent downward slipping. Again, a gap is left on the front of the knee.*

*18, 19. The final layer is elastic tubing, usually Tubigrip, size D, below the knee, but the shaped variety, SSB, size D–F, is used if bandaging extends onto the thigh, as in this patient.*

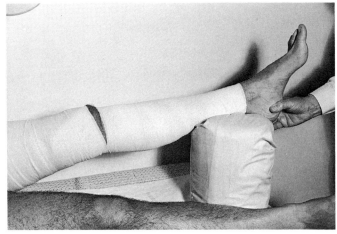

c17

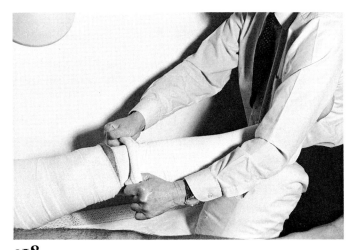

c18

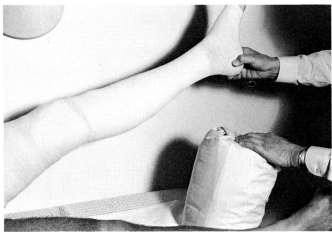

c19

disposal of needles and syringes in suitably designed containers.

*Application of the compression bandage*

The patient remains in the same position, lying flat with the limb elevated.

The object of compression bandaging is to flatten the veins to prevent entry of blood and to hold the walls in apposition so that they may seal together. It also serves the purpose of preventing leakage of blood from needle punctures when the patient first stands. Cotton dental pads are taped (0.25 in Micropore) in position over the injection sites (Figure 19.4(j)) (pads of rubber or plastic foam may be preferred, especially if a large varicosity is to be compressed, but these give a bumpy appearance and occasionally cause allergic skin reaction). Do not apply the tape with any tension as this may drag off surface layers of skin to cause blistering. It is not practical to place a continuous compression pad over the entire length of the varicosities and it is sufficient to put pads over the injection sites and over any particularly large veins, especially in the thigh, where effective compression is not easy to achieve.

**The first layer of bandage** Elastic crepe bandage (4 in, 10 cm) is wound onto the limb from the ankle (or foot if there have been injections to this level) to the upper calf (Figure 19.4(k)) or, if appropriate, to above the uppermost thigh injection site. This is applied quite firmly and if it crosses the knee a small gap is left over the patella so that the bandage is not disrupted by bending of the knee; each turn should overlap half of the turn below.

**The second layer of bandage** The next layer is elastic adhesive bandage and is used to lock the underlying layer of crepe (Figure 19.4(l)). It is applied with a slight stretch, with each turn slightly overlapping the previous one and angled to the crepe to give a crossply strengthening effect. Elastic adhesive bandage can give rise to unpleasant skin reactions so do not allow it to make contact with skin except, possibly, for a 2 in (5 cm) band above the crepe in the upper thigh to stop it rolling down; no skin contact at all is needed if the bandage ends in the upper calf where the shape keeps it in position. No skin contact with adhesive bandage should be allowed if there is any history of reaction to adhesive plasters but few patients show any reaction where the crepe bandage intervenes between the adhesive and the skin. The combination of crepe and the overlying elastic adhesive bandage bind together to provide a firm, but inelastic, encasement of the elevated limb so that the veins cannot fill on standing (inelastic containment).

**The third and final layer of bandage** The outermost layer of bandage is tubular elastic bandage (Figure 19.4(m)) (or, if preferred, a medium-weight elastic stocking but this tends to be less comfortable and requires more accurate fitting). This gives steady pressure to stop filling of the veins whether the patient is lying or standing; it also has the advantage of giving a smooth contour and better appearance. It should always include the foot (to counter-act any tendency to oedema from the compression bandage above) and runs either to the upper calf, to just above the knee or to the upper thigh where it can be supported by a suspender if necessary. When the thigh is included a shaped (tapered) tubular bandage (Tubigrip SSB) is very suitable; with a slender thigh this may stay in place satisfactorily but on a bulky thigh a suspender belt will be required. Tights may be worn over this so that the final appearance is acceptable and, of course, many women will wish to conceal it all by trousers.

Figure 19.5 gives a serial photographic record of an actual injection procedure and the eventual result. The diagrams in Figure 19.6 show positions of hands and fingers that may be used when inserting a needle and sclerosant-containing syringe into a vein.

### Policy of exercise whilst wearing compression bandage

When bandaging is completed the patient is asked to walk for 20 minutes to disperse any unfixed sclerosant. The usual work pattern may be resumed immediately afterwards but the patient is asked to have at least six walks of 15 minutes duration, or more, at intervals during the day and to move the feet frequently whilst sitting. If standing is necessary for any length of time, the patient should keep some movement going by gently rising on the toes and this action does not have to be unduly conspicuous; during leisure sitting, for example, when reading or watching television, the feet should be elevated on a settee, again with frequent foot movement. If the limb is uncomfortable this is best relieved by a further walk and the patient must understand that the policy is one of active movement and that prolonged 'resting' of the limb is unwise. If there are any real doubts the patient should return for advice.

The bandage is left undisturbed, if possible, for 3 weeks. If the thigh portion collapses during this time the patient may fold down the elastic outer layer and cut away the loose underlying bandage to just below the knee, and then replace the elastic layer. Effective thigh compression is difficult to achieve for long and by this stage the elastic support alone is probably sufficient.

### General hygiene whilst wearing the bandage

Instructions to the patient should include the reminder that having a bath or shower will require some arrange-ment to avoid soaking the bandage. A shallow bath is possible by stepping in with the good limb and lying down with the bandaged limb supported on an upturned basin; a shower is easy enough by standing alongside it with a plastic bin-liner over the bandage. In this way general hygiene should not be a problem.

### Removal of the bandage

At the end of 3 weeks the entire bandage is removed with strong scissors, together with the pads. A new elastic tubular bandage, or equivalent light elastic stocking, is now applied to include the foot and up to the knee or thigh according to the extent of the injections; it may be taken off at night but should be reapplied first thing in the morning. This is maintained over the next 6-8 weeks and the patient is seen again at the end of this time.

When the compression bandage is first removed the limb is carefully inspected. The signs of a successful response to the injections are a grey discolouration out-lining the affected vein which can be felt as a knotty cord. Ideally this response is only just discernible but depends on such factors as the size of the vein, how near the surface it is and the effectiveness of the compression bandaging. It may be very pronounced and the patient should be warned that it will take many months to clear (one reason why winter is a good time for sclerotherapy) but that it will eventually disappear and should be regarded as a signal of success. However, in the worst case the vein is bulging, tender and fluctuant, with the overlying skin discoloured dark brown. There may be several such areas, each due to the vein being filled with trapped blood and the skin heavily stained with the break-down product, haemosiderin. It is important to evacuate each of these since otherwise they will take a long time to subside, cause the patient discomfort and are very unsightly (Villavicencio et al., 1985).

### Evacuation of blood trapped in veins following sclerotherapy

The blood is usually in a sufficiently fluid state to be sucked out with a small syringe and 18 gauge needle. A 2 ml size plastic syringe is suitable and the suction must be prolonged and powerful, using the thumb as a strut against the crossbar of the barrel; whilst maintaining suction, firm pressure is given to squeeze blood in the neighbouring portions of vein towards the point of the needle (Figure 19.7(a)). This usually produces several milli-litres of blood in the syringe with collapse of the bulge, immediate relief of discomfort and rapid improvement in appearance. Sometimes the blood is too viscous to suck out in this fashion and then an alternative technique is

**Figure 19.6**   *Details of hand and finger position during insertion of needle and sclerosant-containing syringe into a varicosity.*

*(a)  Left index finger steadies skin so that it does not run before the needle; point of needle is lifted as it is passed through the skin in order to open up vein.*

*(b)  Left index finger transferred to hub of needle or barrel of syringe to hold it in place. Right hand carries out a minimal test suction to confirm needle point is in vein lumen.*

*(c)  Small test injection to clear aspirated blood from needle.*

*(d)  The middle left finger can be extended over the needle point to detect extravasation during test injection.*

*(e)  Left index finger continues to support syringe whilst right hand removes adhesive tape from left hand and uses it to fix syringe to skin.*

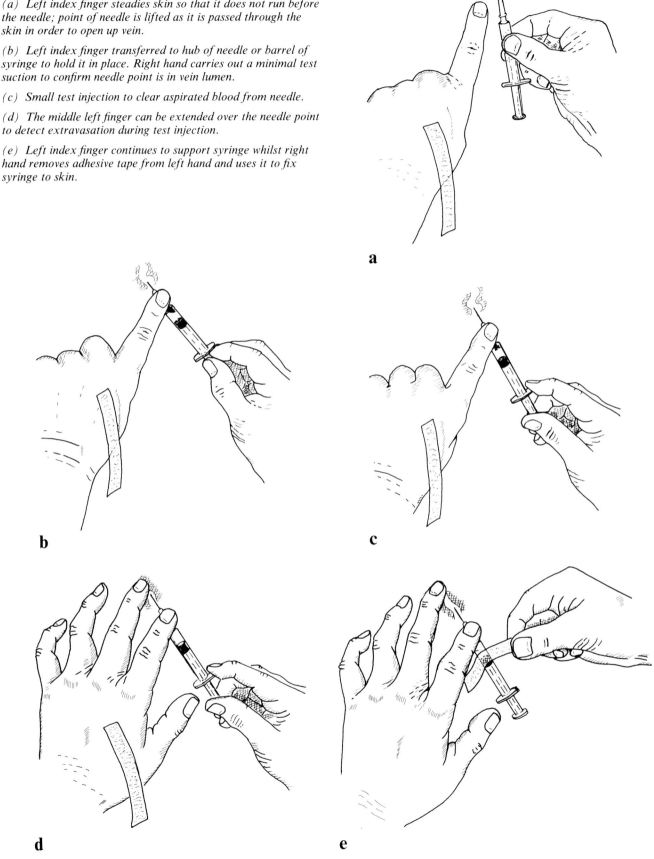

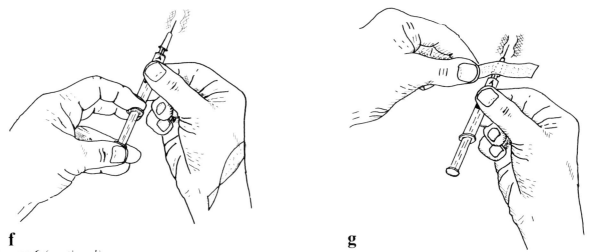

**f**          **g**

**Figure 19.6** (continued)

(f) Alternative hand arrangement. After stage (a) the right hand continues holding the barrel and the left hand operates the syringe plunger. This is often convenient if the varicose vein has an oblique lie but does not allow a finger to overlie the vein during test injection.

(g) Taping syringe to skin follows this

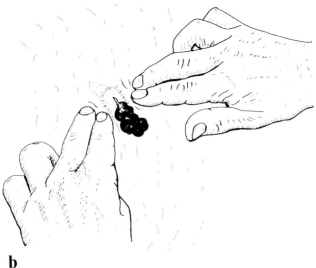

**b**

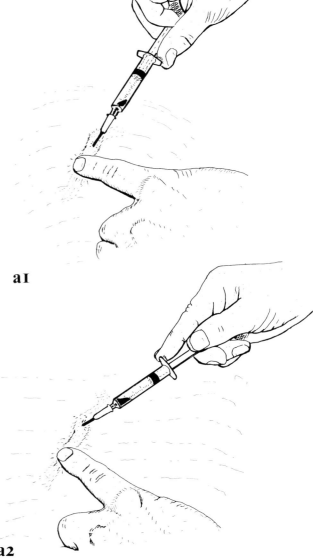

**a1**

**a2**

**Figure 19.7** Removal of excessive clot found trapped in a varicosity at follow-up.

(a) Clot trapped in an injected varicosity can usually be sucked out through a No. 18 needle or larger. Prolonged, powerful suction is applied by syringe, using the fingers and thumb of one hand to push the barrel away from the piston, whilst the needle is slowly withdrawn through the vein; the forefinger of the other hand squeezes clot towards the needle point. Alternative finger arrangements for single-handed suction are shown.

(b) If suction fails the clot can be extruded through a small stab incision made into a spot of local anaesthetic; firm finger pressure 'milks' clot towards the aperture to ensure complete evacuation

**Figure 19.8**   *Intradermal venules suitable for treatment by micro-injection.*

*(a)   A small venous flare such as this, on the calf or thigh, may respond well to a single injection into its lumen.*

*(b)   1. Telangiectasia, shown here in close-up view, responds well but will need multiple injections at various points; much can be achieved at one session but a large area may require several sessions.*
   *2. General view of same patient after one session. The venules in the lower part are indurated and brown in colour, indicating a satisfactory response.*

*(c)   Typical spider veins behind the knee of woman of 42 years and very obvious even through a stocking. Moreover they caused an unpleasant stinging discomfort at menstruation. The appearances before and after two sessions of multiple microinjections are shown; the symptoms ceased with disappearance of the venules*

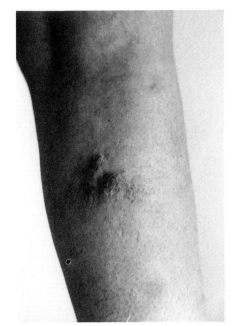

**a**

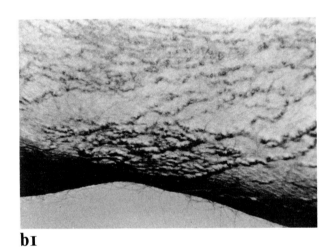

**b1**

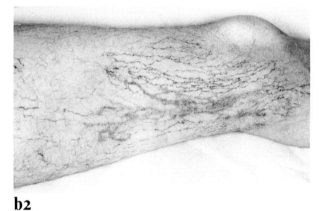

**b2**

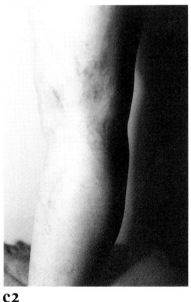

**c1**

**c2**

used. A spot of local anaesthetic is put into the skin and a small (2 mm) stab incision made into the vein. The blood and clot within can then be squeezed out from the vein by firm finger pressure for some distance either side of the incision (Figure 19.7(b)). This does not require suturing but may seep some old blood for a while and the patient should be reassured that this is not a haemorrhage and only simple renewal of the dressing is required.

The patient is seen again at the end of 2 months (or sooner if veins on the opposite limb are to be injected). At this stage discolouration and knottiness will still be obvious but the patient can be reassured that from now on these changes will slowly recede. If there are further veins on either limb to be injected these can be seen to or an arrangement made for the future.

*Policy for the future care of the patient*

Clinics specializing in treating extensive veins by sclerotherapy will often advise the patient to return every year or two so the the treatment may be 'topped up'. Others, who use surgery as the mainstay of treatment for a large set of veins and only inject lesser veins, will be content to leave return visits to the patient's discretion in the belief that the results will stand the test of time. The policy followed will depend upon the outlook of the doctor concerned and the nature of the individual problems of the patient. The author's own policy is to try to take treatment to a stage where the limb should be self maintaining for a long time to come and only to ask patients to come back regularly if it is clear that the venous state is unstable and will benefit from renewed attention or, in some unduly nervous patients, to reassure them that the veins are remaining in a satisfactory state.

## Sclerotherapy for spider veins, small venous flares or telangiectasia; microinjection

Sclerotherapy can be very effective for unsightly small venules (Figure 19.8) lying intradermally or immediately beneath the skin but the technique has to be scaled down appropriately for these diminutive veins. The first requirement, however, is to check that they are not the surface expression of a larger, but less visible, pattern of superficial incompetence and varicose veins underlying them (Figure 19.9) and, if so, these should be treated first as this may eliminate the surface venules. The following description only applies to the treatment of venules in the skin.

Injection of superficial venules is a delicate procedure, requiring a steady hand and good sight, perhaps aided by magnification. The needles used should be very fine (27 or 30 gauge), with short bevels on their points so that they can enter a small lumen without penetrating the far side. The sclerosant should be at reduced strength (for

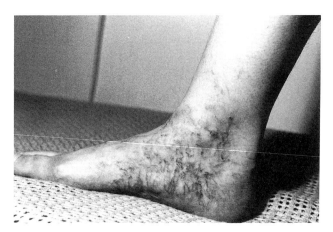

**Figure 19.9** *Numerous intradermal veins forming flares at the ankle in a patient of 45 years. Their presence indicates stress and congestion in the superficial veins at the ankle, usually caused by superficial vein incompetence. There is not necessarily any severe accompanying venotension but it may well be present. Treating these venules will not be very effective without prior treatment by surgery or sclerotherapy to the superficial vein incompetence that accompanies it. This patient was treated by sclerotherapy to superficial veins and the venules, with a good result*

example 1% STD, or use of polidocanol at 0.5% or 1.0%) because a stronger solution too easily causes necrosis of the skin if it is injected intradermally. A 2 ml syringe is best because the piston moves with less resistance than the narrow-bore smaller 1 ml size and, contrary to popular belief, there is less pressure generated by a similar force on the piston. In this way, the 2 ml syringe gives a more sensitive 'feed-back' on meeting resistance, if the needle point should shift intradermally outside the venule.

The amounts injected into very superficial or intradermal venules should be quite small, 0.2 ml at the most, and important confirmation of successful injection is seen when the venule and neighbouring branches 'clear' as the injection fluid passes through them. This is an essential signal of success and, if it is not seen after an initial small quantity, further injection should cease as it is likely to be outside the venule. If a larger feeding vein lying subcutaneously beneath the venules has been chosen then this clearing effect may not be seen and cannot be relied upon in the same way.

As soon as the injection is completed, pressure is applied through a small pad, and the needle withdrawn. To allow further injections nearby, pressure is maintained by taping the pad into place or by two turns of cohesive (e.g. Coban) bandage, but often the patient is happy to participate and apply pressure whilst the next injection is being carried out. There is no reason why a single syringe, containing 1.5 ml of dilute sclerosant should not be used with the same needle for up to six injections at different sites. This means that a number of blemishes can be treated quickly and easily.

As with sclerotherapy of larger veins, every surgeon

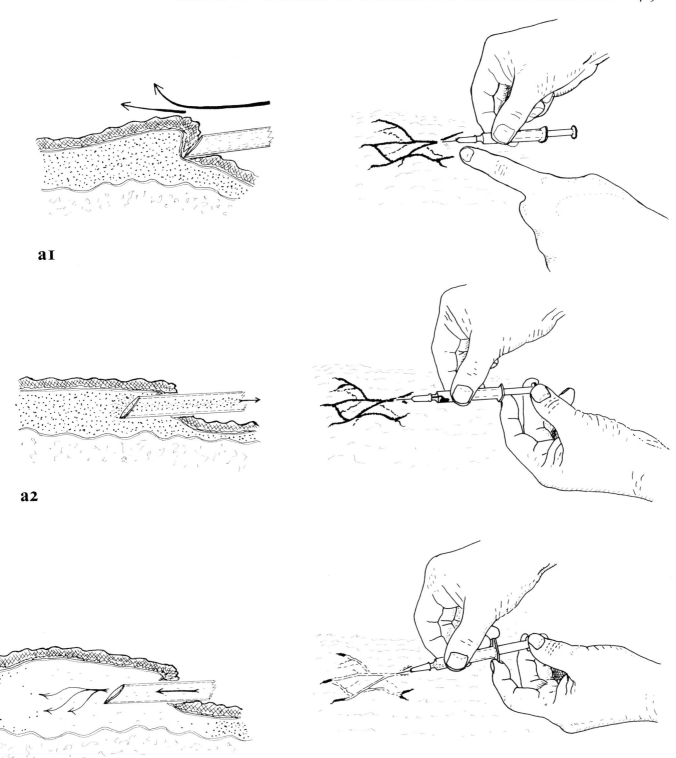

**a1**

**a2**

**a3**

**Figure 19.10**   *Steps in microinjection of intradermal venules; positioning of the needle point, greatly enlarged, is shown for each step.*

*(a)  1. Needle is inserted with a lifting action to open up lumen of venule. Left index finger steadies skin.*
*2. Syringe held immobile by right hand resting against the skin whilst left hand gives test suction to check that needle point is in lumen. Plunger is withdrawn by extension of left index finger against syringe barrel to minimize syringe displacement which is likely to occur with a two-handed action.*
*3. Sclerosant is injected by hooking index finger under crossbar of syringe to depress plunger held by middle finger and thumb. This single-handed action minimizes syringe movement. The venules are seen to clear as blood is replaced by sclerosant fluid. Only 0.2 ml is injected at any one site.*

**Figure 19.10** *(continued)*

*(b) Alternative hand position adopted after step (a)1 when lie of the syringe is across the limb.*

*1. Left hand grips hub and locks syringe against skin; this allows lowermost syringe barrel to be seen and right hand transferred to plunger for test aspiration to be carried out.*

*2, 3. Fingers and thumb of right hand are used to inject sclerosant. Two good positions are shown; pushing right hand against the left hand to depress plunger may displace needle point from lumen of venule.*

*(c) Alternative method. Placing needle point in lumen of venule by transfixion technique.*

*1. Needle is deliberately inserted obliquely through the venule to emerge from far side.*

*2. Needle is slowly withdrawn in steps, sucking at each pause until blood is aspirated. Injection can then be made*

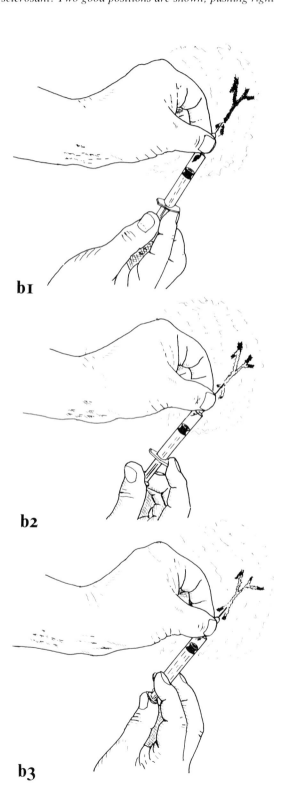

b1

b2

b3

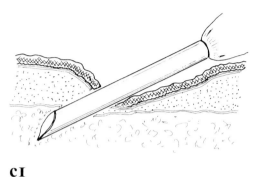

c1

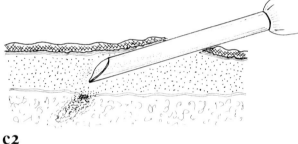

c2

will evolve his own detailed technique but the author finds the following points helpful (written for a right-handed person):

- The venules should be kept filled by the patient sitting upright with the legs over the side of the couch and remaining in this position until the injections have been completed.
- The venule chosen should be seen and felt as a small elevation in the skin surface; this indicates that it has sufficient calibre to be entered (cannulated) by a fine needle.
- It is essential to remember that intradermal venules are an integral part of the skin and move with it.
- With the left index finger, the skin is drawn slightly towards the approaching needle to prevent puckering as it is penetrated; the other hand, holding the syringe, directs the needle into the venule (Figure 19.10(a)1). The skin must not be allowed to deform because this distorts the venule so that it cannot be entered or, once entered, elastic recoil of skin can easily pull the venule off the needle, or cause it to puncture outwards; this is a common cause of failure.
- The needle is inserted with a slight lifting action in order to keep the lumen open (Figure 19.10(a)1), since

otherwise the skin, resisting needle puncture, flattens the venule and the needle passes right through it. The fingers holding the syringe are kept in contact with the skin, partly to steady the right hand and partly to prevent the skin recoiling as the next step is carried out.

- As soon as the needle point is judged to be in the lumen, syringe and needle must be held immobile against the skin so that there is no shift of one relative to the other. This may be achieved in one of two ways depending on the lie of the syringe:

  (1) If the right hand is comfortably supported against the skin, it should remain immobile, locking the syringe in this position, and the left hand is transferred cautiously to the plunger of the syringe to give, first, test suction, and then, to deliver the sclerosant (Figure 19.10(a)2,3).

  (2) If the right hand is not in contact with skin (for example, because the syringe and needle are lying transversely, across the curved circumference of the leg), then the left hand, so far used to steady the skin, is transferred to take a strong grip with finger and thumb on the needle hub, and at the same time in close contact with the underlying skin to prevent any shift (Figure 19.10(b)1). Once the syringe and needle are securely locked into position in this way, the right hand can be moved to take hold of the syringe plunger (Figure 19.10(b)2). During this sequence of movements great care must be taken to avoid any movement of the needle point which can be so easily displaced from the delicate venule.

- Continuing to keep the needle and syringe immobile, cautious suction is applied to the syringe (Figure 19.10(a)2,(b)1). As soon as a trace of blood appears in the syringe the action is reversed to give slow injection and as this proceeds the venule is watched for two possibilities:

  (1) The venule clears of blood as the solution enters it and, in this case, up to 0.2 ml is put in (Figure 19.10(a)3,(b)2,3).

  (2) A small white, raised area appears at the needle point and there is no clearing of the vein; in this case injection should cease, so that skin necrosis by intradermal injection is minimized.

- If there is difficulty in finding the lumen, then the needle may be advanced further, deliberately to transfix the venule (Figure 19.10(c)1), and then withdrawn in a series of 1 mm steps, testing by suction after each step, until blood appears in the syringe (Figure 19.10(c)2).

- Having completed all injections, the patient is asked to lie flat on the couch and a small pad of cotton wool or lint is placed over each site and compressed gently with cohesive bandage (Coban) applied only at that level of the limb; full length bandaging and elastic compression is not necessary for these very localized procedures.

Many variants in technique are advocated by different authorities, such as deliberate transfixion of the venule with the patient lying down, use of a froth created by shaking syringe contents with indrawn air, or use of a fine gauge butterfly needle relying on blood appearing as soon as the vein is entered. The author has tried these methods but finds that the single syringe and fine needle technique described above is the most adaptable to all circumstances and allows a number of lesions to be treated in quick succession. For injection into these very fine intradermal venules, the main 'tricks' are: to prevent skin distortion and recoil displacing the venule from the needle; to lift the skin slightly with the point of the needle as it enters, and, once in position, to lock the needle and adjacent skin immobile together whilst test aspiration and injection proceed.

The procedure should be virtually painless but is followed by a slight stinging or burning sensation, and a flushing of the skin in this locality. If compression is not applied, the venules may become engorged and skin oedema develops in the immediate vicinity, within a minute or so. Obvious pain indicates that something is amiss, in this instance usually intradermal injection, and the procedure should cease.

## References

Cockett, F. B. (1986) Arterial complications in treatment of varicose veins. *Phlebology*, **1**, 3–6.

Conrad, P. (1975) Sclerostripping – a 'new' procedure for the treatment of varicose veins. *Medical Journal of Australia*, **2**, 42–44

Eklof, B. (1988) Modern treatment of varicose veins. *British Journal of Surgery*, **75**, 297–298

Fegan, W. G. (1960) Continuous uninterrupted compression technique of injecting varicose veins. *Proceedings of the Royal Society of Medicine*, **53**, 837–840

Fegan, W. G. and Pegum, J. M. (1974) Accidental intra-arterial injection during sclerotherapy of varicose veins. *British Journal of Surgery*, **61**, 124–126

Fegan, W. G. (1967) *Varicose Veins: Compression Sclerotherapy*. William Heinemann, London

Goren, G. (1988, 1989) Sclerotherapy for truncal varicose veins. The concomitant high ligation and single session perfusion-compression method. Vein Disorders Center, Encino, California, USA (personal communications)

Goren, G. (1991) Injection sclerotherapy for varicose veins: history and effectiveness. *Phlebology*, **6**, 7–11

Hadfield, G. (1971) Thromboembolism in patients under injection treatment. In *Stoke Mandeville Symposium. The treatment of varicose veins by injection and compression*. Pharmaceutical Research, London, p. 52

Hobbs, J. T. (1974) Surgery and sclerotherapy in the treatment of varicose veins. *Archives of Surgery*, **109**, 793–796

Hobbs, J. T. (1978) Compression sclerotherapy of varicose veins. In *Venous Problems* (eds J. J. Bergan and J. S. T. Yao), Year Book Medical, Chicago

Jakobsen, B. H. (1979) The value of different forms of treatment for varicose veins. *British Journal of Surgery*, **66**, 182–184

Mac Gowan, W. A. L., Holland, P. D. J., Browne, H. I. and Byrnes, D. (1972) The local effects of intra-arterial injections of sodium tetradecyl sulphate (S.T.D.) 3 per cent: an experimental study. *British Journal of Surgery*, **59**, 101–104

Oesch, A., Mahler, F. and Stirnemann, P. (1986) Acute ischaemia of the foot following sclerotherapy. In *Phlebology '85* (eds D. Negus and G. Jantet), John Libbey, London, pp. 122–124

Villavicencio, J. L., Collins, G. J., Youkey, J. R. *et al.* (1985) Nonsurgical management of lower extremity venous problems. In *Surgery of the Veins* (eds J. J. Bergan and J. S. T. Yao), Grune and Stratton, New York, pp. 323–345

## Bibliography

(These references are not necessarily referred to in the text but their relevance is clear from the titles of each publication; some are included to help in the evaluation of alternative viewpoints not expressed in this chapter.)

Callum, M. J., Ruckley, C. V., Dale, J. J. and Harper, Dr (1987) Hazards of compression treatment of the leg: an estimate from Scottish surgeons. *British Medical Journal*, **295**, 1382.

Conrad, P. (1987) Injection of varicose veins and spider veins. *Australian Family Physician*, **16**, 451–454

Hobbs, J. T. (1977) The treatment of dilated venules. In *The Treatment of Venous Disorders* (ed. J. T. Hobbs), MTP Press, Lancaster, pp. 399–413

Hobbs, J. T. (1977) A random trial of the treatment of varicose veins by surgery and sclerotherapy. In *The Treatment of Venous Disorders* (ed. J. T. Hobbs), MTP Press, Lancaster, pp. 195–207.

Hoerdegen, K. M. and Sigg, K. (1988) Injection-compression sclerotherapy of the greater saphenous vein with proximal incompetence (crosse insufficiency) as an alternative treatment to surgery. *Phlebology*, **3**, 41–48

Hoyte, P. (1987) Hazards of injections. *Journal of the Medical Defence Union*, Summer, 9

Jakobsen, B. H. (1979) The value of different forms of treatment for varicose veins. *British Journal of Surgery*, **66**, 182–184

Keddie, N. C. (1987) Medico-legal problems from the treatment of varicose veins. *Journal of the Medical Defence Union*, Winter, 8–9

McFarland, R. J., Scott, H. J., Kay, D. N. and Scott, R. A. P. (1988) High injection sclerotherapy for varicose veins in the presence of femoro-saphenous reflux. *Phlebology*, **3**, 49–54

MacGowan, W. A. L. (1985) Sclerotherapy – prevention of accidents: a review. *Journal of the Royal Society of Medicine*, **78**, 136–137

Marks, C. G. (1974) Localised hirsuties following compression sclerotherapy with sodium tetradecyl sulphate. *British Journal of Surgery*, **61**, 127–128

Neglen, P., Einarsson, E. and Eklof, B. (1986) High tie with sclerotherapy for saphenous vein insufficiency. *Phlebology*, **1**, 105–111

Neglen, P., Jonsson, B., Einarsson, E. and Eklof, B. (1986) Socio-economic benefits of ambulatory surgery and compression sclerotherapy for varicose veins. *Phlebology*, **1**, 225–230

Ouvry, P. A. and Davy, A. (1986) Traitement sclerosant de la saphene extern variqueuse. In *Phlebology '85* (eds D. Negus and G. Jantet), John Libbey, London, pp. 115–118

Ouvry, P. A. and Davy, A. (1986) Sclerotherapie apres stripping. In *Phlebology '85* (eds D. Negus and G. Jantet), John Libbey, London, pp. 125–128

Stother, I. G. Bryson, A. and Alexander, S. (1974) The treatment of varicose veins by compression sclerotherapy. *British Journal of Surgery*, **61**, 387–390

Thompson, The Hon. Mr Justice (1975) *Transcript of Proceedings. Judgement* (*revised*). Queen's Bench Division, 15 July, 74/NJ/3104

Tournay, R. (1990) How should resistant varicose veins be sclerosed? *Phlebology*, **5**, 151–155

Various authors of several nationalities (1977) Techniques of sclerotherapy. In *The Treatment of Venous Disorders* (ed. J. Hobbs), MTP Press, Lancaster

Wallois, P. (1980) Indications et techniques de la sclerose des varices. *Bulletin d'Actualite Therapeutique* **XXV**, 2485–2495

*References upon aspects of compression bandaging with sclerotherapy*

Batch, A. J. G., Wickremesinghe, S. S., Gannon, M. E. and Dormandy, J. A. (1980) Randomised trial of bandaging after sclerotherapy for varicose veins. *British Medical Journal*, **281**, 423

Fraser, I. A., Perry, E. P., Hatton, M. and Watkin, D. F. L. (1985) Prolonged bandaging is not required following sclerotherapy of varicose veins. *British Journal of Surgery*, **72**, 488–490

Raj, T. B., Goddard, M. and Makin, G. S. (1980) How long do compression bandages maintain their pressure during ambulatory treatment of varicose veins? *British Journal of Surgery*, **67**, 122–124

Reddy, P., Wickers, J., Terry, T. *et al.* (1986) What is the correct period of bandaging following sclerotherapy? *Phlebology*, **1**, 218–220

Scurr, J. H., Coleridge-Smith, P. and Cutting, P. (1985) Varicose veins: optimum compression following sclerotherapy. *Annals of the Royal College of Surgeons*, **67**, 109–111

Shouler, P. J. and Runchman, P. C. (1989) Varicose veins: optimum compression after surgery and sclerotherapy. *Annals of the Royal College of Surgeons of England*, **71**, 402–404

# 20

# Treatment of varicose veins and other manifestations of superficial vein incompetence. 3. Surgery

The essential principle in active treatment of incompetence in the superficial veins, that is to say, the cause of simple or primary varicose veins, is to eliminate the pathway of incompetence as completely as possible. Obliteration of the pathway by sclerotherapy has been discussed in Chapter 19 and the purpose of the present chapter is to consider technical aspects of surgical treatment. There are four components to this:

1. Elimination of the source of incompetence. This usually involves ligation, flush with the deep vein from which it arises, of the source of retrograde flow, usually the termination of a long or a short saphenous vein.
2. Removing the principle pathway of incompetence. This is usually a long single channel, such as one or other of the saphenous veins, which is removed by stripping for much of its length.
3. Removing the varicosities (tributaries in pathway of incompetence) as far as possible. Varicose veins often do not lend themselves to stripping, and then, a commonly employed method is to use multiple dissections through small incisions.
4. Elimination of perforating veins when this is appropriate. There is much misunderstanding about the role of perforating veins in superficial incompetence and this has been considered in Chapter 11. In most cases of simple incompetence in the superficial veins, the perforators are doing no more than carrying out their normal function of allowing inward flow from superficial to deep veins and do not need special attention. However, in a minority of cases one or two perforating veins become excessively enlarged and are associated with heavy surge, in and out, with each contraction of the leg muscles; these veins are usually easily identified, especially those arising from the arcuate branch of the saphenous vein, and are best eliminated in case they should become a source of continuing downflow to the foot. In the mid-thigh perforating veins connecting with the long saphenous vein, and similarly with the

short saphenous vein in mid-calf, may provide a new source of incompetence if the saphenous vein is not stripped. A specific form of perforator incompetence, leading to forceful outflow, from the gastrocnemius and soleus perforating veins, posteriorly on the calf, may require individual elimination, but often this is achieved incidentally during the course of stripping a short saphenous vein and dissection of its varicosities (and see comment later in this chapter in the section on 'Perforating veins as a primary source of superficial vein incompetence').

*Combination of surgery with sclerotherapy*

In this chapter the emphasis will be upon full surgical treatment of all the aspects summarized above. Nevertheless, there are occasions when the surgeon may complete treatment by sclerotherapy, either at the time of operation or subsequently. This is not infrequently done when conspicuous varicosities have inadvertently survived an operation, or have been too fragile for surgical removal, but some vein clinics, specializing in short-stay or outpatient treatment, may deliberately restrict surgery to removing the source, perhaps also stripping of a saphenous vein, and completing treatment by sclerotherapy as a routine policy (van der Stricht *et al.*, 1986). This combination of surgery with sclerotherapy has been considered in Chapter 19 and will not be referred to again here.

*Should contraceptive pill be stopped*

This is discussed in Chapter 16, with the general conclusion that contraception with oestrogen-containing pills should be suspended for several weeks before surgery and restarted at the next convenient period 2 weeks afterwards. Some surgeons consider this is being overcautious (Sue-Ling and Hughes, 1988) when a progestogen pill with very low oestrogen content is being used and the patient is to be mobilized immediately. In any case it is wise to have a policy on this agreed between surgeon and the physician advising the patient on contraception.

### Anaesthesia for surgical treatment

If full, uninhibited surgery is to be carried out, then light general anaesthesia provides by far the best circumstances for the surgeon and is probably kindest for the patient. A detailed operation may take over an hour for each limb, and following this at least a 24-hour stay in hospital is advisable. The author's practice is to admit the patients 2 hours before the operation and to discharge them 2 or 3 days later, so that there is no overnight wait in hospital before operation, and the patient returns home fully confident, freely mobile and independent of medical care.

In certain circumstances, such as excessive fear of general anaesthesia or severe cardiac and respiratory disease, the operation may been carried out satisfactorily with spinal or extradural anaesthesia. This can form the basis of a routine surgical procedure provided the specialized skills are available, but most clinics keep these methods in reserve to be used only in the unusual case where general anaesthesia has to be avoided. The relatively long interval after operation without active movement of the lower limbs is a theoretical disadvantage but there is no convincing evidence of increased incidence of deep vein thrombosis caused by this.

As regards local anaesthesia, there is no difficulty in using this for surgery to a single site, such as high ligation of the long saphenous vein, but it is more difficult to obtain satisfactory anaesthesia for the wide area usually covered in full stripping of a saphenous vein and dissection of varicosities. This can be done either by extensive local infiltration of the areas involved (Nabatoff, 1953) or by a regional nerve block, for example, into the femoral nerve to anaesthetize long saphenous territory (Taylor et al., 1981; Bishop and Jarrett, 1986; Jakobsen, 1986). These methods can be made to work well by those who have gained experience in them and perhaps have the advantage of allowing a surgeon to do the operation unaided by an anaesthetist but this would seem time consuming and only appropriate for rather special circumstances. Goren and Yellin (1991) describe a method under local anaesthesia, followed by immediate ambulation, that permits high saphenous ligation, with removal of the incompetent portion of the saphenous vein and all the outlying varicosities through multiple stab incisions. They recommend this as being a low cost procedure with minimal inconvenience to the patient.

Intravenous regional anaesthesia (Fagg, 1987) in the lower limb requires prolonged use of a tourniquet and is associated with an occasional deep vein thrombosis. It may have a place in orthopaedic surgery but is not recommended for surgery to the veins.

In the description that follows it must be assumed that general anaesthesia is employed. Laryngeal intubation is not strictly necessary unless the patient is to be positioned face down. Since the operation is almost entirely subcutaneous, muscle relaxants are not required and best avoided.

### Preoperative marking out of the veins and instruction of the patient

The detailed planning of the operation should have been made, and fully noted, at the time of outpatient consultation. However, the superficial veins cannot be reliably identified when the patient is lying horizontally with all the veins collapsed and it is essential to mark out the pathway of incompetence immediately preoperatively with the patient standing; a felt-tipped pen is suitable for this and the marking must include the pattern of varicose veins and the likely positioning of incisions at strategic points (Figures 20.1, 20.24 (c)). On the operating table, the veins may be detectable as hollows and grooves and this is a useful ploy if for some reason marking has proved inadequate. The author believes it is important that the surgeon himself should mark out the veins and this should include final confirmation of the suitability of the proposed operation.

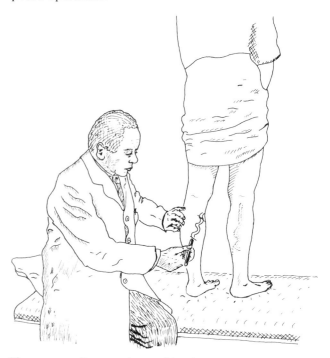

**Figure 20.1** *Preoperative marking, by surgeon or experienced deputy, of veins and likely incisions is essential and can only be carried out with the patient standing*

### Postoperative programme of activity

Having marked out the veins, it is a good moment to give the patient simple instructions on the programme to be followed postoperatively. The patient is asked to carry out frequent foot movements (full sweeps at the ankle), for example, a series of six foot movements every 5 minutes, and accompanied by one or two deep breaths 'to turn over the vein circulation and to avoid any unwanted clotting'. This should start as soon as the patient awakes from anaesthesia. Next morning, in addition to the foot and other movements, the patient should get up 'every hour – on the hour' and walk steadily in the corridor for 5 minutes, without sitting or standing still; during any short pause on the walk, movement should be maintained by marking time or rhythmically rising on the toes. Thus, the patient will be expected to spend 55 minutes in the hour on the bed, using it as a couch, with repeated foot movements, alternating with 5 minutes of active walking before returning to the bed. The patient may, of course, get up and go to the lavatory whenever required.

*Other postoperative details*

The foot of the bed is raised 45 cm, with a cage over the feet to allow free movement, and the patient may sit or lie in any position found comfortable, changing this whenever it is wished. The legs will have been bandaged with crepe in theatre to give moderate support and this will be retained over the stay in hospital. Provided that skin closure is by unknotted subcuticular stitches (see later in this chapter, under 'Obtaining good cosmetic results') or by adhesive strip, the patient suffers little

discomfort and may be assured beforehand that walking soon after the operation will not cause any difficulty. The only postoperative analgesia usually needed is a mild oral agent, such as co-proxamol, but often the patient declares that they 'do not require any tablets'.

## Surgical technique

### Incompetence in the long saphenous system

The best results will require:

- High ligation of long saphenous termination, flush with the common femoral vein.
- Stripping of the long saphenous vein, usually down to the upper calf but sometimes to the ankle.
- Removal of all visible varicosities, marked pre-operatively when the patient was standing.
- In some cases, location and interruption of one or more perforating veins

### High, flush ligation of the long saphenous termination

*Some anatomical points* (Figures 20.2–20.5)

*Note:* Although the operation is commonly referred to as 'Trendelenburg's', this eminent surgeon advised ligation

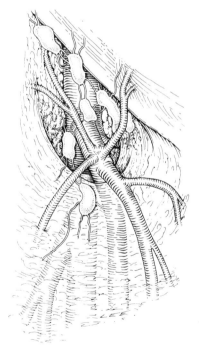

**Figure 20.3** *Double saphenous vein. Occasionally the long saphenous vein forms two channels, so that the more superficial vein is mistakenly assumed to be the only saphenous vein, and the larger, deeper component, more likely be the main pathway of incompetence, is left intact. The small size of the more superficial vein should arouse suspicion and its termination displayed with particular care; this will reveal that it lacks the usual complement of branches and joins a deeper vein, which in turn joins the common femoral vein and has the usual saphenous terminal branches. A syringe test will, of course, indicate which channel is incompetent, or if both are at fault*

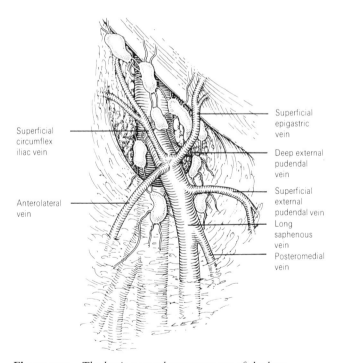

Superficial circumflex iliac vein

Anterolateral vein

Superficial epigastric vein

Deep external pudendal vein

Superficial external pudendal vein

Long saphenous vein

Posteromedial vein

**Figure 20.2** *The basic normal arrangement of the long saphenous termination and its branches. The details of this vary considerably and some of these variants are also illustrated later. These branches are always present in some form and may come off the vein separately, or, with two or more originating from one common stem*

**Figure 20.4** *Relationship of long saphenous termination to superficial external pudendal artery.*

*(a) Often it lies posterior to the vein and may not be noticed.*

*(b) Commonly, it runs in front of the saphenous vein and has to be divided and ligated, or, at a later stage, the saphenous vein is divided between clamps and drawn from under it. A small vein runs with it which should also be ligated. Haemostasis in the groin should be meticulous since otherwise haematoma occurs all too readily and avulsion techniques should not be used here*

below mid-thigh and the benefits of this were soon lost by the development of enlarged veins joining the upper saphenous with the original varicosities; his description (1891) did not include high ligation, with elimination of the uppermost tributaries, nowadays considered essential to minimize 'anatomical' recurrence of the source. W.T. Thomas in 1896 was the first to recommend ligation at the 'highest available point' (Dodd and Cockett, 1976).

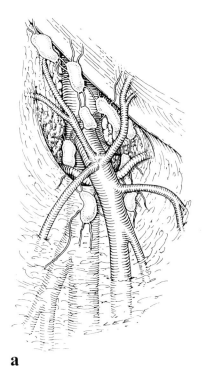

**a**

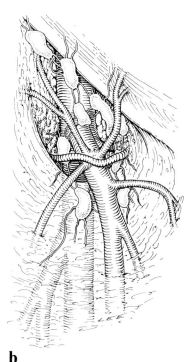

**b**

**Figure 20.5** *(a)–(e)   Some anatomical variants and abnormal findings in the vicinity of saphenous termination. These include:*

*(a)  A large saccule (saphena varix) lying below an incompetent uppermost saphenous valve.*

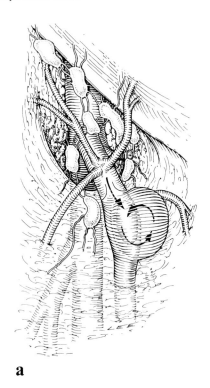

**a**

*(b)  An incompetent anterolateral branch giving rise to varicose veins on the front of the thigh.*

*(c)  An anterolateral vein, sharing origin with the superficial circumflex branch, and giving rise to varices running down the outer thigh and leg.*

*(d)  An incompetent anterolateral vein predominating the circumflex branch and giving rise to an accessory saphenous vein, as large as the main saphenous and sweeping down to rejoin it in the lower thigh or upper calf.*

*(e)  A variant of this is a massive anterolateral accessory saphenous vein which is incompetent and has a saccule beneath its upper valve; the true saphenous vein is undersized but competent. Failure to remove this accessory saphenous vein will leave behind a massive source of incompetence with inevitable persistence or recurrence of the varicosities arising from it.*

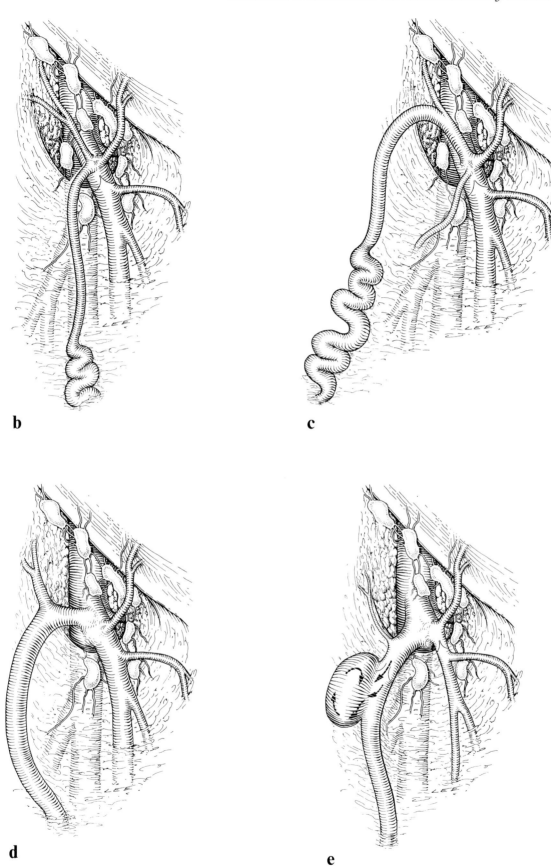

**b**

**c**

**d**

**e**

**Figure 20.5** *(continued)*

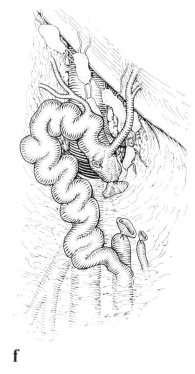

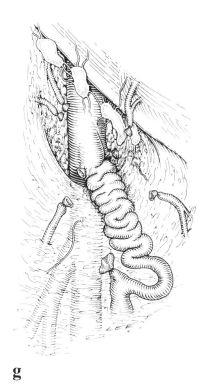

**f**                                   **g**

**Figure 20.5** *(continued)*
*(f), (g) Incompetent branches from the saphenous termination may allow downflow to bypass competent uppermost saphenous valves and empty into an incompetent saphenous vein below this level. This can give a false impression of saphenous competence on syringe testing (see later). Two high-level examples are shown here, from actual findings at operation after division of the saphenous vein, but any of the incompetent veins, shown in illustrations (b)–(e), can bypass saphenous valves in this fashion by interconnection at various levels in the thigh*

**Figure 20.6** *Placing the incision and avoiding lymphatics. The incision is centred upon a point 3 cm outside, and 3 cm below, the pubic tubercle, and adjusted to be slightly below the skin crease but parallel with it; this usually avoids lymphatic glands. Five centimetres in length is sufficient if hand-held retractors allow free mobility of the wound but a self-retaining retractor, immobilizing the approach, will require a larger incision. If lymphatic glands are encountered, they should be skirted by moving to one side and driving obliquely under them. Unnecessary damage to lymphatic channels should always be avoided; they can often be recognized and should be displaced rather than cut. This is facilitated by the fatty tissue over the saphenous vein which is easily brushed aside and sharp dissection is only necessary for incision of skin and the investing layer of fascia. If lymphatic channels are divided, they should be ligated whenever possible; a collection of lymph or a lymph fistula are tedious complications that can follow heavy-handed surgery in this region. Finesse is needed and a massive approach 'to improve recognition of the veins' is seldom required, provided the anatomical landmarks suggested above are followed. Operating through scar tissue, as in saphenous recurrence, will, however, require sharp dissection and is particularly prone to damage lymphatics enmeshed in it (and see later section on 'Lymph collection and lymph fistula after dissection in the groin')*

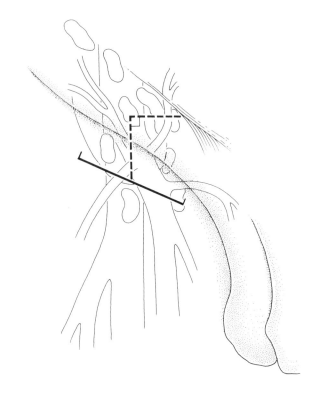

*Surgical technique in high ligation* (Figures 20.6–20.11)

The technique of high saphenous ligation given in Figures 20.6–20.11 tends to remove the uppermost saphenous valve with the saphenous stump and a modification of the syringe test will be required if it is particularly wished to check this valve. The test described, however, is usually sufficient to determine whether the thigh portion of saphenous vein has significant incompetence or not.

**Figure 20.7** *Displaying the saphenous termination.*

*(a) The incision is deepened to the investing layer of superficial fascia and a small opening in this is stretched apart by retractors.*

*(b) The underlying fat is gently parted to reveal the long saphenous vein which is progressively cleaned to display the characteristic branches at its termination.*

*(c) The dissection is continued to display the saphenous termination running through the fossa ovalis and into the common femoral vein. The latter is cleaned sufficiently to see its surface both above and below the termination*

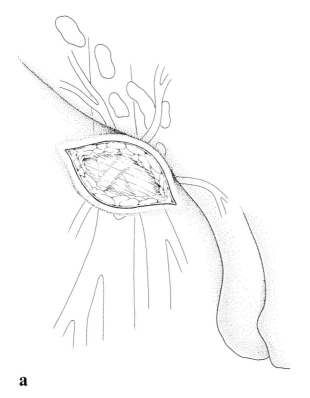

a

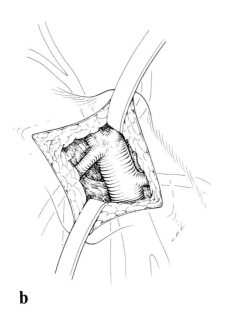

b

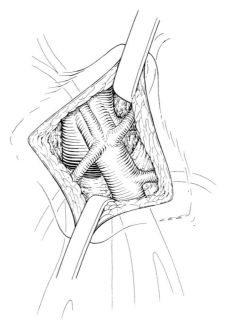

c

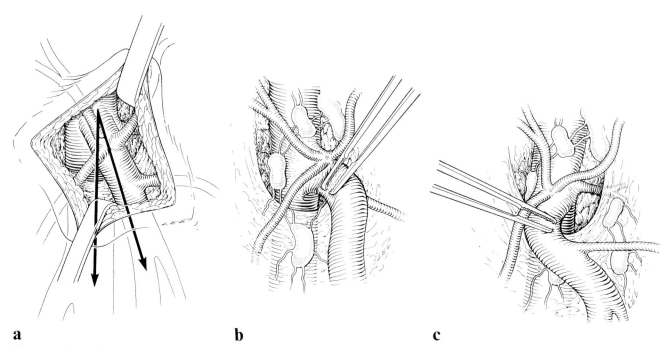

**a**                                    **b**                                    **c**

**Figure 20.8**   *At this point there should be a conscious pause whilst the accurate identification of the structures is double checked before any sizeable veins are divided. Even experienced surgeons are occasionally surprised to find that they have mobilized the common femoral vein and are poised to divide it; this is particularly likely to happen in a thin patient. Division of a common femoral vein is a surgical disaster, only retrievable by considerable skill. Size alone is not an adequate criterion, particularly as the surgeon is accustomed to finding a saphenous vein often as large as the deep vein when it is first exposed and before it contracts down. The following should be verified:*

*(a)   At least two characteristic branches should be seen arising from the saphenous termination and running upwards.*
   *The saphenous vein should be seen to make a definite angle medially, whilst the common femoral vein follows the axis of the limb.*

*(b), (c)   The saphenous termination is gently pushed first medially and then laterally to see beyond doubt that it joins the deep vein in characteristic fashion. In doing this the vein presumed to be the saphenous is not traumatized (hence the open forceps shown in the illustrations) just in case it is in fact the deep vein. If all the tests just given are entirely satisfactory, a final test is to pull upwardly upon the saphenous vein to confirm that this transmits a corresponding movement to the skin on the medial aspect of the upper thigh*

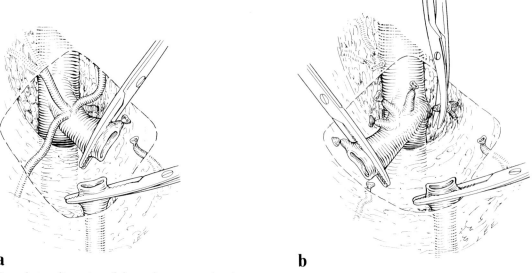

**a**                                    **b**

**Figure 20.9**   *Completing dissection of the saphenous termination.*

*(a)   Now that the identity of the long saphenous vein has been confirmed beyond doubt it may be divided between clamps, about 2 or 3 cm down, in order to facilitate the full mobilization and flush ligation of the termination. Handle the saphenous termination gently and do not use excessive traction which may damage the deep vein.*

*(b)   All terminal branches are ligated and divided. The uppermost point of union between saphenous and deep vein is fully visualized to ensure that all terminal branches have been dealt with. The inner aspect of the common femoral vein is inspected for the deep external pudendal branch; if this is present it should be ligated with or without division*

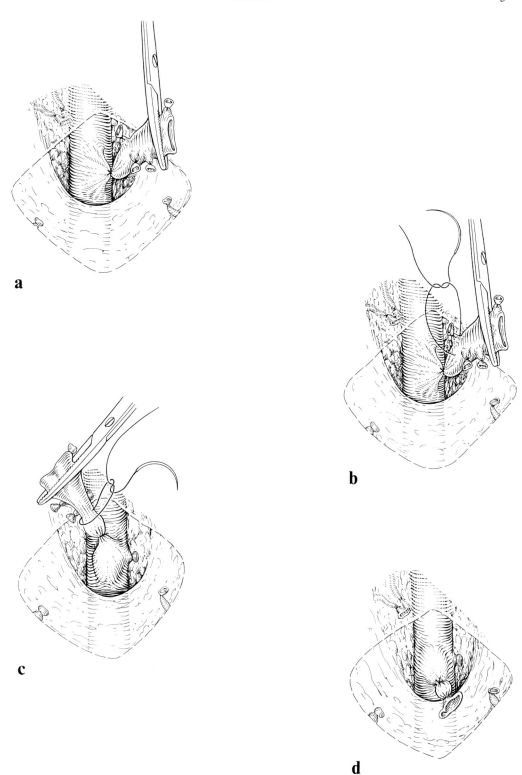

**Figure 20.10**   *Ligation of the long saphenous stump.*

*(a)  The long saphenous termination is now raised up and ligated, without tranfixion, flush with the common femoral vein (author's choice is 60 gauge linen).*

*(b), (c)  A transfixion stitch is now placed just superficial to the first ligature, to give double security in sealing the saphenous stump. This double ligature may also help to prevent recurrence by revascularization of the stump. A single ligature, especially with catgut, is NOT recommended for closing this large vein.*

*(d)  The excess saphenous stump is now trimmed away and attention turned to checking the correct identity of the pathway of incompetence by the syringe test*

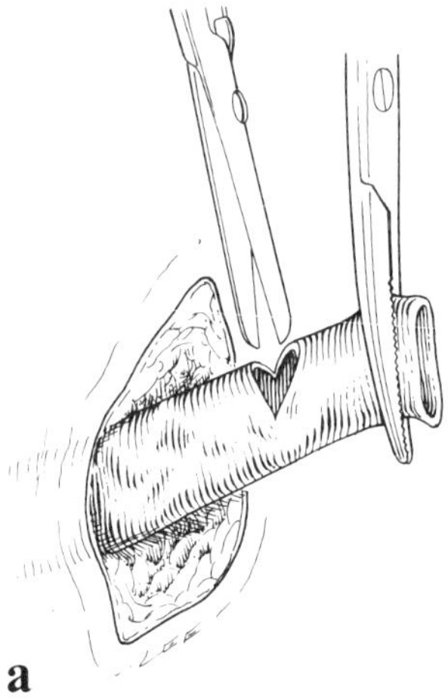

a

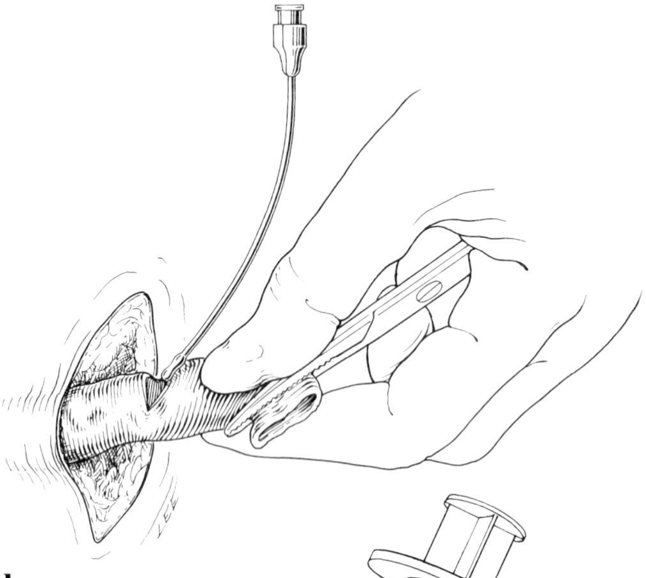

b

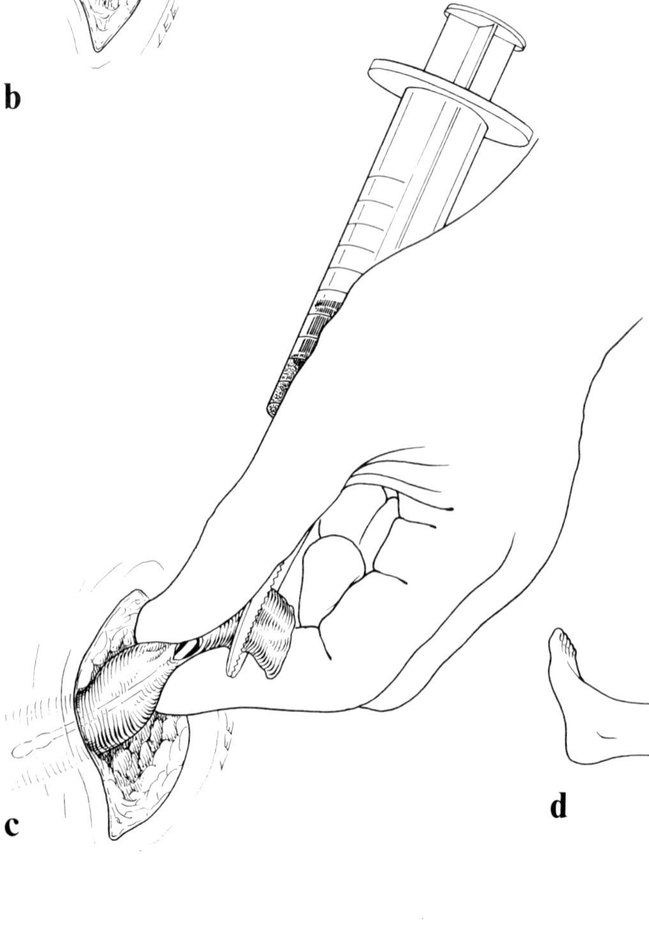

c

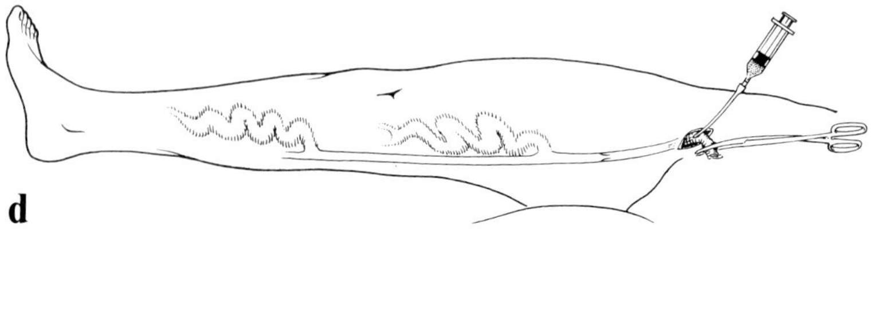

d

**Figure 20.11** *The syringe test. The purpose of this is to test the competence of the valves in the saphenous vein or any major downward-running tributaries.*

*(a), (b) A small opening is made into the side of the divided downward portion of saphenous vein, just below the clamp, and a 50 ml syringe, filled with normal saline, with suitable cannula attached, is inserted into this.*

*(c) Simple pressure between finger and thumb usually provides an adequate seal without having to tie the cannula in.*

*(d) The syringe is emptied down the saphenous vein with a steady, but not forceful, pressure. The following circumstances may be encountered:*

- *Usually there is no resistance at all and the varicosities in lower thigh or upper leg can be seen to give a slight bulge. This indicates complete lack of any competent valves within the vein between syringe and the first varicosity, or beyond.*
- *There may be partial resistance that yields within a few seconds, due to a partly contracted vein expanding up to full size and causing valve rings to dilate, so that partial becomes full incompetence.*
- *There is complete resistance to emptying the syringe. It is possible that the cannula end is jammed into a valve cusp and it should be withdrawn as far as possible and the test repeated. If full resistance is still encountered, without yielding to steady pressure, it is evident that there is one or more competent valves below the syringe so that the vein, at least in its upper part, is not the pathway of incompetence and another pathway must be looked for. This will usually be an enlarged downward-running branch from the saphenous termination, an anterolateral or anterior accessory saphenous vein, which will probably have already declared itself as a likely pathway of incompetence by its obvious size. The syringe test is applied to this and confirmation given by lack of resistance and bulging of varicosities on the front of thigh. This pattern of incompetence may, in fact, bypass one or two competent valves in the upper saphenous vein by rejoining this vein below these valves (Figure 20.5 (b)–(d), (f), (g)); in this case, there will be resistance on the syringe testing to the upper part of the saphenous vein even though its lower part is incompetent and taking over the pathway of incompetence started by the anterolateral varicosity. With this state, it is usually simplest to strip the entire thigh portion of saphenous vein*

## Stripping the long saphenous vein (Figure 20.12)

Having confirmed the identity of the pathway of incompetence by the syringe test, the vein is now removed. If the test has shown this to be an anterolateral branch this is removed by stripping and the thigh varicosities arising from it removed by multiple dissections or avulsion (see below). More usually the long saphenous vein will be at fault and should be stripped. Near the ankle this vein is in close proximity to the saphenous nerve and branches of this surround the vein, so that stripping from this level may damage the nerve, giving rise to cutaneous anaesthesia, or worse, to an unpleasant traction neuritis persisting for many months. For this reason stripping from the ankle is only carried out if there is a clear indication of heavy incompetence in the vein down to this level. Commonly, the arcuate branch is involved and the varicose and perforating veins arising from this can be removed by a combination of stripping and local dissection (it is here that careful preoperative marking is so important).

It is always more satisfactory to pass the stripper up the vein from below (Figure 20.12 (b)–(i)) so that it does not catch on valve cusps (incompetent valves often have quite large cusps), nor does it tend to enter branch veins as it will if passed from above. When marking out the veins, it is important to locate the saphenous vein in the upper calf and mark it clearly so that there is no difficulty in finding it and passing the stripper upwards. The stripper may be caught by entering a saccule but, usually, by withdrawing it slightly, rotating it to alter the alignment of the tip, and gently probing upwards, perhaps with intermittent hand pressure over the tip, it can be persuaded to pass this point. Force must not be used and if necessary a small incision is made over the end of the

**Figure 20.12**

*(a) A safe level from which to take saphenous stripping is in the upper third of the calf, where the vein is not so closely related to the nerve.*

*(b) Exposing the saphenous vein in the upper calf.*

*(c) A small side opening is made into the upward-running portion of saphenous vein.*

*(d) The stripper is passed into this and passed up to the groin.*

*(e) A strong tie is placed around the saphenous vein to prevent the stripper head from slipping into the lumen and failing to strip; it also prevents bleeding. A double ligature is used in a large vein to help avoid invagination and possible breaking of the vein as it is stripped.*

*(f), (g) The tip of the stripper is made to emerge through a small side hole in the upper end of the saphenous vein.*

*(h) The upper end is most easily sealed, to prevent blood loss, by artery forceps applied across the lumen but not including the stripper, which is pushed to one side.*

*(i) The saphenous vein is now stripped by a slow, strong pull on the upper end. As side branches are pulled taut, the overlying skin dimples and at this stage there should be a pause for 15 seconds to allow the branch to contract down before breaking it off, and, in this way, bleeding from it is minimized. The process of stripping should be a controlled one, carefully watched throughout. Great force should not be used without checking to ensure that it is impeded by no more than an extra-strong branch which can be felt as a tight cord and seen to be dimpling the skin. A sudden loss of resistance means that the vein has invaginated and either is splitting up its length, or has snapped, usually where a major tributary joins it. If the vein has broken and part is retained, the portion on the stripper can be stretched out to act as a measure to locate the end of the retained portion. The vein on the stripper should always be stretched out and examined for completeness of stripping and for evidence of incompetence, such as saccules. It is instructive to open the vein throughout its length to see the state of the valves. Cusps are commonly seen even though the valves have been shown to be incompetent by the syringe test*

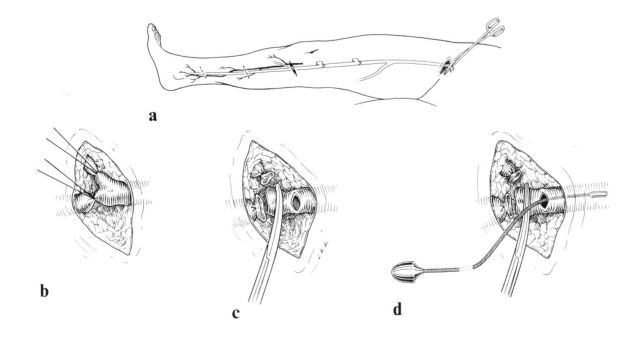

a

b

c

d

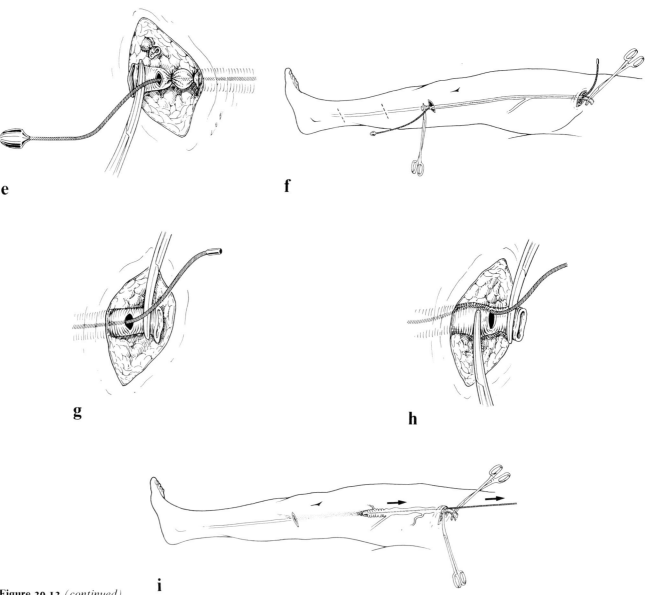

**Figure 20.12** *(continued)*

stripper, easily palpated, in order to guide its tip beyond the irregularity, or to strip the vein already traversed and reinsert the stripper again at the point of interruption.

The direction of stripping is often debated but no conclusive advantage has been shown for either direction, although, possibly, stripping from above downwards below the knee is less likely to damage the saphenous nerve. If the stripper has been passed upwards to the groin, or vice versa, there need be no hesitation to carry out the actual stripping in this direction.

*Clearing clot from the track of the stripped saphenous vein, skin suture and bandaging*

After stripping, clot usually accumulates in the track of the vein, due to blood coming from disconnected tributaries. The amount varies from insignificant to a con-siderable quantity that causes discomfort and extreme ecchymosis appearing over the next few days. This is minimized by clearing the track of clot but is best delayed until a late stage in the operation, when haemostasis in disconnected veins is well established; the saphenous incisions are left open until all the peripheral vein dis-sections have been carried out and sutured, and then the track is cleared by one of the means illustrated in Figure 20.13. Suture of the remaining incisions and bandaging are shown in Figure 20.14.

**High ligation and stripping of the short saphenous vein (saphenopopliteal ligation)**

The broad principles of high ligation and stripping of the short saphenous vein are similar to those already described for the long saphenous vein. Certainly, there is a similar need to understand the anatomy and the

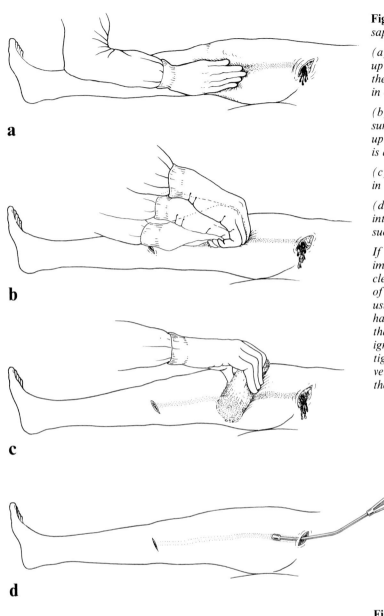

**a**

**b**

**c**

**d**

**Figure 20.13** *Clearing clot from the track of a stripped saphenous vein.*

*(a) Pressure applied with the flat of the hand, successively up the length of the track. This may not press out clot in the mid-portion and a rolling technique is more effective in clearing the full length.*

*(b) The back of semiflexed fingers and knuckles of the surgeon's hand are used as a roller, moving successively up the thigh to drive out clot through the upper end; this is a very effective method.*

*(c) A roll of bandage is firmly run up and down the thigh in the line of the track.*

*(d) With suction temporarily off, a sucker end is introduced down the track. When it is well positioned, the suction is turned on and the sucker withdrawn slowly.*

*If bleeding at any stage is troublesome, whether immediately after stripping, or by starting again after clearance of the track, firm pressure applied with the flat of the hand and forearm over the track for 2 minutes is usually effective. The policy of clearing clot after giving haemostasis time to take full effect is more satisfactory than stripping with a thigh bandage already in place and ignoring any clot that may then accumulate. A bandage tight enough to prevent bleeding will constrict the deep veins and cause a most undesirable venous congestion in the limb*

**Figure 20.14** *Suture of main incisions by subcuticular stitch: bandaging of the limb. An 'unfixed', subcuticular stitch, unlike a conventional transverse stitch or clip, causes no pain and does not create any reaction. If a monofilament, such as Prolene, is used, its eventual withdrawal is completely painless and no foreign material is left behind. No stitch marks are caused and, cosmetically, subcuticular suture is by far the best method to use on any part of the limb. It is kept in place by 2.5 cm (1 in) adhesive strips (Steri-Strip or Micropore) along the length of the incision and extending beyond it, without any other fixation or covering. This method is more fully illustrated in Figure 20.22. Tight bandaging must be avoided and a 10 cm or 15 cm (4 in or 6 in) inch cotton crepe bandage, giving moderate support, evenly applied up to mid-thigh, is sufficient. It should include the foot and should only be lightly applied to the thigh, for fear of causing constriction to the underlying deep veins. Early movement and walking is an invariable routine. Closure of stab incisions used for removal of outlying varicose veins is described presently and illustrated in Figure 20.24(j)–(l)*

variations in level and mode of termination of the short saphenous vein at its upper end. Its termination into the popliteal vein is closely surrounded by major nerves, arteries and veins, and the relationship to these has much individual variation. Inept surgery damaging the popliteal deep vein has consequences even more severe than damage to the common femoral vein. Some important anatomical points are considered in Figure 20.15.

Both patterns of upward extension of short saphenous vein given in Figure 20.15 (c)1, 2 may become major collateral channels compensating for post-thrombotic occlusion or severe deformity in the deep veins (Figures 8.2 (c), 8.6). In these circumstances, they can become so large that they may be mistaken on phlebography for the original deep vein. The great enlargement of the vein renders their valves incompetent and they are then a

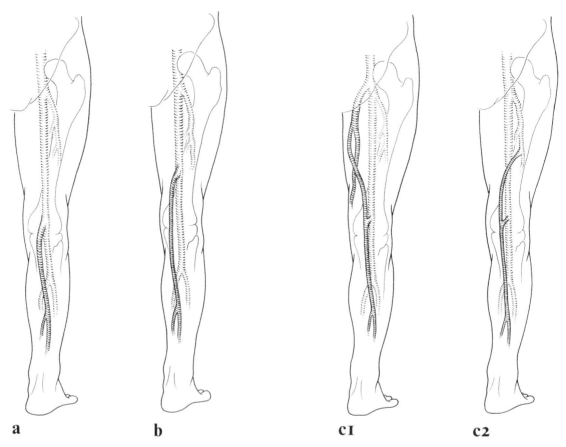

**a**  **b**  **c1**  **c2**

**Figure 20.15** *Level and mode of short saphenous termination.*

*(a) The short saphenous vein usually terminates in the mid-popliteal fossa slightly above the level of the knee joint by joining the popliteal vein (see Figures 1.5(c)2,3, 4.22 (a)1, 4.23, 20.24 (b)). At this point it is closely related to medial and lateral popliteal nerves, and the popliteal artery directly underlies the popliteal vein.*

*(b) The level of termination is variable; occasionally, it may enter the popliteal vein in its lower part, or, more commonly it terminates at a higher level than usual, well above the knee joint, illustrated here (and see Figure 1.5 (c)4). This may lead to ligation at too low a level, below branches which may form a renewed source of incompetence (see Figures 5.25 (a), (b), 5.26, 5.32 (b)).*

*(c) It is commonplace for the short saphenous vein to have an upward extension given off near the sapheno-popliteal junction (Figures 4.24, 5.8 (c)2, 5.9 (b) (right and left limb), 5.11(d). The size of this upward extension varies from a slender branch of no great significance, to a large vein which may have no competent valves and appears to be an upward continuation, rather than a branch, of the short saphenous vein. A large incompetent vein of this sort can easily act as a renewed source of incompetence even if it is interrupted by high ligation and stripping of the short saphenous vein below this level. It is this upward extension, so often unrecognized, that commonly causes an operation to be inadequately performed (Figure 10.5 (b), (c)).*
*The upward extension may take one of two courses, illustrated in (c)1 and c (2).*

*1. It may wind round the posterior thigh subcutaneously to its medial aspect where it joins the upper part of the long saphenous vein, often linking with its posteromedial branch. This can be an important pathway of incompetence taking origin in the long saphenous but transferring this to the short saphenous system. An occasional variant of this is a long channel running posteriorly up the thigh to join veins emerging from the pelvis via pudendal or gluteal veins.*
*2. The upward extension may continue as a large channel, deeply placed, and in direct continuity with profunda femoris vein. This is usually adequately valved but not necessarily so and can be a source of incompetence*

major cause for a component of 'deep vein' incompetence in the post-thrombotic syndrome. When an upward extension is present, even when it appears as a direct continuation of the saphenous, there is always a communication with the popliteal vein, corresponding with the usual sapheno-popliteal junction, but very variable in size and disposition. A large saccule (varix or venous aneurysm) is often present in this vicinity.

*The importance of phlebography for short saphenous surgery*

Because of the considerable variation in the level and mode of saphenopopliteal termination, and the real possibility of an upward extension, it is important to have precise information by phlebography or ultrasonography before surgery (Hobbs, 1980). The author's preference is to carry out phlebography a few days before the operation and this causes little disturbance to the patient. More than just anatomical outlining of the termination should be aimed at. Functional phlebography (see Chapter 22), which requires the active cooperation of the patient, should be carried out to determine the precise anatomy of the saphenopopliteal junction, the branches and the pathway of incompetence; if an upward extension is present this is followed to its termination so that, if necessary, it may be removed at surgery, for example, an incompetent posteromedial vein running to the upper long saphenous vein. This method is greatly to be preferred to a peroperative venogram carried out on the operating table, which provides only limited information and may not visualize important branches.

It is probable that future development of ultrasonography will supersede functional phlebography for this important examination (A. Nicolaides *et al.*, 1989). Whichever method is used, ultrasonography or phlebography, it is highly desirable that the surgeon should have a clear guide to the anatomy and function of the veins in this region before surgery is carried out.

*Aspects of technique in high ligation of the short saphenous vein* (Figures 20.16–20.17)

Although phlebography will have displayed the saphenous vein and its branches, it cannot give warning of unusual arrangements of major nerves and arteries. The medial popliteal nerve and its sural branch lie close to the saphenous termination and may actually embrace it. Other nerve variants are possible and the only safe rule is to keep close to the short saphenous vein, to displace neighbouring structures, and not divide anything more than trivial fibrous bands. The medial popliteal nerve may be encountered before the short saphenous vein and may be mistaken for it because it is similar in size and colour to a contracted saphenous vein empty of blood. The proximity of popliteal nerves and branches must never be forgotten and there should be no hesitation in consciously checking that the structure about to be divided is the saphenous vein and not a nerve. Distinguishing between the two will be helped by:

- Careful visual inspection will show that a nerve has a texture of longitudinally running fibres with a characteristic pattern of blood vessels; a saphenous vein in a contracted state will appear as a light grey structure of uniform texture and without the distinctive vascular markings.
- On gently feeling the structure between finger and thumb, a vein becomes a flat ribbon but a nerve is felt as a firm cord.
- In extremis, a small longitudinal incision, sufficient to enter a vein lumen, can be made to ensure that the structure is not made up of longitudinal bundles.
- A nerve stimulator, if available, would identify a motor nerve but only the most unusual circumstances would require this. The greatest safeguard is remembering this possible confusion and critical inspection should then quickly resolve any doubts.

(Sheppard (1986) described a condition of phlebectasia of nerves in the popliteal fossa, in which a sizeable vein may actually run into a plexus of small veins mingled with a major nerve. In these circumstances injury to the nerve could easily occur but this condition is rare and the author has only seen one possible case shown on phlebography.)

**Branches of the upper short saphenous vein – gastrocnemius veins** An upward extension from short saphenous to long saphenous or profunda femoris veins has already been

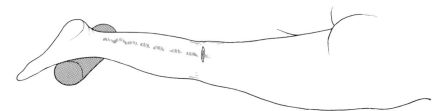

**Figure 20.16**    *The patient is positioned face down with the foot comfortably supported. The incision to the popliteal fossa will usually be transverse, close to the skin crease, but this must be varied if prior phlebography, or ultrasonography, show that a higher level will be required*

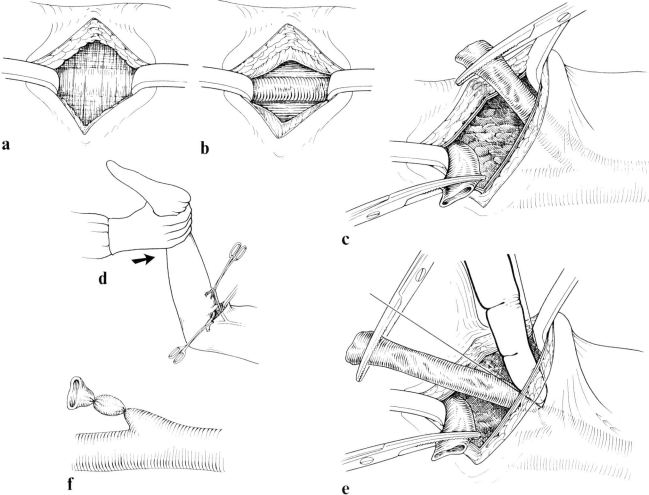

**Figure 20.17**    *Exposing the short saphenous vein.*

*(a)  The incision is deepened down to the deep fascia.*

*(b)  The fascia is incised transversely, in line with its fibres, to enter the popliteal fossa. If the incision has been properly centred, the saphenous vein is usually immediately apparent, lying directly beneath the deep fascia.*

*(c)  The vein is carefully dissected free from its surroundings and divided in order to facilitate further dissection. However this should only be done if the vein lies directly under the fascia and conforms exactly with the X-ray appearances; if the vein has only been located after deep dissection it should not be damaged in any way until its identity has been clarified by:*

- *Further dissection showing that it plunges deeply to join the underlying deep vein.*
- *That pulsation of the popliteal artery does not directly underlie it, but is remote.*
- *By following the vein downwards to check that the saphenous termination is not below this level (but phlebography should have given forewarning of this).*
- *By locating the saphenous vein in mid-calf and using the small end of a stripper as a probe passed up this to ensure direct continuity with the vein exposed in the fossa. This may also be used as a method for locating the short saphenous vein in obese patients when it is hard to find. However, it must be remembered that the 'probe' could have entered the popliteal vein by a termination low in the popliteal fossa (again, phlebography should have excluded this).*

*(d)  Following the short saphenous vein upwards, as it retreats more deeply into the popliteal fossa, is greatly helped by flexing the knee to a right angle, so that the incision moves upwards and the wound margins are slackened.*

*(e)  Dissection up to its termination in the popliteal vein proceeds with care, keeping close to the vein itself and brushing away surrounding fatty tissue rather than using sharp dissection.*

*(f)  Having freed the short saphenous vein up to its junction with the popliteal vein, ligation is carried out close to the deep vein and reinforced by a second ligature, preferably by transfixion distally. At this level a saccule beneath a valve may be encountered and will require careful separation from its surroundings. This final stage of the operation is not easy; appropriate retractors are essential and use of a strong headlight is invaluable. Haemorrhage, particularly from a ruptured saccule, may be very troublesome but can usually be controlled by packing with gauze for several minutes; this also gives time to think out an appropriate strategy before a renewed attempt is made to secure the bleeding point. Moreover, the bleeding may not be renewed once the pack is removed and such prompt natural haemostasis indicates that a difficult search for the torn vein deep in the popliteal fossa is probably unnecessary and it is best to accept this good fortune. Blind use of artery forceps must never be resorted to for fear of damaging major nerves in the vicinity. A skilfully used sucker is essential but this may lead to rapid, concealed loss of blood and the anaesthetist should be asked to keep a close watch on the amount accumulating in the sucker chamber!*

referred to above. One or more gastrocnemius veins commonly join the short saphenous vein. These may be quite large but are not necessarily abnormal or incompetent. Small veins may be ligated but a large one should not be automatically sacrificed. If phlebography has shown that it is likely to be heavily incompetent and perhaps with its lower end emerging as a perforator in mid-calf (see Chapter 11), then it should be ligated and divided. If there is no evidence of incompetence and it can be seen to run deeply into gastrocnemius muscle then it is reasonable to preserve this vein by ligating the saphenous vein below this level, and checking that there are no further branches above this that run superficially. This can be a difficult decision, best made from study of the phlebograms beforehand. The author has qualms about taking away a major channel of venous outflow from the muscle, particularly as some patients have undoubted calf pain, on walking, for some days after this, but it must be admitted that no lasting harm has been seen. It is another reason for gathering all possible information by phlebography before operation. A paper by Hobbs (1988) has an excellent discussion around this topic.

**Stripping short saphenous vein – care of sural nerve** (Figures 20.18, 20.20 (b))

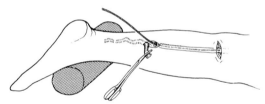

**Figure 20.18** *A syringe test is now carried out (Figure 20.11) to the downward portion of the short saphenous vein as a final check that this is the source of calf varicosities. The saphenous vein is then exposed at a lower level, either mid-calf or just above the ankle, and a stripper passed up from here much as described in the preceding section on long saphenous stripping. In the lower part, near to the ankle, the sural nerve is very close, and often adherent, to the short saphenous vein and particular care should be taken to identify this nerve and separate it before the vein is divided and stripping is carried out (Figure 20.20 (b)). Following stripping, the peripheral varicosities are removed by one of the methods described in the next section*

**Closing the popliteal fossa** The deep fascia behind the knee is a strong layer which should be closed by a few interrupted stitches. This will prevent fatty protrusion here and may play an important part in preventing recurrent varicosities by recanalization of haematoma (see Chapter 5, section on 'Recurrent varicose veins by anatomical routes or by re(neo)vascularization of saphenous stump'). The skin is closed by subcuticular stitch.

## Peripheral dissection of varicose veins

### Obtaining good cosmetic results

Undoubtedly appearance is important to the patient and so often the main reason for having surgical treatment. It is inherent in varicose vein surgery that great care must be taken to obtain the best cosmetic result, not only by complete elimination of varicosities, but also by ensuring that the surgical scars are as inconspicuous as possible. The following points will help to ensure this:

- The incisions should be parallel to the skin elasticity, Langer's lines, and suitable alignment of incisions is illustrated in Figure 20.19. In many parts of the limb this is not critical, but in the groin and behind the knee it is important to keep the incision close to and parallel to the skin creases.

- As far as is consistent with safe surgery, the incisions are kept as small as possible. At certain key points, such as exposing a saphenous termination, or where a large stripper head has to be admitted, an adequate incision has to be made. Where numerous small incisions to remove varicose veins (Rivlin, 1975) are required it is remarkable how well the vein can be removed through these and how inconspicuous the scars eventually become. With very small stab incisions the alignment matters little and often a vertical incision is convenient for access and gives an inconspicuous scar (Goren and Yellin, 1991).

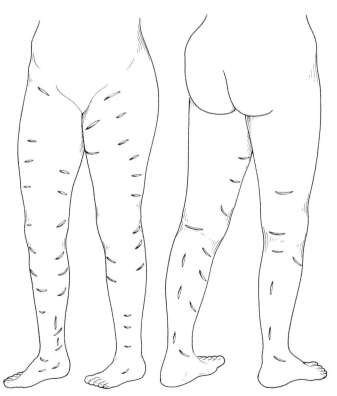

**Figure 20.19** *Alignment of incisions in the lower limbs, parallel with Langer's lines*

- Conventional interrupted stitching, across and encircling the skin edges, often gives a rim of necrosis under each stitch and should never be used; not only does this cause appreciable pain but it gives an ugly cross-hatching of stitch scars along the incision. Metal clips are no better and certainly the older designs cause pain, local necrosis and leave a permanent imprint. A subcuticular stitch (Figure 20.22 (b), (c)) is far superior but it should not be locked in any fashion; it is kept in place by only an adhesive covering so that it can yield before any oedema without cutting into the skin. With small stab incisions the edges can be drawn together by an adhesive strip without any stitch, but the author finds that a mini-subcuticular stitch, with only one bite on each side, gives a better result and is worth the brief time it takes for anything more than a minimal stab.
- Subcutaneous fat must not been removed or damaged because this may leave an ugly hollow, particularly on the inner and front aspect of the leg. Fat should be carefully preserved in the vicinity of the wound.
- There is much individual variation in the skin's healing and scar formation after an incision. Some patients are the surgeon's delight but others defeat the best of efforts, but nevertheless those in the latter category will be far less disappointing if good cosmetic principles have been followed.

*Avoiding damage to cutaneous nerves* (Figure 20.20)

Where it is known that an important cutaneous nerve is close to the vein an adequate size of incision must be used to ensure that the nerve is not damaged.

*Caution*

A number of sizeable branches of saphenous and musculocutaneous nerves run across the front of the ankle and are very vulnerable if avulsion of varicose veins through stab incisions is carried out here. If the varicose vein is not immediately apparent and cleanly delivered, there must be no blind groping with artery forceps in the hope of finding the vein because these nerves may be picked up instead. It is wiser to enlarge the incision so that the vein can be clearly seen and, fortunately, transverse incisions near the ankle give minimal scars.

**Techniques in removing varicose veins**

Branch veins leading down to varicosities are often long and straight so that a stripper can easily be passed up them and they should be dealt with by this means using a small-headed instrument. However, the varicosities themselves are often too tortuous to allow a stripper to be passed. The surgical technique used to remove these veins will vary according to their size and for descriptive purposes three grades are recognized here:

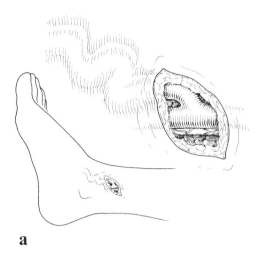

**a**

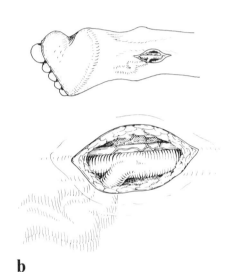

**b**

**Figure 20.20** *Avoiding damage to cutaneous nerves.*

*(a) The saphenous nerve runs parallel with the saphenous vein from knee level downwards (Figure 20.12 (a)), but near the ankle the two structures are in close proximity so that it is easy to pick up the nerve together with the vein and both are divided. This gives rise to an area of anaesthesia on the dorsum of the foot that worries the patient and should not be allowed to occur. If it is necessary to strip the long saphenous vein from ankle level, then great care must be taken to identify the nerve and gently separate it from the vein for as far as the incision allows. Only then should the vein be divided and a stripper inserted. Even so, it is possible for the stripper head to drag on the nerve or its branches and for this reason a small sized stripper head should be used at this level and stripping recommenced with a larger head in the upper calf.*

*(b) The sural nerve runs parallel and close to the short saphenous vein throughout its course but in the lower part, near the ankle, it is closely applied to it and easily lifted up with the vein. Damage to this nerve gives rise to extensive anaesthesia of the outer and lower aspects of the foot and is much resented by the patient. Moreover the sural nerve is quite large and, if divided, may develop a painful neuroma at its end, or, by traction along its length, develop an unpleasant and persistent neuritis. In the lower leg this nerve should always be positively identified and well separated from the vein before the vein is divided and stripped. Even in mid-calf care must be taken not to pick up this nerve*

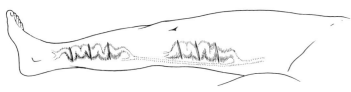

**a**

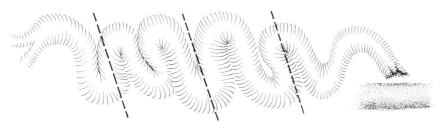

**b**

**Figure 20.21** *Removal of a cluster of massive varicosities.*

*(a), (b) The long saphenous vein has been stripped and two clusters of varicosities on the thigh and inner leg are to be removed. Over each cluster several parallel incisions, each 2–3 cm in length, are made.*

*(c) The underlying vein is often adherent to the skin and may require sharp dissection to free it. The vein is lifted up and unravelled by a combination of stretching with artery forceps and sharp dissection. The uppermost end of vein, detached when the saphenous vein was stripped, is delivered and dissection continued downwards by tunnelling under the skin towards the next incision.*

*(d) A similar process is followed at the next incision and at a suitable stage the vein is divided to facilitate dissection.*

*(e) The vein between each incision is freed by sharp dissection with scissors dividing the fibrous bands between vein and skin*

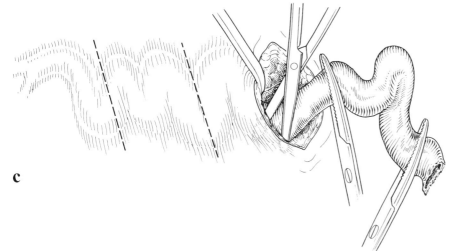

**c**

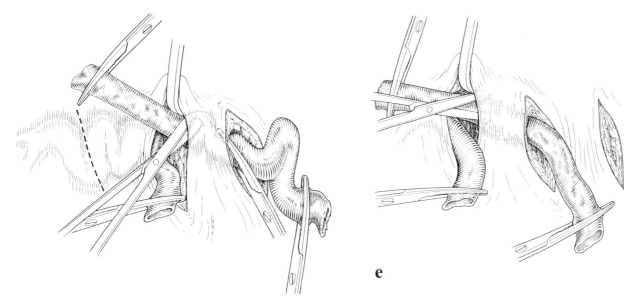

**e**

**d**

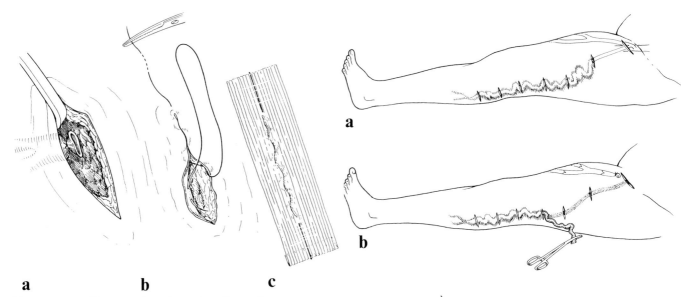

**Figure 20.22** *Haemostasis and suturing of wounds.*

*(a) The process is continued down to the lowest part of the varicose cluster and any vein continuing onwards from here is delivered as far as possible and, if it is large, ligated. Lesser veins may be avulsed and given a short period of pressure by the assistant whilst the surgeon continues to work nearby; this almost invariably gives good haemostasis.*

*(b) The incision is closed by a subcuticular stitch using monofilament, for example, Prolene.*

*(c) To complete closure, the stitch is pulled tight and an adhesive strip (Micropore or Steri-Strip) is laid over it along its length and including about 3 cm of the outstretched stitch at each end. It is useful to double over one end of the adhesive strip to act as a lifting tab when the stitch is removed*

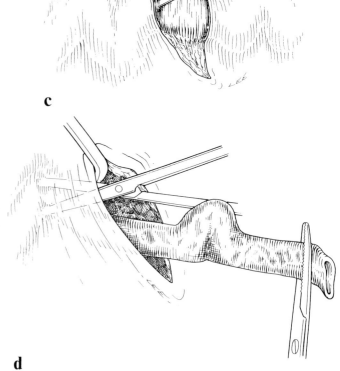

**Figure 20.23** *Removal of moderate-sized varicose veins running the length of the limb. When marking out the veins preoperatively, special marks should be made to indicate any divisions of the vein so that these key points are adequately removed.*

*(a), (b) An anterolateral branch of the long saphenous meandering down the front and outer aspect of the thigh and leg. This vein may be quite substantial, perhaps 1.0 cm across, and require more than stab incisions to remove it. A number of incisions are made across the vein at intervals, perhaps a hand's breadth apart, and each incision 0.5–1.0 cm in length (No. 15, Swan Morton blade).*

*(c), (d) At each incision the vein is exposed, lifted out and divided in order to facilitate further dissection. Each arm of the vein is followed by a combination of stretch and sharp dissection. At each tortuosity the vein is likely to be adherent to the skin and this will show by the vein resisting further delivery and the skin puckering at the point of adhesion. These adhesions can either be broken down by stretching with fine artery forceps or divided with round-ended scissors with their flat surface close to the undersurface of the skin. This process of multiple dissection of the varicosities is continued as far as necessary down the limb. It is often possible to get complete removal for its entire length*

1. Massive, clustered varicose veins, sometimes termed a 'bunch of grapes', are usually one continuous vein grotesquely coiled upon itself. These are best removed by a series of incisions perhaps 3 cm in length and placed reasonably close together so that the varicosities may be tunnelled out from one incision to the other (Figures 20.21, 20.22). A small series of parallel

incisions of this sort, closed with subcuticular stitches, gives a good cosmetic result and is less obvious than one long incision.

2. Moderate sized varicosities, more than 1 cm across when distended. These veins may prove too large for diminutive stab incisions, and then incisions 0.5–1.0 cm in length are made at intervals along the varicose vein (Figure 20.23). These larger incisions allow a greater length of vein to be removed reliably, so that they need not be placed quite so closely along the vein as with the stab technique. When closed with a subcuticular stitch the scar becomes insignificant within a few weeks.

3. Long meandering varicosities up to 1 cm in width when fully distended. These can usually be removed through a series of stab incisions, about 2–3 mm across, through which the varicose vein is extracted (Figure 20.24 (d)–(l)). At each stab incision the vein is coaxed out as far as possible and avulsed. This gives a series of interruptions in the vein but not necessarily a complete removal of its entire length. Nevertheless, if the incisions are placed every few centimetres along the vein it is unusual to find any vein that has survived and the cosmetic result with such small incisions is excellent.

**Figure 20.24**  *An example of the use of multiple stab incisions and avulsion of varicosities in a case of short saphenous vein incompetence.*

*(a)  General appearance of varicosities arising from the short saphenous vein and encircling the upper leg.*

*(b)  1–2. The preoperative phlebograms for this patient showing the termination of the short saphenous vein and the varicose vein encircling the upper leg to join the long saphenous vein. Both functional phlebography and Doppler flowmetry showed that the flow pattern after exercise was down the short saphenous vein, into the varicose vein, round the outer leg and across the front to flow down the long saphenous vein before dispersing by various perforators into the deep veins of the leg.*

*(c)  1–3. Preoperative marking. The intended incision over the popliteal fossa is shown together with marking of the short saphenous vein, palpable in the upper calf; a saccule easily felt in its upper part is noted. The varicosities arising from this vein extend round the outer side and front of the leg to join the long saphenous vein. (Compare these markings with the phlebogram.)*

*(d)  At a late stage in the operation, after the short saphenous vein has been ligated flush with the popliteal vein and stripped to mid-calf and on to near-ankle level. Two calf incisions to expose the saphenous vein have been sutured by subcuticular stitches and can be seen in the background. Removal of the varicosity is proceeding by multiple stab incisions and dissection-avulsions. The vein held in the artery forceps has just been delivered.*

*(e)  The portion of vein displayed between artery forceps has been removed from the interval between the incision and the track of stripped saphenous vein. The knife (No. 15, Swan Morton scapel blade) is poised to make a further stab incision to remove the next section of vein.*

*(f)  Incision being made immediately alongside skin marking of vein.*

*(g)  The vein has been picked up with fine mosquito forceps and will be freed sufficiently to divide it so that the upper portion can be coaxed out.*

*(h)  The upper portion of vein has been further freed of any attachments by gently stretching and teasing with the points of artery forceps and is being progressively delivered.*

*(i)  The complete run of vein has now been freed back to the previous incision and is being drawn out of the lower incision. This process is continued from one incision to the next until all*

*the varicose vein has been removed. Where necessary, if the far end is not accessible, the vein is avulsed with artery forceps placed as far down it as possible. Haemostasis is achieved by a short period of pressure through folded gauze.*
*(j)  The skin is closed by adhesive strips (Steri-Strip or sterilized Micropore). In the background, the stitches of the mid-calf incisions have been drawn taut and kept in place by adhesive strips. One of the stab incisions is being closed with adhesive strip alone, without any stitch. The strip has been stuck to one side of the incision and is being drawn forward to close the skin edges.*
*(k)  When skin edges are together the adhesive strip is smoothed into position. The eventual scar is always least conspicuous when the skin edges are brought together rather than left open.*
*(l)  A further adhesive strip being laid into position. All the stab incisions are closed this way, right round the leg*

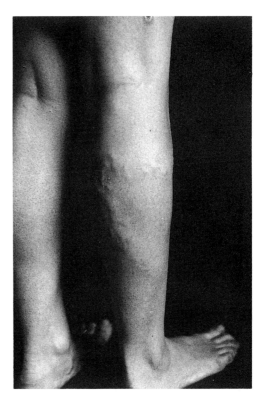

**a**

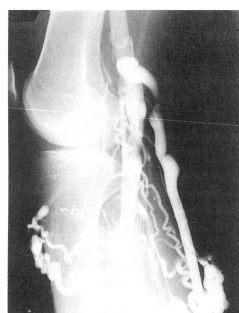
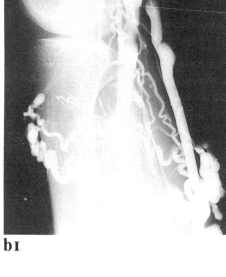

**b1**

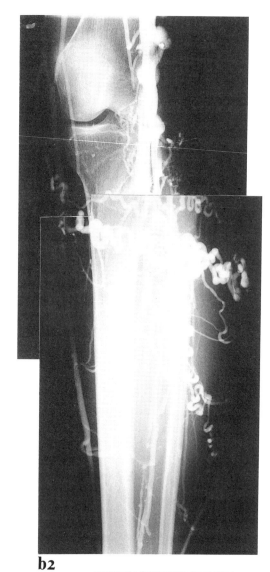

**b2**

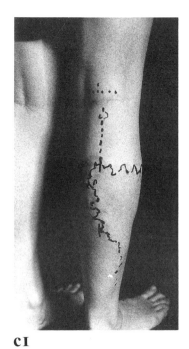

**c1**

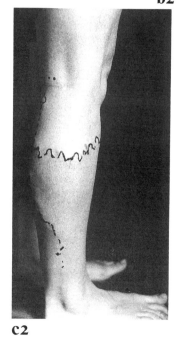

**c2**

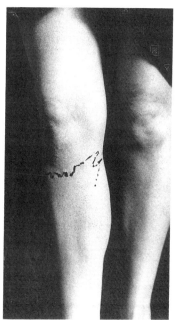

**c3**

**Figure 20.24** *(continued)*

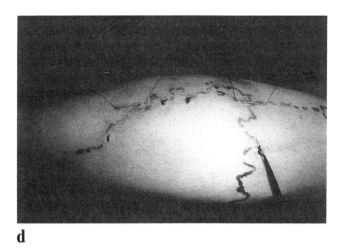

**d**

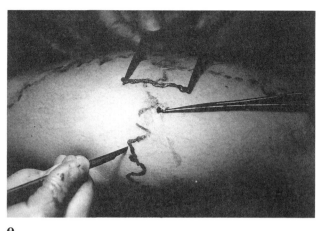

**e**

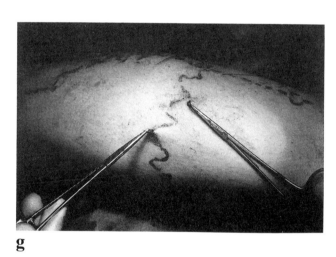

**f**

**g**

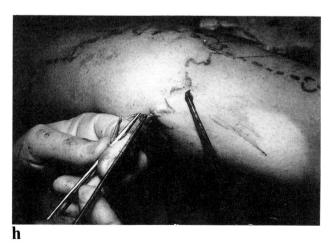

**h**

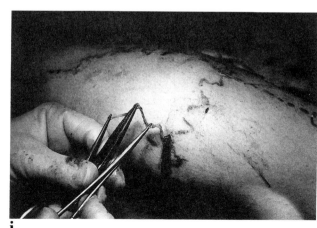

**i**

**Figure 20.24** *(continued)*

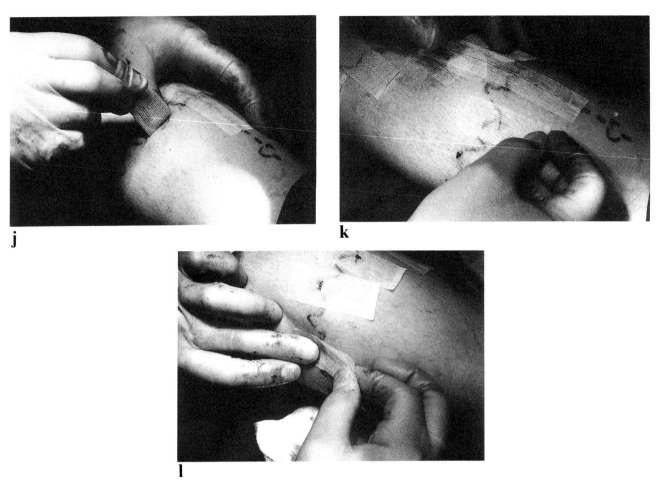

**Figure 20.24** *(continued)*

## Surgery for recurrent varicose veins

Surgery for varicose veins that recur after long or short saphenous vein ligation, with or without stripping, presents two particular difficulties:

1. *Identifying the source.* This is discussed in Chapter 5 and it is essential to distinguish between, persisting varicose veins due to incorrect identification of the source, and varicosities recurring a year or two after initially successful surgery. Locating the source of a recurrence, that is to say, the point of outflow from deep veins to the surface, will depend upon careful clinical and Doppler flowmeter examination, and its demonstration by phlebography. It commonly arises from important branches at the termination of the saphenous vein that have survived previous surgery, or by revascularization of a saphenous stump (see Chapter 5). Functional and upward trace phlebography is an essential preliminary to surgery for recurrent veins.

2. *Approaching a source through the scar tissue created by previous surgery.* In the description that follows it will be assumed that the recurrent source is the commonest variety, in the groin or popliteal fossa, after long or short saphenous surgery. Invariably the previous surgery leaves scar tissue leading down to the original ligation. Fatty tissue will no longer brush aside and will require sharp dissection in order to gain access.

Usually, large coiled varices, running from the renewed source, lie in amongst the scar tissue and closely adherent to it. Lymphatic channels are also caught in scar tissue and easily divided to cause subsequent lymph collection or fistula. The varicosities have very fragile walls and following them can be difficult, with the field repeatedly obscured by blood. Approaching the underlying deep vein through this puts it in hazard, since this vein cannot be felt and is all too easily damaged. Nevertheless, careful use of fine, round-ended scissors, dividing numerous fibrous strands, retracting and compressing any bleeding points through gauze, will often allow the surgeon to traverse the scar tissue and glimpse the strong walls of a saphenous stump or the deep vein. Once this stage has been reached these structures can be followed by dissection with the scissors to outline the full anatomy. However, there is no doubt that this procedure can be difficult, with some danger, and is only suitable for an experienced surgeon. It must be emphasized again that the surgeon will depend upon phlebograms obtained beforehand clearly outlining the saphenous stump, the veins arising from it and the deep vein itself, This examination will require the patient's cooperation and is best done, as an outpatient, a day or two before operation. Assuming this essential information is available, the policy illustrated in Figure 20.25 is suggested for surgery to a recurrent source in a long saphenous stump. A set of vascular instruments, suitable for repair of veins, including small, narrow-bladed vascular clamps and fine gauge suture material such as Prolene 7-0 gauge, can be invaluable and must be immediately available.

**Injury to the deep vein** The common femoral vein cannot be felt but only recognized visually by its appearance, so often confused by overlying fibrous tissue, or by heavy bleeding if it is breached, and injury to it is a real possibility for which the surgeon must be fully prepared; as stated above, a set of vascular instruments, suitable for

repair of injury to the femoral vein, should be immediately available. The following points may prove helpful:

- Venous bleeding is at low pressure, easily controlled by light pressure. A single finger over a venous bleeding point can usually control it whilst dissection proceeds alongside.
- Sharp dissection with curved scissors, with the tissues gently stretched and the flat of the blades against the vein wall, is effective and least likely to enter the vein.
- Use of suction to define the point of bleeding may lead to heavy, concealed blood loss, directly into the sucker. Nevertheless, at certain stages the sucker can be essential, but it must be raised repeatedly to judge the rapidity with which blood is coming, and the anaesthetist must be asked to give warning if the suction chamber fills with blood.

**Figure 20.25** *Recurrent varicose veins: locating a long saphenous stump through scar of a previous operation.*
*(a) An incision is made parallel with the skin crease and over the saphenous stump as described earlier in this chapter. This is deepened and any large veins are followed. When more room is required an incision into the scar tissue is made in the long axis of the limb to minimize damage to lymphatics. Not infrequently, the varicosities can be followed without undue difficulty to the saphenous stump which is then dissected free. The underlying deep vein is displayed sufficiently to make sure that any surviving branch vein of the saphenous termination is recognized. The sapheous stump is then double ligated in the usual way flush with the deep vein and above any branches.*

*(b) If this approach proves too difficult and is defeated by repeated haemorrhage from varicosities, it is best to locate the common femoral artery by its pulsation and redirect the approach towards this, again obtaining adequate room by incising scar tissue in the axis of the limb. This will soon enter a plane free of scar tissue and when the front of the femoral artery has been exposed, the overlying structures are lifted up and dissection directed medially, deliberately to expose the common femoral vein. The anterior surface of this is then shown sufficiently to see the saphenous stump which is then progressively freed. This may be doubly ligated, or clamped with a narrow-bladed vascular clamp and closed with a continuous suture of 7-0 gauge Prolene. Once this vessel is controlled there should be no undue problems in removing the overlying varicosities. Haemostasis at the end of the operation must be meticulous, since otherwise postoperative haematoma is likely. The author recommends this approach for any surgeon who is uncertain how best to proceed.*

*(c) An alternative approach, which can be adopted from the outset, is to expose the inguinal ligament and find the common femoral vein just below this, so that it is approached without having to cross the troublesome scar tissue and varices; it does not, however, eliminate the possibility of creating a lymph fistula. The superficial tissues are lifted up to allow the vein to be followed down until the saphenous termination is reached. This approach is favoured by many surgeons but there is great variation in the circumstances encountered whatever approach is used and the importance of reconnaissance by phlebography is again emphasized*

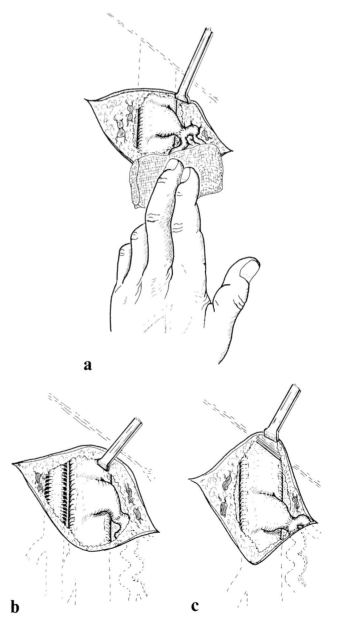

a

b          c

- Allis' forceps can be invaluable for temporarily sealing an aperture in fibrotic vein wall whilst a new plane of dissection is found.
- The vein wall is progressively exposed until it is possible to apply a vascular side clamp that isolates the bleeding point and allows it to be sutured with 7-0 Prolene (Figure 20.26).

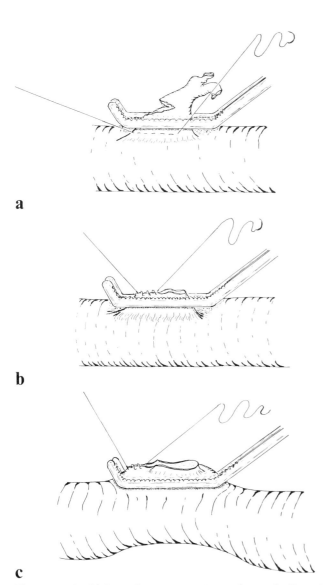

**a**

**b**

**c**

**Figure 20.26** *If the saphenous stump is too short to be ligated a vascular clamp can be applied in the following ways:*

*(a) Close to the base of the stump, so that a stitch can be applied back and forth beneath the clamp.*

*(b) At the base, with the suture used to close the remnant of the stump protruding above the clamp.*

*(c) To include the neighbouring portion of the deep vein if it has been injured or a tear in the stump has extended into it. In this way the deep vein need not be occluded and a continuous suture of 7 × 0 monofilament is used to repair the defect and close the stump without any narrowing or deformity of the femoral vein. It is of course essential that this vein is preserved intact*

In spite of the setbacks just given the common femoral vein and saphenous stump should be adequately exposed so that, at the finish, there is no doubt that the saphenous stump and its branches have been completely removed. In all probability there will be no better opportunity to succeed than the present one and the attempt should not be abandoned without good cause.

In closing the wound the scar tissue is brought together by a few interrupted sutures and the skin closed as usual by a subcuticular stitch. Open drainage should not be used for fear of introducing infection. The majority of wounds after re-exploration of the groin heal well without any form of drainage, but closed suction drainage with a fine bore tube would seem reasonable if the surgeon is particularly uneasy. This will not, however, prevent haematoma and must not be used as a substitute for good haemostasis, with all vein ends ligated.

*Recurrence from the short saphenous vein*

Similar principles to those just described apply and in the case of the short saphenous vein it must be stated that it would be folly to tackle recurrence here without phlebograms displaying precisely the nature and the position of the recurrence (Figures 5.21 (b), (c), 5.25, 5.26, 5.28 (b)1, 5.32(a), (b)). The approach to a short saphenous stump has more formidable difficulties than the long saphenous operation because of the major nerves that overlie the vein (lateral and medial popliteal and sural nerves) and the fact that the important landmark of the popliteal artery lies under the vein rather than alongside it. Fortunately there is usually a moderately substantial vein leading down to the saphenous stump and, with care, this can be followed satisfactorily. Dissection must keep very close to the vein and the surgeon must not be deterred by one or two episodes of breaching this vein on the way. The skin incision is, of course, placed at an appropriate level according to the phlebogram. A transverse incision through the skin and fascia is best, with an adequate exposure of the fossa; if necessary the popliteal and sural nerves should be deliberately displayed. The saphenous stump is ligated at high level, close to the popliteal vein, and all branches disconnected. An upward extension of the saphenous vein is often present, and will have been shown on the phlebograms; if there is no doubt that this vein runs subcutaneously to join the long saphenous vein a stripper may be passed up it to the upper thigh so that it may be removed.

*Caution*: Interconnection between superficial and deep vein make it possible for a stripper to enter the deep veins and its passage upwards should be checked visually, as a ripple under the skin, and by palpation, to be certain that it is lying subcutaneously; when its upper end is located, the vein in which it is lying must be checked most carefully to confirm that it is a superficial vein before it is opened and stripped!

A deep extension to profunda femoris vein will usually be ligated at the highest practical level, according to phlebogram appearances. Any remnants of long or short saphenous vein and recurrent varicosities running down the limb should not present any undue difficulty and are removed in the usual way.

## Lymph collection and lymph fistula after dissection in the groin

Re-exploration through scar tissue in the groin is particularly prone to divide lymphatic channels and cause either a collection of lymph or a lymph fistula. A lymph collection usually becomes evident in the second or third week as an indurated swelling causing some discomfort. If this is fluctuant it is best aspirated with a needle to confirm the diagnosis of seroma or lymph fluid and, as a precaution, a sample should be sent for microscopy and culture. The swelling is emptied as far as possible and the needle withdrawn. It is likely that the swelling will reappear within a few days and at this stage it is best left to absorb spontaneously. This may take several weeks but is better than trying any drainage procedure that may convert it into a fistula.

A lymph fistula may become evident within the first few weeks after operation, perhaps preceeded by discomfort, swelling and induration. The fistula will then continue day after day as a source of embarrassment to the patient, releasing up to half a litre of fluid each day. The author has experienced three such cases and all were cured by application of a lymph fistula sponge (Figure 20.27). Avoiding this unpleasant complication is important and extensive transverse incisions through scar tissue in the groin must not be used. As stated above the skin incision should be oblique and the underlying tissues opened in the long axis of the limb, parallel with lymphatics, as far as possible. If lymphatic glands are exposed it is permissible to transect them if this appears to offer least damage to lymphatic channels.

## Choice of instrument used for stripping superficial veins

The instrument used for stripping incompetent superficial veins, such as the saphenous vein, was evolved in the early part of this century and many versions are available. A saphenous vein may be stripped by two basic methods:

### Extraluminal stripping

This entails passing a ring outside the vein and along its length so that all its branches are disconnected either by a cutting edge or avulsion according to the configuration of the ring. The stripper most widely used in the early part of this century was the Mayo (1906) stripper which was essentially a ring on the end of a slender rod.

### Intraluminal stripping

This was first described by Keller (1905) using a wire passed up the vein and inverting it as it was stripped. Another early version of this was the Babcock stripper (1907) which consisted of a slender rod, rounded into a probe at one end and expanded into a small head at the other. The rod was passed up the lumen of the vein and a ligature passed around the vein to fix it to the stripper rod, near the head. When the rod was pulled upon the vein was progressively inverted and its branches snapped off in turn as the stripper moved along. The next stage in the development of the stripper was to replace the inflexible rod with a flexible cable and to use a larger head designed to prevent inversion of the vein; this was introduced by Myers (1957), whose stripper became widely used and is still perhaps the most popular version today. In essence, its stem is a strong, stranded cable or piano wire, with a small, rounded probe at one end, which is used to introduce it along the vein. At the other end there is a substantial head that does not enter the vein lumen and against which the vein is bunched as stripping proceeds. A ligature is placed around the vein, just beneath the head to prevent it from sliding up the lumen; even so, with a large vein, it can invert the vein, as with the older Babcock stripper, and then the vein may break so that stripping is incomplete. The flexible wire can be any length but is usually about 70 cm so that it can reach from ankle to groin if required. It is made in a range of head sizes and lengths of stem. Many variants of the Myers stripper have been suggested:

- The probe and head are attached by a screw fitting so that different sizes of head can be attached, or the head and probe ends can be interchanged after introduction of the stripper, to give a choice of direction in stripping. The same screw attachment can be used to fix on a toggle-shaped handle to provide an easy means for pulling on the stripper.
- The head may have various shapes and may include a ring to which a long thread can be attached that trails up the track left by stripping the vein. This can then be used, in certain circumstances, to draw the head back, through the original incision of entry, rather than make a 2 cm incision for it to emerge, for example, when stripping from groin down to upper calf. It can also be used to reposition the head at any level if the vein has invaginated and snapped so that stripping is incomplete.

### Intraluminal stripping by invagination

With this technique, as with the original Babcock technique, a small head is used and tied into place in the same fashion. Due to its small size and shape it slips into the lumen, progressively inverting the vein, rather like a coat sleeve being turned inside out. The advantage is that it

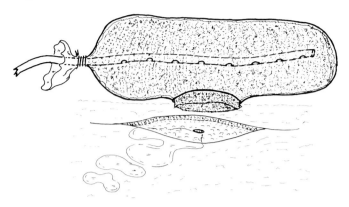

**a**

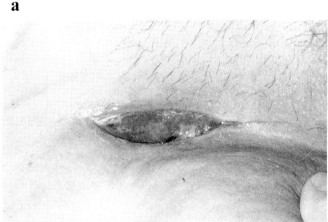

**b**

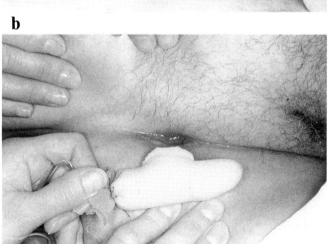

**c**

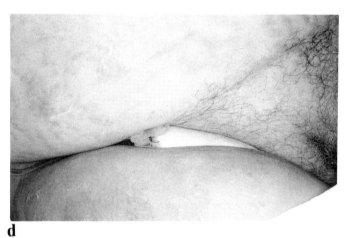

**d**

**Figure 20.27**

*(a) Lymph fistula suction sponge. This sponge is a small block of plastic sponge material and its apertures must interconnect so that it is highly absorptive (some materials are not). It is enclosed in an impervious sheath with a 2 cm opening on its undersurface and running through its centre is a perforated tube to which continuous suction is applied. The opening of the sponge is placed over the fistula opening so that the fluid is soaked up by capillary action into the sponge, but as soon as it collects there it is sucked away by the suction tube. This not only keeps the patient dry but, if well applied, sucks the fistulous track flat so that it is able to contract down and eventually close off. This principle is invaluable for any lymph fistula following surgery, particularly of the thoracic duct following exploration of the supraclavicular fossa. The diagram corresponds with the improvised suction sponge used in (b)–(d), but its shape and size will be varied according to the cavity and body contour it is to overlie.*

*(b), (c) Lymph fistula suction sponge in use. (b) An unhealed groin incision in a patient with a lymph fistula continuously discharging 3 weeks after surgery for recurrent saphenous incompetence.*

*(c), (d) A fistula sponge improvised from a rubber glove finger and shaped to fit into the fold of groin. With continuous suction this kept the patient completely dry, and after 3 days the fistula had ceased to discharge and did not recur*

is most unlikely to damage the saphenous nerve or its branches in the lower leg where it is most vulnerable. A drawback is that the inverted vein may snap, particularly where it is joined by a major branch that proves stronger than the saphenous vein itself. For this reason a trailing thread attached to the head is used, following up the track. If the vein should break it is then easy to reposition the head so that it may be exposed through a small incision and the unstripped vein tied back to the instrument so that stripping can be completed (van der Stricht, 1963).

*Combined extraluminal and intraluminal stripping*

Many most ingenious strippers have been designed to improve the effectiveness, and the series of instruments suggested by Umansky (1977) are representative of this category, including an extraluminal stripper that can be used to remove retained vein when the vein has broken during intraluminal stripping.

Various papers by K. Loftgren (1958, 1978) describe the evolution of the stripper, in which the Mayo Clinic played such a prominent part. The flexible Myers' stripper remains the most popular basic design. Many small variations are available, for example, there is a version in nylon, with a corkscrew probe end to facilitate passage through irregularities in the vein, with a range of detachable heads in different sizes. Nevertheless, the surgeon's skill of application is more important than the precise details of design and the essential features of a good stripper are:

- A flexible stem of adequate length and strength for its purpose, with a rounded probe end for passing along the vein.
- A head of sufficient size to prevent easy invagination of the vein; it is an advantage if the stripper head is detachable so that an appropriate size may be chosen for the particular vein to be stripped. The alternative is to have a set of, say, three or four strippers, each with a different size of head. In addition a small-headed, short length stripper is very useful for lesser veins.

Strippers of stranded or piano-wire cable require care and should not be wound round the hand to gain purchase when pulling strongly upon, because this will put a permanent kink in the wire. With such usage the stripper soon becomes deformed and difficult to steer past irregularities in the vein. Gripping between forefinger and thumb of both hands is usually sufficient and if resistance is offered by a particularly strong branch the assistant is asked to join in by giving a controlled pull in similar fashion. Sudden force should never be used and often a strong branch vein resisting the stripper will yield if given a steady, firm pull over 30 seconds rather than resorting to a violent jerk.

*Dangerous errors when stripping a vein*

It is possible for a stripper to pass from the saphenous vein into the deep vein and to be located here in mistake for the superficial vein, with disasterous consequences. Even worse is the entry of a stripper into an artery, for example, the posterior tibial, and passed up this to be located in the femoral artery in the groin. Several cases have been recorded, where the arterial tree has been stripped in this way by inexperienced surgeons (Cockett, 1986). Errors of this magnitude are hard to imagine but they have actually occurred and must be recognized as a possible danger. Surgery involving high ligation and stripping of a saphenous vein has some very serious potential dangers if the person operating has not had adequate training.

*Is use of a tourniquet permissible?*

From time to time papers appear giving the advantages of using an exsanguinating tourniquet during varicose vein surgery in order to minimize blood loss (Farrands

*et al.*, 1987; Corbett and Jayakumar, 1989). No doubt a number of surgeons do employ this but one's instinct is strongly against the use of a potential hazard without considerably more justification than avoiding a small inconvenience to the surgeon and the loss of perhaps 100 ml of blood. The blood loss should not ordinarily be greater than this and, if it is, perhaps the surgeon should reappraise his technique or even consider elevating the limb during surgery to eliminate venous pressure and bleeding from the veins (Lawrie, 1960). Admittedly harm from use of a tourniquet in surgery to the superficial veins has not been reported but at least a possible danger is referred to by exponents of this method (McDonald *et al.*, 1989), who point out that cyanotic toes may be observed 1–2 hours after operation. They state 'As the leg has been exsanguinated, normal bandaging leads to excessive pressure when the tourniquet is removed' and that the nurses should be instructed to loosen the bandage if cyanosis is seen. This comes as a reminder that use of a tourniquet requires special care and there must be considerable reserve about its use in this fashion (Klenerman, 1982; Fletcher and Healy, 1983). We do not recommend it.

## Surgery for perforating veins

It has already been explained in Chapter 11 that there are several different categories of perforating veins, communicating between superficial and deep veins, that take part in venous disorders, each requiring individual thought. Some are primarily at fault but most are incidentally involved. There is no single policy that is suitable for all of them and even when one is known to have valvular incompetence, that is, allowing substantial outward flow from deep to superficial veins, its removal may not be appropriate.

The 'incompetent perforator' is frequently invoked as an explanation for severe venotensive change and ulceration, but often a concealed superficial vein incompetence is being overlooked and the primary fault is not in the perforator. If incompetence in perforators is present, it may be a secondary consequence of deep vein obstruction and, although an aggravating factor, is also a compensatory mechanism not to be interfered with lightly. The diagnosis of 'incompetent perforator' should never be made without detailed understanding of the individual problem.

### Indications and contraindications for surgery to incompetent perforating veins

Numerous perforating veins are widely present over the lower limbs. This is the normal state and there is nothing to be gained in removing such veins unless they are demonstrably incompetent. An incompetent perforator may be suspected if there is an enlarged vein at one of the sites where this is known to occur (see Chapter 11), but this is not easy to confirm. A hollow palpated in an elevated limb is often incorrectly interpreted as a deficiency in the deep fascia through which an enlarged perforator emerges when, in fact, it is no more than the space occupied by a large varicosity. A directional Doppler flowmeter over a suspicious varix, or an enlarged vein leading to it, may give useful evidence of substantial outflow emerging to the surface, but by far the best evidence is given by functional phlebography which can display a perforator and give a good understanding of the role it is playing. A perforating vein may be enlarged for one of several reasons:

1. Because flow in the normal inward direction is greatly increased by incompetent superficial veins above it.
2. Because it is the source of superficial vein incompetence and is providing heavy downflow to the varicosities beneath it.
3. Because there is surge back and forth within it with each calf muscle contraction; this occurs when gross incompetence of superficial veins is combined with a weak set of deep vein valves (see Chapter 7). The valveless syndrome is a more extreme form and produces the same effect but more severely.
4. Because it is carrying heavy outward and upward flow as part of a collateral mechanism compensating for deep vein obstruction.

### Enlarged perforating veins in simple incompetence of superficial veins

It is commonplace to find one or more perforating veins considerably enlarged below incompetence in long or short saphenous systems as a response to the heavy downflow they are transmitting inwards to the deep veins of the leg. Here they are not acting as a source of incompetence but are handling the consequences of incompetence in superficial veins above this level; they are not primarily at fault. Nevertheless, such enlargement may have caused the valves guarding the veins to become incompetent and a possible source for renewed varicosities to the foot. For this reason, if detected, an enlarged perforator should be removed through a small incision when the peripheral varicose veins are dissected or stripped. However, this is not a primary objective in the usual case of varicose veins.

In more severe cases, an obvious element of perforator outflow may be detected by Doppler flowmeter examination. The predominant flow is inward and follows muscular contraction, but there is a short phase of outward flow during actual contraction or when the foot is put down. In this case the superficial veins show significant surge of blood when examined during exercise by Doppler flowmetry or functional phlebography. This

is seen in extreme form in the valveless syndrome (see Chapter 7 and below). To this extent one or more perforators is incompetent and when detected, it is best removed as part of the general procedure, to make sure that it does not survive as a source of renewed downflow to the foot. Such veins are commonly removed or disconnected incidentally during peripheral dissection of varicosities but if approached individually should not require any more than a small incision, at most 1–2 cm in length.

### Valveless syndrome

In Chapter 7 a valveless state in superficial and deep veins was described and attributed to an inborn weakness or deficiency of valves. Similarly a syndrome of weak veins was referred to, in which failure of valves readily occurs because of inadequate strength in the vein walls and at the valve rings. These two groups are not clearly defined and merge with patterns of superficial incompetence combined with poorly valved deep veins at the far end of the spectrum of valve deficiency (see Chapter 7). If functional phlebography confirms that the deep veins are widely open, then surgery to the superficial veins and enlarged perforating veins may bring some benefit without any likelihood of causing harm. However, it may prove disappointing and the patient's expectations should not be raised too far. Conservative management by a policy of elevation whenever possible and the use of strong, graduated, one-way-stretch elastic stockings, up to the knee, may be best.

## Perforating veins as a primary source of superficial vein incompetence

### Perforators from venous sinuses in the calf muscles (gastrocnemius and soleal perforating veins)

Venous sinuses within muscle, such as those in the gastrocnemius and soleal muscles, commonly communicate with the superficial veins and normally accept intermittent flow from them. Occasionally, one or more of these perforators becomes incompetent so that blood flows out to the superficial veins. Although this may be suspected clinically, it can only be satisfactorily proved by functional phlebography or ultrasonography. During phlebography it is commonplace to see inflow from surface veins into the musculovenous sinuses as a normal phenomemon and in order to diagnose incompetence it is necessary to see a phase of outflow from a venous sinus to the overlying varicose veins during or after contraction of the muscle (see Chapter 11). A connection of this sort is often removed incidentally when clearing away varicose veins but if its presence is known beforehand then an adequate incision should be made to ensure that it can found without difficulty. Another way of meeting the problem of the incompetent gastrocnemius venous sinus is to ligate the corresponding gastrocnemius vein in the popliteal fossa.

**Ligation of a gastrocnemius vein** This has been discussed ealier in this chapter from the standpoint of decisions to be made during short saphenous high ligation. If suitable functional phlebography or Duplex ultrasonography have shown undoubted incompetence in a major gastrocnemius vein, allowing reflux back into one or more venous sinuses and out through incompetent gastrocnemius perforators, then ligation of this vein may bring overall benefit to the limb (Hobbs, 1988). Ligation of this vein can cause a period of venous claudication but usually this subsides. There are few comprehensive reports of this procedure and it should be used with caution until more detailed experience and long term follow-up are available and have clarified its role. A minimal requirement should be functional phlebography showing strong downflow from popliteal or saphenous vein through an enlarged, 'baggy' gastrocnemius vein and sinus, with no functioning valves, and out via an incompetent perforator to overlying superficial varices.

*Mid-thigh perforators causing recurrent varicose veins*

Renewed incompetence after surgery to the long saphenous system may arise from a mid-thigh perforating vein communicating with femoral or profunda femoris veins. Again, functional phlebography and varicography is the most reliable way to demonstrate this. In the thigh, direct connection between a perforator and the long saphenous vein is usual and a recurrence taking source from this is most likely when the long saphenous vein has not been stripped adequately or a double long saphenous vein has had only one portion removed. An advantage of stripping the long saphenous vein is that it usually eliminates the mid-thigh perforator as a possible source of recurrence. By contrast, below the knee, the perforators on the inner aspect of the leg usually join the posterior arch (arcuate) vein and are not disconnected when the long saphenous alone is stripped. Enlarged perforating veins below the knee are an occasional cause for varicosities persisting in the lower leg and on the foot, but undetected incompetence in the short saphenous system is a more likely source.

*Perforators from a saphenous stump causing recurrent varicose veins*

A special example of a perforator source to recurrent varicose veins may arise from a stump of long or short saphenous vein, due to inadequate surgery or revascularization of the stump creating, in effect, a substantial perforator which connects with remnants of the incompetent saphenous system. Again, functional phlebography and varicography is the most reliable way of identifying this with certainty. The particular problems of operating to remove this form of recurrence have been discussed earlier in this chapter.

*Technique of removing enlarged perforating veins*

On the inner side of the leg near the ankle a perforating vein is exposed by a small incision; it is often obscured by sizeable varicosities connecting with it and these should be dissected free and removed as far as the incision allows. During the course of this the perforator is found 'anchoring' the varicosities and running down to its fascial aperture. It is gently lifted up so that it may be followed through the aperture. Care is required because it leads down to tibial veins, artery and nerve which may be exposed with surprising ease. It should be ligated close to the underlying deep veins and divided.

In other situations, for example, a gastrocnemius perforator, the vein runs into a venous sinus without any underlying artery or nerve and it should be delivered as far as possible and ligated as deeply as the exposure will allow.

If the deep fascia has been divided this should be restored with a few interrupted sutures but otherwise it is not usually possible to close a fascial aperture satisfactorily and, fortunately, this does not seem necessary.

*Incompetent perforators in post-thrombotic (postphlebitic) syndrome*

Obstructed or severely deformed deep veins following thrombosis will be associated with collateral outflow to the surface veins. Usually this is from multiple small perforating veins which are not individually detectable. However, one or more perforators may become grossly enlarged so that it is obvious on clinical examination or clearly seen on phlebography. These veins are likely to be providing a valuable collateral pathway, compensating for the loss of deep veins and their removal may not bring benefit to the limb but cause harm. If there is any history of previous deep vein thrombosis, or of circumstances that may have caused this, such as a major fracture, and especially if a Doppler flowmeter shows continuous upflow in superficial veins, accentuated by exercise, then it is essential to evaluate the venous state by functional phlebography. If this confirms the collateral role of the perforator then surgery is contraindicated unless most careful assessment has shown otherwise. As an example of this, sometimes a particular perforator carries such forceful flow that it gives severe venous hypertension in its immediate vicinity. Removal of this vein may redirect collateral flow elsewhere to give a more favourable distribution of venous pressure and so bring relief to the worst affected area. Proof of the possible benefits to be gained in removing such a vein may be obtained by plethysmography showing an improved response to exercise when the perforator indentified by phlebography is temporarily occluded by localized pressure with finger or thumb (not an encircling band). In this case, removal of the perforator through a small incision is justified, but it would be most unwise also to carry out extensive removal of superficial veins, such as the saphenous vein, without knowing what other means of collateral return were available to the limb. There is no set rule here and each case must be assessed individually and the importance of the superficial veins in collateral flow clearly understood. A sapheous vein, shown by phlebography to be well valved, should never be removed; its contribution can only be beneficial.

## Procedures locating incompetent perforating veins by surgical exploration through a long incision in the leg

In the treatment of venous ulceration, various procedures have been advocated by Linton (1938), Cockett & Elgan Jones (1953), Cocket (1955), Dodd & Cockett (1976), Dodd (1964), Negus and Friedgood (1983) and Negus (1985) to locate incompetent perforators by extrafascial

**Figure 20.28**

*(a) Linton's incision through the deep fascia, with exploration beneath it, is shown here. Raising up the deep fascia allows any enlarged perforators emerging alongside the tibia to be easily seen and appropriately removed; the accompanying artery should be preserved if possible. Cockett advised extrafascial dissection and this is suitable for a more limited exposure. Extensive subcutaneous exposure may lead to necrosis of skin edges and Cockett emphasized that the perforators in the lower leg connect with the posterior arch (arcuate) vein and the incision should be positioned in a straight line over this in order to minimize undercutting the skin.*

*(b) As an alternative, a long incision on the posterior calf and lower leg, deepened through the fascia, has been recommended by Dodd (1964) and Negus (1985). The deep fascia can be raised extensively to expose the perforating veins beneath it and this has the advantage of allowing perforating veins to be seen on the posterior aspect of the calf as well as those on the medial side of the tibia; the latter may be approached without crossing the difficult terrain of large veins embedded in fibrotic subcutaneous tissue so often present on the inner aspect. Negus commonly removes a long or short saphenous vein at the same time but whilst this could be virtually curative in ulceration caused by gross saphenous incompetence, it would be most unwise in true post-thrombotic syndrome without strong preoperative evidence that the limb would not be harmed by loss of a valuable collateral vessel*

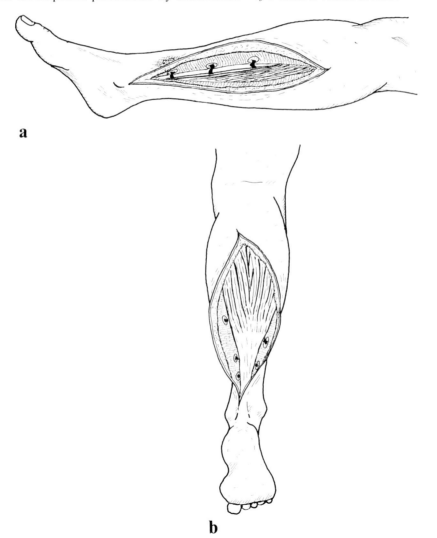

a

b

or subfascial exploration (Figure 20.28). It is probable that in the past these operations have been frequently used in the wrong circumstances and many have brought disappointing results, particularly in the post-thrombotic syndrome. In this book, it has been stressed that incompetent perforators are not a single entity and there is no single general purpose procedure by surgical exploration that will give satisfactory results. Each case must be carefully assessed along the lines given above and in Chapter 11. In this way the significance of a perforator may be determined, so that it may be decided whether it is performing a normal function, or it is abnormal, and in this case, whether its removal will bring benefit or do possible harm. Clinical diagnosis alone is not a sufficient preliminary to surgery here because much more accurate localization and prediction of the outcome to surgical removal is now possible by the techniques available to us, notably Doppler flowmetry, functional phlebography and ultrasonography. Incompetent perforators demonstrated and localized by these means are best removed by a small incision 3 cm or less in length, directly over the perforator. There are few circumstances that will require a long incision on the inner aspect of the leg or at the back of the calf.

## References

Babcock, W. W. (1907) A new operation for the extirpation of varicose veins of the leg. *New York Medical Journal*, **86**, 153–156

Bishop, C. C. R. and Jarrett, P. E. M. (1986) Outpatient varicose vein surgery under local anaesthesia. *British Journal of Surgery*, **73**, 821–822

Cockett, F. B. (1955) The pathology and treatment of venous ulcers of the leg. *British Journal of Surgery*, **43**, 260–278

Cockett, F. B. (1986) Arterial complications during surgery and sclerotherapy of varicose veins. *Phlebology*, **1**, 3–6

Cockett, F. B. and Elgan Jones, D. E. (1953) The ankle blowout syndrome. A new approach to the varicose ulcer problem. *Lancet*, **i**, 17–23

Corbett, R. and Jayakumar, K. N. (1989) Clean up varicose vein surgery – use a tourniquet. *Annals of the Royal College of Surgeons of England*, **71**, 57–58

Dodd, H. (1964) The diagnosis and ligation of incompetent perforating veins. *Annals of the Royal College of Surgeons of England*, **34**, 186–196

Dodd, H. and Cockett, F. B. (1976) *The Pathology and Surgery of the Veins of the Lower Limb*, Churchill Livingstone, Edinburgh, p. 106

Fagg, P. (1987) Intravenous regional anaesthesia for lower limb orthopaedic surgery. *Annals of the Royal College of Surgeons of England*, **69**, 274–275

Farrands, P. A., Royle, G., Najmaldin, A. and Webster, J. H. H. (1987) Varicose veins surgery: effect of a tourniquet on intraoperative blood loss and postoperative cosmesis. *British Journal of Surgery*, **74**, 330

Fletcher, I. R. and Healy, T. E. The arterial tourniquet. *Annals of the Royal College of Surgeons of England*, **65**, 410–417

Gorin, G. and Yellin, A. E. (1991) Ambulatory stab evulsion phlebectomy for truncal varicose veins. *American Journal of Surgery*, **162**, 166–174

Hobbs, J. T. (1980) Per-operative venography to ensure accurate sapheno-popliteal ligation. *British Medical Journal*, **2**, 1578

Hobbs, J. (1988) The enigma of the gastrocnemius vein. *Phlebology*, **3**, 19–30

Jakobsen, B. H. (1986) Out-patient radical operation for varices performed under local analgesia. In *Phlebology '85* (eds D. Negus and G. Jantet), John Libbey, London, pp. 193–195

Keller, W. L. (1905) A new method of extirpating the internal saphenous and similar veins in varicose conditions: a preliminary report. *New York Medical Journal*, **82**, 385–389

Klenerman, L. (1982) The tourniquet in operations on the knee; a review. *Journal of the Royal Society of Medicine*, **75**, 31–32

Lawrie, R. (1960) Limb suspension in varicose-vein surgery. *Lancet*, **ii**, 797

Linton, R. R. (1938) The communicating veins of the lower leg and the operative technic for their ligation. *Annals of Surgery*, **107**, 582–593

Loftgren, K. A. (1958) An evaluation of stripping versus ligation for varicose veins. *AMA Archives of Surgery*, **76**, 310–316

Loftgren, K. A. (1978) Management of varicose veins: Mayo Clinic Experience. *In Venous Problems* (eds J. J. Bergan and J. S. T. Yao), Year Book Medical, Chicago

McDonald, P. J., Webster, J. H. H., Royle, G. T. and Sutton, G. (1989) Comment. *Annals of the Royal College of Surgeons of England*, **72**, 271

Mayo, C. H. (1906) Treatment of varicose veins. *Surgery, Gynecology and Obstetrics*, **2**, 385–388

Myers, T. T. (1957) Results and technique of stripping operation for varicose veins. *Journal of the American Medical Association*, **163**, 87–92

Nabatoff, R. A. (1953) A complete stripping operation of varicose veins under local anaesthesia. *New York Journal of Medicine*, **53**, 1445

Negus, D. (1985) Perforating vein interruption in postphlebitic syndrome. In *Surgery of the Veins* (eds J. J. Bergan and J. S. T. Yao), Grune and Stratton, New York, pp 191–204

Negus, D. and Friedgood, G. (1983) The efficient management of venous ulceration. *British Journal of Surgery*, **70**, 623–627

Nicolaides, A., Christopoulos, D. and Vasdekis, S. (1989) Progress in the investigation of chronic venous insufficiency. *Annals of Vascular Surgery*, **3**, 278–292

Sheppard, M. (1986) The incidence and management of sapheno-popliteal incompetence. *Phlebology*, **1**, 23–32

Sue-Ling, H. and Hughes, L. E. (1988) Should the pill be stopped preoperatively? *British Medical Journal*, **296**, 447–448

Taylor, E. W., Fielding, J. W., Keighley, M. R. and Alexander-Williams, L. (1981) Long saphenous vein stripping under local anaesthesia. *Annals of the Royal College of Surgeons of England*, **63**, 206–207

Trendelenberg, F. (1891) Uber die unterbindung der vena saphena magna bei unterschenkelvaricen. *Beitrag Z Clin Chir*, **7**, 195–210

Umansky, S. (1977) New instruments in the treatment of varicose veins and dilated vessels from South America. In *The Treatment of Venous Disorders* (ed. J. T. Hobbs), MTP, Lancaster, pp. 389–398

van der Stricht, J. (1963) Saphenectomie par invagination sur fil. *La Presse Médicale*, **71**, 1081–1082

van der Stricht, J., van Dale, P., van Bellingen, N. and Bertrand, A. (1986) Long-term results of associated surgery and sclerotherapy for primary varicose disease. *Phlebology '85* (eds D. Negus and G. Jantet), John Libbey, London, pp. 189–191

## Bibliography

Aitenhead, A. R. (1990) Prudence with the pill. *Journal of the Medical Defence Union*, **6**, 62–64

Clinton, O. and Negus, D. (1990) Suitability for day-care varicose vein surgery. *Phlebology*, **5**, 277–279

Corcos, L., Peruzzi, G. P., Romeo, V. and Procacci, T. (1989) Preliminary results of external valvuloplasty in saphenofemoral junction insufficiency. *Phlebology*, **4**, 197–202

Daseler, E. H., Anson, B. J., Reimann, A. F. and Beaton, L. E. (1946) The saphenous tributaries and related structures in relation to the technique of high ligation. *Surgery, Gynecology and Obstetrics*, **82**, 53–63

Fullarton, G. M. and Calvert, M. H. (1987) Intraluminal long saphenous vein stripping: a technique minimizing perivenous tissue trauma. *British Journal of Surgery*, **74**, 255

Gaylis, H. (1968) Subcutaneous implantation of varicose veins for future arterial grafting. *Surgery*, **63**, 591–593

Juhan, C., Haupert, S., Miltgen, G., Barthelemy, P. and Eklof, B. (1990) Recurrent varicose veins. *Phlebology*, **5**, 201–211

Li, A. K. C. (1975) A technique for re-exploration of the saphenofemoral junction for recurrent varicose veins. *British Journal of Surgery*, **62**, 745–746

McMullin, G. M., Coleridge Smith, P. D. and Scurr, J. H. (1991) Objective assessment of high ligation without stripping the long saphenous vein. *British Journal of Surgery*, **78**, 1139–1142

Robinson, G. E., Burren, T., Mackie, I. J., Bounds, W., Walshe, K., Faint, R., Guillebaud, J. and Machin, S. J. (1991) Changes in haemostasis after stopping the combined contraceptive pill: implications for major surgery. *British Medical Journal*, **302**, 269–271

Sheppard, M. (1978) A procedure for the prevention of recurrent saphenofemoral incompetence. *Australian and New Zealand Journal of Surgery*, **48**, 322–326

Vandenriessche, M. (1989) The association between gastrocnemius vein insufficiency and varicose veins. *Phlebology*, **4**, 171–184

Zamboni, P. and Liboni, A. (1991) External valvuloplasty of the sapheno-femoral junction using perforated prosthesis. *Phlebology*, **6**, 141–147

# 21

# Surgery to the deep veins: repair of venous injury; surgery in post-thrombotic syndrome and in valve deficiency states

The surgeon specializing in the treatment of varicose veins may seldom see injury to the deep veins but nevertheless should be prepared to meet this whether it is caused by surgery itself or by external violence. Circumstances leading to injury of a deep vein are too varied to consider further here and only the main principles will be discussed.

## Repair of deep vein injury

### General considerations

Injury to a deep vein may bring the immediate danger of haemorrhage but also the longer term consequences of losing an important channel of venous return. The control of haemorrhage by ligation of a severed vein may seem the simplest course but, in each case, the long-term effects of losing the affected vein must be weighed up; having located the vein ends, repair of a deep vein may be little more difficult than ligation and only take slightly longer. There are some situations where it is virtually mandatory to repair the deep veins if this is in any way possible. In the lower limb there are certain venous bottlenecks, notably the popliteal and common femoral veins, where permanent loss of the vein will be the cause of lasting disability in the limb. Here a maximal effort to obtain high quality repair must be made and by far the best opportunity is immediately after the injury before infection and fibrosis make it a much more difficult procedure, with less prospect of success. This is especially true when there is an accompanying arterial injury and then it is obligatory to repair the vein alongside before the artery is restored. Without this, severe venous congestion will occur as soon as the artery is re-opened and will jeopardize success or leave the limb unnecessarily impaired.

### Initial assessment

In cases of major trauma, assessment must include the likelihood of injuries elsewhere, such as to the abdomen, thorax or head; a fracture in the injured limb may be present. The patient should be checked for evidence of haemorrhagic shock which will require appropriate transfusion before he/she can be properly assessed or surgically treated. If there is accompanying ischaemia in the limb, so that arterial injury seems likely, an arteriogram to assess this is advisable. When there is a major fracture of the bone alongside the vascular injury, orthopaedic help should be called in to fix the fractured bone as a preliminary to vascular repair. The possibility of nerve injury should be considered and any problems of skin coverage assessed.

### Partial injury to a deep vein

This, on its own, may be caused by mishaps during surgery or by localized trauma, for example, in a stab wound. The sequence at operation should be as follows:

- Expose the vein by an adequate incision.
- Haemorrhage must be controlled to allow the vein injury to be seen. Do not use suction for prolonged periods as this can swiftly exsanguinate the patient. Methods of control of haemorrhage are illustrated in Figure 21.1.
- Free the vein sufficiently to apply either soft-faced vascular clamps across it, above and below the laceration, or a single curved clamp partially across the vein and isolating the opening.
- Before applying clamps any clot within the vein should be gently extracted and the vein flushed in both directions with heparin-saline solution (2000 units of heparin to 1 litre of normal saline). Balloon catheters are best avoided because they may easily damage the vein interior and, of course, valves oppose their passage in a peripheral direction.
- Haemostasis is obtained by applying the clamps and stay sutures of 7-0 Prolene are inserted into each end of the laceration.

**Figure 21.1** *Repair of laceration in major vein.*

*(a)* *The sucker should not be used to give a prolonged view of an actively bleeding aperture in a vein. It can exsanguinate the patient quickly and silently. Other means to control bleeding must be used.*

*(b)* *1. The simplest way is to place a finger over the point of bleeding and gently free the vein above and below so that clamps may be applied.*
*2. The assistant's fingers straddling the injury and compressing the vein on either side to give a dry field.*
*3. Gauze pads held in Allis' forceps used by the assistant to compress the vein above and below the bleeding point.*
*4. Isolating the bleeding point by a metal ring (Shen's ring) on a handle. This can be improvised from strong malleable wire if necessary.*

*(c)* *1. Having obtained a dry field and good view, the aperture of the laceration is picked up in an angled vascular clamp and the edges sutured.*
*2. Allis' forceps can be used to give temporary control of the aperture and allow positioning of a less traumatic vascular clamp*

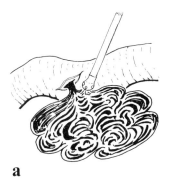

**a**

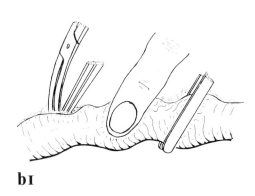

**b1**

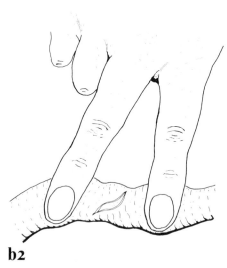

**b2**

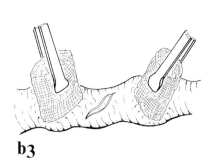

**b3**

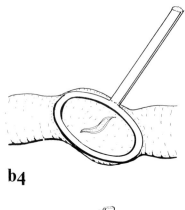

**b4**

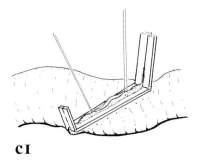

**c1**

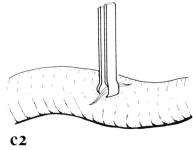

**c2**

- The stay sutures are gently drawn upon to stretch the margins of the opening so that it may be inspected.
- If it is a clean incision, it may be directly sutured with continuous or interrupted stitches of Prolene or PTFE (Figure 21.2).

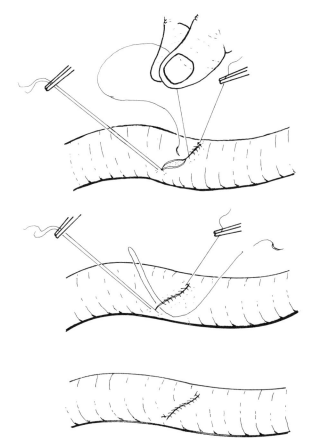

**Figure 21.2** *A clean laceration may be closed by a continuous suture of Prolene or PTFE (clamps omitted in diagram)*

- If the edges are ragged they should be trimmed back to healthy vein with a shining endothelial interior. This must be done with delicacy to avoid unnecessary creation of a serious deficiency in the vein wall. Suturing may then proceed as described above.
- Vein wall is very thin tissue which dries and dies rapidly. Throughout the procedure care must be taken to keep the vein moist with normal saline, particularly the exposed endothelial surface.
- The vascular clamps may now be removed and venous flow restarted. If it is assessed that the endothelial interior of the vein has suffered little damage and the vein concerned is a major one, and seen to fill well swiftly, without deformity, then there is a good prospect of a successful result. Support by a temporary arteriovenous fistula should not be necessary.

*Complete division of a major vein*

- If necessary an accompanying fracture should be fixed by an internal pin as a first step.
- The injured blood vessels are exposed by an adequate incision.
- Define and free the ends of the divided vein. (If arterial injury is present, similarly free the injured artery from its surroundings and apply clamps if there is bleeding.)
- Insert a pair of stay sutures symmetrically into each vein end so that they may be gently stretched for inspection.
- Excise any tattered and devitalized vein. Gently clear clot from the mouth of the vein and obtain good backbleeding from below. If necessary, compress the calf sharply to expel any clot.
- Flush out the vein ends with heparin-saline and apply soft-faced vascular clamps well clear of the vein ends. Approximate the clamps by loops of thread around them to bring the vein ends together.
- Four stay sutures are then placed with care to unite the vein ends as evenly as possible. Two neighbouring stay sutures are then lifted up to raise the vein edges between them and a series of interrupted 7-0 Prolene sutures inserted. This process is repeated until the entire circumference is closed with interrupted sutures. Veins are very thin walled and require a different technique from arteries. Interrupted sutures are to be preferred because they allow maximum circumference to the anastomosis without any purse-string effect and are not liable to separation, with inward collapse of the vein ends, that so easily occurs with long runs of continuous suture in these highly elastic vessels (Figure 21.3).

(If arterial injury is also present, this is now repaired by cleaning and trimming the arterial ends, gently extracting clot with a Fogarty catheter if necessary, flushing with heparin-saline and anastomosis with continuous 6-0 Prolene. The arterial circulation is not allowed to run until the venous clamps have been removed (Figure 21.4).)

- The venous clamps are now removed (followed by arterial clamps). If a satisfactory arterial circulation is present, the vein should be seen to swell up quickly with no deformity or narrowing. Bleeding from a venous anastomosis is usually small and easily controlled by finger touch or the lightest of pressure with gauze. Care must be taken not to impede venous return.

The greatest problem is when there is a serious deficiency of deep vein at the site of injury, as may arise in wounds caused by a high velocity missile taking away a portion of vein and this is likely to be accompanied by arterial injury. A determined effort must be made to reconstruct vein and artery if the limb is to be saved. The best prospect for the venous repair is by grafting with autogenous vein but no vein of matching calibre can be spared from

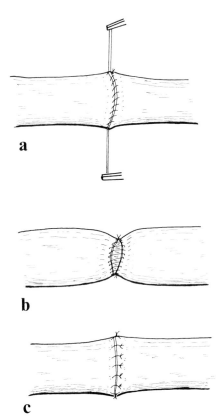

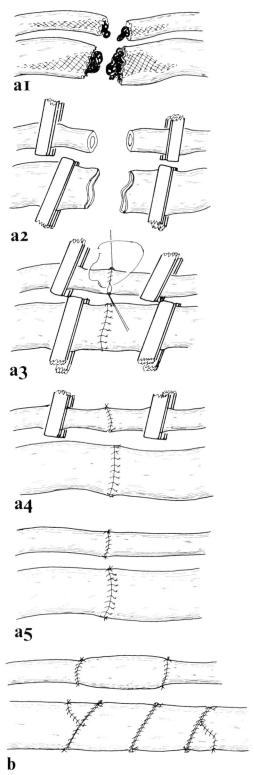

**Figure 21.3** *When end-to-end anastomosis is required for complete division of a vein, a continuous suture suitable for arteries may not prove appropriate for the thin wall of a vein.*

*(a) When the vein is well stretched by stay sutures anastomosis appears satisfactory.*

*(b) When the stay sutures are cut the edges may pull apart with the continuous stitch pulling in the anastomosis, which bleeds heavily and is severely narrowed.*

*(c) It is better to use interrupted sutures which avoid the possible drawstring effect of a continuous suture. The best result is obtained by commencing the anastomosis with four symmetrical stay sutures and then adding no more than two or three interrupted sutures between each of these; greater density of sutures is not necessary and is undesirable*

**Figure 21.4** *Repair after traumatic division of major artery and vein in a limb. It is essential to repair the vein as well as the artery.*

*(a) 1. Both artery and vein will require clot removing from the open vessel ends, with clearing of adherent tissue and adventitia to give a clear view so that ragged edges may be trimmed away.*
*2. Heparin solution is instilled into the vessels and clamps applied.*
*3. The vein is anastomosed with interrupted sutures and the artery with a continuous suture.*
*4. When the anastomoses are completed the clamps are removed from the vein first and after it has filled without deformity the arterial clamps are removed. This avoids an undesirable period of severe venous congestion.*
*5. Both vein and artery have been repaired. Repairing the vein only takes a few extra minutes and greatly improves the prospect of a good limb without venous problems.*

*(b) Bridging a deficiency in vein and artery following severe damage to the vessels. A graft of the patient's own saphenous vein, reversed so that the valves do not oppose flow, is a good match for popliteal and superficial femoral arteries and should be used by end-to-end anastomosis as illustrated. However, the saphenous vein is too narrow to match the corresponding vein but it may be used to fashion a graft of suitable calibre as shown in Figure 21.5. Here a spiral graft is illustrated*

elsewhere. However, it is possible to use a portion of saphenous vein to fashion a length of composite vein of adequate calibre. A saphenous vein without such modification will almost certainly be too narrow and would jeopardize success. This fashioning process is best carried out over a glass or plastic tube. An adequate portion of saphenous vein is removed from the thigh, cleaned of excess tissue, and divided up its length. The interior is kept moist and inspected for valves which are trimmed away. It is then cut across to give two or three panels which can be sewn longitudinally to give an adequate circumference (Figure 21.5(a)1–7). Alternatively, a single length of opened saphenous vein may be sutured in spiral fashion to give a graft of adequate width and length (Figures 21.4(b), 21.5(b)); a continuous suture with 7-0 Prolene is suitable. The graft tissue must not be allowed to dry out, particularly the endothelial surface, and it is repeatedly moistened with saline. When this graft has been prepared it is interposed between the two vein ends and anastomosed into position with interrupted sutures. This form of autograft is greatly to be preferred to any synthetic graft which should only be used as a last resort.

(Arterial repair by reversed saphenous vein graft should be carried out, if necessary. Saphenous vein from the thigh is usually an adequate match for popliteal to common femoral arteries (Figure 21.4(b)).)

Injury to major nerves should be repaired, or at least the ends approximated, if possible.

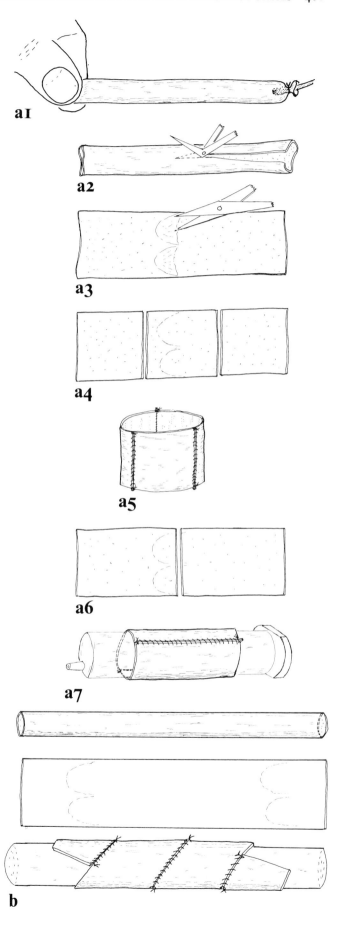

**Figure 21.5** *Fashioning a large calibre vein graft from autogenous saphenous vein.*

*(a)  1. A suitable length of saphenous vein is removed and distended with saline.*
*2. It is opened up along its length.*
*3. Valve cusps are removed.*
*4. It is cut into three panels.*
*5. The panels are sewn together to form a wide vein graft.*
*6. Alternatively the vein may be cut into two panels to give a longer but slightly narrower graft.*
*7.  Shaping the graft over glass or plastic tubing, or the barrel of a syringe, ensures a regular outline of appropriate width.*

*(b)  If a longer vein graft is required this may be fashioned from saphenous vein, opened up and sutured over a tube in spiral fashion.*

*As a rough guide to the length of donor saphenous vein required: to give a graft twice the original, distended saphenous diameter, twice the length of gap to be bridged will be required, and if three times the saphenous diameter is required, three times the length of the gap will be needed; this applies to both panel and spiral grafts, but with a spiral graft there is some wastage at the ends so that an excess of donor vein should be removed*

*Use of temporary arteriovenous fistula to improve venous flow*

In some circumstances the success rate of surgery reconstructing veins is improved by using a temporary arteriovenous fistula between a neighbouring artery and the repaired vein. A suitable branch artery is swung into position below the repaired portion of vein in order to give local increase in venous pressure and flow (Figure 21.6(b)4, (c)). This will distend the anastomosis and prevent its collapse, and also, by the speed of flow, diminish the likelihood of thrombus building up to occlude the vein. In most cases of vein injury, where the vein interior is relatively undamaged, it is not necessary to add this. In procedures such as venous thrombectomy, where there is an extensive area of severely damaged or absent endothelium, there is a strong case for using this supporting measure. In any case, it should only be used if the surgeon is confident in his ability to place the fistula and eventually close it without creating increased difficulties in the management of the patient.

## Operations to reconstruct deep veins and valves

A large number of people suffer moderate to severe disability from deep vein impairment, typified by pigmentation of skin near the ankle, oedema, induration and eventually ulceration. For many years this state was regarded as being post-thrombotic (postphlebitic) but more recently it has been realized that many cases do not have any evidence of previous deep vein thrombosis and appear to arise either by an inborn deficiency in the number and durability of valves, or from a general weakening of vein structure causing their dilatation and progressive loss of valve function. Various terms have been given to these states: Gruss (1988b) refers to a 'dilating venopathy' and an 'idiopathic valvular insufficiency'; Taheri *et al.* (1985) refer to 'the recent discovery of congenital redundancy of the valve leading to venous hypertension' and suggest the term 'venous insufficiency syndrome'; Kistner (1980, 1985) refers to 'primary valve incompetence' with 'valve prolapse' and distinguishes this from postphlebitic damage to valves; Tibbs and Fletcher (1983) referred to the 'valveless syndrome' and in this book the same term and 'weak vein syndrome' have been used to describe venous insufficiency without evidence of preceding deep vein thrombosis. The essential failure, whether post-thrombotic or by some form of valve deficiency, is a severe impairment of the venous pumping mechanism but in the post-thrombotic group also accompanied by the effects of obstruction and deformity in major veins. Reconstruction of the deep veins and valves to restore their lost function is the most prized objective sought after by present-day phlebologists and the progress made towards this so far gives some encour-

agement. The search for this 'holy grail' continues endlessly by the leading exponents.

Below the inferior vena cava and iliac veins the construction of a valveless conduit is not enough and valves must be included in some fashion. The post-thrombotic state all too often has a complex arrangement of obstructed and deformed deep veins with compensatory mechanisms of greatly expanded collateral veins which have lost all valve function. In most cases the failure is far too extensive to lend itself to methods at present available but, in some, it may be sufficiently localized to allow some form of rearrangement of the veins to improve function and these methods are discussed in this chapter. They are important because the principles used may form the basis for progress in the future.

## Suitability of patients for deep vein and valve reconstruction

Certainly in the post-thrombotic state there is a great capacity for compensatory mechanisms to develop and in most patients it will not be possible to improve the state of the limb by present-day methods. Mild clinical disability does not justify the uncertainties of reconstructive surgery. Only those who are severely handicapped should be considered.

When post-thrombotic obstruction is present, it is most unlikely to succeed unless there is to be a vigorous flow through the reconstructed veins and preoperative investigation should verify that venous pressure in the vein below the intended reconstruction is substantially higher than in the vein beyond it, that is to say, a significant pressure gradient exists. This will also confirm the existence of a severe venous dysfunction that should be relieved if possible. In the non-obstructed 'valveless' states, pressure studies should give evidence of heavy reflux indicated by an excessive swing of pressure with each muscular contraction and a very brief reduction in venous pressure after exercise. Functional phlebography plays an essential part in demonstrating obstructed or deformed veins, but, equally important, may show widely open deep veins lacking valves, or valves with cusps that leak heavily. It should also be used to display competent valves, for example, in a long saphenous or a profunda femoris vein, because these may form a good basis for reconstruction.

Reconstructive surgery should only be considered if phlebography has shown a clear opportunity of bringing benefit to the limb by one of the following ways:

- Providing a simple conduit bypassing an obstruction (as in common iliac vein occlusion).
- Rearranging veins in some fashion to overcome a blockage and utilizing a vein with at least one undamaged valve.
- In non-thrombotic conditions, repair of heavily

leaking valves or transposition of the vein concerned into a venous channel that possesses good valves.

- When valvular incompetence from any cause is the main fault, the insertion of a segment of valved vein, taken from elsewhere, and interposed as a graft to provide a functioning valve. Identifying a suitable donor valve from an upper limb or saphenous vein of the opposite side will, of course, be essential.

In all cases the principal deep veins of the limb up to the inferior vena cava must be visualized. This is especially important in post-thrombotic cases where the damage is usually more extensive than the clinical findings might suggest and for this reason often precludes reconstructive surgery (see various phlebograms in Chapter 8). There is little point in carrying out a reconstruction if the veins leading to it, or away from it, are damaged and inadequate.

Gruss (1988b) points out that in deep vein reconstruction concomitant incompetence of superficial and perforating veins should be rectified beforehand, for example, in the valveless syndrome it would be pointless to transpose the superficial femoral vein to a valved profunda femoris but leave a massively incompetent long saphenous vein (Figure 21.9(b)).

Reconstructive surgery to the deep veins should not usually be considered in the acute phase of venous thrombosis and at least a year should have elapsed without evidence of continuing activity. This interval will allow the patient to have reached a stable state with maximal improvement and is an appropriate stage for the assessment of residual disability. It will also allow a long-term appraisal of the significance of the thrombotic episode.

## Notes on technique in reconstructive surgery to deep veins

Veins must be handled with care. Any trauma that damages the endothelium will cause deposition of thrombus. Such trauma includes:

- Crushing with unsuitable vascular clamps; only the lightest pressure should be used with broad, soft-surfaced clamps or by use of silastic rubber slings lightly applied.
- Handling the interior with metal instruments or abrading it by use of gauze against the endothelial surfaces.
- Allowing the exposed interior to dry. If left exposed, the endothelial surfaces must be kept moist with normal saline repeatedly sprayed on with a syringe.
- Excessive traction. This may rupture the intima and create thrombogenic areas.

Suture materials should be of gauge 6-0, 7-0 or 8-0 in monofilament of Prolene or PTFE. Both these materials are virtually non-thrombogenic and non-reactive with the tissues. The gauge of suture is judged by the width of vein and thickness of wall but the lightest suture consistent with adequate strength should be used.

If the veins are shut off for any length of time, heparin solution (2000 units to 1 litre of normal saline) should be instilled into the stagnant vein, or in some cases the patient should be systemically heparinized before applying any clamps. Heparinization postoperatively for several days, under strict control, is permissible but may cause a haematoma which could impede venous flow. Alternatively, if heparinization is to be maintained for some days, this can be achieved locally by continuous drip through a fine catheter inserted into a side branch of the vein beneath the reconstruction, delivering a dosage insufficient to affect systemic coagulation. Anticoagulation can be extended further, if required, by warfarin orally for a further 3–6 months. As an additional measure against thrombus deposition, intravenous dextran can be used postoperatively for several days.

A temporary arteriovenous fistula may be employed to increase flow through the reconstructed veins. This will diminish any tendency for thrombosis by stasis and will help to distend the veins and their anastomoses. Undoubtedly this can improve the results in many cases and will be referred to again in the appropriate sections later.

Employment of a synthetic prosthesis may be permissible in some circumstances, particularly above the inguinal ligament, but in general, below this level it is inferior to finding some way of using the patient's own veins and should be avoided. At the time of writing, the prosthesis of choice is a PTFE graft with external spiral or ringed support to maintain a wide lumen that cannot easily be compressed or obstructed by kinking. A temporary arteriovenous fistula and postoperative anticoagulation with heparin initially and warfarin over the following months is advisable.

## Operations for the post-thrombotic states

### Common iliac vein occlusion (Palma's operation)

If occlusion is limited to common and external iliac veins, without any significant thrombotic damage below the inguinal ligament, and the patient is severely handicapped by swelling, then Palma's operation, or some variant of it, may well be appropriate. In its simplest form, the long saphenous vein from the opposite limb is divided in the lower thigh, mobilized and swung across suprapubically to be anastomosed end to side with a suitable vein in the groin of the affected limb (Figure 21.6(a), (b)1–3). Flow from this side will pass through the saphenous vein, unopposed by valves, and across to the contralateral common femoral vein. This arrangement will then act as a substantial collateral which can only be to the betterment of the limb.

Often the common femoral vein on the affected side is not suitable because it has sustained some thrombotic damage and in this case the mobilized saphenous vein may be anastomosed to the front of the profunda femoris vein, or to the long saphenous vein if this is of good size and in free communication with the deep veins (Figure 21.6(b)2,3). Incompetence in the transposed long saphenous vein should not prevent it being used. If no saphenous vein is available on the opposite side, it may be possible to use the long saphenous vein from the affected limb mobilized in reverse fashion, but here, of course, its valves will tend to oppose flow and will have to be destroyed with a suitable valvulotome. Moreover, the saphenous vein in the affected limb may be serving a valuable collateral function and should not be sacrificed unless it is clear that popliteal and superficial femoral veins, or profunda femoris vein, are providing a good alternative venous outlet. Often this is not so and not only would the operation be likely to fail because of inadequate flow, but any advantage gained could be lost by the limb being deprived of a collateral upon which it was dependent.

More recently Gruss (1988a, b) has recommended the use of a spirally supported PTFE prosthesis (0.8–1 cm in width) anastomosed to a suitable vein in the groin of the affected side, tunnelled under the inguinal ligament, and crossing extraperitoneally, deep to the abdominal muscles and pubes, to be anastomosed end to side with the external iliac vein of the opposite limb (Figure 21.6(c)). This procedure is supported by localized heparin given by a catheter into a branch of the superficial femoral vein (also allowing postoperative phlebography a week later), oral anticoagulation is substituted after a few days and maintained for at least 6 months. In addition, Gruss advocates the use of an arteriovenous fistula using a branch of the saphenous vein on the affected side, anastomosed to the neighbouring superficial femoral artery and maintained for 3 months.

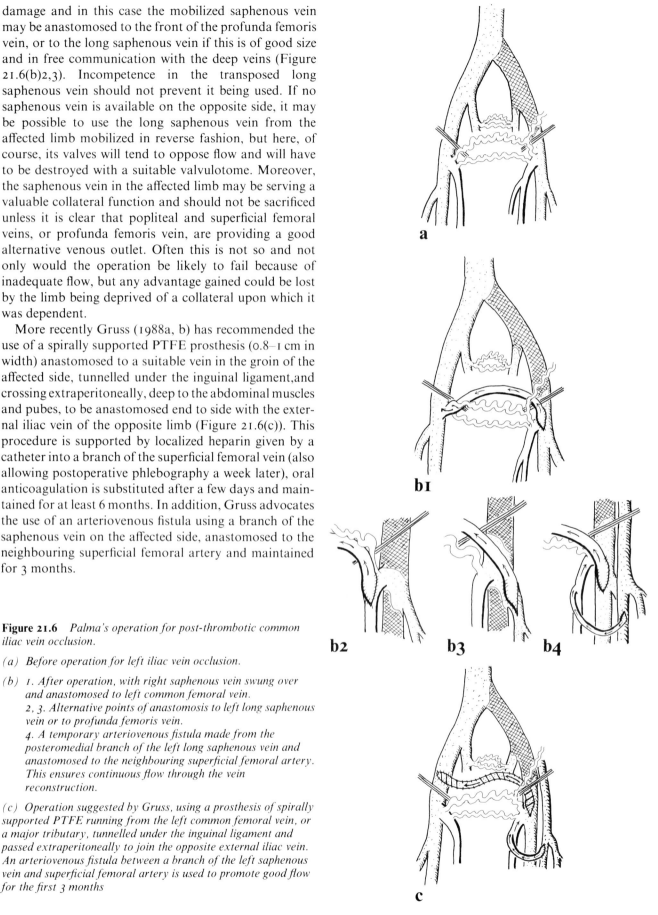

**Figure 21.6** *Palma's operation for post-thrombotic common iliac vein occlusion.*

*(a) Before operation for left iliac vein occlusion.*

*(b) 1. After operation, with right saphenous vein swung over and anastomosed to left common femoral vein.*
*2, 3. Alternative points of anastomosis to left long saphenous vein or to profunda femoris vein.*
*4. A temporary arteriovenous fistula made from the posteromedial branch of the left long saphenous vein and anastomosed to the neighbouring superficial femoral artery. This ensures continuous flow through the vein reconstruction.*

*(c) Operation suggested by Gruss, using a prosthesis of spirally supported PTFE running from the left common femoral vein, or a major tributary, tunnelled under the inguinal ligament and passed extraperitoneally to join the opposite external iliac vein. An arteriovenous fistula between a branch of the left saphenous vein and superficial femoral artery is used to promote good flow for the first 3 months*

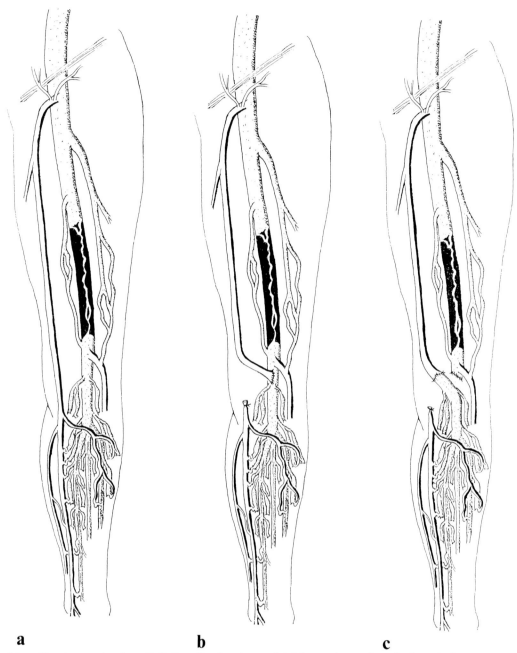

**a**                    **b**                    **c**

**Figure 21.7**   *May–Husni operation for relief of popliteal and superficial femoral post-thrombotic occlusion.*

*(a)  The state before operation showing a long saphenous vein filling by multiple perforator outflow and acting as a collateral to the occluded deep veins.*

*(b)  The saphenous divided and its upper portion anastomosed, end to side, with popliteal vein.*

*(c)  Alternative arrangement with saphenous vein anastomosed, end to side, with a divided popliteal vein.*

*In either of these reconstructions a temporary arteriovenous fistula can be made by dividing the long saphenous vein near the ankle and anastomosing its leg portion, end to side, to the posterior tibial artery nearby. This is not illustrated but the postoperative diagrams show how arterial flow into the leg portion of the saphenous vein will enter the deep veins by multiple perforators to enhance flow through the reconstruction. Dividing the saphenous vein avoids possible venous hypertension in the foot caused by the fistula*

### Transposition of internal jugular vein for subclavian occlusion

A similar principle of swinging in a neighbouring vein to provide a venous conduit is used to restore flow past an occluded subclavian vein and is described in Chapter 15. The internal jugular vein is divided at high level and brought down to anastomose with the axillary vein below the obstruction.

*Post-thrombotic occlusion and deformity of superficial femoral vein (May–Husni operation)*

If post-thrombotic damage is confined to the superficial femoral and upper popliteal veins, and an otherwise satisfactory musculovenous pump below the knee is impeded by having only indirect collateral outflow, then it may be possible to bring considerable improvement by the May–Husni operation. In this, the long saphenous vein is rerouted to take flow directly from the popliteal vein by dividing the saphenous vein and anastomosing its upper portion to the popliteal vein, either above or below the knee. This may done by end-to-side anastomosis (Figure 21.7(a), (b)) or by dividing the popliteal vein to form an oblique end-to-end anastomosis between the two vessels and giving a better alignment (Figure 21.7(c)). Gruss (1988a, b) suggests that a temporary arterio-venous fistula should be added to this by dividing the long saphenous vein just above the medial malleolus and anastomosing its upper part to the posterior tibial artery. The arteriovenous fistula created gives increased flow via perforating veins into the tibial veins and so up to the poplitosaphenous anastomosis at knee level. This fistula apparently closes easily when a firm bandage is placed over it in 3 months time.

## Operations for incompetence in popliteal and superficial femoral veins

*Transposition of deep vein into a valved vein near by*

When the most significant defect is due to gross incompetence in popliteal and superficial femoral veins, without any obstruction above this level, it may be possible to utilize a good valve often present in either profunda femoris vein or in the upper portion of the long saphenous vein. The superficial femoral vein is divided near its upper end and the upper residue closed off by a continuous stitch, care being taken not to deform the profunda femoris termination. The lower portion is then anastomosed, end to side, below a valve demonstrated by previous phlebography in the profunda femoris vein or a major branch of it (Figure 21.8(a), (b)1, 2); alternatively the divided superficial femoral vein may be anastomosed, end to side, into the long saphenous vein in the upper thigh if this has a functioning valve above this level (Figure 21.8(c)1, 2). By these means at least one good valve can be interposed at the outlet of the superficial femoral vein.

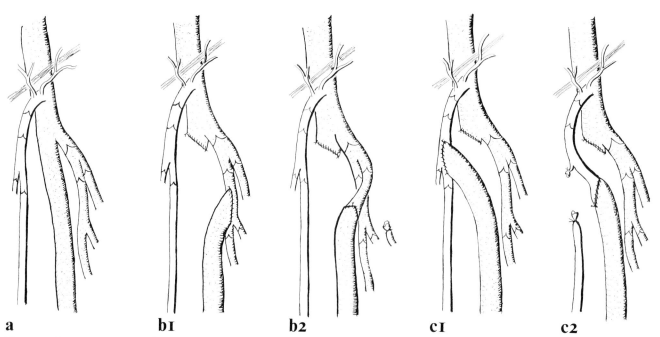

**a**    **b1**    **b2**    **c1**    **c2**

**Figure 21.8**  *Transposition of a valveless deep vein into a valved vein.*

*(a)  The state before operation with the superficial femoral and other deep veins below this fully patent but deficient in valves.*

*(b)  1. The superficial femoral vein has been divided near its upper end and is inserted, end to side, into a well-valved portion of the profunda femoris vein.*
*2. Alternative arrangement with end-to-end anastomosis to a valved branch of profunda femoris.*

*(c)  1. Anastomosis, end to side, with a well-valved long saphenous vein.*
*2. Alternative arrangement when the long saphenous vein lacks valves below the point of anastomosis. It has been divided to give an oblique end-to-end anastomosis with the superficial femoral vein; this prevents retrograde flow down the valveless portion of the saphenous vein*

*Transplantation of a segment of valved vein (Taheri)*

This procedure has been described by Taheri et al (1982a, b, 1985a, b) who report good results in over 40 patients. The main indication is similar to that described above, gross incompetence in the popliteal and superficial veins caused either by previous thrombosis or a valve deficiency state. The intention is to utilize a segment of the vein containing a valve taken from one of the few sites in the body where this can be spared without causing undue harm. An axillary or brachial vein often proves a suitable donor site or possibly the upper end of the long saphenous vein in the opposite limb. The best place for inserting this

is in the upper popliteal vein; the vein is divided here and the valved graft inserted by end-to-end anastomoses (Figure 21.9). Taheri *et al.* (1985a, b) more recently advise that the graft should be wrapped in PTFE mesh in order to prevent its eventual dilatation with loss of valve function, which is seen in some cases.

*Repair of valves to restore competence (Kistner)*

Kistner (1985) has demonstrated that chronic insufficiency arises in some patients because valves in popliteal and superficial femoral veins have become defective

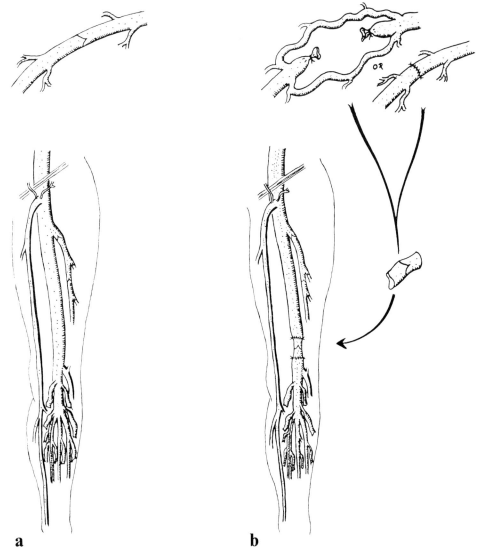

**a**                                                        **b**

**Figure 21.9**  *Taheri's operation for valve deficiency in the deep veins. A portion of vein with a good valve is transposed from brachial or axillary vein and is inserted into the popliteal vein.*

*(a)  The state before operation. The upper part illustrates a good valve identified in brachial or axillary vein, and the lower part shows the deep veins, which are widely open but deficient in valves.*

*(b)  The portion of brachio-axillary vein containing a valve has been resected and the donor vein is either ligated, with venous return continuing by collateral circulation, or it may be possible to restore continuity by end-to-end anastomosis. The valved graft is inserted into the upper popliteal vein. In the illustration, the long saphenous vein is shown as valveless and in this case reflux down it should be prevented by removing it, but if well valved it should be retained. The transposed portion of vein may be wrapped in PTFE net or prosthesis in order to prevent its eventual expansion and failure of the valve*

with one cusp elongated and prolapsing beneath the other (Figure 21.10(a)). This group corresponds with those patients we have described in Chapter 7, with the valveless syndrome and weak vein syndrome. In these states, the few valves present are poorly formed and incompetent or there is generalized weakening and dilatation of the veins so that the cusps separate and become ineffective. In Kistner's operation suitable valves, selected by phlebography, are exposed by an incision into the vein, with great care being taken to avoid any damage to the cusps. Stitches are then placed at each end of the cusps to take up excessive length and to restore symmetry (Figure 21.10(b), (c)). The vein is then closed and the competence of the valve tested by opening the upper clamp to see if the segment of vein below the valve remains empty.

It must be emphasized that few patients are suitable for the procedures described above. There is no point in doing any of these operations if the veins above or below the reconstruction are themselves severely damaged. In valve deficiency states it remains to be proved that vein transposition or valve transplantation is justified by the benefit given. In most cases it seems unlikely that, however well placed, the interposition of one or two valves will make any appreciable difference. The defects often seem far too widespread for this. The number of reported cases having this form of surgery is small and the follow-up time limited. Nevertheless, reconstructive surgery of veins will not advance unless experts in this field are tentatively exploring its possibilities. The average surgeon, who perhaps is not able to give this subject the careful study and detailed work-up that is required for each patient, would be well advised to visit one of the recognized exponents before attempting it. Certainly, the excellent account of venous reconstruction given by Gruss (1988a, b), with a most comprehensive bibliography, should be consulted.

### Construction of an external popliteal valve by silastic sling (Psathakis)

This procedure (Psathakis, 1968; Psathakis and Psathakis, 1985) uses a sling attached to flexor muscles of the knee and placed around the popliteal vein. The intention is that the sling tightens around the vein, preventing reflux in it, when the flexor muscles of the knee contract as the foot is raised off the ground with each footstep. Thus, initially, with knee straight and calf muscle contraction causing maximal upward pumping, free flow occurs, but in the final phase, as the knee bends and the foot is raised off the ground, upward pumping ceases and the contracting flexor muscles tighten the sling, so preventing popliteal reflux. In the original operation the gracilis tendon, detached distally and joined across the popliteal fossa to biceps femoris muscle, was used; subsequently a silastic artificial tendon was employed to give more length and passed round the vein to provide a sling between biceps femoris laterally and a detached flexor tendon medially.

This is certainly an ingenious solution when the predominant failure is reflux in the popliteal vein but although arousing much interest has been little used in spite of the originator's impressive results, possibly because at first sight it seems somewhat improbable to succeed. Psathakis and Psathakis (1985) have never-

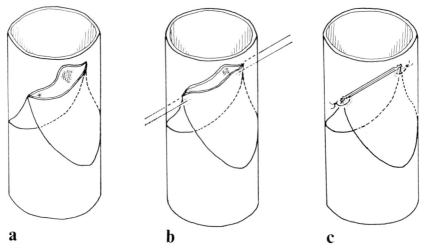

**a**        **b**        **c**

**Figure 21.10** *Kistner's operation to restore competence in a valve with slack cusps.*

*(a) Representation of the valve's original state showing loose cusps with one prolapsed beneath the other and allowing heavy leakage.*

*(b) The valve is exposed so that stitches may be placed at each end to shorten the redundant cusp edges.*

*(c) The stitches are tied to give equally aligned cusps that meet effectively to give a competent valve*

theless persisted and report over 200 cases with good results. McMullin *et al.* (1990) point out that it is difficult to evaluate this work because the procedure has often been accompanied by surgery to the superficial veins and, in order to give independent evaluation, they have carried out the procedure on its own in twelve selected patients with undoubted deep vein reflux. They report that in six out of eight patients there was complete healing of an ulcer, with improvement in the others; in two, ambulatory venous pressures improved but there was no improvement of venous refilling times judged by photo-plethysmography in any patient. Duplex scanning showed that all popliteal veins remained open post-operatively but there was one death from massive pulmonary embolism.

This operation cannot be dismissed but clearly should not be carried out without careful investigation and a familiarity with the experience of others with a special interest in this procedure.

## Can vein and valve reconstruction be developed further? Author's comment

Present achievements in deep vein reconstruction have underlined how limited is our ability to replace veins and valves. Synthetic prostheses fall far short of the exquisite, delicate structure of a natural vein, with its highly elastic and contractile walls, lined with an endothelium designed to eliminate a thrombus by lysis if it should form, and with feather-light valves responding instantly to the slightest movement of blood, but yet capable of resisting strong pressures. It is hard to envisage a man-made prosthesis that can emulate these features. Nevertheless, if one's imagination strays it is not inconceivable that valves of synthetic gossamer-thin net, precoated with the patient's own endothelial cells and introduced by transluminal endoscope, can be developed for valveless syndrome. Even today there would be little difficulty in developing endoscopic methods for performing the repair of leaking valves in veins, equivalent to Kistner's procedure. On the other hand the increasing capability in tissue culture and genetic engineering give reason to believe that it should be possible biologically to prepare tubes of living tissues with all the right qualities. Meso-thelial-derived tissues possess an endothelium very like that in veins and possessing similar thrombus-resisting properties. With this in mind, in Oxford during 1968–69, a small number of experimental grafts were carried out using autogenous canine peritoneum fashioned into tubes and inserted into the inferior vena cava. Care was taken to oppose endothelial surfaces accurately without any inversion, using microclips in some preparations and fine Mersilk in others, but without using any systemic anti-coagulation. Only a small number of good results were obtained (Figure 21.11), but these gave some indication of what might be attainable with a living autogenous

graft using tissue with endothelium closely similar to vein itself. More recently, other workers, with more refined techniques, have also obtained encouraging results using tubes of peritoneum to replace veins (Nicholson *et al.*, 1984; Louagie *et al.*, 1986; Bull *et al.*, 1988; Ribbe *et al.*, 1988a, b). This method in itself may find a place but, if nothing else, points the way to the preparation of living vein grafts, antigenically compatible with the host, and with valves grown or constructed at intervals along their length. The preparation of such vein substitutes may be attainable in the not-too-distant future and should give a reliable replacement of major veins. By conducting and holding blood pumped up from below without reflux, it would make an 'ideal' valved outlet above a relatively undamaged musculovenous mechanism. However, persisting collateral channels, lacking effective valves and allowing heavy reflux, would probably require eliminating since otherwise the advantages of the new vein would be invalidated.

In the reconstruction outlined above, another more serious problem would be that in many cases the pumping mechanism within the muscles is also severely defective so that little would be achieved. Extensive damage by thrombosis of the intricate venous pumping mechanisms within the muscles, or by a widespread inborn deficiency of valves guarding the venous sinuses, may prove impossible to repair in the foreseeable future. Elastic stockings, or any other form of external support at present available, cannot fill this role; they may bring some improvement in the effectiveness of a damaged musculovenous pump but certainly cannot substitute for an active pumping mechanism. For these reasons a different, but important, technical principle should be explored. This entails the development of an ultralightweight, externally applied, pumping device fitting over the leg. Simple versions of this have already been described (Holan, 1971; Holan *et al.*, 1976; Gardner & Fox, 1983) and improvised versions tried by the author have certainly given encouragement that such a device is entirely feasible and could be of great value in treating, for example, the post-thrombotic limb, especially if combined with a surgical reconstruction providing a suitably valved main conduit; similarly, it could be highly effective in the valveless syndrome. By present techniques and materials, it should be possible to construct a garment, not much more bulky than a strong elastic stocking, that fits over the leg up to the knee and gives a ripple of sequential pressure passing up the limb with each footstep. This could be powered at each step by body weight on the underside of the feet or by an external source of power (electropneumatic or hydraulic) for a patient having to perform prolonged tasks with little movement. Such a device, together with the venous outlet provided by a biological valved graft, could substitute for a grossly defective musculovenous pump.

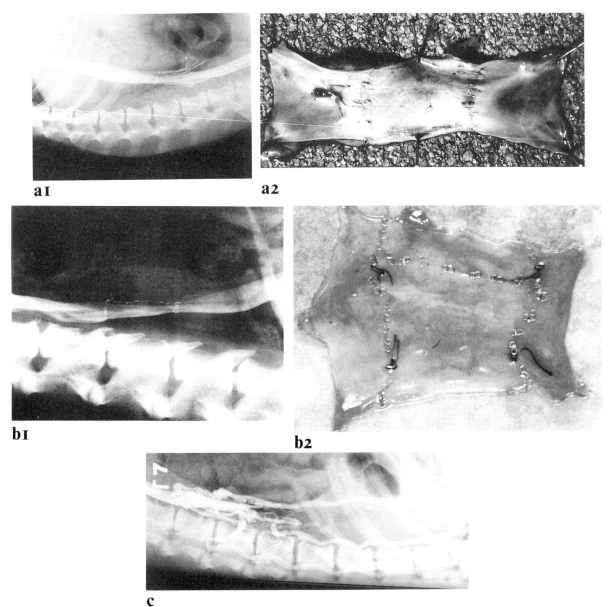

**Figure 21.11** *The potential of mesothelial tissue as a substitute for vein. Examples from a series (M. Keynes and D. Tibbs, 1967–69, unpublished) of canine autografts, using tubes fashioned from peritoneum of the anterior abdominal wall to replace a 2–3 cm segment of inferior vena cava. These were left in place between 1 and 9 months. The results were as follows:*

- *Four grafts were fully patent and with either no or minimal adherent thrombus within; in clinical circumstances a satisfactory functional result likely.*
- *Two grafts had moderate narrowing, with some collateral vein formation evident on phlebography and some thrombus at one anastomosis, but with survival of a functioning vein substitute; in clinical circumstances might have given a useful result.*
- *Nine grafts gave bad results, with occlusion and large collateral veins on phlebography. Nevertheless, in two grafts partial survival of an endothelialized lumen was found on opening. In two cases it was known that the original preparation was imperfect.*

*Neither postoperative anticoagulation nor arteriovenous fistula was used in these preparations and it is possible that a higher success rate might have been achieved by these means. The reasons for such variable results are uncertain, but even a few good results imply that a method using living tissue, antigenetically acceptable and lined with thrombus-resisting endothelium, might be capable of development to give dependable results.*

*The illustrations from two 'successful' preparations show:*

*(a) 1. Phlebogram at 2 months with some narrowing of peritoneal graft by external fibrosis, and a few small collaterals.*
*2. The graft, retrieved soon afterwards, opened to show a good lumen and smooth endothelial surface but with a small adherent thrombus at one anastomosis.*

*(b) 1. Phlebogram of another preparation 3 months after insertion.*
*2. Interior of graft; stitches and microclips are easily seen through transparent endothelium and appear to have been well accepted.*

*(c) Typical appearances on phlebogram in unsuccessful preparation with total occlusion and large collateral veins*

# Thrombectomy

## Iliofemoral thrombectomy with temporary arteriovenous fistula

It is well recognized that the best way to protect a patient with iliofemoral thrombosis from the imminent danger of pulmonary embolus and eventual post-thrombotic syndrome is by early removal of the thrombus (Mavor and Galloway, 1969; Mavor, 1971; DeWeese, 1978). At this stage the vein wall has not reacted extensively and the thrombus is not adherent so that it is easily removed and the wall less likely to precipitate recurrent thrombosis. Whether achieved by thrombolysis or thrombectomy, treatment is most effective when applied in the first 5 days to a non-adherent (non-obstructive) thrombus in the iliofemoral veins, the venous outlet of the limb. But even so, until recently the advantages have not been sufficient to persuade most surgeons to change from the simpler policy of heparin-coumarin anticoagulation; both methods give a similar, relatively high incidence of post-thrombotic disability. However, over the last few years greatly improved results have been reported from several sources (Eklof, Einarsson and Plate, 1985; Zetterquist et al., 1986; Eklof et al., 1987; Gruss, 1988a) when early thrombectomy has been backed by a temporary arteriovenous fistula to ensure rapid flow is maintained through the vital area of thrombectomized venous outlet. This has now become a valid option in centres where the necessary skill and experience are available. It is not proposed here to discuss thrombectomy in great detail and only the main principles of active intervention for venous thrombosis are outlined below.

### Intentions of thrombectomy

To remove early thrombus in iliofemoral veins before it becomes adherent in order:

1. To minimize likelihood of pulmonary embolus, potentially massive and fatal.
2. To prevent progressive damage to the venous outlet of the limb.
3. To minimize the damage to the lumen and valves in the major veins and musculovenous pumping mechanisms lower down the limb.
4. To forestall full development of phlegmasia caerulea dolens, the forerunner of venous gangrene and possible loss of the limb.
5. To relieve the severe symptoms of acute venous thrombotic obstruction.

### Preliminary assessment

Phlebography is essential to outline the state and extent of thrombus. This must include the affected limb, the iliac veins of both sides and the inferior vena cava; chest X-ray and lung scans for evidence of pulmonary embolus should be obtained. The likely cause for venous thrombosis must be investigated, particularly to exclude hidden malignancy (computer-assisted tomography to the abdomen is very helpful here) or any abnormality in coagulation.

Heparin infusion is started immediately these preliminary investigations have been completed.

## Indications for thrombectomy and alternative treatments

Thrombectomy with temporary arteriovenous fistula is particularly indicated in a young patient with a history of onset over the previous few days and demonstration by phlebology of non-adherent thrombus in the iliofemoral veins. An alternative here is treatment by thrombolysis, depending on the prevailing policy in the hospital concerned.

If the thrombus is comparatively old (over 7 days) and extensively adherent at any level in the limb, thrombolysis or thrombectomy offer little advantage over heparin-coumarin anticoagulation and, since it is the least troublesome, this should be used.

If loose thrombus is seen in iliac veins or inferior vena cava at any stage (it may be a recent, late development), its extraction by thrombectomy and/or restricting the vena cava above this level by ligation, venous clip (DeWeese, 1978) or internal filter device (Greenfield et al., 1973, 1981) is indicated in order to prevent embolism. The Greenfield filter is also indicated if pulmonary embolism occurs in spite of treatment by anticoagulants or thrombectomy.

If thrombus is confined to the popliteal and calf veins treatment at any stage by simple anticoagulation is as effective as any and should be employed. However, Bartels and Gruss (1986) have reported favourable results in 55 patients treated by thrombectomy to popliteal and crural veins; this was combined with arteriovenous fistula between the posterior tibial vessels in some cases where thrombectomy was incomplete.

### Contraindications

In the presence of an irreversible cause, such as malignancy, thrombectomy is contraindicated. In longstanding, extensively adherent thrombus, thrombectomy will not be successful and should not be employed; a bypassing procedure with Teflon prosthesis may be suitable here. In the presence of a known obstruction to the left common iliac vein, either by a spur within or from external pressure by overlying iliac artery, there is little point in thrombectomy unless it is to be combined with a procedure relieving the obstruction; however, loose clot lying above this level may require active intervention.

## Technical points

Precautions against dislodging embolus during the procedure must be taken. General anaesthesia is preferred, with endotracheal tube so that positive pressure ventilation is possible. The patient is given a moderate head-up tilt to encourage downflow in the inferior vena cava when required; in this way loose clot can be swept down the vena cava to the opened vein. Care is taken to avoid putting a clamp across a vein containing thrombus and breaking off a portion that may eventually drift upwards as a pulmonary embolus. If clamps are to be used at all they should have soft cushioned faces to minimize damage to the vein interior.

The common femoral vein on the affected side is exposed and opened by a transverse incision. Thrombus is expelled from the veins below this level by systematic two-handed pressure up the limb and by use of an Esmarch's bandage wound on firmly from the foot upwards.

## Use of a balloon (Fogarty) catheter

A balloon catheter has become indispensable in removing recent thrombus and clot from arteries and veins (Fogarty et al., 1963; Fogarty, Dennis and Krippaehne, 1966). It is introduced from above, through the clot, with the balloon deflated, and withdrawn with it inflated so that it acts as a piston pushing out clot ahead of it. However, it should not be forced downwards against the valves during its introduction. Instead a small opening is made into the lower popliteal vein, approached medially just below the knee; a silicone tube is then passed up the vein and delivered in the groin; here the tip of a balloon catheter is passed into its end so that the catheter with balloon deflated can be drawn downwards without being caught on valve cusps. When it has reached the popliteal vein the balloon is inflated appropriately and the catheter withdrawn upwards, displacing clot out of the groin incision and not opposed by valves; the silicone tube is left attached to its tip so that the process can be repeated several times. Various versions of 'tailed' catheters are available, designed to facilitate their introduction past the valves, much as just described.

Thrombus in iliac veins and the inferior vena cava is now expelled by raising intrathoracic pressure via the endotracheal tube (or by a Valsalva manoeuvre if the patient is conscious). With the intrathoracic pressure kept slightly raised the procedure is completed by passage of a large balloon catheter to obstruct the vena cava above any likely thrombus whilst a second balloon thrombectomy catheter is used to sweep down any remaining thrombus from lower vena cava and iliac veins. If thrombus is present in the iliac veins of the other side these are similarly cleared by a balloon catheter introduced through a small incision in the groin of that side.

Completeness of thrombectomy is checked by phlebography on the operating table and, if need be, further extraction of clot carried out. Desjardin's forceps can be valuable to remove areas of adherent thrombus but the comparative fragility of the veins must be kept in mind.

## Construction of an arteriovenous fistula

When all thrombus has been satisfactorily removed an arteriovenous fistula is constructed in the groin by anastomosis of a good sized branch, or the long saphenous vein itself, to the neighbouring femoral artery, or, less satisfactory, an arterial branch to the femoral vein. This is fashioned in a way to facilitate closure of the fistula some months later. Ecklof et al. (1987) close it 6 weeks later by occlusion with a detachable balloon introduced through the femoral artery under local anaesthetic. Postoperatively, heparin is continued until coumarin anticoagulation has reached satisfactory levels a few days later, and this is maintained for at least 6 months.

This is not an operation for beginners but the exponents are reporting favourable results, with an acceptably low complication rate. It is well worth reading the original papers referred to in this section. These papers also trace the development of venous thrombectomy with appropriate recognition of the contribution made by many other workers in this field. The treatment of acute deep vein thrombosis is well discussed by Browse, Burnand and Lea Thomas (1988).

## Phlegmasia cerulea dolens

(Note. Caeruleus is the Latin term used to describe the dark blue colour of the sky (caelum), and hence the English word of similar meaning, cerulean.)

Ideally iliofemoral thrombectomy will be carried out sufficiently early to prevent deterioration into the warm and swollen, blue, painful limb universally referred to by phlebologists as phlegmasia cerulea dolens (strangely, very few medical dictionaries include it). This state indicates severe obstruction to venous outflow and any further deterioration may lead to ischaemic venous gangrene (Haimovici, 1985). With this severe state, massive sequestration of blood and oedema fluid may cause hypovolaemic shock with failure of peripheral perfusion and possibly death.

With phlegmasia cerulea dolens it is likely that phlebography will show obstructive, adherent thrombus filling the iliac veins so that thrombectomy is unlikely to succeed and the opportunity to use this technique has passed. In this circumstance thrombolysis followed by prolonged anticoagulation probably offers the best prospect or, if everything points to onset more than 10 days previously, treatment by anticoagulation alone. If thrombectomy is carried out on a late case then an arteriovenous fistula should not be used since it could prove an adverse factor in limb survival if the venous outlet above is obstructed by renewed thrombosis, as is probable. Thrombectomy at this late stage should only be used to remove loose, floating thrombus detected by phlebography above the main obstruction.

With venous gangrene appropriate resuscitation to restore the blood volume may be necessary. Fasciotomy, decompressing fascial compartments above and below the knee, may be highly desirable but this should not be done if the patient is receiving thrombolytic treatment for fear of persistent haemorrhage: however, it is possible with heparin therapy alone because this can be quickly reversed by protamine sulphate if bleeding is a problem.

Every major hospital should have a team, including a surgeon, fully prepared to advise and treat this serious emergency when it arises. Such a team should have a clear policy, frequently reviewed and rehearsed; there is so much that is controversial that every centre must evolve its own policy according to local understanding and skills. The specialist in venous disorders must decide whether he is part of this team, but at least he should ensure that a suitable vascular surgical group within the hospital is acknowledged as the experts to be called upon for those cases of acute deep vein thrombosis where surgery may be desirable. A dynamic approach is needed with physician, radiologist, haematologist and surgeon all familiar with the requirements so that early assessment by phlebography and a decision upon policy of treatment can be agreed and acted upon without delay. In this way considerable morbidity and appreciable mortality can be avoided; in the light of present understanding anything less than this is inadequate.

## References

Bartels, D. and Gruss, J. D. (1986) Operative treatment of acute thrombosis of popliteal vein. In *Phlebology '85* (eds D. Negus and G. Jantet), John Libbey, London, pp. 510–511

Browse, N. L., Burnand, K. G. and Lea Thomas, M. (1988) *Diseases of the Veins*, Edward Arnold, London, pp. 501–541

Bull, H. A., Pittilo, R. M., Dury, J. *et al.* (1988) Effects of autologous mesothelial cell seeding on prostacyclin production within Dacron arterial prostheses. *British Journal of Surgery*, **75**, 671–674

DeWeese, J. A. (1978) Iliofemoral venous thrombectomy. In *Venous Problems* (eds J. J. Bergan and J. S. T. Yao), Year Book Medical, Chicago, pp. 421–435

Eklof, B., Einarsson, E. and Plate, G. (1985) Role of thrombectomy and temporary arteriovenous fistula in acute iliofemoral venous thrombosis. In *Surgery of the Veins* (eds J. J. Bergan and J. S. T. Yao), Grune and Stratton, New York, pp. 131–144

Eklof, B., Einarsson, E., Endrys, J. *et al.* (1987) Surgical treatment of iliofemoral venous thrombosis. *Phlebology*, **2**, 13–22

Fogarty, T. J., Cranley, J. J., Krause, R. J. *et al.* (1963) A method for extraction of arterial emboli and thrombi. *Surgery and Gynecology and Obstetrics*, **116**, 241–244

Fogarty, T. J., Dennis, D. and Krippaehne, W. W. (1966) Sur-

gical management of iliofemoral venous thrombosis. *American Journal of Surgery*, **112**, 211–217

Gardner, A. M. N. and Fox, R. H. (1983) The venous pump of the human foot – preliminary report. *Bristol Med-Chir J.*, 109–112

Greenfield, L. J., McCurdy, J. R., Brown, P. P. and Elkins, R. C. (1973) A new intracaval filter permitting continued flow and resolution of emboli. *Surgery*, **73**, 599–606

Greenfield, L. J., Peyton, R., Crute, S. and Barnes, R. (1981) Greenfield vena caval filter experience. *Archives of Surgery*, **I**, 1451–1455

Gruss, J. D. (1988a) Venous reconstruction. Part I. *Phlebology*, **3**, 7–18

Gruss, J. D. (1988b) Venous reconstruction. Part 2. *Phlebology*, **3**, 75–87

Haimovici, H. (1985) Treatment of ischemic deep vein thrombosis. In *Surgery of the Veins* (eds J. J. Bergan and J. S. T. Yao), Grune and Stratton, New York, pp. 165–187

Holan, V. (1971) Die luftpolsterkompresse in der therapie des ulcis cruris. *Der Hautarzt*, **22**, 345–347

Holan, V., Jiraskova, M. and Pankova, E. (1976) Hydrostatic compression – a new treatment of leg ulcers. *Vasa*, **4**, 355–359

Kistner, R. L. (1980) Primary venous valve incompetence of the leg. *American Journal of Surgery*, **140**, 218–224

Kistner, R. L. (1985) Venous valve surgery. In *Surgery of the Veins* (eds J. J. Bergan and J. S. T. Yao), Grune and Stratton, New York, pp. 205–217

Louagie, Y., Legrand-Monsieur, A., Remacle, C. *et al.* (1986) Morphology and fibrinolytic activity of canine autogenous mesothelium used as a venous substitute. *Research in Experimental Medicine*, **186**, 236–247

McMullin, G. M., Coleridge Smith, P. D. and Scurr, J. H. (1990) Evaluation of Psathakis' silastic sling procedure for deep vein reflux; a preliminary report. *Phlebology*, **5**, 95–106

Mavor, G. E. (1971) Surgery of deep vein thrombosis. *British Journal of Hospital Medicine*, December, 755–764

Mavor, G. E. and Galloway, J. M. D. (1969) Iliofemoral venous thrombosis. Pathological considerations and surgical management. *British Journal of Surgery*, **56**, 45–59

Nicholson, L. J., Clarke, J. M. F., Pittilo, R. M. *et al.* (1984) The mesothelial cell as a non-thrombogenic surface. *Thrombosis and Haemostasis*, **52**, 2511–2514

Psathakis, N. D. (1968) Has the 'substitute valve' at the popliteal vein solved the problem of venous insufficiency of the lower extremity? *Journal of Cardiovascular Surgery*, **9**, 64–70

Psathakis, N. D. and Psathakis, D. N. (1985) Rationale of the substitute 'valve' operation by technique II in the treatment of chronic venous insufficiency. *International Angiology*, **4**, 397–412

Ribbe, E. F. B., Alm, P., Hallberg, E. and Norgren, L. E. H. (1988a) Evaluation of peritoneal tube grafts in the inferior vena cava of the pig. *British Journal of Surgery*, **75**, 357–360

Ribbe, E. F. B., Jonsson, B. A., Norgren, L. E. H. *et al.* (1988b) Platelet aggregation on peritoneal tube grafts and double velour grafts in the inferior vena cava of the pig. *British Journal of Surgery*, **75**, 81–85

Taheri, S. A., Lazar, L., Elias, S. M. *et al.* (1982a) Surgical treatment of postphlebitic syndrome with vein valve transplant. *American Journal of Surgery*, **144**, 221–224

Taheri, S. A., Lazar, L., Elias, S. M. and Marchand, P. (1982b) Vein valve transplant. *Surgery*, **91**, 28–31

Taheri, S. A., Heffner, R., Meenaghan, M. A. *et al.* (1985a) Technique and results of venous valve transplantation. In *Surgery of the Veins* (eds J. J. Bergan and J. S. T. Yao), Grune and Stratton, New York, pp. 219–231

Taheri, S. A., Heffner, R., Meenaghan, M. A. *et al.* (1985b) Vein valve transplant. *International Angiology*, **4**, 425

Tibbs, D. J. and Fletcher, E. W. L. (1983) Direction of flow in superficial veins as a guide to venous disorders in lower limbs. *Surgery*, **93**, 758–767

Zetterquist, S., Hagglof, R., Jacobsson, H. *et al.* (1986) Long-term results of thrombectomy with temporary arteriovenous fistula for iliofemoral venous thrombosis. *Phlebology*, **1**, 113–117

## Bibliography

Clarke, J. M. F., Pittilo, R. M. and Machin, S. J. (1984) A study of the possible role of mesothelium as a surface for flowing blood. *Thrombosis and Haemostasis*, **51**, 57–60

Dale, W. A. (1979) Reconstructive venous surgery. *Archives of Surgery*, **114**, 1312–1318

Gardner, A. M. N. and Fox, R. H. (1989) *The Return of Blood to the Heart: Venous Pumps in Health and Disease*, John Libbey, London

Husni, E. A. (1970) In situ saphenopopliteal bypass graft for incompetence of the femoral and popliteal veins. *Surgery, Gynecology and Obstetrics*, **130**, 279

Husni, E. A. (1978) Clinical experience with femoropopliteal venous reconstruction. In *Venous Problems* (eds J. J. Bergan and J. S. T. Yao), Year Book Medical, Chicago, pp. 485–491

Ijima, H., Hirabayashi, K., Sakakibara, Y., Tsutsui, T., Mitsui, T. and Hori, M. (1990) Results of femoro–femoral vein bypass grafting with temporary arteriovenous fistula for femoro-iliac venous thrombosis: differences between operations in the acute and chronic phases. *Phlebology*, **5**, 237–244

McMullin, G. M., Coleridge Smith, P. D. and Scurr, J. H. (1990) Evaluation of Psathakis' silastic sling procedure for deep vein reflux: a preliminary report. *Phlebology*, **5**, 95–106

May, R. (1972) Der femoralisbypass beim postthrombotischen zustandsbild. *Vasa*, **1**, 267

May, R. (1972) Venentransplantation beim postthrombotishen zustandsbild. *Actuelle Chir*, **7**, 1

May, R. and Nissl, R. (1979) The post-thrombotic syndrome. In *Surgery of the Veins of the Leg and Pelvis* (ed. R. May), Saunders, Philadelphia; Georg Thieme, Stuttgart, pp. 135–157

Psathakis, N. D. and Psathakis, D. N. (1986) The substitute valve operation by technique II and venous pressure measurements. In *Phlebology '85* (eds D. Negus and G. Jantet), John Libbey, London, pp. 704–706

Psathakis, N. D. and Psathakis, D. N. (1986) Substitute valve operation by technique II in post-thrombotic syndrome. In *Phlebology '85* (eds D. Negus and G. Jantet), John Libbey, London, pp. 707–710

Psathakis, N. D. and Psathakis, D. N. (1988) Surgical treatment of deep venous insufficiency of the lower limb. *Surgery, Gynacology and Obstetrics*, **166**, 131–141

Shen, D. (1989) A new haemostatic instrument: Shen's ring-form haemostatic compressor. *Phlebology*, **4**, 55–56

Sottiurai, V. S. (1991) Incompetent transplanted arm vein valves: surgical correction and result. *Phlebology*, **6**, 41–46

Thompson, J. N., Paterson-Brown, S., Harbourne, T. *et al.* (1989) Reduced human peritoneal plasminogen activating activity: possible mechanism of adhesion formation. *British Journal of Surgery*, **76**, 382–384

Wilson, N. M., Rutt, D. L. and Browse, N. L. (1991) Repair and replacement of deep vein valves in the treatment of venous insufficiency. *British Journal of Surgery*, **78**, 388–394

Wilson, N. M., Rutt, D. L. and Browse, N. L. (1991) In situ venous valve construction. *British Journal of Surgery*, **78**, 595–600

Vohra, R., Thomson, G. J. L., Carr, H. M. H., Sharma, H. and Walker, M. G. (1991) Comparison of different vascular prostheses and matrices in relationship to endothelial seeding. *British Journal of Surgery*, **78**, 417–420

# 22

# Functional phlebography in venous disorders of the lower limbs

The value of phlebography in venous disorders of the lower limbs has been transformed by a number of factors in recent years. These include: an increased understanding of the patterns of venous disorder and how to display them; the prolonged viewing possible with an image intensifier; the use of non-irritant low osmolar contrast medium which allows larger volumes to be used in safety. Highly sophisticated techniques based on digitalized, computerized venography are being developed and alternative techniques for imaging veins, such as duplex scanning and colour flow ultrasonography, are improving all the time. This account cannot include the complete range that is available and each radiologist will have to develop his technique according to the apparatus available to him. The basic fact is that it is now possible, with safety and virtually no discomfort to the patient, to outline the veins and their valves in the lower limb, and by watching the patterns of flow in various circumstances obtain a good demonstration of overall function. Satisfactory results can be obtained with standard X-ray equipment available in most medical centres and the description that follows is based upon our experience using such apparatus. If more sophisticated apparatus is available, then the principles that are described will be equally applicable but with the advantage that detailed information will be more easily obtained. All current techniques suffer from the disadvantage of giving either a very limited area of detailed viewing at any one moment, or a much bigger field but lacking detail, for example, by gamma camera venography. Detail is essential in most cases and the radiologist has to view the quickly changing scene at venography through a number of 'windows' by re-centring his apparatus repeatedly. In this way a series of views are seen on the screen and a permanent record is provided, either by a number of static films or as a videotape, to give very comprehensive information. It does, however, require good judgement by the radiologist to choose his 'windows' suitably and there is considerable variation in the density with which neighbouring veins are recorded due to changes in the concentration of contrast

medium with flow. Future development of computerized techniques should allow a complete view of both lower limbs so that repeated changing of the field is not necessary, but until this is available functional phlebography requires constant readjustment of the viewpoint to match the changing phases of flow. However, the information gives a very rewarding understanding of the state of the veins. The examination must be conducted in an orderly fashion and according to certain principles if good results are to be obtained. It is entirely suitable as an outpatient procedure and is usually completed within 30 minutes.

## The principles of functional phlebography

The examination proceeds by three phases: the first is a filling phase, during which the patient stands still and, in the normal patient, the deep veins fill steadily; in the second phase the pumping mechanism is activated by the patient moving several times and demonstrates the way in which venous blood circulates in the limb. This will not, however, give much information upon the distribution of valves and so, in the third phase, the patient is tilted to near-horizontal and back again in order to swill opacified blood upwards and then downwards against the valves in the now deflated veins. Other special manoeuvres can also be carried out at this phase.

Certain principles are of fundamental importance if this rather complex examination is to be successful and these will now be considered.

### Briefing the radiologist

It is unreasonable to expect the radiologist to give a comprehensive demonstration of the veins when the examination so often only gives one opportunity for a brief view of an essential flow pattern before it is submerged by a general outlining of all the veins in the vicinity. Repeating a manoeuvre may be possible but only if this does not require an unacceptable quantity of contrast medium to be used. The radiologist has to concentrate on the most likely phenomena in that particular patient. He must know the nature of the venous problem and those aspects upon which the surgeon particularly wants clarification. The clearest of briefings should be given to the radiologist but, perhaps best of all, the surgeon should be present together with the radiologist during functional phlebography. In this way the limited duration of the examination is used to best advantage and priority can be given to looking for defects in the venous system that explain the findings on clinical examination, Doppler flowmetry and plethysmography.

### Use of a low osmolar contrast medium

Contrast media of low osmolality are non-irritant to veins, so that their use causes virtually no discomfort and subsequent phlebitis is rare; at moderate concentration, a relatively large volume can be used, allowing both limbs to be viewed at the same session. These features, together with a low incidence of reaction by the patient, make this type of medium an essential choice for phlebography. Further details are given below in the section on 'Technical aspects'.

### Use of the image intensifier

The electronic image intensifier has given a great improvement in phlebography over the last few years. It permits prolonged viewing of the patient without risk of radiation overdosage and in this way all stages can be monitored almost continuously. The steady filling of the veins with opacified blood and the patterns of flow, either passive or in response to exercise, can be closely observed and the best moment for static film exposures chosen. The sequence of events during phlebography moves so quickly and is so detailed that it certainly cannot be reliably remembered and a permanent record of key events must be obtained. Careful study and piecing together of the static films after the examination often reveals extra details and is a clear reminder of events. Videotape can also be used but the frequent change in the area under view can make it difficult to interpret later on unless it is accompanied by some system of location with each new situation. This can be by simultaneous recorded commentary or by visual markers but it is to be hoped that new techniques will be developed giving a large area of viewing and provide an ideal combination with videotape. In the meantime a series of static film shots gives an adequate record of the essential findings.

Although the image intensifier is essential for functional phlebography and removes the need for much guesswork, it does suffer from the limitation of viewing a large area through a series of small windows. This is overcome to a considerable extent by constant movement of the viewing screen to keep the entire limb under observation and to pick up special events for more prolonged viewing and recording.

### Avoidance of constricting bands or tourniquets

Any form of constricting band or tourniquet is avoided during the examination, except as a final manoeuvre in special circumstances. In the recent past there has been widespread use of constricting bands in phlebography (Figure 22.1), but this is not compatible with functional venography. A band can only derange the usual venous function, conceal many abnormalities and distort venous anatomy. Its use is only acceptable when all aspects of venous function have been fully assessed by the earlier parts of the examination. In this connection a distinction must be made between functional phlebography and a

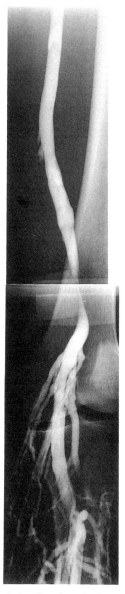

**Figure 22.1** *Constricting band applied just above knee level during phlebology. Its effect is evident and this is not compatible with any study of the usual venous function in that limb*

passive outlining of clot within deep veins with the patient lying horizontally.

## Positioning the needle

In most cases any readily accessible vein on the leg below the knee may be used, with some distension given by a moderate head-up tilt. This will usually be a saphenous vein or one of its branches; varicosities may be used but their shape is irregular and the walls fragile so that the needle is easily dislodged and it is preferable to use a more robust vein. If it is known from Doppler examination that deep vein impairment is likely then a foot vein may give the best opportunity to outline the deep veins. Similarly, if it is clear at an early stage of the examination that the deep veins are not being filled and all the contrast medium is passing up the saphenous vein, the needle should be changed to the foot. Calf veins are usually chosen for the first insertion because they are easier targets and less sensitive than foot veins which also can be very elusive; moreover they allow demonstration of superficial downflow in response to exercise. Certainly, there is no difficulty in outlining unobstructed deep veins from a superficial calf vein.

## The upright position

Venous problems only become significant when the patient is upright and it is essential that the patient is examined in this position. Valves have virtually no function in the lying position and their state cannot be satisfactorily assessed in the horizontal limb. When the patient is upright the influence of gravity is maximal and any failure of venous return will become evident; vein walls and valve rings are fully distended by venous pressure so that the valves are being tested under the conditions most likely to reveal any weakness. For the purposes of functional phlebography, it is sufficient to use a near-upright position with the patient resting securely against a table inclined to, say, 60 degrees or more (Figure 22.2). In this way patterns of abnormal flow that would not otherwise occur will be seen.

## Exercise to cause venous return

When the patient is upright but remaining still, the deep veins will fill to maximal capacity with a slow upward drift of blood. Contrast medium will outline the anatomy and general form of the veins but little is learnt about the function. For venous return to occur blood must be displaced by muscular contraction and, in the normal state, valves will prevent it from falling back. Many patterns of abnormal flow, especially those derived from valve failure, will not occur unless there is some muscular activity or change in posture in the lower limb. It is an essential part of functional phlebography that at some

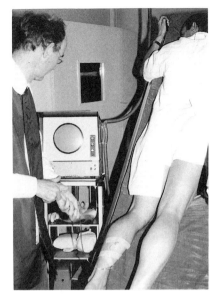

**Figure 22.2** *Functional phlebology being carried out with the patient in a near-upright position. The spread of opaque medium is watched on the image intensifier and key features are recorded by static X-ray film*

stage the patient should be asked to move, usually by rising up on the toes and down again several times. At this moment the examination passes from being a simple anatomical demonstration to one showing both normal and abnormal function within the venous system. Moreover, a much more complete anatomical demonstration is obtained as opacified blood is shifted into previously static veins.

## The swill test for valves

Exercise by the patient is stopped before too much contrast medium is dispersed from the limb; the table is then lowered quickly to a near-horizontal position until the major veins in the upper part show distinct reduction in width due to the fall in venous pressure. At this stage the table is quickly brought up again to 60 degrees or more so that there is a sharp downward movement of blood against the valves throughout the limb. In this way the valve cusps in a considerable part of the venous system will be shown clearly with a good indication of their competence. This phase soon passes as an upward drift of blood recommences and presses the valve cusps back to become invisible against the vein walls. However, there is time enough to make a series of static exposures down the limb for permanent record.

Other manoeuvres may be carried out, such as upward trace varicography or, in special circumstances, the application of localized compression used to close off selected veins and direct blood into veins suspected of not filling with the manoeuvres carried out so far. These will usually be abnormal veins made virtual cul-de-sacs by obstruction higher up. However, any selective compression of this sort must be left to the very end of the examination because it will cause a distortion of the usual flow patterns within the limb which may disguise the true state of affairs. This is permissible when all other information has been gathered and there are special reasons for it. It can be a valuable addition to the technique of examination and further reference will be made to this later.

## Indications for functional phlebography

Functional phlebography is usually carried out to give the surgeon guidance along the following broad lines:

- To confirm that the condition is surgically curable, for example, simple superficial incompetence.
- To give guidance over the details of surgery, for example, disposition of a short saphenous termination.
- To ensure that the surgeon is not missing an opportunity to help the patient, as in concealed saphenous incompetence.
- To confirm that it is a post-thrombotic state and unlikely to benefit by surgery. This is an important decision that must be backed by good evidence.

If the problem is one of uncomplicated varicosities from superficial vein incompetence, phlebography is seldom necessary. Here, the clinical examination, supported by special diagnostic tests, will usually give a clear diagnosis of superficial vein incompetence. However, when severe venotensive changes with threatened or actual ulceration are present then phlebography is usually desirable, or indeed essential, for one or more of the following reasons:

1. To confirm that the deep veins are widely open without any deformity due to previous thrombosis and that surgery to the superficial veins is therefore unlikely to do harm.
2. To confirm that massive superficial incompetence, as shown by gravitational downflow, is present.
3. To identify the source of this downflow. This is of particular importance in recurrent varicosities.
4. To ensure that a clinically concealed state of saphenous incompetence is not being overlooked.
5. To know the valve state of the deep veins as this may have considerable bearing upon future management, for example, the use of elastic stockings after surgery.
6. To know if the predominant diagnosis is one of valveless deep veins; here surgery to superficial veins may achieve little.
7. To estimate the extent of pooling within the foot and the importance of varicosities running onto the foot.
8. To detect obstruction in the deep veins, usually the result of deep vein thrombosis in the past. Here the surgeon may do harm by removing superficial veins and the important decision to be made is whether a cure can be offered to the patient, or only a system of rather tedious conservative care for life.

9. To identify any case suitable for deep vein reconstruction and to plan the appropriate operation. Very few patients fall into this category and the operation should only be carried out by a specialist in this field.
10. To ensure that active thrombosis, with recent clot, is not present. If it is, then surgery is usually contraindicated and the significance of thrombosis will require full assessment.

During the investigation of oedema it may be necessary to exclude venous obstruction as a cause. Phlebography can be very effective but it should not be a routine examination in all cases; simpler examinations, such as photoplethysmography, can usually indicate if phlebography is advisable (see Chapter 14) or if assessment of the lymphatics by radioactive isotope uptake is a more appropriate next step.

## Technical aspects

### Apparatus required

- Standard X-ray equipment with image intensifier, suitable for prolonged viewing, and having the ability to take static films or video recordings.
- The table must be able to tilt from horizontal to vertical and have a good longitudinal movement.
- The X-ray head must be capable of mobility from the subject's feet up to the pelvis and over the full width of both limbs.
- A platform, fixed to the table under the patient's feet, to give support when in a vertical position; this should allow the patient to exercise by rising on the toes and to turn in either direction for rotated views.
- No. 18 or 20 'butterfly' needle and connecting tube, with an additional 1 m length of extension tubing from this to the syringe.
- Two 50 ml syringes for contrast medium; filling quill; Micropore adhesive tape for fixing 'butterfly' needle and anchoring its tubing.
- Heparinized normal saline (1000 units to 500 ml) and 25 ml syringe for use with this.

### Contrast medium

This should be low osmolar and known to be trouble free. The authors' preference is iohexol (Omnipaque, Nycomed (UK) Ltd); a concentration of 240 mg l/ml is most suitable and usually up to 150 ml will be required per limb; if both limbs are examined a total of 350 ml should not be exceeded.

**Precautions** The patient should be fit and well hydrated. Pregnancy should be excluded. A history of allergy or of any previous reaction to contrast media should be enquired for; if present, and phlebography is considered essential, give 100 mg of hydrocortisone slowly intravenously beforehand, or, at least, ensure hydro-cortisone and antihistamine are available for immediate use intravenously. Although a severe general reaction is very rare the means for resuscitation should be close by, including endotracheal tube, larynogoscope and suction.

### Insertion of the needle

During insertion of the needle the patient is tilted to 45 degrees to give moderate distension of the veins. If difficulty is found in locating a suitable vein, the foot and ankle should be immersed in a basin of warm water for 5 minutes. Any convenient vein on the calf may be used and should either be entered from one side, or, from the front with a definite lifting action so that the vein is not flattened by the point which then passes right through it instead of entering the lumen. When the needle is satisfactorily placed it is taped in position; care is taken not to fix it with its bevel pressed against the inner aspect of vein wall since this will not allow free flow, especially when aspirating, and will easily puncture its way out of the vein. It is often convenient to use a varicose vein but its irregular outline and fragile walls make the needle prone to pierce its way out of the vein so that extra care will be required.

### Abortive needle puncture

Puncturing a vein but failing to enter its lumen satisfactorily will cause extravasation of blood into the perivenous adventitia and local contraction of the vein. This will certainly narrow, or even completely block, the vein temporarily so that, with reinsertion of the needle nearby, demonstration of flow patterns by opaque medium in the superficial veins nearby is spoiled (Figures 22.3, 22.7(f), 22.21(c)). Often this is of no great consequence but clean entry into a vein without transfixion is desirable.

### Elimination of air

A small air bubble may be harmless (Figure 22.4) but complete elimination of air in the injection system should be carried out as a consistent routine at all stages; only in this way can the possibility of accidental massive injection of air be minimized.

### Extravasation of opacified blood at site of venepuncture

The injection of saline or of contrast medium should not cause any pain, nor should it raise any bulge locally. If the patient complains of pain whilst medium is being injected, check by the X-ray screen to see if contrast is collecting around the vein (Figure 22.5); in this case the only satisfactory remedy is to change the needle to a separate vein several inches away if possible. Extravasation around a vein will narrow its lumen to give an

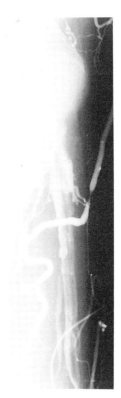

**Figure 22.3**  *Effect of abortive needle puncture in branch of long saphenous vein of upper calf. Infiltration of blood around the vein and contraction of its muscle have almost blocked the lumen and this portion of vein cannot be relied on to show its usual flow patterns*

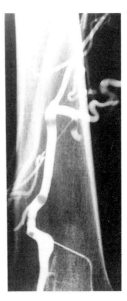

**Figure 22.4**  *Air bubbles inadvertently injected during phlebography. The amount shown here may be harmless but should be avoided. Constant vigilance is necessary to safeguard against air embolism and elimination of all air in the injection apparatus must be carried out as a routine at every stage*

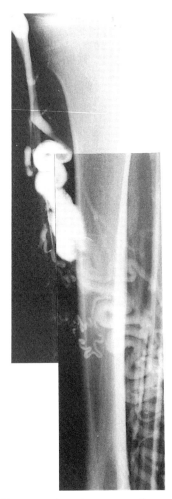

**Figure 22.5** *Extravasation of opaque medium outside the vein. The patient complained of discomfort and the varicosity into which the needle was inserted had become unnaturally dense, with a fuzzy outline. Once this has happened it is best to abandon this site and reintroduce the needle elsewhere*

abnormal appearance which must be allowed for if it is visualized by re-entering the same vein at a different level.

*Effect of exercise*

Remember that when the patient exercises the contrast medium is rapidly dispersed. This can either lead to insufficient contrast to display veins, or by spreading into multiple veins, give a very confused picture. Instructions to exercise must therefore be concise in the number of times it is to be repeated and no unnecessary movement is requested. It is best to rehearse this with the patient before injection begins.

*The sequence of examination in functional phlebography*

This is summarized diagrammatically in Figure 22.6 together with an indication of some of the main flow patterns likely to be seen. These and other features are described in more detail in the next section.

## Features to be looked for during functional phlebography

*Preliminary check on direction of flow in a superficial calf vein*

The needle is usually inserted in an accessible vein in the calf region. This may well be an abnormally enlarged or varicose vein and after an initial injection of 5 ml of contrast medium a check is made upon the direction of flow within the vein at rest and in response to calf muscle contraction. When the patient is standing still, the medium will drift downwards, largely because its specific gravity is greater than that of blood (Figures 22.7(a), 22.20), but when the patient gives a single movement the blood moves rapidly downwards and may be seen entering, through perforating veins, the deep veins lower down (Figure 22.7(b)–(f)). This is diagnostic of simple incompetence in the superficial veins. On the other hand upward flow in a superficial vein, whether it is the saphenous vein itself or a branch, suggests preferential flow up that vein because it is being used as a collateral past an occluded deep vein (Figure 22.8). In this case exercise will cause a rapid acceleration of blood up the superficial vein.

**Outlining the deep veins by passive filling** After using only a small quantity of medium to show the direction of flow in superficial veins, the patient is asked to stand still whilst 100–150 ml of contrast medium are infused steadily. In most cases this will give an ascending outline of the deep veins right up to the pelvis (Figure 22.9). This moves only slowly and remains unchanged for quite a prolonged period, provided the patient does not move. When this column has fully developed and includes the iliac veins, then a series of static film exposures are made up the length of the limb to record the outline of the deep veins. If the deep veins are widely open throughout, so that there is no impedence to blood travelling up them, then few branches will be shown, the valve cusps will not be evident and superficial veins will be shown only in the lower leg. This phase gives a demonstration of the state of the deep veins and will confirm that they are either widely open, or deformed and possibly obstructed, usually by post-thrombotic changes (Figure 22.12). Failure of the principal deep conduit veins to fill is strongly suggestive of obstruction in them and this is particularly so if at this stage the long saphenous vein is outlined by flow travelling up it in preference to the deep veins.

*Abnormality indicated by shape*

**Tortuosity** This is the most common visible manifestation of abnormality in veins, both at clinical examination

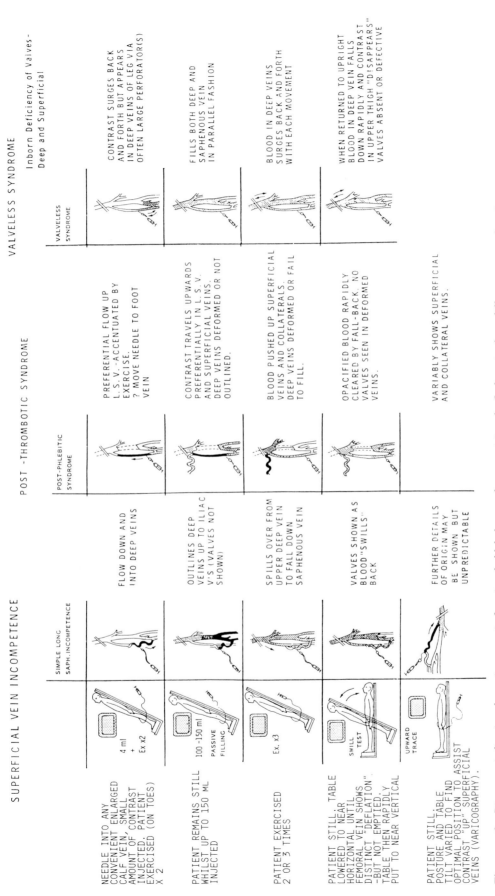

**Figure 22.6** *Diagrams indicating the main stages in functional phlebology and summarizing the findings in three different venous disorders*

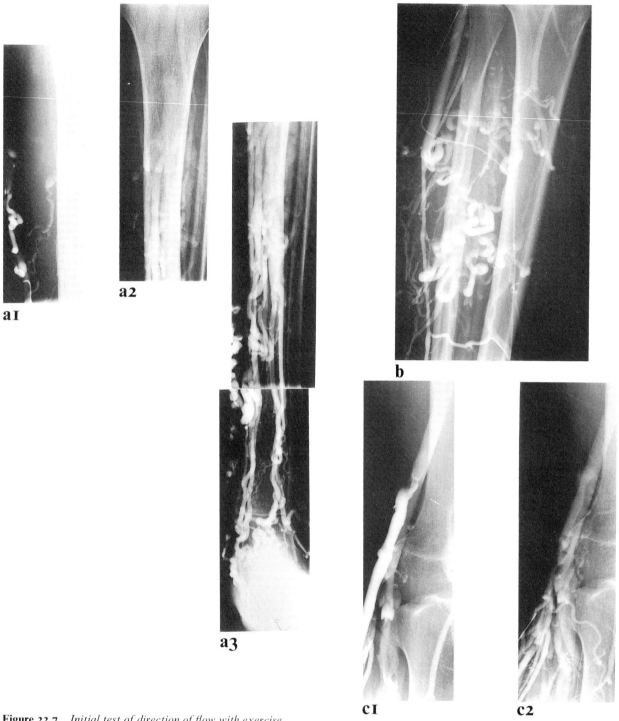

**Figure 22.7**   *Initial test of direction of flow with exercise.*

*(a)  1. A small quantity of opaque medium has been injected into a long saphenous varicosity on the leg and because of its higher specific gravity it tends to drift downwards.*
*2. After one exercise movement, rising on the toes, it appears in the tibial veins.*
*3. With further injection and a movement the medium has moved swiftly down and is seen entering deep veins through a perforator and also running down superficial veins to the foot. Such downward and inward flow is characteristic of superficial vein incompetence; flow runs to low pressure areas beneath any pumping mechanism, including the foot.*

*(b)  Injection needle is in a short saphenous vein in the upper part of the picture and about 8 ml of medium has been injected, followed by an exercise movement. This has swept the opacified blood through the varicosities and it can be seen beginning to appear in the deep veins in mid-leg.*

*(c)  1. Short saphenous vein well outlined by medium with patient standing still.*
*2. After a single movement the saphenous vein has emptied with a corresponding increase in the deep veins outlined.*

**Figure 22.7** *(continued)*

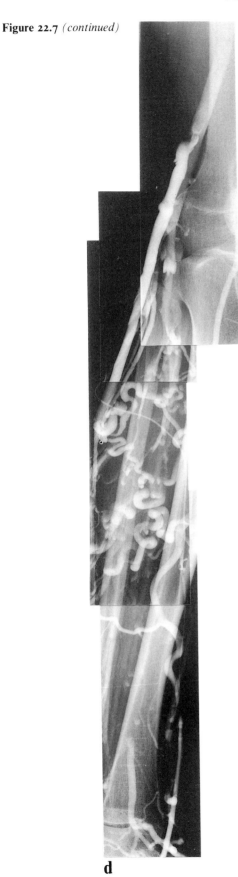

**d**

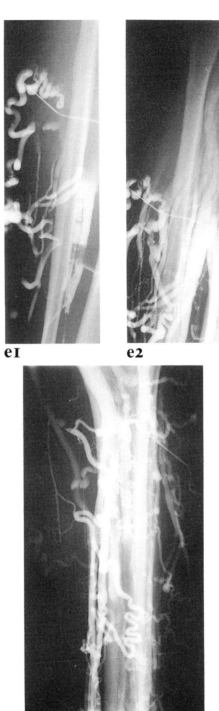

**eI**          **e2**

**f**

*(e)   Short saphenous varicose veins in two phases of filling. The inward flow from the superficial to deep veins through a paired perforator is clearly outlined.*

*(f)   Long saphenous varicosities on the front of the leg. The saphenous vein itself is showing only faintly because the branch running to it has been obstructed by an abortive needle puncture (in upper left of picture). The needle has been transferred to a vein nearby (near top central) and medium injected here has flowed down varicosities on the front of the leg and into paired posterior tibial and other deep veins.*

*In all these illustrations the inward flow through perforators to deep veins is a normal phenomenon and does not indicate that the perforators are at fault*

*(d)   A composite phlebogram giving a display of the short saphenous termination, the varicosities arising from it and running down to the foot. This gives valuable guidance to the surgeon.*

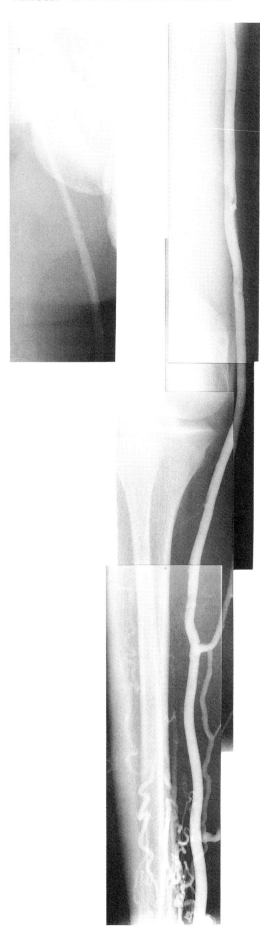

**Figure 22.8** *Preferential upflow in superficial veins in extensive deep vein occlusion due to recent acute deep vein thrombosis. Opaque medium has been injected into a prominent vein on the foot and shows strong preferential upflow in the long saphenous vein without any tendency to enter the deep veins, even with active exercise. The long saphenous vein is shown from ankle to mid-thigh and, in the smaller picture, near to the groin again shows the same strong upflow without any filling of the deep veins (see Figure 24.6 for further details)*

and on phlebography (Figure 22.10(a)). It indicates the presence of one or a combination of these factors:

- Intermittent or constant flow in reverse to the natural direction.
- Exposure to unnaturally high pressure either constantly or as intermittent peaks.
- Inherent weakness in the veins.

It is usually accompanied by valve failure which may be either the cause or the result of unnatural flow. The strongest superficial veins, the saphenous veins, seldom develop tortuosity, nor do the major deep veins. When tortuous 'deep' veins are seen they are likely to be lesser veins that have taken on a collateral role, compensating for obstruction in a neighbouring major deep vein.

**Deformity in veins** An irregular, narrowed lumen is usually the result of previous thrombosis in that vein and may be seen in either superficial or deep veins (Figures 22.10(b), 22.12(a)–(d)). The thrombosis is likely to have damaged valve cusps in the vicinity so that it is usually accompanied by incompetence.

**Saccule formation** This is commonly seen in the saphenous veins immediately below a heavily leaking valve cusp (Figure 22.10(c)–(e)). Whether this is cause or effect is not certain but its presence indicates incompetence in the valves of that vein. It is also seen in states of inherent weakness of the vein wall. Any varicose vein shows 'sacculation' when straightened out and this is discussed under pseudosacculation in Chapter 1.

*Response to exercise*

**1. Spillover from deep to superficial veins** If the deep veins are widely open a rapid viewing of the full width of the limb is made at this stage to observe the degree of filling in superficial veins. The patient is then asked to exercise three times whilst the uppermost termination of the long saphenous vein is kept in view. At this stage spillover of blood from the common femoral to the long saphenous vein may be seen (Figure 22.11(a), (b)) and may continue downwards to outline varicosities. The contrast medium will be diluted considerably by the blood already in the saphenous vein and will often outline only weakly, but this spillover phenomenon is characteristic of long saphenous incompetence. It may, of course, be seen at other sites, for example, at a large perforator in mid-thigh (Figure 22.11(c)), in the short saphenous vein (Figure 22.7(b)), from pelvic veins (Figure 22.11(d)), or from any combination of these sources (Figure 22.11(e)), and

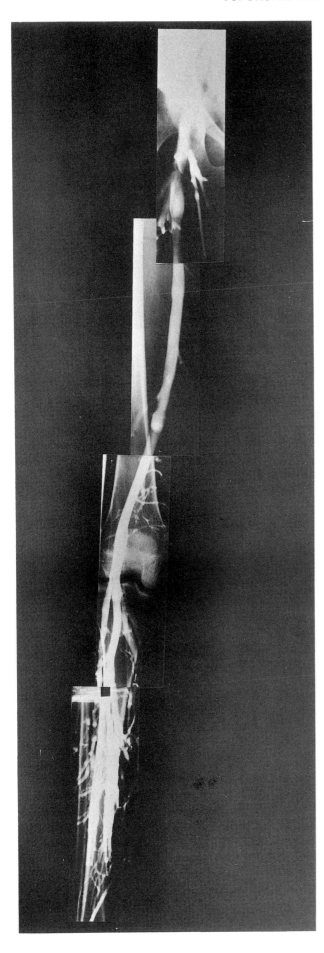

**Figure 22.9.**  *Passive filling of the deep veins. With the patient remaining still, at a head-up tilt of 60 degrees, 100 ml of opaque medium has been injected into a calf vein. This has progressively filled the principal deep veins up to the iliac region. In this position, without movement, filling of the major deep veins will always occur provided they are normal, without deformity or obstruction. They fill by a passive upward drift of blood and this is not dependent on valves. With a normal set of deep vein valves any movement rapidly expels the opacified blood upwards. The valves can be displayed by a subsequent manoeuvre, the swill test, shown in later figures*

**Figure 22.10**  *Abnormality indicated by shape.*

*(a) Tortuosity, shown here in a vein interconnecting between a short saphenous stump and long saphenous system. This developed within 18 months of an inadequately performed ligation of the short saphenous vein. Tortuosity such as this indicates intermittent or continuous flow in the reverse to natural direction for that vein; peaks of excessively high pressure may have the same effect. It is by far the commonest evidence of abnormal function in a vein seen on clinical examination or at phlebography.*

*(b) 1. A deformed and sacculated short saphenous vein in the popliteal fossa. Just before it enters the popliteal vein it is seen to be sacculated but below this its outline is grossly irregular.*
*2. The same vein opened after surgical removal. The upper part is sacculated (possibly a form of early tortuosity – see Chapter 1, section on 'Pseudosacculation in tortuous veins'), a change often found near the termination of an incompetent short saphenous vein. Beneath this, the vein shows an irregular interior with synechiae bridging the lumen; this type of deformity suggests that at some stage this portion of the vein has been thrombosed but recanalized (see page 286).*

*(c) 1. Opaque medium has been injected into a short saphenous vein just below the knee. This has outlined the vein and a varicosity arising from it. In its lower part a large saccule is present.*
*2. The same vein opened after surgery to show the interior*

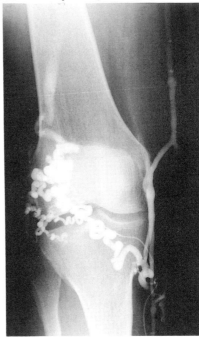

**a**

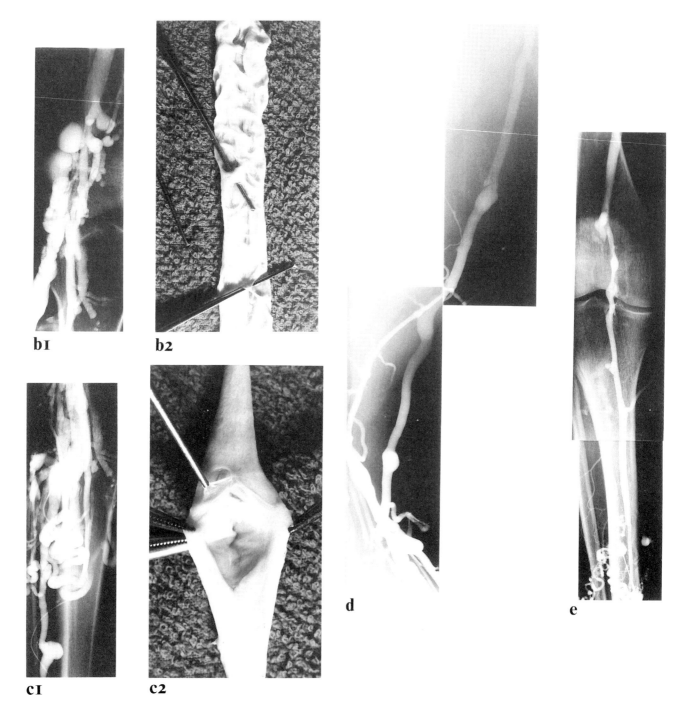

bi          b2

ci          c2

d                                    e

**Figure 22.10** *(continued)*

    *of the saccule and neighbouring vein. The saccule has collapsed to give a folded appearance; this lies beneath a pair of valve cusps, one of which is lifted by forceps. Such saccules are commonly found beneath an incompetent valve in a saphenous vein and confirm its incompetence.*

*(d) Saccules in the long saphenous vein. In the upper one, in the mid-thigh, a single valve cusp has been caught in profile and can be clearly seen with the saccule beneath it. Its corresponding second cusp is not evident and such loss of symmetry is in keeping with incompetence. Towards the lower part of the saphenous vein another saccule is seen but its details are obscured by the density of medium within it.*

*(e) A saccule on the short saphenous vein just below the knee. Within the saccule a thin curved band is seen but this is likely to be the mouth of the saccule rather than a cusp. Further sacculation is present behind the knee, and in the lower part of the picture varicosities can be seen arising from the saphenous vein. This picture was obtained by varicography with the patient near horizontal and is therefore not demonstrating function but does display typical features of incompetence. Transferring the patient to near vertical and requesting an exercise movement would immediately show the typical downflow of superficial incompetence, a demonstration of function*

**Figure 22.11**   *Response to exercise in upright position. Spillover from a high-level source.*

*(a)  Spillover from deep to superficial veins seen at the long saphenous termination.*

> *1. The patient is near vertical and the deep veins have been allowed to fill passively. An exercise movement has just been carried out and the saphenous vein is showing faintly.*
> *2. With a second movement, opacified blood has moved up the deep veins and can be seen streaming down the long saphenous vein which is now well outlined. This spillover is characteristic of a source of incompetent superficial downflow.*

*(b)  A further example of spillover from common femoral to saphenous vein.*

> *1. A picture taken after passive filling of the deep veins.*
> *2. After two exercise movements opacified blood has moved up the femoral vein and can be seen spilling over and down an enlarged long saphenous vein, eventually outlining varicosities in the lower thigh.*

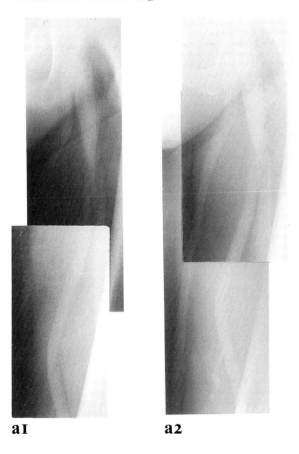

**a1**          **a2**

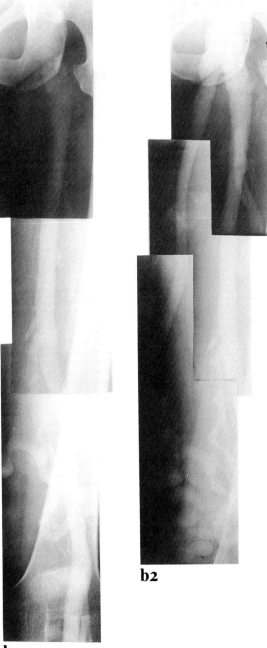

**b1**

**b2**

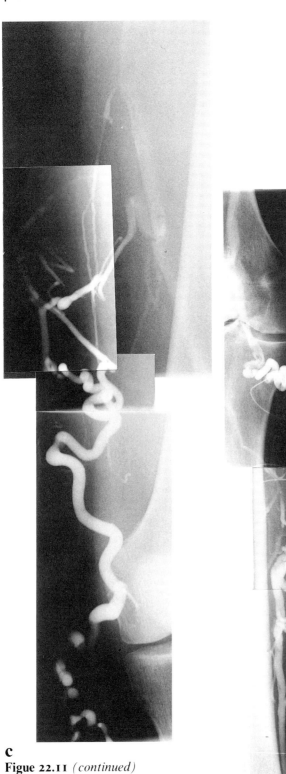

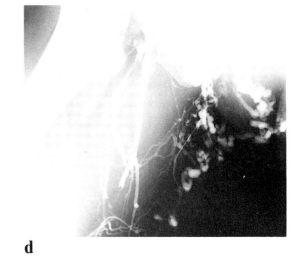

**d**

**c**

**Figue 22.11** *(continued)*

**e**

*(c) Spillover from a mid-thigh perforating vein entering varicose remnants of a long saphenous system left by a previous operation.*

*(d) Less usual sources of incompetence. Clinical examination suggested the source of incompetence in this patient was the internal pudendal vein. This picture was obtained by varicography and shows inflow to the internal pudendal vein, but when given a head-up tilt, downward movement of the opacified blood, in keeping with the suspected diagnosis, was evident.*

*(e) Filling from two sources is less usual but certainly occurs. This patient had massive varicose veins on the inner aspect of the calf which were shown to fill from the short saphenous vein. However, Doppler flowmetry had also shown downflow after exercise in the long saphenous vein in the thigh; during phlebography this was looked for and the spillover down this vein is shown in the upper picture. Both saphenous veins are acting as sources of incompetence to the same varicose veins*

clinical examination beforehand will usually have given a clear indication of the likelihood of this, so that X-ray examination is specifically directed to the most likely sites for spillover to occur. In the case of recurrent varicosities, tortuous veins filling by the same spillover phenomena may be seen connecting with remnants of the saphenous system (Figure 22.11(c)). Other indications of saphenous incompetence will be the presence of gross sacculation positioned immediately below valve cusps and signifying their incompetence; the cusps do not necessarily show up well at this stage (Figure 22.10(c)–(e)).

**2. Accentuation of preferential upflow in superficial veins** This strongly suggests that they are acting as collaterals because of deep vein obstruction. This will be supported by failure of the deep veins to fill at some level or gross deformity in them (Figure 22.12). With normal deep veins there is no difficulty in filling and outlining them throughout the limb, using the technique described. If these veins have not filled, and are not outlined by the swill test that follows, then a final effort to display them must be made by use of local compression or a constricting band (Figure 22.12(b)–(d)) over the principal superficial collateral veins, but this may interfere with underlying deep veins so that its positioning requires thought. Further exercise may be carried out at this stage.

**3. Surge with little upward propulsion** This is seen in an overall deficiency of deep vein valves (valveless syndrome) and is often accompanied by a filling of the long saphenous veins in parallel with the deep vein during the preceding phase of passive filling. With calf muscle contraction the blood in the deep veins, particularly in the upper part of the limb, can be seen to surge upwards and then fall back again as the muscles relax. The sign of 'disappearing contrast', seen in the swill test, described presently, is often found in these patients. The superficial veins may share the valveless state and in the leg a powerful surge out through perforators into the superficial veins is often seen on exercise, with a rapid return flow on relaxing (Figure 22.13). The veins, both superficial and deep, are usually oversized, giving the impression of weak walls that have yielded under venous pressure (Figure 22.14). This state is typically found in patients with severe ulceration but without any history of thrombosis. However many less well defined examples are seen and it appears to be the far end of a spectrum of inborn deep valve deficiency which includes many examples of simple varicose veins in its centre portion and varicosities with normal deep valves at its near end (see Chapter 7).

**The swill test to show valves** The distribution and competence of deep vein valves may now be determined by the swill test described above. This is done whilst there is still sufficient contrast medium in the lower limb; the patient is rapidly positioned to near-horizontal by tilting the table and then brought up to the near-vertical again. Competent valves will be thrown into sharp relief with a column of blood above them (Figure 22.15) and this may,

of course, prevent proper display of valves below this level. In other circumstances valve cusps are shown with no suggestion of blood being retained above them and implying that they are poorly competent, or, again, there may be a widespread deficiency of valves and any that are shown may be defective with, for example, only a single cusp. Some care must be used in interpreting apparently defective or deficient valves because satisfactory demonstration will depend upon the amount of contrast available to reflux down the limb when the patient is returned to vertical and the time interval between this and the moment of viewing or taking static films. It is a manoeuvre that needs to be carried out quite briskly,

**Figure 22.12** *Response to exercise in upright position. Preferential upflow in superficial veins (see pages 490 and 491).*

*(a) This patient was known to have had a deep vein thrombosis on the left side 3 years previously. Strong preferential upflow could be seen in the long saphenous vein; this was also particularly marked in the short saphenous vein and a large upward extension from it, which can be seen curving round the back of the thigh to join the long saphenous vein near the groin. This collateral vein is commonly seen on phlebography in post-thrombotic syndrome. The popliteal vein appears open but other deep veins have failed to show or are only represented by thin deformed channels. A large tortuous collateral vein can be seen crossing the pubes in keeping with iliac vein occlusion.*

*(b) A patient known to have had a deep vein thrombosis in the past. There was strong preferential upflow in the long saphenous vein (seen in its upper part). Opacified blood was persuaded to enter the deep veins by use of a constricting band at the ankle. The only deep veins seen show gross irregularity and deformity in keeping with previous thrombosis. The iliac vein appears open.*

*(c) This patient sustained a severe deep vein thrombosis following a fracture of the hip and prosthetic replacement. Again preferential upflow in the long saphenous vein is evident and partly shown in this composite phlebogram. Compression bands at the ankle and knee succeeded in driving some blood into the deep veins of the leg where they are very deficient and, in the thigh, show gross narrowing and deformity.*

*(d) This patient presented with an uncomfortable leg and enlarged superficial veins. He had previously had an operation to the short saphenous vein which was complicated by haemorrhage and the limb had been troublesome since then.*

> *1. Phlebography shows strong preferential upflow in the long saphenous vein with little outlining of the deep veins.*
> *2. Use of an ankle tourniquet gave some improvement in filling of the deep veins but these are still very deficient and those seen are severely deformed. The patient gave no history of deep vein thrombosis and it is not known whether the operation on the short saphenous vein was mistakenly carried out in a post-thrombotic syndrome or whether, in fact, it caused a deep vein thrombosis. The patient was advised against further surgery and instructed in conservative management.*

*(e) The same patient showing preferential saphenous upflow near the groin. The first view (1) is taken from posteriorly, with the saphenous view close to the X-ray source, and the second view (2) after the patient has been turned with the saphenous vein now more distant from the X-ray source. The magnifying effect of the first position is evident (and see Figure 22.16(c))*

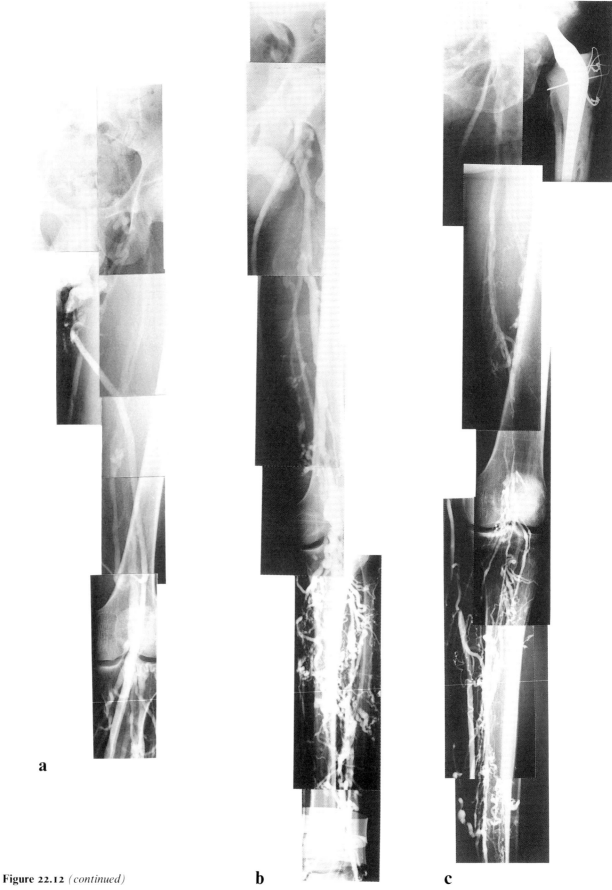

**Figure 22.12** *(continued)*

a

b

c

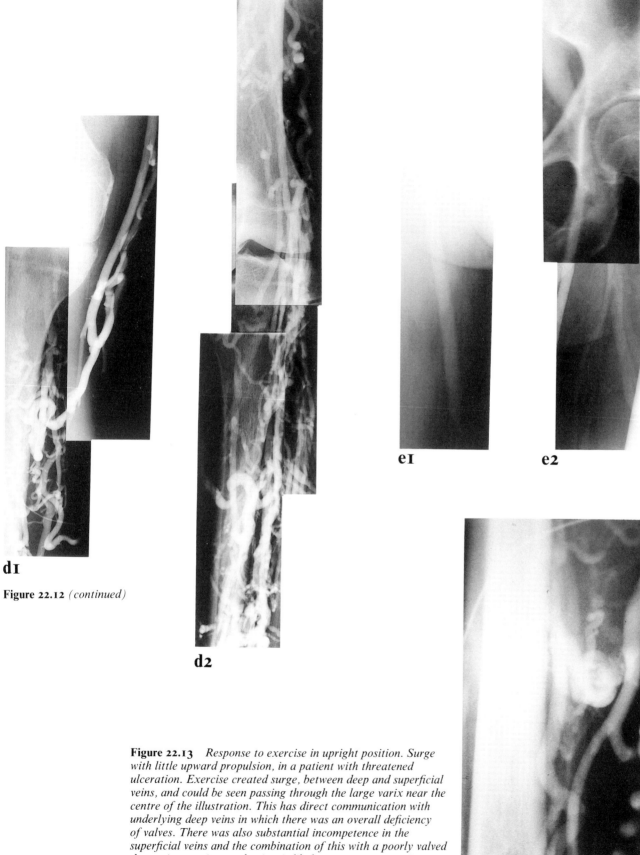

**d1**

**Figure 22.12** *(continued)*

**d2**

**e1**

**e2**

**Figure 22.13** *Response to exercise in upright position. Surge with little upward propulsion, in a patient with threatened ulceration. Exercise created surge, between deep and superficial veins, and could be seen passing through the large varix near the centre of the illustration. This has direct communication with underlying deep veins in which there was an overall deficiency of valves. There was also substantial incompetence in the superficial veins and the combination of this with a poorly valved deep vein pumping mechanism is likely to cause venotensive changes and, eventually, ulceration*

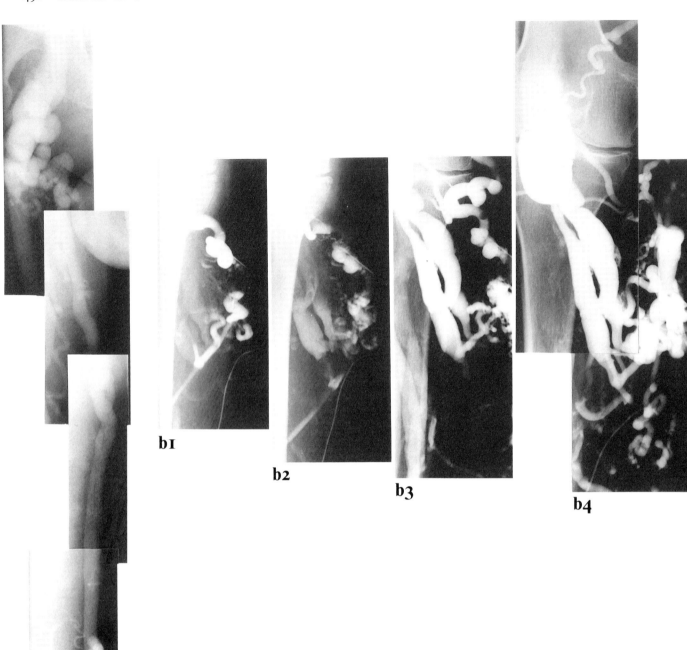

**Figure 22.14**   *Recurrent varicose veins in 'weak vein syndrome'.*

*(a)  This patient developed massive varicosities within a few years of bilateral high ligation of the long saphenous vein but without stripping it. This composite phlebogram shows a large varicose vein running from the right saphenous stump to the unstripped long saphenous vein which has a varicosity arising from it just above the knee. All veins, including the deep veins, seem oversized and expanded.*

*(b)  The same patient, showing filling of gastrocnemius venous sinuses with contrast medium injected into a calf varicosity. These gastrocnemius veins are unusually large and slightly tortuous; they lead into a massive venous saccule lying in the popliteal fossa. Throughout the leg the deep veins were oversized, shapeless and lacking valves; the overall impression was of generalized weakness and overexpansion in the veins. It is perhaps relevant that the patient was obese and had a severe problem with alcohol*

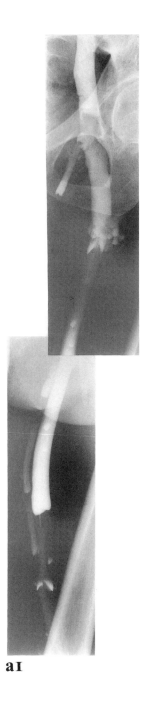

**a1**

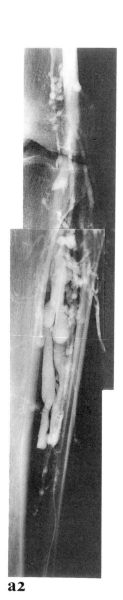

**a2**

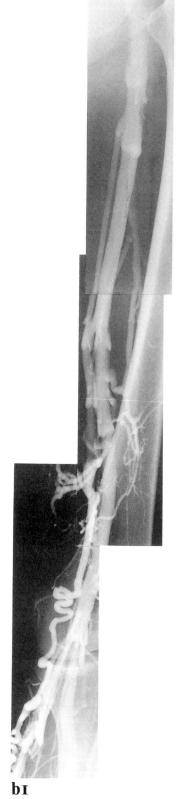

**b1**

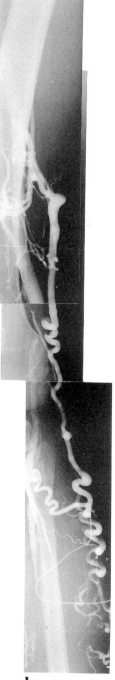

**b2**

**Figure 22.15**  *The swill test to show valves. The patient has been taken from near vertical to near horizontal and back to vertical again.*

*(a)  Valves in thigh (1) and leg (2) shown by the swill test. Note the well-valved long saphenous vein and the relatively normal complement of valves in the veins shown. These phlebograms are from the patient illustrated in Figure 5.11(d)–(f), with varicose veins arising from the internal pudendal vein, and confirm the normality of these other veins.*

*(b)  Composite picture (1) of a patient with recurrent short saphenous varicosities and showing good valves throughout the femoral vein. A rotated view (2) clarifies the origin of the varicose veins from an upward extension of the short saphenous vein not removed at the previous operation*

with no delay in taking static record films, because upward flow reasserts itself within a few seconds so that the valve cusps are soon pushed aside and cease to be visible.

**The disappearing contrast sign** During the swill test, the absence of effective deep vein valve function may give rise to a characteristic sign by abrupt disappearance of the contrast medium from the upper part of the limb as the patient returns to the vertical position. This is caused by a large volume of blood flowing rapidly downwards, unchecked by valves, and sweeping away the contrast medium to the lower reaches of the limb.

**Upward trace by varicography** Some of the other features that may be brought out by upward trace varicography or use of selective compression will be described in a special section later in this chapter.

### Summary of features

The features above will allow the accurate identification of superficial incompetence and its origin, and can give clear assurance that the deep veins are in good order and widely open together with an assessment of their valves. Conversely, it may give clear warning that the deep veins are severely deformed or obstructed with the superficial veins acting as collaterals. In other circumstances the deep veins, although widely open and undeformed, are severely deficient in valves; in these patients this may have been made apparent by movement of the column of blood back and forth as the patient exercises but with little onward progress; in the same way, during the 'swill' test it may be quite clear that opacified blood rushes down the limb unchecked by any valves as the patient returns to the vertical and this gives a characteristic abrupt disappearance of the contrast medium from the upper part of the limb; if a few valves are present, a more prolonged movement may be seen with blood escaping through cusps that fail to meet adequately and delay rather than prevent downflow.

## Special manoeuvres and pitfalls

### Variability in the appearance of veins: magnification in image size: effect of posture on size and flow

#### Magnification of image

Images from conventional X-ray, on screen or film, are always slightly magnified because they are in effect a shadow from a source smaller than the subject. The nearer the subject is to the source the greater this effect will be and considerable magnification of structures close to the X-ray head occurs. Thus, alteration in the apparent size of veins occurs when they are repositioned relative to the source, for example, by changing from supine to

prone position. Veins near the surface and lying close to the X-ray source will appear unnaturally large but when the patient turns over become more typical in size and vice versa (Figures 22.12(e)3, 22.16(c)).

#### Effect of posture on size of veins

It is important to realize the great change that occurs in the appearance of the vein between horizontal and vertical positions (Figure 22.16). In the former, where venous pressure drops to zero, even a large vein may collapse down to insignificance; in the vertical, with full venous pressure, the same vein is fully distended so that its width may now be quadruple that shown in the horizontal position. At times it is hard to believe that one is viewing the same vein and it must be remembered that it is difficult to recognize the size and importance of a vein when it is collapsed in the horizontal position.

#### Effect of posture on flow patterns

The direction in which blood will flow in veins is profoundly influenced by gravity and, hence, by the posture of the patient. For instance, change from upright to lying will alter patterns of longitudinal flow in the limb, and rotation of a horizontal limb will influence flow across the limb. Such a change in the pattern of flow with posture (Figure 22.17) may be used to direct opacified blood to where it is required.

#### Effect of specific gravity on flow

Another important factor in this is that opacified blood has a higher specific gravity and therefore tends to run towards and displace non-opacified blood level with it; this is discussed further and illustrated (Figure 22.20) in the section on varicography later in this chapter.

Needless to say a vein will not show at all unless it is outlined by contrast medium and this will depend entirely upon the prevailing flow patterns which can be very unpredictable in abnormal states. Positive demonstration of the vein is meaningful but apparent absence of a vein cannot be relied upon to exclude an open channel that has failed to fill; the display of surviving deep veins in a post-thrombotic limb is often incomplete because the remaining channels are virtual cul-de-sacs. However, failure of the deep veins to fill, when using the technique described here, strongly suggests that they are abnormal. Venous blood will flow wherever the resistance is least and it will flow much more easily through collateral channels, such as a saphenous vein, rather than thrust its way up a severely deformed deep vein. It is in these circumstances that local compression of the superficial veins acting as collaterals may be used to redirect flow to outline deep veins that are failing to fill.

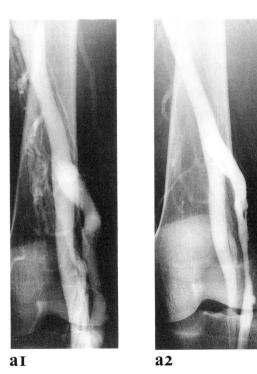

**aI**          **a2**

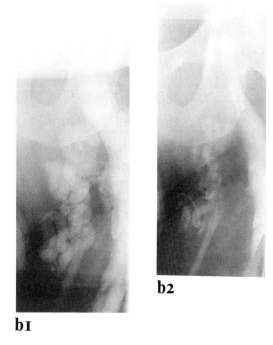

**b2**

**bI**

**Figure 22.16** *Variability in appearance of veins: effect of posture: magnification of image varying with relationship to X-ray source.*

*(a)  1. Short saphenous termination in patient in near-vertical position.*
*2. Reduction in the calibre of veins when patient is put in near-horizontal position.*

*(b)  1. Massive recurrent varicosity arising from a saphenous stump and joining an unstripped saphenous vein, seen with patient in near-vertical position (same patient as in Figure 22.14 but opposite limb).*
*2. With patient in near-horizontal position a great reduction in size is evident.*

*(c)  Massive varicosities lying behind the knee and taking origin from an upward extension of the short saphenous vein.*
*1. Patient in near-vertical position with veins close to X-ray source.*
*2. In near-horizontal position and lying on side with varicose veins well removed from X-ray source. A striking reduction in size is seen, partly due to reduced distension in the horizontal position but also because the change in position of the veins relative to the X-ray source gives less magnification*

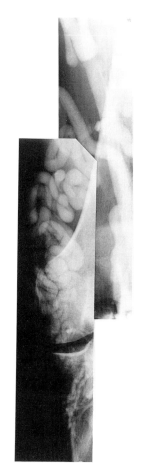

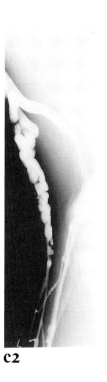

**c2**

**cI**

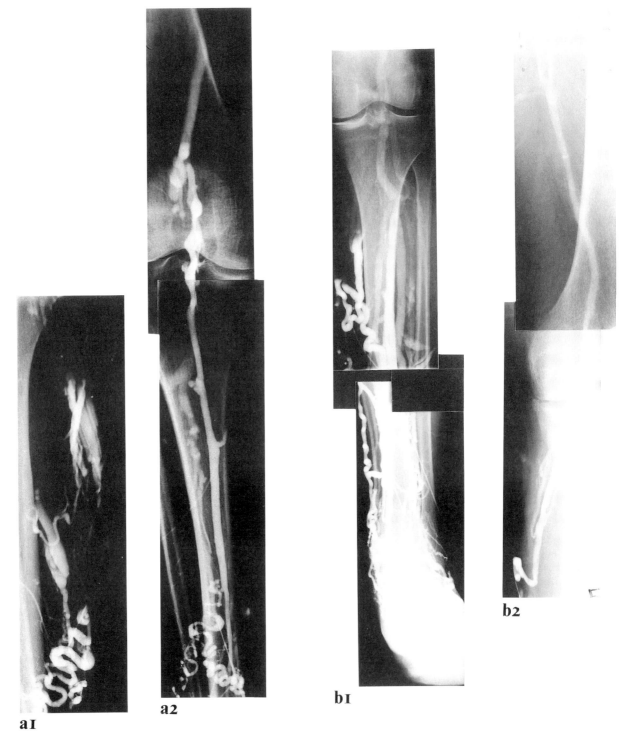

**Figure 22.17**  *Change in pattern of flow with posture.*

*(a)* *1. Contrast medium injected into calf varicosity whilst patient is upright and after one exercise movement; leg in external rotation. Medium has flowed directly into gastrocnemius and soleal intramuscular venous sinuses, a normal phenomenon.*
*2. Procedure repeated with patient in near-horizontal position; leg in mid-rotation. The varicose vein is partially collapsed and flow is now exclusively to the short saphenous vein with none entering the venous sinuses in muscle.*

*(b)* *1. Injection of medium to long saphenous varicosities on inner leg with patient near upright and after two exercise movements. The tibial veins are well outlined but gastrocnemius veins have not shown.*
*2. Procedure repeated with patient in near-horizontal position, flow enters a gastrocnemius vein and on to the popliteal and femoral veins.*

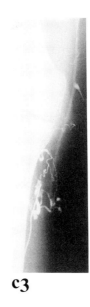

**c3**

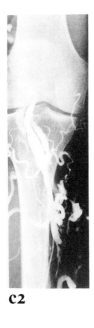

**c2**

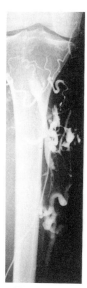

**CI**

**Figure 22.17** *(continued)*
*(c)* *1, 2. Injection of contrast medium into calf varicosities with patient in near-vertical position; progressive filling of gastrocnemius veins occurs.*
*3. Patient in near-horizontal position, the veins around the needle have collapsed and medium now flows into the long saphenous vein.*

*In the upright position, inward flow from superficial veins to intramuscular venous sinuses is a commonplace, normal phenomenon and will occur when these veins have been recently emptied by muscular contraction, or by change of position, and provided effective valves above them have prevented reflux. At that moment they are an area of low pressure into which flow will tend to go, in preference to, say, an incompetent saphenous vein which, in a standing patient, will be at relatively high pressure. Moreover, with exercise, active flow down an incompetent saphenous clears it of any medium; but when the patient is horizontal, pressure in it becomes low, without downward flow, and, as all these illustrations show, flow from varicosities will then tend to be towards it. These considerations are important in understanding the distribution of contrast medium during functional phlebography*

*Use of compression to occlude superficial veins and redirect flow*

This will prevent the blood from following its preferred course in superficial veins and force it to use channels, such as remnants of the deep vein, that would not ordinarily be used as a main pathway of venous return. Although this creates an artefact that changes the usual functioning of the veins it does give a useful outline of the deep veins, confirming deformity or actual obstruction in them. If the needle is in the foot, a band placed just above

the ankle is usually effective in driving contrast medium into the deep veins of the leg (Figure 22.12(b)–(d)); if it is in the calf region, a band at the level of the femoral condyles will compress the long saphenous vein against the medial condyle without undue pressure on the popliteal fossa. The short saphenous vein, often a collateral, can be compressed by a small pad placed over it in the upper calf and a band applied over this but the underlying deep veins are bound to be affected by this. It must be emphasized again that these manoeuvres should only be carried out when all other aspects of the examination have been carried out in correct sequence. Premature use of bands tends to produce a confusing display of veins, which conceals the main flow patterns and is very difficult to interpret. All of these manoeuvres, excepting briefly in the swill test, are carried out with the patient in a near-vertical position.

**Viewing with the limb in rotation**

Because the veins will all be represented on one plane it may be difficult to decide upon the relationship of one vein to another and many misleading effects may be obtained. This can be overcome to a large extent by asking the patient to rotate the limb first outwardly and then inwardly; this gives a near-stereoscopic understanding of the depth and relationship of the veins (Figure 22.18 (a), (b)). Often two veins apparently connected will be seen to be widely separated in a rotated view (Figures 22.15(b), 22.18(c)). The tortuosity of superficial varicose veins tends to lie in one plane and their appearance changes greatly when viewed in different rotations (Figure 22.18(d)). Static film records are obtained at both extremities of rotation, a careful note is made of this, and the patient then returned to the original neutral position. The patient's movements in doing this are equivalent to exercising the limb and will tend to disperse contrast medium which may cause difficulties. Ideally a rotating platform should be used so that the patient remains still without any muscle contraction whilst being rotated first in one direction and then the other. Rotation is an important manoeuvre, particularly when the popliteal and the calf regions are being viewed, and will easily overcome the common difficulty of distinguishing between the short saphenous and the deep veins. Limited use of a videotape during this part of the examination is of great value in recording the changing relationships as rotation occurs. If a rotating platform is not available the manoeuvre should be rehearsed with the patient beforehand so that it can be achieved with minimal muscle contraction.

**Varicography**

This can be a very valuable manoeuvre either as an examination carried out on its own or as an additional phase following or preceding functional phlebography.

**Figure 22.18** *Views of veins in different rotations of the limb.*

*(a) Recurrent long saphenous incompetence.*
*   *1. In external rotation, a long saphenous remnant, common femoral and profunda veins are all superimposed so that it is difficult to interpret.*
*   *2. In mid-rotation the principal veins are beginning to separate and can be well defined.*
*   *3. In internal rotation of the limb the saphenous stump and the vein arising from it are now shown. This vein is in fact a lateral accessory saphenous vein and ligation had been carried out distal to its origin.*

*(b) Views of short saphenous termination in three rotations.*
*   *1. External rotation.*
*   *2. Mid-rotation.*
*   *3. Internal rotation. These pictures have been combined with the swill test and give comprehensive guidance to the surgeon.*

*(c) Recurrent varicosities in the lower thigh.*
*   *1. A direct connection with the underlying femoral vein looks possible.*
*   *2. With external rotation the varix has separated from the deep vein and its origin seems likely to be from an upward extension of the short saphenous vein. Paired perforating veins, of slender calibre and normal in appearance, also communicate with the varicosity but do not seem likely to be its source. Surgical removal of the varicosity should remove the source (a pseudo-perforator) and deep dissection does not appear necessary*

*(d) In different rotations varicose veins may become almost unrecognizable as being the same veins.*
*   *1. Postero-anterior view. The varicosities in the lower part of the picture are seen end-on to the plane of their tortuosity.*
*   *2. Oblique view. The same veins seen face-on to the plane of tortuosity.*

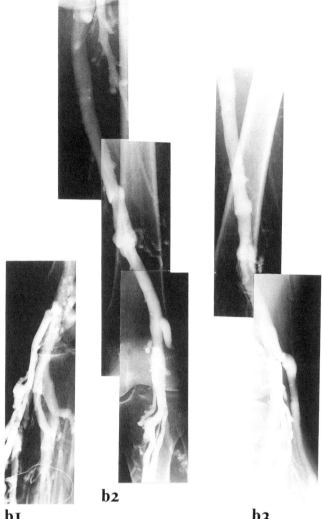

b1　　　b2　　　b3

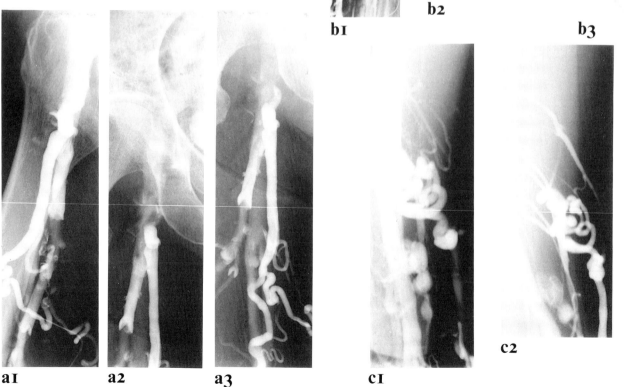

a1　　　a2　　　a3　　　c1　　　c2

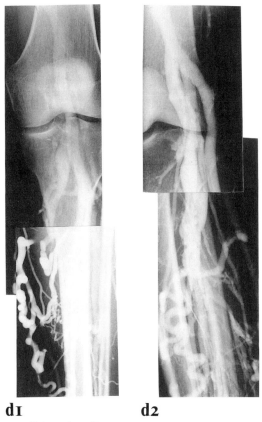

**d1**    **d2**

**Figure 22.18** *(continued)*

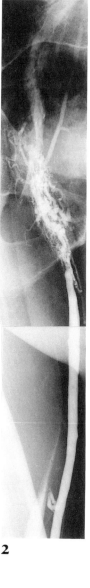

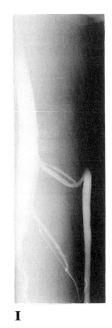

**1**

**2**

The contrast medium is injected into the problem varicosity and its upward connections are traced by this means. This will be no more than an anatomical display and will not show function which can only be implied by the apparent origin and size of vessel. Since flow in varicose veins is usually downwards in the upright patient, the contrast will not move 'upwards' unless the patient is in a near-horizontal position. However, this position has the serious drawback that the reduced venous pressure causes the veins to collapse and their significance cannot be assessed. Moreover, the varicosity is usually filled from above and unaccustomed flow from below does not necessarily follow the same channels but will, as usual, take the line of least resistance, often determined gravitationally. Thus the contrast medium may suddenly divert into a normal perforating vein to join the deep veins and fail to reveal the principal channel that in fact continues on upwards, above the perforating branch, to the true origin much higher up (Figure 22.19). This combination of veins collapsed to near insignificance and the unpredictable path followed in the upward direction can give misleading results. The following measures will however help to overcome these difficulties.

1. Often the best results are obtained with a slight head-up tilt of about 10 degrees which may allow good filling without undue collapse of veins, and is worth

**Figure 22.19** *Diversion of flow in varicography.*

*1. Patient near horizontal, lying face up; the saphenous vein is well outlined in mid-thigh with normal looking paired perforating veins running to the femoral vein. Does the saphenous vein end here?*
*2. The patient has now been repositioned, lying on the left side so that the saphenous vein is on the underside of the limb. Flow now runs easily to the groin where a varicose spongework connects it with the femoral vein; the appearances are those of a non-anatomical recurrence due to revascularization connecting the saphenous stump with an unstripped saphenous vein.*

*In varicography, a sudden diversion of flow can be misleading and repositioning the patient so that gravity counters flow into the diversion can often succeed in giving a full demonstration*

initial trial. A horizontal position, or a head-down tilt, may cause such rapid loss of contrast in an 'upward' direction or into a neighbouring deep vein that little is achieved. Trial and error, varying tilt or lateral posture, may be needed to find the position of optimal filling.

2. Because of the slight upward tilt injected contrast medium will tend to gravitate down into the voluminous varicosities below the needle and it is the upward connections that are to be demonstrated. This difficulty can be countered by using a firm bandage applied round the limb from foot to, say, 2 in (5 cm) below the needle. This prevents pooling of a large quantity of contrast in the lower levels but will prevent any demonstration of gravitational downflow in response to exercise.

3. Contrast medium, 50 ml or more, should be injected fairly rapidly and its progress watched on the image intensifier. It may be an advantage to use medium diluted by 50% with normal saline so that its viscosity is reduced and the contrast dose minimized. This dilution will give satisfactory outlining.

4. The movement of opaque medium, which has a higher specific gravity than blood, is strongly influenced by gravity. Rotation of the limb to change the direction of gravitational pull across the limb may cause the medium to outline a completely different set of veins, for example, short instead of long saphenous vein (Figure 22.20). Differing rotations should be employed to show alternative pathways.

5. As soon as the vein is adequately outlined static films are taken without delay because the contrast may disperse quickly. If necessary, more contrast medium is injected to ensure that a maximal demonstration has been obtained and further exposures of static films made.

6. Further value from the examination can often be obtained at this stage by positioning the image intensifier in the vicinity of the needle and the veins below it. The bandage is now removed and the patient asked to exercise two or three times. This will usually give a downward demonstration of the varicosity and show how the veins disperse either by flowing into deep veins through communicators and/or running to the underside of the foot.

Varicography is best carried out as a separate procedure as an outpatient before surgery. Patients do not seem to be in any way disturbed by being asked to have this examination either a day or two before the operation or, on the day of admission, an hour or two before the operation. It is not really satisfactory to do this in the operating theatre as a preliminary to the operation itself. The best information can only be obtained when it is carried out in a fully equipped X-ray department and with the cooperation of the patient. Moreover, there is a

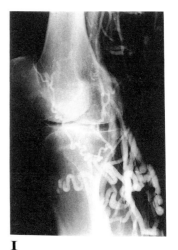 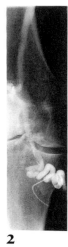 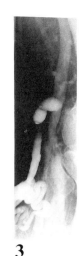

**1**　　　　**2**　　　　**3**

**Figure 22.20** *The effect of specific gravity in directing flow. Contrast medium gives blood a higher specific gravity so that in conditions of equal pressure opacified blood will choose to flow gravitationally downwards. These pictures, taken during varicography, with the patient near horizontal, illustrate this. (Left leg, with needle into posterior calf varicosity.)*

　　*1. Patient lying on right side and long saphenous system therefore on lower aspect of limb. Medium injected into calf varicosity persistently outlines long saphenous vein and varicosities arising from it.*
　　*2. Patient lying face down (mid-rotation). The direction of flow changes and a large communication with the short saphenous vein becomes apparent.*
　　*3. With rotation internally contrast medium flows exclusively into the short saphenous vein, its termination and the popliteal vein.*

*It was clear that the medium ran to the gravitationally lowest point, its greater weight displacing blood that lay beneath it. (This is the same patient as Figure 22.11(e), with both long and short saphenous veins acting as sources of incompetent flow)*

better opportunity to modify the method to improve the display if the first attempt is inadequate. The examination is not really complete until the surgeon has sat down with the various static records and joined these together to give a full view of the veins that have been outlined. These can be combined with films obtained from functional phlebography to give a very revealing composite picture (Figures 22.15(b), 22.22(b)). This is best done by photographing the best static phlebograms and using the prints to build up a complete picture. For this purpose Polaroid prints may be used but prints made from ordinary colour negative film, mass developed and printed at low cost, prove very satisfactory; however, these will require sending out to a quick service processing unit nearby.

### The short saphenous vein

Varicography is of particular value in displaying the upper termination of the short saphenous vein (Figures 22.18(b), 22.21) and many surgeons believe that it is desirable that this should be done in all cases when

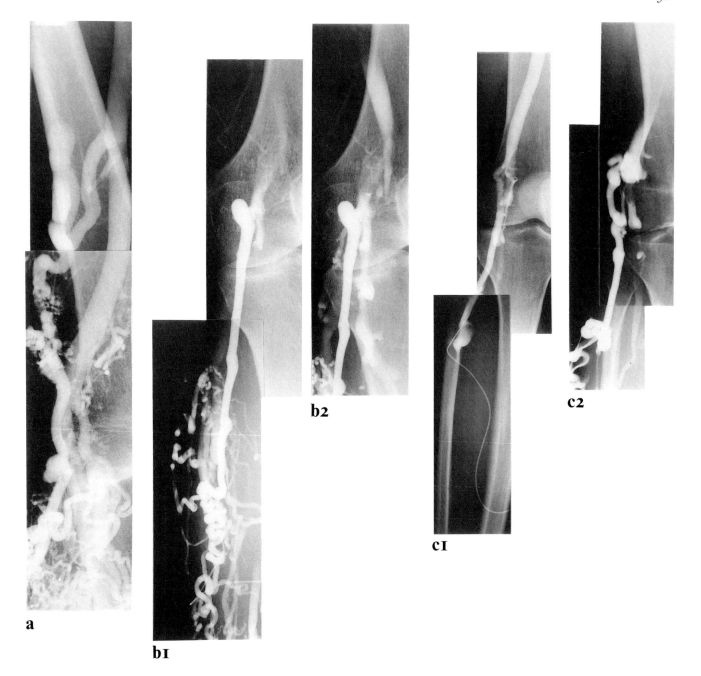

**a**

**b1**

**b2**

**c1**

**c2**

**Figure 22.21** *Termination of the short saphenous vein is very variable and deeply placed amongst complex anatomy. It is important that the surgeon should have clear guidance on this.*

*(a) Composite phlebogram illustrating high-level termination which takes a meandering course, doubling back on itself in the lower thigh. There is gross irregularity suggesting possible recanalized thrombosis just above the knee joint and below this is a large saccule, confirming incompetence in this vein. In the lower part of the picture varicosities arising from the saphenous vein can be seen. Ultrasonography might have difficulty unravelling this.*

*(b) Two phases in filling of a sacculated short saphenous vein terminating at the commonest level. Just before it joins the deep vein a large valved gastrocnemius vein joins it. The surgeon decided to preserve this vein by ligating the short saphenous vein immediately above the saccule; the remainder of the saphenous vein was stripped with multiple dissections of varicosities. (More details of this patient are shown in (g)).*

*(c) Two views of a short saphenous vein terminating at the usual level but showing marked irregularity and apparently joined by a gastrocnemius vein. At operation two well-valved gastrocnemius veins were found to join it and these were both preserved. Note that the downward outlining of the short saphenous vein ends abruptly just below the needle. This was due to an abortive first attempt at insertion of the needle, causing temporary block in the vein. The needle was reintroduced into a neighbouring varicosity, as the rotated view shows. The abortive puncture has nevertheless spoilt demonstration of the downward distribution of the short saphenous vein. (Continued on pages 502 and 503.)*

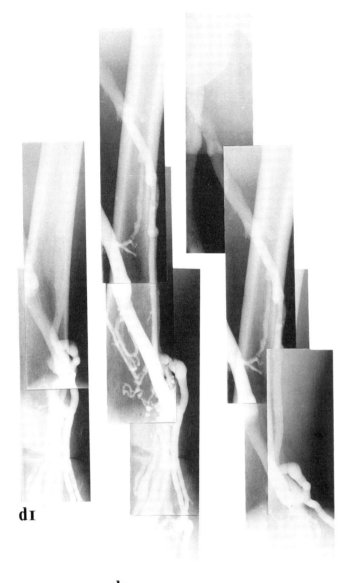

**d1**

**d2**

**d3**

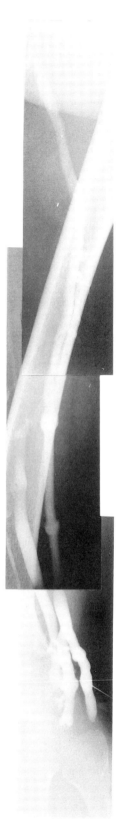

**e**

**Figure 22.21** *(continued)*
*(d)  A complex termination of the short saphenous vein with a large upward extension, shown by composite pictures in various phases of filling, in different rotations and knee flexion. It shows a rather bulbous communication with the popliteal vein and a double channel running up from this unites to form a large vein in continuity with the profunda femoris vein. Without this demonstration the findings at surgery could have been puzzling but the surgeon was able to decide beforehand the points of ligation and portions of vein to be removed. The deeper channel of the upward extension was left intact because it appeared harmless, but the more superficial portion was removed together with the short saphenous vein and its termination.*

*(e)  Another example of massive upward extension in continuity with profunda femoris vein. Note the way in which this lies close to the edge of the mid-shaft of the femur which often conceals it during phlebography. This upward extension is well valved and was left intact by ligation and division of the short saphenous vein flush with it.*

*examination had shown downflow, after exercise in the upright position, in both the long saphenous remnant and in the short saphenous vein; pressure over the short saphenous termination controlled both these downstreams. At phlebography no spillover in the groin could be seen and the composite phlebogram shown here explains the pattern of flow. An upward extension from the short saphenous termination runs vertically to mid-thigh where it winds round to the medial aspect to join the upper part of the unstripped long saphenous vein. Not only is typical short saphenous incompetence present but the upward extension is sending flow to the long saphenous vein where it changes direction to run down to the varicose veins arising from it; the source of its incompetent flow is the short saphenous via its upward extension. As explained in (b), the short sapheous vein was ligated immediately above the sacculation in order to preserve a gastrocnemius vein. At this stage the upward extension was easily recognized and a stripper passed up it; this could be felt running superficially, posteromedially round the thigh to join the long saphenous vein in its upper part. The stripper was delivered here, the upward extension stripped and the stripper reintroduced to strip the long saphenous down the thigh, together with dissection of its varicosities. The surgeon was fortunate to have such clear guidance upon which a plan of action could be based before, rather than during, the operation. This superficially running sapheno-saphenous extension is common and often left intact at short saphenous surgery so that it gives rise to puzzling recurrences (see page 504).*

*(h)  A further variant of upward extension of the short saphenous vein, here running as a reduplication of the femoral vein, the two veins merging in the upper thigh. It would not be a practical procedure to attempt removing this even though it could possibly cause a recurrence by a perforating branch seen arising from it. A reasonable policy would be to carry out flush ligation of the short saphenous and the lower end of the upward extension, together with stripping the short saphenous vein (see page 504)*

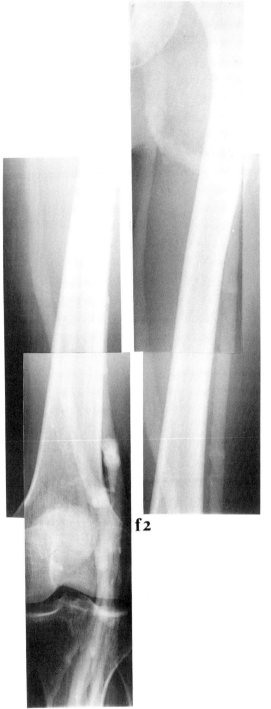

**f2**

**f1**

**Figure 22.21** *(continued)*
*(f)  1.  A further example of upward extension in continuity with profunda femoris vein, illustrating its concealment by the outer edge of the shaft of the femur.*
*2.  The limb has been rotated in the upper picture to separate the vein from the shaft.*

*(g)  A complex arrangement of veins at saphenous termination. This patient has already been shown in (b), but further details are given here. The patient had previously had high ligation of the long saphenous vein without stripping it. Doppler*

surgery to the short saphenous vein in the popliteal fossa is planned. There is all manner of variety in the level and complexity of its termination, and it is important that the surgeon should be forewarned (Figure 22.21(a)). The examination will usually be carried out from the back of the limb (Figure 22.2).

When demonstrating the short saphenous vein it is important to identify whether gastrocnemius veins are entering it instead of the popliteal vein (Figure 22.21(b),(c)). The surgeon should know of the presence of this in order to consider whether to preserve the gastrocnemius vein together with the saphenous vein continuing above this point, or whether they should be sacrificed and flush ligation carried out. Much will depend upon the importance of the gastrocnemius vein(s) concerned (see Chapters 11 and 20) and any further branches, possibly the origin of potential varicosities, above this level.

Another important possibility is an upward extension of the short saphenous vein continuing up the thigh to join profunda femoris or upper long saphenous vein (see Figures 1.5(c)4, 4.24, 5.9(b), 22.21(d)–(h)). An upward extension of this sort (Giacomini vein) is often present and it may be the principal source of incompetence that needs to be interrupted or removed up to a high level in

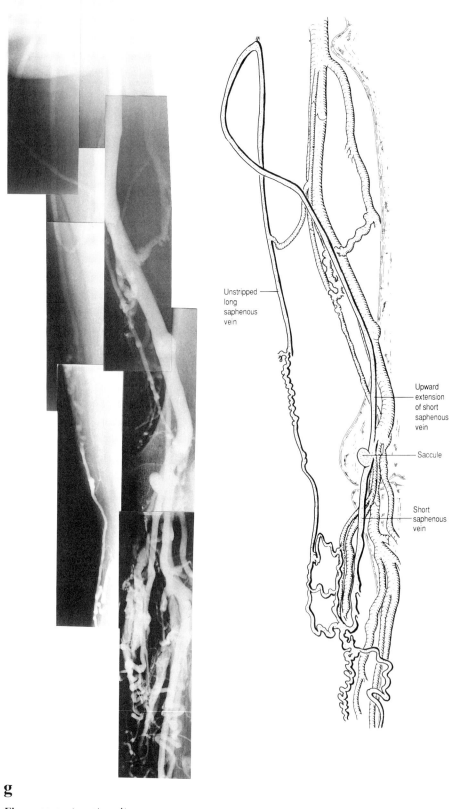

Unstripped
long
saphenous
vein

Upward
extension
of short
saphenous
vein

Saccule

Short
saphenous
vein

**g**

**Figure 22.21** *(continued)*

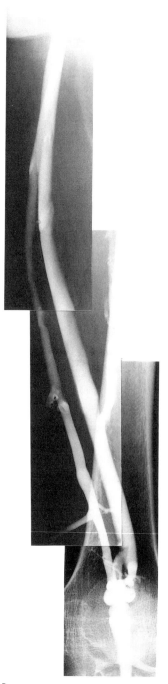

**h**

**Figure 22.22**  *Varicography for long saphenous recurrence. Many examples are shown in this chapter and elsewhere in this book, but two further illustrations are given here.*

*(a)  In this illustration the right saphenous vein remains intact after previous surgery and its upper end has a single substantial communication with the common femoral vein. The opposite limb (not illustrated) had not had a previous operation and surgery to this side found a superficial accessory saphenous vein of substantial diameter. This gave every appearance of a normal saphenous termination with the usual upward branches and its own fossa ovale. Further dissection showed that a larger and deeper principal saphenous vein lay beneath it. Syringe testing showed that the superficial component was well valved but the deeper vein was incompetent. The findings on the right side were in keeping with the previous operation having only ligated and stripped a superficial component identical to that just described; dissection of the surviving deeper vein showed little evidence of previous disturbance and flush ligation was carried out. Venous anatomical variants are often identical on the two sides in this fashion.*

*(b)  This patient had had high ligation, without stripping, of the right long saphenous vein. Eight years later he came for advice with massive varicosities on the inner aspect of the right knee and calf, with marked venotensive changes near the ankle. Doppler flowmetry showed characteristic downflow after exercise in the long saphenous vein of the upper leg and this was completely controlled by pressure at one point in the mid-thigh; pressure in the upper thigh did not give control although Doppler downflow was detected here. Recurrence from a large mid-thigh perforator was diagnosed.*

*The composite phlebogram shows a large varicosity in the groin arising from a saphenous stump and communicating with an intact long saphenous vein showing faintly in the upper half of the thigh. In the mid-thigh a massive varicosity (a pseudo-perforator) arises from an upward extension of the short saphenous vein and joins the long saphenous vein which shows strongly below this level. The coiled varicose veins at knee level, arising from the long saphenous, are evident; this part of the picture was obtained in the near-horizontal position by varicography but the upper thigh was obtained by spillover during functional phlebology. Combining the best of both examinations can give a very informative picture. At surgery both sources, the long saphenous stump and the mid-thigh 'perforator', were removed by dissection, the long saphenous vein stripped to mid-leg and the varicosities removed by multiple dissections*

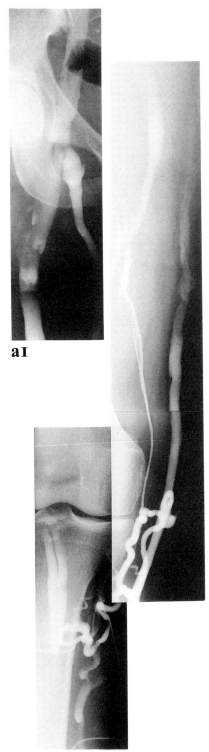

**a1**

**a2**

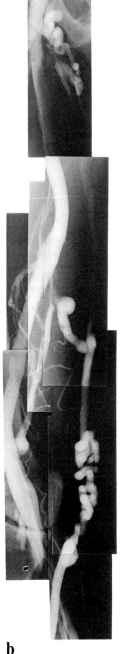

**b**

the thigh. When detected at phlebology special measures should be taken to display and understand its significance. Reduplication of popliteal vein, short saphenous vein or an upward extension of it can give a surprisingly complex arrangement best displayed before surgery.

A number of variable factors have been referred to above and it is part of the skill, and the challenge, of functional phlebography to allow for these and by a brisk, disciplined sequence to make sure that the 'moment of truth' is not lost.

*Examination for recurrent varicose veins*

Varicography is also of value in identifying the source of recurrent varicose veins (Figures 5.24–5.29, 22.19, 22.22).

The findings will complement and probably clarify those of functional phlebography in which spillover may have been detected at the origin of a renewed pathway of incompetence. As stated above, when comparing the film records taken by the two methods one must be prepared for the considerable difference in calibre between films taken in the near-upright and the near-horizontal positions. It may be clear that an apparently insignificant vessel outlined by varicography is in fact much more impressive when viewed in its fully distended state during functional phlebography; the combined information of the two examinations may reveal that it is of real importance (Figure 22.22(b)).

### Gastrocnemius and soleal intramuscular sinuses and veins

Direct inflow from superficial veins to gastrocnemius and soleal intramuscular venous sinuses is, of course, normal and is frequently seen during functional phlebology and varicography when the medium is introduced by superficial veins on the calf (Figure 22.23); in itself it does not indicate abnormality. It does however produce some puzzling appearances that are liable to be misdiagnosed

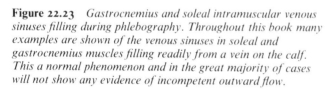
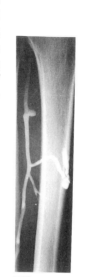
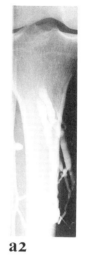
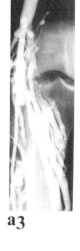
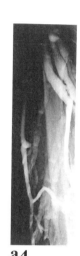

a1  a2  a3  a4

**Figure 22.23** *Gastrocnemius and soleal intramuscular venous sinuses filling during phlebography. Throughout this book many examples are shown of the venous sinuses in soleal and gastrocnemius muscles filling readily from a vein on the calf. This a normal phenomenon and in the great majority of cases will not show any evidence of incompetent outward flow.*

*(a) The example shown here has interconnections between a calf varicosity, gastrocnemius veins, short and long saphenous veins.*

> *1. Needle in varicosity at right-hand edge of picture. Early phase of filling to short saphenous and an upward-running vein.*
> *2. Further filling now outlining gastrocnemius veins.*
> *3. Further filling showing an extensive set of gastrocnemius veins joining the popliteal vein; tibial veins are also showing faintly.*
> *4. The leg has been rotated to include the long saphenous vein, on right-hand edge of picture, which has also filled.*

*The sacculation on the short saphenous vein indicates incompetence in this vein and the varicosity was probably caused by this. The surgical procedure here was limited to local removal of the varicosity and neighbouring short saphenous vein because the patient's main problem was in the opposite limb (Figure 22.21(d)).*

*(b) An unusually clear example of contrast medium injected into a varicose vein on the posterior calf directly communicating with and filling a gastrocnemius sinus; note intercommunication between this and the neighbouring sinus.*

*(c) A chance demonstration of paired perforating veins running from superficial varicosities to a tibial vein and to a gastrocnemius sinus, both well valved. A gastrocnemius sinus showing in this fashion may be mistaken for a short saphenous vein but this can be clarified by further filling and taking rotated views*

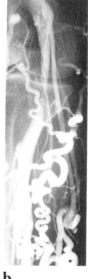

b

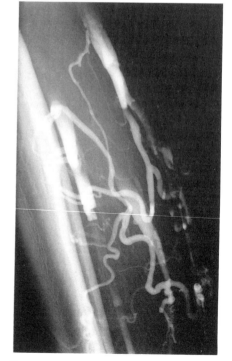

c

by those not aware of the numerous communications between superficial veins and the venous sinuses in all the leg muscles. Usually it is an entirely normal phenomenon but if there is doubt further observations can be made at the time of exercise and during the swill test to see if there is incompetent outflow here from deep to superficial veins and to assess its magnitude and to localize the actual point of leakage (Figure 11.30). Static films of this will, of course, be of considerable importance to the surgeon. The response of gastrocnemius and soleal veins to exercise or the swill test will show if their valves are defective (see Figures 5.32(b), 11.22) and, if so, may show substantial perforator outflow to superficial veins. It must be admitted that functional phlebography gives only a brief glimpse of this, so that it may easily be missed. In this respect, colour flow ultrasonography is greatly superior, by allowing repeated viewing of deep veins in the popliteal fossa and upper calf, whilst the patient exercises.

## Perforating veins

Perforating veins are discussed at length in Chapter 11 and here it is sufficient to emphasize that inward flow, from superficial to deep, is normal and only heavy outward flow is proof of abnormality, either at high level, as a source or superficial incompetence, or in the leg, often as part of an important collateral compensatory mechanism. Unnaturally created outward flow, by use of constricting bands or tourniquets, cannot give meaningful information upon function but only an anatomical outlining of the vessels involved. However, the size and shape of the veins may clearly imply abnormal function (Figure 22.24).

## Varicosities to the foot

Large varicose veins running to the foot should be demonstrated as far as possible and some estimation made of the degree of pooling of contrast medium in the foot. The elimination of these varicosities may be of some importance in the surgical treatment of large varicose veins on the leg, especially when threatened or actual venous ulceration is present (Figure 22.25).

## Unexpected connections

Varicography performed in varying positions can often be very rewarding in showing unexpected connections and one example is shown in Figure 22.26.

## The texture of veins

Further observations of value may be made upon the outline of the veins seen in full distension. In some of the most formidable problems, both in terms of the size of

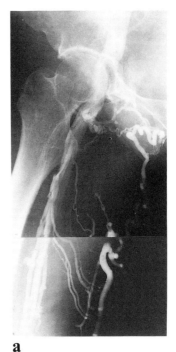

a

b

**Figure 22.24** *Perforating veins are commonly seen at functional phlebography and it must not be too readily assumed that they are abnormal.*

*(a) Recurrent long saphenous varicose veins in the thigh can be seen communicating by two pairs of perforating veins with the profunda femoris vein. These perforators are slender with regular outline and almost certainly not at fault. Further examination showed substantial recurrence at the saphenous stump.*

*(b) Recurrent long saphenous varicosities in mid-thigh with a somewhat enlarged, irregular perforator running from the femoral vein directly into the varicosities, which in turn join the unstripped long saphenous vein. This degree of abnormality is in keeping with it being a significant source of incompetence*

varicosities and in venous stasis associated with them, it can be seen that the superficial and deep veins are oversized and often with rather irregular lumens so that they

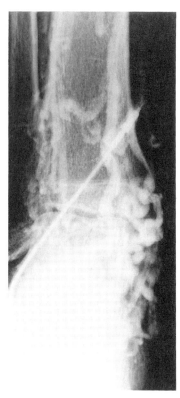

**Figure 22.25** *In long and short saphenous incompetence the varicose veins arising from this commonly extend onto the foot and an example is shown here. It was obtained in the near-vertical position by injection of contrast medium in mid-calf and after raising the foot once to allow flow to its underside. Foot varicosities are easily diagnosed clinically but the surgeon will welcome this confirmation of their significance if it is conveniently obtained during phlebography for other reasons*

appear baggy and possibly weak walled. A lasting surgical cure in such patients may be difficult to achieve and any improvement brought about by surgery should perhaps be backed by external support with calf-length elastic stockings. It is helpful for the surgeon to be forewarned of this so that he can advise the patient accordingly (Figure 22.14).

Another form of irregularity in venous outline is caused by a previous thrombosis but this is usually accompanied by narrowing so that it is possible to distinguish this from 'weak-walled' veins. However, veins that have undergone extensive deep vein thrombosis may show many changes of a disorganized venous system, with some veins deformed because they have recanalized after thrombosis, whilst others are enlarged and distorted by a compensatory hypertrophy so that it is not possible to give a precise interpretation of the appearances beyond their being in keeping with post-thrombotic changes. The full diagnosis will depend on the overall pattern of flow.

## Pelvic veins

During functional phlebology it is usually possible to

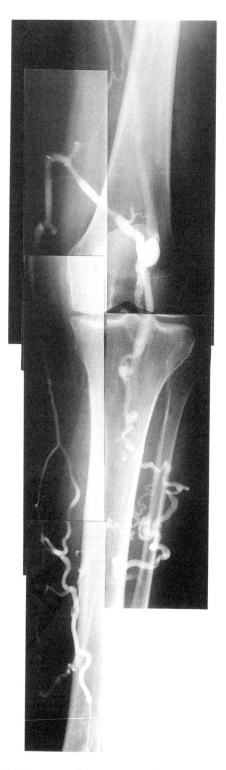

**Figure 22.26** *Unexpected connections. This composite phlebogram is from a patient with recurrent long saphenous varicose veins. Contrast medium injected into a remnant of the long saphenous vein on the lower leg has flowed up this, across to the short saphenous vein and run down it to enter varicosities on the back of the calf. The appearances are in keeping with unsuspected short saphenous incompetence with an interconnecting branch to a long saphenous remnant*

outline the external and common iliac veins and the lower inferior vena cava. However, the contrast by this stage is well diluted, easily dispersed and weak in outline; putting the patient in horizontal position will rapidly clear these vessels. Thus failure to show an iliac vein is not proof that it is occluded and a key sign to be looked for is the presence of tortuous collaterals crossing the pelvic region, indicating a strong likelihood of post-thrombotic occlusion in an iliac vein (Figure 22.27). If the external

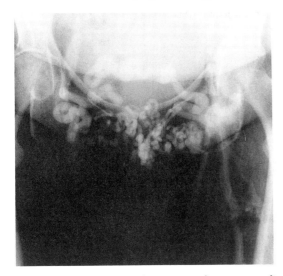

**Figure 22.27**   *Pelvic veins. With injection of contrast medium in the calf or foot, the concentration of contrast medium reaching iliac veins and inferior vena cava is often very thin so that failure to outline these large veins cannot be regarded as evidence of their occlusion. However, collateral veins compensating for occlusion are far more readily shown and usually run from one side of the pelvis to the other, either suprapubically or internally within the pelvis. The illustration shows an example of this with large tortuous pubic veins crossing from the left common femoral to the right femoral vein and up the external iliac vein. Usually such veins are evident on clinical examination but not infrequently are first detected at functional phlebography which should always include inspection of the pelvic region at an appropriate stage*

and common iliac veins do not show clearly there should be close scrutiny of the screen for collaterals crossing the pelvis; static X-ray films should be taken for subsequent examination which may well reveal their presence although screening failed to detect them.

Some other aspects of pelvic veins are discussed in Chapters 5 and 9. Special techniques, such as transfemoral catheterization of ovarian veins, may be needed to demonstrate incompetence in these veins and their relationship to tortuous veins in the pelvis (see Chapter 5).

## Phlebography augmented by digital subtraction angiography

With this computerized digital technique it is possible to enhance the image by subtraction of unwanted back-

ground structures, such as bone. It is sufficiently sensitive to visualize arteries outlined by contrast medium on its first passage through the arterial system after injection into a vein, and it is commonly used for this, including pulmonary and limb arteries. When used for phlebography a low dose of medium injected peripherally can give strong and detailed outlining of the veins, free from skeletal interference. However, it is necessary for the patient to remain still because any displacement will cause subtraction to be ineffective and this prevents its use in demonstrating functional abnormality in the veins of the lower limb, only possible with exercise in a near upright position. Fortunately, phlebography for deep vein thrombosis does not require movement and digital subtraction angiography is being used increasingly for this. It is particularly effective in the upper limb when axillo-sub-

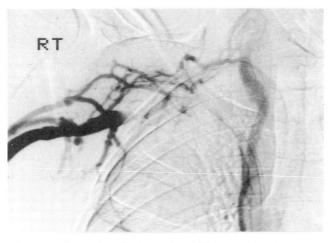

**Figure 22.28**   *A digital subtraction phlebogram, showing occlusion of axillary and subclavian veins, with a group of collaterals crossing the subclavian region to join the superior vena cava*

clavian vein thrombosis is suspected (Figure 22.28) (Hughes, Dixon and Fletcher, 1987). Only a small volume of contrast medium at low osmolality is required and this is helpful in renal or cardiac disease; moreover, it allows an inexpensive medium to be used with considerable saving in cost. Images at two frames a second build up a dynamic picture, recording all the details of the medium's passage through collaterals to the superior vena cava; usually no more than a single injection is needed and one hard copy is sufficient. This technique is of importance in the management of central lines, used for parenteral nutrition or chemotherapy, or in cardiac pacemakers, where thrombosis in the upper extremity may be a problem requiring treatment by anticoagulants.

## Reference

Hughes, D. G., Dixon, P. M. and Fletcher, E. W. L. (1987) Augmentation of upper limb venography with digital subtraction. *Phlebology*, **2**, 125–127

# Bibliography

Ackroyd, J. S., Lea Thomas, M. and Browse, N. L. (1986) Deep vein reflux: an assessment by descending phlebography. *British Journal of Surgery*, **73**, 31–33

Browse, N. L., Burnand, K. G. and Lea Thomas, M. (1988) *Diseases of the Veins*, London, Edward Arnold, pp. 103–134

Corbett, C. R., McIrvine, A. J., Aston, N. O. *et al.* (1984) The use of varicography to identify the sources of incompetence in recurrent varicose veins. *Annals of the Royal College of Surgeons of England*, **66**, 412–415

Corcos, L., Peruzzi, G., Romeo, V. and Fiori, C. (1987) Intraoperative phlebography of the short saphenous vein. *Phlebology*, **2**, 241–248

Craig, J. O. M. C. (1977) Investigation of the leg veins by venography. In *The Treatment of Venous Disorders* (ed. J. T. Hobbs), MTP, Lancaster, pp. 83–95

Dow, J. D. (1951) Venography of the leg with particular reference to acute deep thrombophlebitis and to gravitational ulceration. *Journal of the Faculty of Radiologists*, **2**, 180–205

Ferreira, J. A., Villamil, E. J. F. and Ciruzzi, A. O. (1951) Dynamic phlebology. *Angiology*, **2**, 350–373

Fletcher, E. W. L. and Tibbs, D. J. (1986) Functional phlebology in chronic venous disorders of the lower limbs. In *Phlebology '85* (eds D. Negus and G. Jantet), John Libbey, London, pp. 51–54

Gardner, A. M. N. and Fox, R. H. (1989) *The Return of Blood to the Heart: Venous Pumps in Health and Disease*, John Libbey, London

Giacomini, Giorn, di Accad. di Med. Torini 1893; 14: (as quoted by Vandendriessche, 1989)

Grainger, R. G. (1984) Low osmolar contrast media. *British Medical Journal*, **289**, 144–145

Grainger, R. G. and Dawson, P. (1990) Low osmolar contrast media: an appraisal. *Clinical Radiology*, **42**, 1–5

Hobbs, J. T. (1988) The enigma of the gastrocnemius vein. *Phlebology*, **3**, 19–30

Katayama, H. (1987) Clinical survey on adverse reactions of iodinated contrast media. In *Advance and Future Trends of Contrast Media* (Proceedings of the International Symposium of Contrast Media, Tokyo); No. 6, 7.

Lea Thomas, M. (1982) *Phlebography of the Lower Limb*, Churchill Livingstone, Edinburgh

Lea Thomas, M. and Mahraj, R. P. M. (1988) A comparison of varicography and descending phlebology in clinically suspected recurrent groin and upper thigh varicose veins. *Phlebology*, **3**, 155–162

May, R. and Nissl, R. (1979) The post-thrombotic syndrome. Roentgenologic aspects. In *Surgery of the Veins of the Leg and Pelvis* (ed. R. May), Saunders, Philadelphia, pp. 134–139

Neiman, H. L. (1985) Venography in acute and chronic venous disease. In *Surgery of the Veins* (eds J. J. Bergan and J. S. T. Yao), Grune and Stratton, New York, pp. 73–87

Palmer, F. J. (1988) The RACR Survey of intravenous contrast media reactions, final reports. *Australasian Radiology*, **32**, 426–428

Perrin, M., Bolot, J. E., Genevois, A. and Hiltbrand, B. (1988) Dynamic popliteal phlebography. *Phlebology*, **3**, 227–235

Starnes, H. F., Vallance, R. and Hamilton, D. N. H. (1984) Recurrent varicose veins: a radiological approach to investigation. *Clinical Radiology*, **35**, 95–99

Thornbury, J. R. and Fischer, H. W. (1989) Issues in uroradiology. *Current Imaging*, **1**, 3–9

Vandendriessche, M. (1989) Association between gastrocnemial vein insufficiency and varicose veins. (With invited comment by Nicolaides A. N., Christopoulos, D., Vasdelis, S.) *Phlebology*, **4**, 171–184

Vasdekis, S. N., Clarke, G. H., Hobbs, J. T. and Nicolaides, A. N. (1989) Evaluation of non-invasive and invasive methods in the assessment of short saphenous vein termination. *British Journal of Surgery*, **76**, 929–932

# 23

# Alternative imaging techniques and special investigations

**Tarik F. Massoud** MB, BCh., BAO, FRCR and **Basil J. Shepstone** MA, DPhil., MD, DSc., FRCR
*Department of Radiology, Oxfordshire Health Authority and University of Oxford, John Radcliffe Hospital and Radcliffe Infirmary, Oxford*

Since its introduction over fifty years ago contrast venography has remained the 'gold standard' amongst the modalities available for assessing veins of the lower limbs. The search for non-invasive alternatives and the wish to overcome the limitations of venography (Albrechtson and Ollson, 1976; Bettman and Paulin, 1977; Albrechtson and Ollson, 1979; Roddie, 1989) has encouraged recent development of several alternative techniques for imaging veins. These include ultrasonography, radionuclide or isotope scintigraphy, thermography, computed tomography, and magnetic resonance imaging. At present, these other methods play a minor role in the day-to-day assessment of patients with venous disorders of the lower limbs and they have been mainly employed either in selected patients or as part of a general study of their suitability in the detailed assessment of veins, including the display of venous anatomy, patterns of venous flow, overall venous pumping capability, diagnosis of pathological process such as thrombosis, and in distinguishing venous from lymphatic causes of oedema.

## Diagnosis by ultrasound

Ultrasound is any high frequency sound wave that cannot be detected by the human ear, that is, more than 20 KHz, and, as used diagnostically in medicine, has a frequency between 1 and 15 MHz. The generation of high frequency sound waves depends on the property of certain crystals to respond to stress by producing an electric current or, conversely, to change its dimension in response to an electric signal, the piezoelectric effect (Dendy and Heaton, 1987i). Such a crystal can be used to produce ultrasound waves by application of a continuous wave or pulsed electric current, and the same crystal can convert the 'stresses' of sound waves it receives into electric signals. In this way an ultrasound transducer containing a piezoelectric crystal can emit high frequency sound waves and also receive them to give corresponding electric frequencies. Although many natural crystals are piezoelectric, the material used most commonly for ultrasound transducers is lead zirconate titanate, a synthetic ceramic. Separate emitting and receiving transducers are usually employed; these are disc shaped and the resonant frequency is determined by size and thickness. At high frequencies the ultrasound beam is absorbed by tissue very rapidly and frequencies of around 10 MHz can only be used for superficial investigations. At 5 MHz the useful penetration depth of tissue is approximately 8 cm and at 2.5 MHz it is about 15 cm. A coupling agent of fluid or jelly is always interposed between probe and skin as any intervening air will not transmit ultrasound satisfactorily.

The two main applications of ultrasound techniques in vascular work are, the detection of speed and direction of blood flow by use of the Doppler effect, and real-time imaging:

### Doppler flowmetry (velocimetry)

Doppler flow detection depends on the principle that the frequency of a sound wave reflected from a moving object is changed in proportion to the speed of movement of the reflecting object. The frequency change can be used to detect direction of movement, towards or away from the probe, and to measure its velocity. To obtain the Doppler effect, the ultrasound beam must be angled to the direction of movement (blood flow), so that this is either towards or away from the probe. In a simple directional Doppler ultrasound velocimeter (flowmeter) the results are expressed by one or more of the following means:

- An audible signal (created by reflected frequencies now in the audible range due to Doppler shift) which may be stereophonic to convey direction of movement.

- An instrument or array of lights that indicate direction and velocity of flow.
- A chart recorder that provides a permanent record of variations in direction and velocity of flow.
- A computerized analysis of flow giving a sophisticated display and printout, including a sound spectrum analysis of reflected Doppler-shifted audiofrequencies, proportionate to velocity of flow, from which many characteristics are immediately apparent or may be computed (mostly used in arterial examination).

Directional Doppler ultrasound may employ either continuous wave emission, as in a simple velocimeter, or it may be pulsed when combined with duplex real-time ultrasound scanning.

### Ultrasonography – imaging by ultrasound

Ultrasound is reflected back by tissue interfaces of changing density and it is from this, received by the transducer, that information of the underlying tissue is derived. To ensure that the air–skin interface is satisfactorily crossed, a coupling agent, a jelly, is always used. The body tissues reflect ultrasound at fractional time intervals varying with their distance away and at an intensity depending on the physical qualities of the soft-tissue layers; this is scanned and displayed electronically to give a detailed image in differing shades of brightness (hence B mode), termed the grey-scale. Certain tissues or structures, such as bone or calculi, absorb the ultrasound so completely that only an opaque area is shown and little can be learnt. Fluid transmits ultrasound well but only reflects it at interfaces or where there is a change of consistency, for example, well-established blood clot. Red cells in blood, having high density compared with surrounding plasma, are reflective and the movement of numerous reflecting surfaces can set up a Doppler shift of ultrasound frequency which is put to good use in the detection of blood flow. Gas, however, has no such compensation and transmits ultrasound poorly so that intestinal gas acts as a barrier beyond which little is seen and creates a dark area on the display screen. In general, a 7.5 MHz probe is used to examine superficial veins generally and the deep veins above the knee, and a 5 MHz probe is used for the deep veins below the knee. The 5 MHz probe is a very practical frequency for most purposes, applicable to most veins in the limbs and to the iliac veins in the lower abdomen, if intestinal gas does not obscure them. At lower frequencies the resolution of the image is progressively reduced so that greater penetration is gained at the expense of image detail. Variable focus transducer probes are produced by arranging transducer elements into a number of concentric rings (annular probe), or by using a linear array of small elements that can be fired individually or in a group (linear array probe). If the probe depends on sweeping the beam to and fro the image will be wedge shaped but a linear array gives a rectangular image.

In B-mode real-time imaging, pulsed ultrasound is beamed across a section of the limb and scanned to give a display on an electronic screen. This may be used to study the morphology and movement of blood vessel wall and valves; the image represents a tomographic cut through tissues which may be longitudinal, cross-sectional or any obliquity in between, according to the positioning of the probe. The ultrasound pulses are scanned fast enough to give a flicker-free image which is updated so rapidly that movement is immediately shown and a picture of the tissues is presented in multiple tones of grey, conveyed by varying degrees of brightness in the screen, the B-mode or grey-scale.

Most real-time scanners now include a facility to carry out pulsed Doppler measurement of flow in any selected area of the screen with the same probe and, in recognition of this dual function, are referred to as duplex scanners (Figure 2.12). The source of the 'sample' volume giving a Doppler shift is accurately selected on the image by moving a cursor over it; the Doppler ultrasound beam must be appropriately angled to flow and an indicator line on the screen will show the alignment of the beam relative to the blood vessels so that maximum efficiency can be attained. Without proper angling, the Doppler effect will not be achieved and misleading results will be obtained. The width of the Doppler beam is adjustable and this may be used to provide a gate limiting the area sampled to the vessel lumen. As the width of the lumen can be measured, its cross-section may be calculated and, knowing the mean velocity, the volume of blood flowing through per unit of time can be arrived at by a suitably linked computer software program. This allows the volume of blood moving in a channel, such as a popliteal vein, to be estimated, for example, the amount of venous blood expelled from the leg by each exercise movement, or the volume of blood refluxing after a movement. This is proving of great value, not only in research, but in the practical assessment of venous problems in patients. For instance, the volume expelled per contraction of the musculovenous pump of the leg may be calculated to assess its efficiency or the severity of reflux estimated. It has been shown that there is a direct relationship between the latter and the development of venostatic changes such as pigmentation, induration and ulceration (Nicolaides, Christopoulos and Vasdekis, 1989; Vasdekis, Clarke and Nicolaides, 1989a).

Colour Doppler ultrasound is a more recent development that provides a combination of real-time imaging with a dynamic colour image of vascular flow (Mitchell, 1990). This consists of colour-encoded Doppler information superimposed on a real-time B-mode grey-scale image. There are numerous strategies for encoding the frequency, variance and amplitude of Doppler shifts into colour. Typically, red indicates flow in one direction and blue in the other (see Colour Plate 24); green is often used as a third colour to encode further information. The particular advantages offered by colour Doppler in the venous system (Zwiebel and Priest, 1990) include:

1. An additional means for the rapid recognition and following of veins, particularly in the calf where the profusion of veins makes this difficult.
2. The ability to visualize flow in veins directly, even when they are otherwise obscured by soft tissue, oedema or excessive depth from the transducer.
3. The ability to detect venous reflux immediately without the need for tedious placing of a cursor over a vessel to obtain the direction of its Doppler flow; arteries are quickly distinguished by their pulsatile colour flow away from the heart.

Nicolaides *et al.* (Nicolaides, Christopoulos and Vasdekis, 1989b,c) state that the use of colour flow imaging has reduced the time required to scan the popliteal fossa from 10 minutes, by duplex alone, to 2 minutes. A consistent method of examination must be established by each ultrasonographer to ensure that examinations are comprehensive and accurate. Zwiebel and Priest (1990) and Nicolaides *et al.* (Nicolaides, Christopoulos and Vasdekis, 1989b,c) give detailed protocols for examination of veins in the lower extremity.

## Ultrasound in normal veins

The main features of normal veins examined by ultrasound in the lower limb are summarized below.

### Doppler ultrasound

- Spontaneous flow is evident in medium or large deep veins even when the limb is dependent and without movement. In superficial veins and lesser deep veins this feature is variable and may not be evident.
- Phasic flow is found in the principal deep veins as the velocity changes in response to normal quiet respiration. This is evident by audible signal, flowmeter instruments or a computed flow analysis spectrum.
- Strong Valsalva manoeuvre causes abrupt cessation of flow in medium and large deep veins.
- Manual compression of the extremity distal to the site of Doppler examination, or flexion/extension movement of the foot, increases or 'augments' venous flow in the main deep veins.
- Flow is unidirectional, and blood flows only towards the heart because valves prevent retrograde flow. Venous flow away from the heart is abnormal.

### Real-time imaging

- The vein lumen is echo free and therefore translucent but, with colour flow coding, is filled with colour according to direction of flow when any movement occurs.

- Valve cusps and their movement are visible when image quality is good.
- A normal vein is compressible and its lumen can be narrowed or obliterated with a small amount of extrinsic pressure; this feature will be lost if thrombus occupies the lumen.
- Major veins of the extremity are slightly larger than the corresponding artery alongside, particularly if the patient is standing; the identity of arteries can be proved by their pulsatile flow shown on the Doppler facility with duplex scanning or, with colour flow, they are immediately recognizable by the column of pulsatile colour.
- Major veins increase in diameter with deep inspiration and the Valsalva manoeuvre which will arrest flow and also banish its colour image.

## Recognition of venous abnormality by ultrasound

### By Doppler ultrasound (flowmetry)

In essence Doppler ultrasound only detects the direction and velocity of flow but this may lead to immediate recognition of abnormality. Abnormal venous flow due to incompetence of valves in a lower limb occurs by gravity and will not be revealed unless the patient is standing and moving intermittently, or briefly by respiratory effort.

**Reversed direction of flow** Flow in the direction that should be opposed by valves is direct evidence of incompetent or deficient valves. Many examples of this, as Doppler flowmeter chart recordings from superficial veins, are used to illustrate this book and technical aspects are considered in Chapter 24. Such reversed flow is usually gravitationally determined and may only be revealed when the patient is upright. The velocity of such flow may be locally increased or become turbulent at an incompetent valve which acts as a constriction in the retrograde flow.

**Enhanced flow in the natural direction** Strong flow, enhanced by exercise, found in superficial veins which should not show this, may indicate collateral flow past deep vein occlusion or deformity. However, it is not a positive sign in the same way as reversed flow and must be taken in conjunction with other evidence.

**Pulsatile flow in the natural direction** This may be found in the vicinity of an arteriovenous fistula and in certain other circumstances considered in Chapters 12, 17 and 24. However, Haimovici (1985) gives a further reason for 'arterial' pulsation in varicose veins detected by Doppler ultrasound. In a study of 34 patients with varicose veins he found arterial pulsation especially in the veins of the lower part of the leg, and this was accompanied by local heat. He attributes this to arteriovenous shunting which may be an inherent feature of long-standing venous disorder, either primary varicose veins or secondary veins as in the postphlebitic syndrome. He suggests that in chronic venous insufficiency the arteriovenous anastomoses normally present in the microcirculation of the skin become excessively dilated by venous hypertension to cause this manifestation. Certainly arterial pulsation is not infrequently detected during the course of Doppler examination of superficial veins in severe venous disease, often accompanied by local heat, and arteriovenous shunting is a possible explanation; however, Haimovici may be detecting increased flow across the expanded and proliferative capillary bed in areas of skin affected by venous hypertension, rather than the elusive phenomenon of arteriovenous shunting. Nevertheless, in this way, Doppler flowmetry may provide a simple way of detecting when the patient has reached a significant stage of deterioration (and see discussion on arteriovenous shunts in section on 'Haemodynamic appraisal of pathogenesis in varicose veins' under 'Radionuclide scintigraphy' later in this chapter).

*Note.* Heat over varicose veins is commonplace and, as suggested in Chapters 2 and 4, is likely to be due to flow from deep veins, at true body temperature, down to varicosities on the surface, or as part of collateral outflow in deep vein obstruction. Haimovici may be describing an additional phenomenon.

**Absence of flow** Failure to find flow in a principal deep vein where normally it is found readily, such as the femoral vein, or loss of phasic flow with respiration, or failure of augmentation of flow when the limb below is compressed, all point to partial or complete occlusion. Again, this requires interpretation with care as a negative finding of this sort lacks the positive evidence provided by reversed flow.

*By real-time imaging*

Real-time imaging is able to display the outline of veins and valves, and it is possible to deduce abnormality from size and shape, or loss of mobility in these structures. To this will usually be added the advantages of a Doppler flow facility displaying the features described above. Failure to demonstrate a vein lumen or valves may have technical causes and should not be regarded as absolute proof of occlusion or absence.

**Size and shape of veins** An oversized and tortuous vein is almost certain to be incompetent due to loss of valve function or it is acting as a collateral compensating for deep vein obstruction. A saccule, usually just below a valve, is good evidence of heavy leakage in that valve or structural weakness in the vein walls. Deformity in a vein lumen, particularly the deep veins, indicates previous thrombosis now recanalized. This may be accompanied by rigidity of the walls which fail to distend with a Valsalva manoeuvre or when rising from horizontal the ver-

tical. Loss of compressibility of veins occurs when thrombus occupies the lumen.

**The appearance of valves** Normal valve cusps are delicate structures that may be seen to float back and forth, and to meet when challenged by backflow. Post-thrombotic cusps are thickened, adherent to the walls and will not meet. An incompetent valve, undamaged by thrombosis, is difficult to recognize without use of the Doppler flow facility; colour flow imaging can give a dramatic demonstration of incompetence by a strong jet of colour flow down through the leaking valve cusps and merging with poorly coloured turbulent flow below.

## Practical application of ultrasound in venous disorders

In this book the main author (D.J.T.) has concentrated upon the method of using Doppler flowmetry that he finds most valuable in everyday use and in the section that follows a representative selection of other authors' methods and findings are reviewed; also given are points made by various authors based on their experience with duplex real-time imaging and colour flow imaging.

*Demonstration of superficial vein incompetence and its source*

**Early development: Doppler flowmetry** Selecting appropriate treatment for varicose veins, and the best operation if surgery is preferred, requires accurate diagnosis (Myers, 1983). The use of Doppler ultrasound flowmetry for the assessment of the venous system was first proposed in the late 1960s (Strandness *et al.*, 1967) and early 1970s, principally to detect deep vein occlusion (Sigel *et al.*, 1970; Evans, 1971). Soon, its role was extended to the identification of valvular incompetence in both superficial and deep veins (Folse and Alexander, 1970; Miller and Foote, 1974; Meadway *et al.*, 1975; Day *et al.*, 1976). The high degree of accuracy that Doppler flowmetry allows in the assessment of venous reflux soon led to its becoming an important part of the routine examination of all patients with venous pathology (Barnes, 1979). Indeed, in 1983, Myers suggested that every surgeon who operates on varicose veins should consider purchasing a 'Pocket Doppler Stethoscope' to examine all patients, even though this gives only an audible signal, without indication of direction of flow, but nevertheless can be a great help in diagnosis. In 1987, Bladin and Royle demonstrated that the skills needed for the use of directional Doppler ultrasound flowmetry in the assessment of varicose veins could be acquired in a relatively short time and provided valuable information.

Primary varicose veins are most commonly due to saphenofemoral (long saphenous) or saphenopopliteal (short saphenous) incompetence but secondary varicose veins are seen in deep vein occlusion when enlarged superficial veins act as collaterals. It can be difficult to determine the nature of the veins by clinical examination alone but Doppler ultrasound often clarifies the true state and much of this book is concerned with this.

*Saphenofemoral incompetence* Various tests may be applied in the examination of varicose veins but accurate detection of saphenofemoral (long saphenous) incompetence is the main purpose of all these tests. The cough impulse, tapwave and Trendelenburg tourniquet test give good information but are not always sufficient. Hoare and Royle (1984), using a non-directional Doppler with audible signal only, found that 28% of saphenofemoral incompetence was missed by clinical examination alone, especially in obese patients; Chan, Chisholm and Royle (1983) found that Doppler flowmetry improved accuracy by some 20%. Similarly, Zelikovski *et al.* (1981) reported an increased detection rate of up to 50% in their patients. McIrvine *et al.* (1984) studied 161 limbs with primary varicose veins, comparing detection of saphenofemoral incompetence by standard clinical tests with a Trendelenburg tourniquet test in which reflux down the vein on release of the tourniquet was judged by a Doppler ultrasound probe; this combined test was correct in predicting saphenofemoral incompetence, proved at operation, in 82% of patients and was more accurate than any other method of testing. They considered this method of Doppler assessment completely objective, with reflux either detected or not, and more reliable than assessing the refilling of veins visually. In a study of 205 limbs, Large (1984) provided further support for the role of Doppler ultrasound and advised selective ligation of the saphenofemoral junction only when the Doppler flowmeter had given evidence of incompetence at this level. In other cases he advised it should be preserved and more peripheral surgery carried out, thus sparing a well-valved saphenous termination when the source of incompetence is at a lower level.

*Saphenopopliteal incompetence* The success of clinical diagnosis in saphenopopliteal (short saphenous) incompetence is poor in comparison with diagnosis supported by Doppler ultrasound. Failure to recognize saphenopopliteal incompetence by clinical evaluation may account for the high incidence of recurrent or persistent varicose veins in this state and, indeed, in 1981 Doran and Barkat (1981) noted that when surgery for varicose veins was confined to 'groin ties' and stripping of the long saphenous vein, this failed to control varices in 50% of cases and advised the more frequent use of venography. In a series by Hoare and Royle (1984), only 64% of saphenopopliteal incompetence was detected clinically compared with 100% detected by Doppler ultrasound.

Surgical results may be poor if adequate removal of the short saphenous termination is not carried out and it is a great advantage to know before surgery the level of the termination and branches joining it. The variable siting of the saphenopopliteal junction and the difficulty of localizing it preoperatively are major factors in the unsatisfactory results obtained in the past. In support of this Mitchell and Darke (1987) found a 30% recurrence of saphenopopliteal incompetence as compared with 7% in a long saphenous vein group; they concluded that neither clinical nor Doppler ultrasound assessment was entirely reliable in identifying the level of the saphenopopliteal junction but that Doppler ultrasound in the popliteal fossa certainly improved the accuracy of localization. Various authors (Hobbs, 1980; Hoare and Royle, 1984; Sheppard, 1986), using preoperative varicography, demonstrated that the short saphenous junction with the popliteal vein has a wide variation in anatomy and that the junction is at, or within, 2 cm of the popliteal skin crease in only 64% of cases. These authors all recommend that short saphenous venography should be performed before surgery, in order that the incision should be placed accurately, the source of incompetence verified and the anatomy of the short saphenous termination demonstrated. On the other hand, Gilliland, Gerber and Lewis (1987) suggested that Doppler ultrasound is sufficiently accurate to plan the surgical approach in the majority of limbs but when reflux is audible more than 5 cm above the skin crease the accuracy in localizing the saphenopopliteal junction decreases and preoperative venography should be used.

### Duplex scanning and colour flow imaging for the less accessible sources of superficial vein incompetence

*Short saphenous vein incompetence* There is now widespread agreement on the need to display the short saphenous termination accurately before surgery but, although phlebography gives a clear demonstration of this, the search for a simpler, non-invasive method continues. Vasdekis *et al.* (1989) have shown that much greater accuracy is achieved by duplex scanning then by Doppler flowmetry alone. In 64 limbs they found that clinical examination gave 56%, Doppler ultrasound alone 64% and duplex scanning 96% accuracy compared with preoperative phlebography. Causes for failure by duplex scanning were an unusually high termination and termination on the anterior aspect of the popliteal vein.

The ease and accuracy in diagnosis of short saphenous incompetence and display of its termination is improved still further by the use of colour flow imaging; an example of this is shown in Colour Plate 24. Nicolaides *et al.* (Nicolaides, Christopoulos and Vasdekis, 1989b,c) find that in tracing an upward extension of the short saphenous vein (Giacomini vein) it is particularly valuable to use the probe to scan transversely; this is also the best way to detect gastrocnemius vein incompetence.

*Incompetence of a gastrocnemius vein* This is not usually recognized by the average surgeon dealing with varicose veins. It is well described by Hobbs (1988) and Vandenriessche (1989). Nicolaides *et al.* (Nicolaides,

Christopoulos and Vadekis, 1989b,c) provide striking evidence of the value of colour flow imaging in the demonstration of the short saphenous termination and in the diagnosis of gastrocnemius vein incompetence. Colour flow imaging would seem to be the best available method for displaying gastrocnemius incompetence, particularly because it can be repeated as required in a way not possible with phlebography. These authors give warning that acting on this diagnosis by ligating the gastrocnemius vein should only be considered by an experienced surgeon.

### Perforator vein incompetence

Incompetent perforating veins are not easy to find by clinical examination alone. Myers (1983) expressed the view that the tourniquet tests for perforators should be abandoned and described a method of using the Doppler ultrasound flowmeter which he found detected 80% of incompetent perforators. Similarly, Negus (1985) reported using Doppler ultrasound to locate perforators prior to surgery. A different method of localizing incompetent perforators was proposed by Berni *et al.* (1979) and was based on the detection by Doppler ultrasound of arterial pulsation transmitted to the surface through perforator veins when their valves were incompetent; this localization allowed a small incision to be used selectively to ligate the vein. However, there is not universal agreement upon the value of these measures but more recently Nicolaides *et al.* (Nicolaides, Christopoulos and Vasdekis, 1989b,c) have found that duplex and colour flow imaging can locate incompetent perforators and determine whether they are part of a collateral mechanism.

### Incompetence and occlusion in deep veins

**Doppler ultrasound** The deep veins cannot be assessed adequately by clinical means alone and, here, Doppler ultrasound flowmetry is valuable (Myers, 1983). If veins are normal, phasic flow is found in time with respiration and is sharply augmented by squeezing the distal muscles; this will not be found if the deep veins are occluded. When the deep veins are incompetent, reflux is evident during the Valsalva manoeuvre or on proximal compression of the limb. Whilst Doppler ultrasound is able to give an overall diagnosis of deep vein impairment a phlebogram will still be required for a detailed assessment, for example, in the occasional patient who may be suitable for surgical valve reconstruction or venous bypass grafting.

**Duplex real-time imaging** Duplex ultrasound has been shown to be an accurate method of detecting deep vein incompetence by McMullin *et al.* (1989), who compared photoplethysmography, Doppler ultrasound and duplex scanning. They concluded that if a competent valve was found in the popliteal vein the deep vein system could be considered competent, even if reverse flow was present in the femoral vein; but reverse flow in the popliteal vein indicated a diagnosis of deep vein incompetence likely to cause symptoms. By using phlebography to establish the diagnosis they found that duplex ultrasound with colour flow imaging was the most accurate alternative method for detecting deep vein reflux and incompetence in perforating veins. These authors point out that non-invasive methods (plethysmography, Doppler ultrasound, duplex scanning and colour flow imaging) are able to give both anatomical and physiological information and are replacing the invasive method of phlebography.

Duplex ultrasound has other uses, such as that reported by Wales and Azose (1985) who used it to differentiate a saphena varix from other possible swellings in the groin, for example, aneurysm or hernia. The varix gave a non-pulsatile, well-defined, anechoic structure that could be traced through saphenous termination to the common femoral vein, it was separate from the artery and collapsed when the patient lay down. Duplex imaging can also easily recognize a Baker's synovial cyst arising from the hip or knee joint and is particularly valuable in distinguishing a ruptured cyst in the popliteal fossa from deep vein thrombosis.

### Demonstration of deep vein thrombosis by ultrasonography

Deep vein thrombosis continues to cause considerable diagnostic and therapeutic problems in clinical practice. The development of high resolution real-time B-mode ultrasonography has led to its use in studying, non-invasively, venous thrombosis of the lower extremity, alone or in combination with a Doppler flow facility. In an excellent general review of B-mode ultrasound imaging Flanagan, Sullivan and Cranley (1985) recorded a high success rate, improved with experience, in diagnosing deep vein thrombosis in a group of 41 lower limbs also examined by phlebography, and they predicted that this form of examination would supplant venography in 90% of acute or chronic venous disorders. A comprehensive study by Lensing *et al.* (1989) found a sensitivity and specificity of 100% and 99% respectively, after exclusion of patients with a history of deep vein thrombosis within the previous year. Another study, by Mantoni (1989), on 90 inpatients confirmed the high sensitivity and specificity of duplex ultrasound examination, in spite of the difficulties of having to examine seriously ill patients or those in traction. According to this study the number of venograms could be reduced by at least 42% if patients with deep vein thrombosis were treated on the basis of ultrasound diagnosis alone. Only two false positives and four false negatives were encountered.

**Recognition of thrombus** Some sonographic criteria for diagnosis of deep vein thrombosis in the lower limb are more sensitive than others. Visualization (Mantoni, 1989) of thrombus cannot always be achieved. A fresh thrombus may be isoechoic to flowing blood and therefore not visible sonographically, but with increasing age the thrombus becomes more echogenic and can easily be seen. With high resolution transducers, 7.5 or 10 MHz, it should be easier to demonstrate intraluminal thrombus. In normal compressible veins, turbulence can sometimes be seen and may be mistaken for clot, but with the latest colour-coded Doppler flow imaging such confusion is less likely.

**Duplex sonography as a guide to treatment** Based on experience with 90 patients suspected of having deep vein thrombosis, Mantoni (1990) concludes that duplex sonography is useful in monitoring the changes in vein patency during anticoagulant treatment. Compressibility of the vein is an easy, quick test for acute deep vein thrombosis. A vein with a fresh thrombus is often bigger and more circular on cross-section than the opposite leg vein; it is not compressible and the Doppler ultrasound signal, if present, is more continuous, with loss of phasicity. The veins often recanalize with anticoagulant treatment and regain their natural oval shape and normal compressibility. In the acute phase the use of the pulsed Doppler facility to give additional evidence of deep vein thrombosis does not, in fact, improve the overall detection based on duplex scanning alone; it lengthens the examination time, but gives no more than confirmatory data and an increased level of confidence. However, with the Doppler flow facility it is possible to distinguish occlusive from non-occlusive clot, and it is a great advantage to follow the progress of patients by monitoring the changes in flow and modifying therapy accordingly.

Leven and Al Hassan (1989) compared the merits of duplex ultrasound diagnosis with phlebography in 29 patients with suspected iliofemoral venous thrombosis. In seven patients both methods agreed that there was no thrombosis. In three patients thrombosis was confined to the limb; here duplex ultrasound demonstrated thrombus and its upper limit reliably in keeping with phlebography but Doppler ultrasound did not contribute in establishing the diagnosis per se. In 19 patients iliofemoral thrombosis was present and diagnosed by ultrasound but without defining the extent of thrombosis, except for two patients with complete occlusion in whom Doppler ultrasound correctly registered total absence of flow. In the other 17, intestinal gas and inability to apply the compressibility test made it impossible to determine the extent of thrombosis and in one case, with fresh thrombus in the inferior vena cava reaching to the renal veins, real-time ultrasound failed to reveal this and Doppler ultrasound gave the false reassurance of flow. Attempts to decide the age of thrombus were not reliable as judged by findings at subsequent thrombectomy. The authors conclude that although duplex sonography is reliable for the overall diagnosis of iliofemoral thrombosis, defining the upper

end of the thrombus requires contralateral, transfemoral phlebography, especially if operative treatment is contemplated. This study was carried out to see if duplex real-time ultrasound could replace phlebography in a hospital treating recent cases of iliofemoral thrombosis by routine thrombectomy and temporary arteriovenous fistula.

**Colour flow imaging in suspected deep vein thrombosis** Baxter, McKechnie and Duffy (1990) point out that colour flow imaging has the advantage of combining the well-established sonographic technique of flow augmentation by distal compression with a colour display of venous flow in a manner comparable to phlebography. Modern colour-coded scanning machines have certain properties ideal for imaging the deep venous system. These are:

- High sensitivity for low velocity and low volume flow.
- Residual flow around thrombus can be readily used to outline it.
- Improved resolution at greater penetration.

Of the many studies comparing ultrasound with phlebography in the detection of deep vein thrombosis, few have successfully visualized the calf veins (Baxter *et al.* use the term 'calf veins' to cover proximal tibial, peroneal and distal popliteal veins). Many physicians are prepared to withhold anticoagulation when thrombus is present below the knee, provided they have reassurance that the femoropopliteal section is free from this. Nevertheless, other clinicians still advocate anticoagulant therapy for calf deep vein thrombosis, especially in younger patients, and will wish to have reliable reassurance that this is not present. Thus, if ultrasound is to be accepted as a complete diagnostic tool, then at least some information should be available on calf vein patency. The impact of colour Doppler is at present difficult to assess, and with this in mind Baxter and colleagues conducted a double-blind prospective study comparing colour Doppler with phlebography in the lower limbs of 40 patients with suspected deep vein thrombosis.

In 26 patients there was complete agreement by both methods that deep vein thrombosis was not present; in 18 of these colour flow was recognized in the proximal major veins below the knee which were otherwise not visible. In 14 patients the findings were positive for thrombus and 11 of these showed extensive femoropopliteal and upper calf thrombosis; in the latter group, diagnosis by ultrasound was easily confirmed by lack of spontaneous flow, absence or poor distensibility and thrombus visible in proximal segments; localized areas of thrombus were confirmed by ultrasound and colour Doppler showed non-occlusive thrombus outlined by flow. In two cases the proximal calf veins could not be identified but isolated calf vein thrombosis was successfully diagnosed by ultrasound by absence of any flow, and reduced or absent augmentation of flow with distal compression in the patent veins displayed above this level; in a third patient a thrombus shown by phlebography was not detected by ultrasound, probably because excessive obesity caused a poor image.

These authors conclude that colour flow ultrasound gives similar accuracy to phlebography in the diagnosis of femoral and popliteal vein thrombosis; compared with duplex grey-scale imaging, it gives additional information about flow around non-occlusive clots and is particularly helpful in assessing patency in the adductor canal where the femoral vein is relatively inaccessible. Other pathologies giving a similar clinical picture to deep vein thrombosis in the calf, for example, ruptured Baker's cyst, can often be quickly recognized. It shows promise in the assessment of proximal calf vein patency and early experience suggests that it may be useful in the positive diagnosis of calf vein thrombosis, but further clinical trials are necessary.

Baxter *et al.* indicate that colour flow imaging is likely to be a considerable improvement upon previous methods of ultrasonography in diagnosis or exclusion of deep vein thrombosis.

*Duplex ultrasound in assessing the effect of sclerotherapy*

Schadeck (1987) has used real-time ultrasonography and directional Doppler flowmetry to investigate the effect of sclerotherapy on veins at the saphenofemoral and saphenopopliteal junctions in the treatment of varicose veins. The changes included thickening of the wall and decrease in luminal diameter, and, frequently, transient intraluminal thrombus. The main outcome of this was a reduction of reflux, giving more physiological flow, or its complete disappearance. Distal flowmetry and ultrasonography appear to be valuable methods of assessing success or failure of sclerotherapy.

# Radionuclide scintigraphy

Radionuclide studies carried out *in vivo* may be divided into those primarily concerned with counting local concentrations and those which involve imaging. The primary requirement of imaging is to provide information concerning the spatial distribution of radioactivity in the body. The basic requirements of an imaging system are:

1. A suitable radionuclide, of which technetium-99m is the most widely used (half-life of 6 hours).
2. Its incorporation into an appropriate radiopharmaceutical vehicle which will be taken up by the tissue or organ under investigation.
3. A device, such as a gamma camera, supported by electronics, computing facilities and displays, that is able to use the radiation emitted from the body to produce high resolution images presented to the clin-

ician in the manner most suitable for interpretation (Dendy and Heaton, 1987ii).

A technetium-99m phosphate compound at first circulates in the blood stream and can be used to display blood vessels (blood pool image), but later a large part leaves the blood stream to enter the calcium-crystalline lattice in bone (crystal phase) so that it can be used to image the skeleton; the remainder is excreted through the kidneys.

The radiations that are most suitable for *in vivo* imaging are medium energy gamma rays in the range of 100–200 keV. In all commercial equipment currently available, the radiation detector is a crystal of sodium iodide doped with thallium. Interaction of a gamma ray with this results in a light pulse proportional to the gamma ray energy. An array of photomultiplier tubes and appropriate electronic circuits are used to identify the exact position of a scintillation in the crystal and to convert this information into an image.

Dynamic imaging, in which changes in distribution of the radiopharmaceutical are monitored throughout the investigation, has been widely available in general hospitals since the late 1970s. Important information is obtained by numerical analysis of digitized images on a frame-by-frame basis to produce such features as time–activity curves for a region of interest selected by the operator.

Positron emission tomography makes use of cyclotron produced, short half-life positron emitters such as oxygen-15. When an oxygen-15 nucleus disintegrates a positron is released and captured by a negatively charged electron in the tissues. This results in the annihilation of both particles and the production of a pair of photons which are emitted at 180 degrees to each other. The detection of these simultaneously emerging pairs of photons by a ring of detectors is called 'coincidence detection' and enables their site of origin to be determined. In this way, by using emission computed axial tomography, the *in vivo* distribution of the radionuclide can be measured (Gowland Hopkins *et al.*, 1983).

# Demonstration of varicose veins

The superficial venous system of the lower limb can be investigated by technetium-99m red blood cell blood-pool imaging. Lubin *et al.* (1978) have demonstrated the use of this technique in delineating the anatomy of saphenous vein varicosities. Both *in vitro* and *in vivo* methods of labelling red blood cells can be used. The former involves the labelling of previously separated red blood cells with technetium-99m and their subsequent injection into the patient. *In vivo* labelling requires the injection of a preparation containing pyrophosphate and tin chloride, followed 30 minutes later by sodium pertechnetate. Imaging of the blood pooled in the vessels of the limb is performed shortly after, with the patient standing to fill the veins maximally. Lubin *et al.* have stressed that this method is useful in both the demonstration of varicose veins and in their follow-up, where it was found to be an easy and objective means of determining the change in the blood pool after treatment. This method proved particularly useful in visualizing the varicose veins of obese patients in whom it was difficult to obtain sufficient information by clinical means.

Similarly, Oyama *et al.* (1983) used technetium-99m red blood cell injection for the evaluation of varicose veins. Their method of radionuclide angiography also involved the *in vivo* labelling of red blood cells by arterial injection. Blood-pool images showed prominence, tortuosity and dilatation of the superficial veins with anastomosing branches in both lower limbs.

## Demonstration of deep vein thrombosis

Numerous radioisotope techniques have been described to detect the presence of venous thrombosis (Roddie, 1989). These fall into two broad categories (Table 23.1). Indirect or non-specific tests are radionuclide venographic methods using scanning of the blood-pool in the limbs to portray patent and collateral vessels; this aims to identify the presence of thrombus by changes in the pattern of venous blood flow. Direct or specific tests involve radiolabelling constituents of evolving thrombus, thus identifying it by their incorporation into the thrombus itself.

Technetium-99m red blood cell venography (Zorba, Schier and Postituck, 1986; Leclerc *et al.*, 1988) has a sensitivity of 90% and a specificity of 93% compared with contrast venography. If the calf veins are excluded, these parameters rise to 96% and 97% respectively. This method has the advantage of simplicity, portability, easy tolerance by the patient, and simultaneous depiction of the deep veins bilaterally, including the common iliac veins. In addition, it can be repeated without major risk or discomfort to the patient. The main limiting factor in its performance is its poor resolution. This technique may be used to complement contrast venography when it is technically unsatisfactory or equivocal, in patients with a history of contrast reaction, and in bed-bound patients.

Technetium-99m human albumin macroaggregate or microsphere venography is very unreliable in detecting calf or popliteal vein thrombosis, although in the femoral and iliac veins sensitivities of 75% and 100%, and specificities of 99% and 100%, have respectively been found compared to contrast venography (Whitehouse, 1990). An advantage is that a lung scan can be obtained at the same time as the radionuclide venogram and be used to detect pulmonary emboli (Bentley and Kakkar, 1979).

In 1960, Hobbs and Davies reported the successful demonstration of thrombi in rabbits using I-131 fibrinogen. Counting was done with an external scintillation detector. Since then I-125 fibrinogen has provided the basis for a screening test for newly forming thrombi in the form of the fibrinogen uptake test (Kakkar *et al.*, 1970). This does not provide images but the information obtained is displayed graphically as an activity–time curve. The use of I-123 fibrinogen (DeNardo & DeNardo, 1977) enables gamma camera imaging to be performed. The I-125 fibrinogen uptake test has both a high sensitivity (94%) and a high specificity (93%) for thrombi that form in the distal half of the thigh, the popliteal fossa, or the calf (Secker-Walker, 1986). It is unable to detect thrombi in the upper thigh or pelvis due to background radiation, particularly from free isotope in the urine, and the low energy of the isotope. Another disadvantage is that up to 48 hours may be required before a result can be obtained, due to the long residence time of fibrinogen in blood. False-positive results occur with haematomas, surgical incisions, and inflammation. False-negative results also occur when old thrombi cease to take up fibrinogen, or if thrombus forms when most of the radioactive fibrinogen has cleared from the circulation after approximately a week, or when the thrombus is small. Fibrinogen cannot be autoclaved, but since the introduction of small pools of donors, and testing for hepatitis B antigen and the human immunodeficiency virus, the risk of giving a patient a serum-transmitted disease has almost been abolished (Browse, Burnand and Lea Thomas, 1988). Despite this, I-125 human fibrinogen may not be commercially available for much longer. The sole supplier of this radiopharmaceutical in Europe and in the USA is Amersham (Europe: Amersham, UK; USA: Arlington Heights, IL), who plan to stop producing the product as soon as the present stock of human fibrinogen is exhausted. The company has stated that customers will be notified around 6 months before the expected termination of the product (Knight, 1990).

The most promising and exciting development in this field is the development of specific monoclonal antibodies, radioactively labelled, and directed against platelets and fibrin (Peters *et al.*, 1986). The advantages of using monoclonal antibody for *in vivo* labelling are, first, the convenience of avoiding cell separation, and secondly, a higher rate of clearance of tracer from the blood pool with enhanced imaging of the thrombus. This increased rate of disappearance from the blood is particularly evident when specially prepared fragments of anti-fibrin antibody are used (Knight, 1988).

With the exception of the I-125 fibrinogen uptake test, the major problems with the use of radioisotopes in the diagnosis of venous thrombosis concern the scarcity of carefully performed studies on large numbers of patients to determine their accuracy and reliability in comparison with contrast venography, the different technical methods of carrying out these procedures, and the different criteria used in interpreting the results (Secker-Walker, 1986).

## Haemodynamic appraisal of pathogenesis in varicose veins

The pathogenesis and development of varicose veins remains obscure and investigations of the primary causative factors have centred around vein wall weakness, valvular deficiencies, and haemodynamic effects (Scott, 1990).

It is possible with radionuclide methods to unravel some problems related to the pathogenesis of lower limb varicosis. Much work on micro- and macro-haemodynamics in patients with varicose veins has been conducted by Soviet investigators (Frolov and Konstantinova, 1981; Sevelyev et al., 1981; Frolov, Konstantinova and Karalkin, 1982). They found that comprehensive radionuclide appraisal of circulatory changes enables the identification of stages of compensation, transition and decompensation in the evolution of the disease (Frolov and Konstantinova, 1981). Based on such haemodynamic evaluation, the progression to a stage of decompensation has been estimated to require typically a period of 5–10 years (Sevelyev et al., 1981). Frolov, Konstantinova and Karalkin (1982) have suggested that such an interval from the onset of disease should present the optimal period for surgical intervention on varicose veins.

The role of arteriovenous shunts in venous disease is unclear. At present the evidence for arteriovenous anastomosis being the initiating factor in varicose veins remains interesting, but inconclusive (Scott, 1990). Using radionuclide angiography and the method of technetium-99m pertechnetate clearance from an intracutaneous depot, Keralkin et al. (1988) have provided support for the presence of arteriovenous shunting as a type of microcirculatory disturbance in decompensated venous disease. Other workers (Lindemayr et al., 1972; Hehne et al., 1974; Serise et al., 1982) have refuted the existence of such shunting by measuring technetium-99m radiolabelled albumin particles and comparing the percentage ratio difference of activity after intra-arterial and intravenous injection (also see section on 'Pulsatile flow in the normal direction' under 'Diagnosis by ultrasound' earlier in this chapter).

## Assessment of venous pumping ability

The earliest method employing radioisotopes for assessing function of the venous system of the lower extremity was described by Vitek, Huvar and Vrubel (1974). Their technique of functional isotope phlebography was used to distinguish normal function from venous insufficiency with greater sensitivity than contrast phlebography. The patient's foot vein is injected with [131]I-labelled albumin and radioactivity recorded from probes over the calf and thigh. The rate of decay in activity is obtained following exercise of the calf. Three types of functional curves were recognized, indicating: a normal venous system or one with only small varicosities; an impaired muscle pump mechanism due to the effects of deep vein thrombosis; the presence of overall venous insufficiency but with fully patent deep veins. A drawback of this technique is its failure to distinguish between the causes of insufficiency, whether this is produced only by varicosities and perforators, or by insufficiency of the deep venous system.

More recently, the technique of isotope plethysmography was introduced as a more detailed and accurate method for the assessment of calf pump function (Whitehead, Lemenson and Browse, 1983). Red blood cells are labelled in vivo as previously described. The patient stands on an exercise platform and a scintillation counter is fixed to the back of the calf. The calf muscles are exercised to give reproducible results; occluding tourniquets may be applied to the calf and regulated to any desired pressure. Measurements that can be made include the volume of expelled blood, the rate of emptying, and the rate of refilling. Each measurement can be made following continuous exercise, a sustained calf contraction, or passive compression. The advantages of this technique over the other methods of assessing calf pump function are that the results are direct measurements of the intravascular compartments of the calf, not the volume of all the tissues of the calf. Furthermore, the measurements can be obtained in any body position during active exercise, that is, it allows study of the leg in the position in which venous disease causes symptoms – erect and exercising.

Functional assessment of the venous circulation of the lower limb under different circumstances (chronic venous insufficiency secondary to varicosis or venous obstruction, and following Palma's operation) has been studied by Zicot and Guillaume (1986) and Mark et al. (1988) using dynamic radionuclide venography. The minimal transient time (MTT) of a bolus of radiopharmaceutical ([99]Tc[m]-DTPA or [81]Kr[m]) from the injection site in the foot to a region of interest is calculated. Such a dynamic study is considered to be suitable in the selection of patients for operations reconstructing veins and for postoperative monitoring.

## Bone and soft-tissue changes in chronic venous insufficiency shown by scintigraphy

### Bone changes

The development of extensive lower extremity periosteal reaction secondary to longstanding venous insufficiency is easily recognized on plain radiography. The appearance is of thick, undulating periosteal reaction due to periosteal new bone surrounding the shafts of tibia and fibula. Gensburg, Kawashima and Sandler (1988) provided scintigraphic demonstration of such periostitis on conventional bone scanning with technetium-99m methylene diphosphonate (MDP). The distinctive periosteal pattern of increased activity has been termed the 'double stripe' or 'parallel track' sign, and is also seen in hypertrophic osteoarthropathy, pachydermoperiosteosis and thyroid acropachy.

Increased lower limb soft-tissue uptake of $^{99}Tc^m$-MDP on bone scanning is also seen in the presence of chronic venous insufficiency. This increased activity is demonstrated both during the phase of blood pool imaging, presumably secondary to venous stasis (Gensburg, Kawashima and Sandler, 1988), and in the later crystal phase of imaging by the presence of soft-tissue dystrophic calcification (Lucas-Fehm, Makler and Shapiro, 1986).

### Regional tissue function in venous ulceration

The mechanisms which lead to the skin changes of venous disease in the leg are not fully understood but there is evidence that the microcirculation is abnormal with deposition of a pericapillary fibrin cuff as a result of high pedal venous pressures not reduced by exercise. This may impede the passage of nutrients to the skin and cause ulceration. Scintigraphic methods of indirectly measuring the skin blood flow have included isotope clearance rates with $^{133}Xe$ (Kostuik et al., 1976; Daly & Henry, 1980; Corbett, 1990) and the use of labelled albumin microspheres (Siegel et al., 1975). These methods are either difficult to quantify, with poor reproducibility, or are locally invasive. By contrast, the combined use of the oxygen-15 steady-state inhalation technique and positron emission tomography (Gowland Hopkins et al., 1983; Spinks et al., 1985) provides an accurate, non-invasive method to study both regional blood flow and oxygen extraction and thereby study the effects of the diffusion barrier. Scintigrams are performed while continuously inhaling labelled carbon dioxide for blood flow measurements, and molecular oxygen for metabolic studies. Regional tissue blood volumes are measured by scanning after circulating red cells have been labelled by trace amounts of carbon-11 monoxide. The emission data is processed by an on-line computer and the calculations are solved pixel by pixel to produce both images on screen and numerical computer printout to give a map of regional tissue physiology. In patients with venous liposclerosis or ulceration there is greatly increased blood flow, supporting histopathological findings of a vast proliferation of capillaries in the diseased subcutaneous tissues. There is also grossly impaired oxygen extraction in keeping with numerous capillary walls surrounded by fibrin cuffs. These findings indicate a local functional shunting of blood through the abnormal microcirculation of the skin and subcutaneous tissue but without a corresponding nutritional exchange with the tissues; this may be an important factor in the aetiology of the skin changes seen in patients with calf muscle pump failure.

## Lymphoscintigraphy in the differential diagnosis of leg oedema

Oedema is not a common or prominent feature of varicose veins. It is usually mild and only becomes noticeable at the end of the day. If there is marked oedema and the patient complains of swelling of the lower leg as well as the ankle, other causes of oedema, such as deep vein obstruction or lymphatic obstruction, must be excluded. Lymphoedema is the condition most commonly misdiagnosed as venous oedema (Browse, Burnand and Lea Thomas, 1988).

Lymphoedema is diagnosed in the majority of cases on the basis of clinical findings. Direct lymphography with oily contrast medium is contraindicated in lymphoedema because it may cause lymphadenitis with further deterioration of the oedema. However, radionuclide imaging studies can exclude venous obstruction and give objective confirmation of the diagnosis, together with detection of the site of lymphatic malfunction and the presence of lymphatic malignancy, without harm to the patient. Hence, lymphoscintigraphy has become the imaging modality of choice for evaluating lymphoedema (Weissleder and Weissleder, 1988). $^{99}Tc^m$-labelled human serum albumin is injected subcutaneously in the first and second interdigital space of the foot and images are obtained with a large field-of-view gamma camera. The scintigrams are qualitatively analysed to visualize lymph vessels and nodes for evidence of lymphatic abnormality likely to cause oedema. Features of lymphoedema include the presence of dermal backflow, collateral vessels between lymphatics, megalymphatics, hypoplasia/aplasia of peripheral lymphatics and reduced number of lymph nodes. This qualitative image interpretation does not allow reliable differentiation of primary and secondary lymphoedema. On the other hand, quantitative or dynamic lymphoscintigraphy derived from clearance data is sensitive in detecting and grading lymphoedema. It is capable of detecting mild or incipient cases and has only recently been employed in the evaluation of lymphoedema.

## Thermography

Deep vein thrombosis has long been recognized to cause raised skin temperature in a lower limb and delayed cooling on exposure, even when other physical signs are not present (Pilcher, 1939; Cook and Pilcher, 1974). Modern instruments measuring skin temperature have far greater accuracy than clinical judgement and, over the past two decades, have been used to assess the manifestations of venous disease in the limbs, particularly deep vein thrombosis.

Thermography is a technique for analysing the skin temperature by measuring the infrared emissions with an infrared detector. The electrical impulses from the detector (infrared camera) are converted into a video signal so that a screen image is produced for direct examination and recording by polaroid camera (Cooke, 1981). This has to be carried out in temperature-stabilized conditions and is relatively time consuming.

Alternatively, by simpler and less expensive apparatus, a thermotransducer may be used to give temperature profiles over the length of both lower limbs and which can then be compared with each other by an automatically presented display. This feature is often incorporated in thermographic imaging equipment. A positive temperature profile is present if an average temperature difference of more than 0.6°C is found in any of four segments of the limb when compared with the same segments of the normal limb (Stevenson *et al.*, 1990). Because it depends on comparing one limb against the other it is only of value in unilateral conditions.

A third method is by liquid crystal contact sheet thermography, which displays a pattern corresponding to the temperature of the underlying skin (Sandler and Martin, 1985; Whitehouse, 1985). This is easy and inexpensive to use but its reliability is still under trial.

In a thermogram of normal lower limbs, both sides give similar images and temperature profiles, with even distribution of temperature, but cooler distally and over the front aspects of tibia and patellar; not infrequently there is a general mottling by areas of warmth (Cooke and Pilcher, 1974), possibly due to points of arterial blood supply emerging to the skin. Other venous disorders give rise to temperature changes and may cause confusion. When varicose veins are present and have been well filled by standing, a thermogram will show the contour of large varices due to their relatively high heat emission. In chronic venous insufficiency, temperature profiles may be raised in an uneven fashion which distinguishes them from the uniform increase with deep vein thrombosis (Cooke and Bowcock, 1982). Acute thrombosis causes diffusely increased temperature in the skin overlying the thrombosis but many other conditions may give similar changes, for example, inflammatory states such as cellulitis, superficial thrombophlebitis, injury, arthritis or even a ruptured Baker's cyst. These other conditions usually give an easily recognized local increase in heat and although thermography cannot make a strictly specific diagnosis it can indicate a high probability of thrombosis; perhaps its greatest value is in excluding a range of conditions, most importantly deep vein thrombosis.

### Acute deep vein thrombosis

Simple temperature profiles detect the invariable local rise in temperature that accompanies the formation of a thrombus in the leg and would seem to offer an inexpensive and convenient method of investigating suspected deep vein thrombosis. However, a recent study has emphasized the poor performance of leg temperature profiles when used alone as a screening test (Hamberg *et al.*, 1987) and, since then, other workers comparing temperature profiles and conventional X-ray venography have also concluded that there is little to justify using temperature profiles as a screening test for deep vein thrombosis (Stevenson *et al.*, 1990).

Thermographic imaging by infrared camera, compared with X-ray contrast venography, has been shown (Ritchie, Lapayowker and Soulen, 1979; Cooke, 1981) to give an overall accuracy of over 90% and appears to be a valuable method of screening for deep vein thrombosis. The main barrier to its widespread adoption in screening patients and selecting them for more detailed examination by phlebography is the initial cost of the apparatus and the time-consuming, often inconvenient, nature of the examination. In a different approach to see if deep vein thrombosis could be predicted before surgery, Henderson *et al.* (1978) used the thermographic response to exercise carried out preoperatively and found that when this caused an abnormal pattern of linear hot spots there was a greatly increased likelihood of deep vein thrombosis following operation. They believed this response to exercise indicated a defective calf-muscle pumping mechanism which predisposes to postoperative stasis and thrombosis.

A study of liquid crystal contact sheet thermography by Whitehouse (1985) gave widely varying results reflecting inconsistency in this technique. However, Sandler and Martin (1985) were more confident of its value and found 34 out of 35 patients with deep vein thrombosis were correctly identified but there were 17 false positives, mostly due to non-venous causes and including four ruptured Baker's cysts; negative liquid crystal thermography was 96.5% reliable in excluding unilateral thrombosis. They recommended that when contact sheet thermography was positive, confirmation could be most easily obtained by technetium-99m venoscanning and that this would obviate the need for venography by X-ray in almost 80% of cases; negative thermography excluded thrombosis with sufficient reliability to justify withholding anticoagulants.

### Computed tomography

With computed tomography (CT) the image is the result of numerous signals from detectors opposite to an X-ray tube rotated through 360 degrees round the subject. These signals vary with the density of the tissue the X-rays have crossed and are processed by computer to build up a corresponding image representing a slice of the structure under examination (Greek: 'Toma', a cutting).

CT can only give axial images of the lower limbs, and the resulting cross-sectional slices reveal no more than local information about the longitudinally running veins they cross. Moreover, without enhancement by contrast medium, it cannot easily distinguish between the normal blood stream and static thrombus. For these reasons, it is little employed in investigating widespread abnormalities of veins such as varicosis and thrombosis. It may, however, provide useful information concerning the surrounding tissues in the presence of chronic venous disease.

## Chronic venous insufficiency

Kumar, Roper and Guinto (1983) first described the CT demonstration of extensive ossification of the subcutaneous layer of the leg, enveloping the entire circumference, secondary to chronic venous stasis. This subcutaneous location of ossification remains unexplained with the postulate that the low pH of venous stasis causes metaplasia of mesenchymal cells into osteoblasts, and bone is formed in the subcutaneous layer.

More detailed analysis by Schmeller et al. (1989) of CT appearances in legs of patients with chronic venous insufficiency, as found in the post-thrombotic syndrome, revealed widespread changes in the extravascular connective tissues. In subcutaneous fat there is fibrosis, sometimes with ossification that may extend into the Achilles tendon, which is thinned and reduced in density, with circumscribed, hypodense areas that are a sign of degeneration. In muscles, areas of atrophy with lipomatous degeneration can be found; in bones there are signs of increased osteoporosis, and periosteal new bone formation is seen. The extent of these changes correlates with the degree of venous insufficiency.

## Deep vein thrombosis

CT, enhanced with venographic contrast medium, can be used to demonstrate the filling defect caused by thrombosis of veins in the lower limb (Bauer and Flynn, 1988). The indications for this use of CT are very limited, but it is occasionally helpful when other techniques fail to give a definite answer, or in delineating pelvic and upper thigh veins, and in distinguishing extrinsic compression of the vein from intraluminal clot.

## Magnetic resonance imaging

When a substance, including living tissue, is subjected to a very strong magnetic field, the axis of spin of protons within its atomic nuclei becomes aligned with the magnetic field. If this arrangement is disturbed by a pulsed radiofrequency which exactly matches the frequency of proton movement then resonance occurs, resulting in a change in the axis of spin and the emission of a measurable electromagnetic signal; between each pulse, as the protons realign to the magnetic field, this signal declines at rates characteristic for each tissue ($T_1$ and $T_2$ relax-

ation times). The frequency of proton movement varies proportionately to the strength of the magnetic field and this can be arranged as a gradient across the tissue to give a corresponding gradient of frequency to which the protons will respond; from this the position of affected protons can be determined and placed accordingly in building up an image. $T_1$ and $T_2$ components in the rate of decline of the signal generated by resonance depend on the physicochemical qualities of the tissue at that spot and are used to give varying intensities of contrast in each pixel on the image. This is the basis of magnetic resonance imaging (MRI) and the emitted signals are processed to form an image of varying density corresponding with the nature of the tissue, to give a very sensitive representation of the material under examination. The single protons of hydrogen nuclei, universally present in the tissues, are particularly responsive and it is their emission that is used in the imaging of human tissues. The characteristics of this emission will vary according to changes in the pulsed radiofrequency and selection in weighting of relaxation times in order to obtain optimal display. Armstrong and Keevil (1991) give an excellent, simplified explanation of the complex physics involved in MRI.

This new form of imaging is not confined to the axial plane but can give sectional views in any plane and, amongst other advantages, is able to discriminate between normal blood stream and thrombus. Unlike radiology, MRI is thought to be harmless and there is no limit on 'dosage', but the strong magnetic field does require certain precautions, including avoidance of its use in the presence of metallic foreign bodies.

## Chronic venous insufficiency

Assessment of valve competence and pumping ability of the veins in the lower limbs is not possible by MRI because of its inability to examine the upright patient or to provide real-time imaging. However, static images of the horizontal limb can show some of the secondary consequences of chronic venous insuffiency. A report on the use of MRI in chronic venous insufficiency was published recently by Gmelin et al. (1989). Eight patients with this condition showed similar features to those seen when CT is used, that is, subcutaneous fibrosis with or without calcification, non-specific infiltration of the extrafascial planes, and degeneration of the Achilles tendon. MRI was better in delineating the anatomy of the leg, but overall, CT was somewhat superior to MRI in demonstrating the widespread fibrotic changes and calcification present. These authors suggest the use of MRI only in special circumstances.

## Deep vein thrombosis

The non-invasive modality of MRI appears ready to play a major role in the screening and diagnosis of patients with suspected deep vein thrombosis, and, with such rapid technological advances in this field, contrast venography's days as the time-honoured 'gold standard' for this purpose may be numbered. The value of contrast venography is restricted by its invasiveness, possible complications, and limitations in visualizing the proximal extent of the thrombus. Other methods, such as Doppler flowmetry, duplex ultrasound, plethysmography and scintigraphy, do not provide the anatomical detail needed to follow changes in thrombus size during therapy but MRI can do this well.

Several studies have reported the ability of MRI to identify thrombi in veins in experimental models (Erdman *et al.*, 1986; Rapoport *et al.*, 1987) and in patients (Braun *et al.*, 1985). Another preliminary study has also reported an excellent correlation with venography (Spritzer *et al.*, 1988). MRI has several important features which make it suitable for the diagnosis of deep vein thrombosis and for the monitoring of treatment (Francis *et al.*, 1989):

1. It identifies at high resolution the presence or absence of flowing blood, allowing an accurate measure of the extent of thrombus.
2. There is excellent delineation of small anatomical structures due to the high resolution.
3. The method is non-invasive, without use of ionizing radiation, and does not involve the use of contrast medium, thereby facilitating repeated examinations well accepted by the patient.
4. It is able to distinguish between acute deep vein thrombosis and longstanding post-thrombotic changes (Erdman *et al.*, 1990).
5. Its comprehensive display of all tissues may provide an unexpected diagnosis of extravascular soft-tissue states that explain the patient's symptoms, for example, a ruptured Baker's synovial cyst or cellulitis.

The technique has various modes at the control of the operator (operator dependent) to give maximal definition according to the circumstances. Complete examination does take appreciable time, perhaps 30 minutes for both legs. Movement of tissue presents problems by loss of definition. However, in the case of blood flow the altered signal this creates may be used to improve recognition of blood vessels and, where flow is fast (as in arteriovenous fistulae) they may be outlined with great clarity by dark areas due to absence of any signal. Magnetic resonance contrast medium may be used to enhance the intensity of an image. The agent is usually injected intravenously and its paramagnetic qualities change the response to magnetic resonance. The agent most commonly used is gadolinium diethylenetriaminepenta-acetic acid (DTPA) but other materials are being developed and the use of this principle is likely to increase. These substances are, of course, quite different from the contrast media used in radiography.

At present, high relative cost and limited availability are the major obstacles to utilization of MRI as a routine screening technique for all patients suspected of having deep vein thrombosis (Erdman *et al.*, 1990). It may be used with advantage as a screening examination if:

- There is suspicion of pelvic vein thrombosis.
- There is a history of prior deep vein thrombosis, so that it is necessary to distinguish acute thrombosis from the changes of chronic venous disease.
- If other tests are not available.
- It may have a complementary role when results of conventional screening studies are unsatisfactory.

**TABLE 23.1** Methods of imaging thrombus using radio-isotopes

**Indirect**
$^{99}Tc^m$ macroaggregates of albumin
$^{99}Tc^m$ sulphur colloid
$^{99}Tc^m$ red blood cells
$^{99}Tc^m$ DTPA
$^{81}Kr^m$
$^{133}Xe^m$

**Direct**
$^{99}Tc^m$ fibrinogen
$^{131}I$ and $^{125}I$ fibrinogen (non-imaging)
$^{123}I$ fibrinogen
$^{123}I$ fibrin fragment E1
$^{99}Tc^m$ Plasmin, urokinase, streptokinase, heparin
$^{111}In$ platelets
$^{99}Tc^m$ platelets
Antiplatelet monoclonal antibody
Antifibrin monoclonal antibody

## References

Albrechtson, U. and Ollson, C. G. (1976) Thrombotic side effects of lower limb phlebography. *Lancet*, **i**, 723–724

Albrechtson, U. and Ollson, C. G. (1979) Thrombosis following leg phlebography with ionic and non-ionic contrast media. *Acta Radiologica*, **20**, 46–52

Armstrong, P. and Keevil, S. F. (1991) Magnetic resonance imaging – 1: basic principles of image production. *British Medical Journal*, **303**, 35–40

Armstrong, P. and Keevil, S. F. (1991) Magnetic resonance imaging – 2: clinical uses. *British Medical Journal*, **303**, 105–109

Barnes, R. W. (1979) Noninvasive diagnostic techniques in peripheral vascular disease. *American Heart Journal*, **97**, 241–258

Bauer, A. R. and Flynn, R. R. (1988) Computed tomography diagnosis of venous thrombosis of the lower extremities and pelvis with contrast material. *Surgery, Gynecology and Obstetrics*, **167**, 12–15

Baxter, G. M., McKechnie, S. and Duffy, P. (1990) Colour Doppler ultrasound in deep venous thrombosis: a comparison with venography. *Clinical Radiology*, **42**, 32–36

Bentley, P. G. and Kakkar, V. V. (1979) Radionuclide venography for the demonstration of the proximal deep venous system. *British Journal of Surgery*, **66**, 687–690

Berni, A., Donati, R., Merlino, G. *et al.* (1979) Un metodo di localizzazione delle vene perforanti insufficienti con reoscopia ad ultrasuoni. *Annali Italiani di Chirurgia*, **51**, 333–338

Bettman, M. A. and Paulin, S. (1977) Leg phlebography: the incidence, nature and modification of undesirable side effects. *Radiology*, **122**, 101–104

Bladin, C. and Royle, J. P. (1987) Acquisition of skills required for use of Doppler ultrasound and the assessment of varicose veins. *Australian and New Zealand Journal of Surgery*, **57**, 225–226

Braun, I. F., Hoffman, J. G., Malko, J. A. *et al.* (1985) Jugular venous thrombosis. MR imaging. *Radiology*, **157**, 357

Browse, N. L., Burnand, K. G. and Lea Thomas, M. (1988) *Diseases of the Veins: Pathology, Diagnosis and Treatment.* Arnold, London, pp. 77–144, 169–197

Chan, A., Chisholm, I. and Royle, J. P. (1983) The use of directional Doppler ultrasound in the assessment of saphenofemoral incompetence. *Australian and New Zealand Journal of Surgery*, **53**, 399–402

Cooke, E. D. (1981) Thermography. In *Investigation of Vascular Disorders* (eds. A. N. Nicolaides and J. S. T. Yao), Churchill Livingstone, New York, p. 416

Cooke, E. D. and Pilcher, M. F. (1974) Deep vein thrombosis: preclinical diagnosis by thermography. *British Journal of Surgery*, **61**, 971–978

Cooke, E. D. and Bowcock, S. A. (1982) Investigation of chronic venous insufficiency by thermography. *Vascular Diagnosis and Therapy*, **3**, 25

Corbett, C. R. R. (1990) Report on the meeting of the Venous Forum on 27 October 1989 at the Royal Society of Medicine, London. *Phlebology*, **5**, 63–67

Daly, M. J. and Henry, R. E. (1980) Quantitative measurements of skin perfusion with Xenon-133. *Journal of Nuclear Medicine*, **21**, 156–160

Day, T. K., Fish, P. J. and Kakkar, V. V. (1976) Detection of deep vein thrombosis by Doppler angiography. *British Medical Journal*, **1**, 618–620

DeNardo, S. J. and DeNardo, G. L. (1977) Iodine-123 fibrinogen scintigraphy. *Seminars in Nuclear Medicine*, **7**, 245–252

Dendy, P. P. and Heaton, B. (1987) *Physics for Radiologists*, Blackwell Scientific, Oxford, pp. 347–381(i), 218–250(ii)

Doran, F. S. A. and Barkat, S. (1981) The management of recurrent varicose veins. *Annals of the Royal College of Surgeons of England*, **63**, 432–437

Erdman, W. A., Weinreb, J. C., Cohen, J. M. *et al.* (1986) Venous thrombosis. Clinical and experimental MR imaging. *Radiology*, **161**, 233

Erdman, W. A., Jayson, H. T., Redman, H. C. *et al.* (1990) Deep venous thrombosis of extremities: role of MR imaging in the diagnosis. *Radiology*, **174**, 425–431

Evans, D. S. (1971) The early diagnosis of thrombo-embolism by ultrasound. *Annals of the Royal College of Surgeons of England*, **49**, 225–249

Flanagan, L. D., Sullivan, E. D. and Cranley, J. J. (1985) Venous imaging of the extremities using real-time B-mode ultrasound. In *Surgery of the Veins* (eds J. J. Bergan and J. S. T. Yao), Grune and Stratton, New York, pp. 89–98

Folse, R. and Alexander, R. H. (1970) Directional flow detection for localizing venous valvular incompetency. *Surgery*, **67**, 114–121

Francis, C. W., Foster, T. H., Totterman, B. *et al.* (1989) Monitoring of therapy for deep vein thrombosis using magnetic resonance imaging. *Acta Radiologica*, **30**, 445–446

Frolov, V. K. and Konstantinova, G. D. (1981) Radionuclide angiography in varicose veins of the lower extremities. *Meditsinskaia Radiologiia (Moskva)*, **26**, 6–8

Frolov, V. K., Konstantinova, G. D. and Karalkin, A. V. (1982)

Orthostatic blood distribution in varicose disease of the lower extremities. *Khirurgiia (Moskva)*, **2**, 36–39

Gensburg, R., Kawashima, A. and Sandler, C. M. (1988) Scintigraphic demonstration of lower extremity periostitis secondary to venous insufficiency. *Journal of Nuclear Medicine*, **29**, 1279–1282

Gilliland, E. L., Gerber, C. J. and Lewis, J. D. (1987) Short saphenous vein surgery, pre-operative Doppler ultrasound marking compared with on-table venography and operative findings. *Phlebology*, **2**, 109–114

Gmelin von, E., Rosenthal, M., Schmeller, W. *et al.* (1989) Computed tomography and magnetic resonance tomography of the lower leg in chronic venous insufficiency. *ROFO: Fortschritte auf dem Gebiete der Röntgenstrahlen und der Nuklearmedizin (Stuttgart)*, **151**, 50–56

Gowland Hopkins, N. F., Spinks, T. J., Rhodes, C. G. *et al.* (1983) Positron emission tomography in venous ulceration and liposclerosis: study of regional tissue function. *British Medical Journal*, **26**, 333–336

Haimovici, H. (1985) Arteriovenous shunting in varicose veins. Its diagnosis by Doppler ultrasound flow detector. *Journal of Vascular Surgery*, **2**, 684–691

Hamberg, O., Madsen, G., Hansen, P. B. *et al.* (1987) Segmental mean temperature differences in the diagnosis of acute venous thrombosis in the legs. *Scandinavian Journal of Clinical Investigation*, **47**, 191–193

Hehne, H. J., Locker, J. T., Waibel, P. P. and Fridrich, R. (1974) Zur Bedeutung arteriovenoser Anastomosen bei der primaren Varicosis und der chronisch-venosen insuffizienz. *Vasa*, **3**, 396–398

Henderson, H. P., Cooke, E. D., Bowcock, S. A. and Hackett, M. E. (1978) After-exercise thermography for predicting postoperative deep vein thrombosis. *British Medical Journal*, **1**, 1020

Hoare, M. C. and Royle, J. P. (1984) Doppler ultrasound detection of saphenofemoral and saphenopopliteal incompetence and operative venography to ensure precise saphenopopliteal ligation. *Australian and New Zealand Journal of Surgery*, **54**, 49–52

Hobbs, J. T. (1980) Per-operative venography to ensure accurate sapheno-popliteal ligation. *British Medical Journal*, **2**, 1578

Hobbs, J. T. (1988) The enigma of the gastrocnemius vein. *Phebology*, **3**, 19–30

Hobbs, J. T. and Davies, J. W. L. (1960) Detection of venous thrombosis with I-131 labelled fibrinogen in the rabbit. *Lancet*, **ii**, 134

Kakkar, V. V., Nicolaides, A. N., Renney, J. T. G. *et al.* (1970) I-125 labelled fibrinogen test adapted for routine screening for deep vein thrombosis. *Lancet, i*, 540–542

Keralkin, A. V., Konstantinova, G. D., Alexandrova, N. P. and Finklestein, A. V. (1988) Radionuclide assessment of microcirculatory disorders in varicose veins of the lower extremities. *Meditsinskaia Radiologiia (Moskva)*, **33**, 18–22

Knight, L. C. (1988) Imaging thrombi with radiolabelled antifibrin monoclonal antibodies. *Nuclear Medicine Communications*, **9**, 823–829

Knight, L. C. (1990) Radiopharmaceuticals for thrombus detection. *Seminars in Nuclear Medicine*, **20**, 52–67

Kostuick, J. P., Wood, D., Hornby, R. *et al.* (1976) The measurement of skin blood flow in peripheral vascular disease by epicutaneous application of Xenon-133. *Journal of Bone and Joint Surgery. American Volume*, **58**, 833–837

Kumar, R., Roper, P. R. and Guinto, F. C. (1983) Subcutaneous ossification of the legs in chronic venous stasis. *Journal of Computer Assisted Tomography*, **7**, 377–378

Large, J. (1984) Doppler testing as an important conservation measure in the treatment of varicose veins. *Australian and New Zealand Journal of Surgery*, **54**, 357–359

Leclerc, J. C., Wolfson, C., Arzoumanian, A. *et al.* (1988) Technetium-99m red blood cell venography in patients with clinically suspected deep vein thrombosis: a prospective study. *Journal of Nuclear Medicine*, **29**, 1498–1506

Lensing, A. W. A., Prandoni, P., Bromdies, D. *et al.* (1989) Detection of deep vein thrombosis by real-time B-mode ultrasonography. *New England Journal of Medicine*, **320**, 342–345

Leven, H. O. and Al-Hassan, H. (1990) Ultrasonic diagnosis of iliofemoral venous thrombosis: merits and disadvantages. *Phlebology*, **5**, 107–112

Lindemayr, W., Loefferer, O., Mostbeck, A. and Partsch, H. (1972) Arteriovenous shunts in primary varicosis: a critical essay. *Vascular Surgery*, **6**, 9–13

Lubin, E., Zelihovski, A., Trumper, J. *et al.* (1978) Saphenous vein varicosities – the use of Tc-99m RBC blood pool imaging for evaluation and follow-up. *Journal of Nuclear Medicine*, **19**, 1090–1091

Lucas-Fehm, L. M., Makler, P. T. and Shapiro, B. (1986) Technetium-99m MDP uptake in chronic venous insufficiency. *Clinical Nuclear Medicine*, **11**, 803

McIrvine, A. J., Corbett, C. R. R., Aston, N. O. *et al.* (1984) The demonstration of saphenofemoral incompetence; Doppler ultrasound compared with standard clinical tests. *British Journal of Surgery*, **71**, 509–510

McMullin, G. M., Scott, H. J., Coleridge Smith, P. D. and Scurr, J. H. (1989) A comparison of photoplethysmography, Doppler ultrasound and duplex scanning in the assessment at venous insufficiency. *Phlebology*, **4**, 75–82

Mantoni, M. (1989) Diagnosis of deep vein thrombosis by duplex sonography. *Acta Radiologica*, **30**, 575–579

Mark, B., Szabo, M., Nemessanyi, Z. *et al.* (1988) Testing minimal transient time in the venous system of the lower limbs using dynamic radionuclide venography. *International Angiology*, **7**, 231–233

Meadway, J., Nicolaides, A. N., Walker, C. J. and O'Connell, J. D. (1975) Value of Doppler ultrasound in diagnosis of clinically suspected deep vein thrombosis. *British Medical Journal*, **4**, 552–554

Miller, S. S. and Foote, A. V. (1974) The ultrasonic detection of incompetent perforating veins. *British Journal of Surgery*, **61**, 653–666

Mitchell, D. G. (1990) Colour flow imaging: principles, limitations and artifacts. *Radiology*, **177**, 1–10

Mitchell, D. C. and Darke, S. G. (1987) The assessment of primary varicose veins by Doppler ultrasound – the role of sapheno-popliteal incompetence and the short saphenous systems in calf varicosities. *European Journal of Vascular Surgery*, **1**, 113–115

Myer, K. A. (1983) Special investigations prior to surgery for varicose veins. *Australian and New Zealand Journal of Surgery*, **53**, 394–396

Negus, D. (1985) Perforating vein interruption in postphlebitic syndrome. In *Surgery of the Veins* (eds J. J. Bergan and J. S. T. Yao), Grune and Stratton, New York, pp. 191–204

Nicolaides, A. N., Christopoulos, D. and Vasdekis, S. (1989a) Association between gastrocnemial vein insufficiency and varicose veins. Invited comment to paper by M. Vandendriessche. *Phlebology*, **4**, 171–181

Nicolaides, A., Christopoulos, D. and Vasdekis, S. (1989b) Progress in the investigation of chronic venous insufficiency. *Annals of Vascular Surgery*, **3**, 278–292

Nicolaides, A., Christopoulos, D. and Vasdekis, S. (1989c) Progrès dans l'exploration de l'insuffisance veineuse chronique. *Annales de Chirugie Vasculaire*, **3**, 278–292

Oyama, K., Hayashi, S., Oda, M. *et al.* (1983) RI angiographic evaluation of varicose veins. *Japanese Journal of Clinical Radiology*, **28**, 711–724

Peters, A. M., Lavender, J. P., Needham, S. G. *et al.* (1986) Imaging thrombus with radiolabelled monoclonal antibody to platelets. *British Medical Journal*, **293**, 1525–1527

Pilcher, R. (1939) Post-operative thrombosis and embolism. *Lancet*, **ii**, 629–630

Rapoport, S., Sostman, H. D., Pope, C. *et al.* (1987) Venous clots. Evaluation and MR imaging. *Radiology*, **162**, 527

Ritchie, W., Lapayowker, M. S. and Soulen, R. L. (1979) Thermographic diagnosis of deep venous thrombosis. Anatomically based diagnostic criteria. *Radiology*, **132**, 321

Roddie, M. E. (1989) Detection of venous thrombosis. *RAD Magazine*, *15*, **166**, 22–24

Sandler, D. A. and Martin, J. F. (1985) Liquid crystal thermography as a screening test for deep-vein thrombosis. *Lancet*, **i**, 665–668

Schadeck, M. (1987) Doppler and echotomography in sclerosis of the saphenous veins. *Phlebology*, **2**, 221–240

Scott, J. J. (1990) Varicose veins and arteriovenous shunts: a review. *Phlebology*, **5**, 77–83

Schmeller, W., Rosenthal, N., Gmelin, E. *et al.* (1989) Computerized tomography studies of the lower legs of patients with chronic venous insufficiency and arthrogenic venous stasis syndrome. *Hautarzt*, **40**, 281–289

Secker-Walker, R. H. (1986) The use of radioisotopes in the management of venous thromboembolism. *Chest*, **89**, (5 Suppl): 413S–416S

Serise, J. M., Le Heron, D., Le Heron, G. *et al.* (1982) The use of labelled albumin microspheres in the study of arteriovenus shunting in varicosities of the lower limbs. *Journal des Maladies Vasculaires*, **7**, 37–39

Sevelyev, V. S., Frolov, V. K., Konstantinova, G. D. and Karalkin, A. V. (1981) Comprehensive radionuclide appraisal of haemodynamics in patients with varicosity of the lower limbs. *Kardiologiia (Moskva)*, **21**, 71–75

Sheppard, M. (1986) The incidence, diagnosis and management of saphenofemoral incompetence. *Phlebology*, **1**, 23–32

Siegel, M. E., Giargiana, F. A., Rhodes, B. A. *et al.* (1975) Perfusion of ischaemic ulcers of the extremity. *Archives of Surgery*, **110**, 265–268

Sigel, B., Popky, G. L., Mapp, E. M. *et al.* (1970) Evaluation of Doppler ultrasound examination. *Archives of Surgery*, **100**, 535–540

Spinks, T. J., Lammertsma, A. A., Jones, T. *et al.* (1985) Influence of intravascular activity on the determination of blood flow and oxygen extraction in normal and ulcerated legs using the 0–15 steady-state and positron emission tomography. *Journal of Computer Assisted Tomography*, **9**, 342–351

Spritzer, C. E., Sussman, S. K., Blinder, R. A. *et al.* (1988) Deep venous thrombosis evaluation with limited-flip-angle, gradient-refocused MR imaging. Preliminary experience. *Radiology*, **166**, 371

Stevenson, A. J. M., Moss, J. G. and Kirkpatrick, A. E. (1990) Comparison of temperature profiles (Devetherm) and conventional venography in suspected lower limb thrombosis. *Clinical Radiology*, **42**, 37–39

Strandness, D. E. Jr, Schultz, R. D., Sumner, D. S. and Rushner, R. F. (1967) Ultrasonic flow detection. *American Journal of Surgery*, **113**, 311–320

Vandenriessche, M. (1989) Association between gastrocnemial vein insufficiency and varicose veins. *Phlebology*, **4**, 171–184

Vasdekis, S. N., Clarke, G. H., Hobbs, J. T. and Nicolaides, A. N. (1989) Evaluation of non-invasive and invasive methods in the assessment of short saphenous vein termination. *British Journal of Surgery*, **76**, 929–932

Vasdekis, S. N., Clarke, H. G. and Nicolaides, A. N. (1989)

Quantification of venous reflux by means of duplex scanning. *Journal of Vascular Surgery*, **10**, 670–677

Vitek, J., Huvar, A. and Vrubel, F. (1974) Functional isotope phlebography of lower extremities. *Acta Radiologica*, **15**, 161–168

Wales, L. R. and Azose, A. A. (1985) Saphenous varix: ultrasonic diagnosis. *Journal of Ultrasound in Medicine*, **4**, 143–145

Weissleder, H. and Weissleder, R. (1988) Lymphoedema: evaluation of qualitative and quantitative lymphoscintigraphy in 238 patients. *Radiology*, **167**, 729–735

Whitehead, S., Lemenson, G. and Browse, N. L. (1983) The assessment of calf pump function by isotope plethysmography. *British Journal of Surgery*, **70**, 675–679

Whitehouse, G. H. (1985) Liquid crystal thermography. *Radiology Now*, **6**, 3–5

Whitehouse, G. H. (1990) Venous thrombosis and thromboembolism. *Clinical Radiology*, **41**, 77–80

Zelikovski, A., Zamir, B., Hadar, H. and Urca, I. (1981) Saphenofemoral valve insufficiency in varicose veins of the lower limb. *Angiology*, **32**, 807–811

Zicot, M. and Guillaume, M. (1986) The assessment of chronic venous obstructions by non-invasive haemodynamic studies and imaging with Kr-81m venography. *International Angiology*, **5**, 21–25

Zorba, J., Schier, D. and Postituck, G. (1986) Clinical value of blood pool radionuclide venography. *American Journal of Radiology*, **146**, 1051–1055

Zwiebel, W. J. and Priest, D. L. (1990) Color duplex sonography of extremity veins. *Seminars in Ultrasound, CT and MR*, **11**, 136–167

## Bibliography

Bergan, J. J. and Yao, J. S. T. (1991) *Venous Disorders*, Saunders, Philadelphia

Cheatle T. R., McMullin, G. M., Farrah, J., Coleridge Smith, P. D. and Scurr, J. H. (1990) Three tests of microcirculatory function in the evaluation of treatment. *Phlebology*, **5**, 165–172

Coleridge Smith, P. (1990) Noninvasive venous investigation. *Vascular Medicine Review*, **1**, 139–166

Irvine, A. T. and Lea Thomas, M. (1991) Colour-coded duplex sonography in the diagnosis of deep vein thrombosis: a comparison with phlebography. *Phlebology*, **6**, 103–109

Jenson, C., Lomholdt Knudsen, L. and Hegedus, V. (1983) The role of contact thermography in the diagnosis of deep venous thrombosis. *European Journal of Radiology*, **3**, 99–102

Nicolaides, A. N. and Sumner, D. S. (1991) *Investigation of Patients with Deep Vein Thrombosis and Chronic Venous Insufficiency*, Med–Orion, London

Pochaczevsky, R., Pillari, G. and Feldman, F. (1982) Liquid crystal contact thermography of deep venous thrombosis. *American Journal of Radiology*, **138**, 717–723

Richardson, G. D. and Beckwith, T. (1990) Duplex scanning of recurrent varicose veins. *Phlebology*, **5**, 281–284

Richardson, G. D., Beckwith, T. C. and Sheldon, M. (1991) Ultrasound windows to abdominal and pelvic veins. *Phlebology*, **6**, 111–125

# 24

# Investigation by directional Doppler flowmetry, photoplethysmography and other techniques

This chapter is concerned with a range of special investigations, mostly non-invasive, which are of value in diagnosis and understanding of venous problems. There is a considerable variety of such investigations, some much more useful than others, so that it is not practicable to give a comprehensive description and, indeed, might cause confusion. Instead this chapter will concentrate upon giving a description of those believed by the author to be the most useful in practice because of their simplicity and reliability. Alternative investigations will also be referred to briefly, to give an indication of the choice available, and some of these may have advantages over the methods recommended but much will depend upon the outlook of the venous specialist who is to use them. Many surgeons will prefer relatively simple methods which may be used at the time of consultation with the patient. Others will prefer more sophisticated techniques carried out in a well-equipped vascular laboratory employing one or two technicians, but this does not necessarily yield a corresponding increase in the accuracy and detail of the information provided. The non-invasive tests with instruments are often preliminaries giving guidance on whether or not phlebography or duplex ultrasonography are needed in any particular patient.

With many patients thorough examination by clinical means alone can be sufficient, but in all patients it is a great help to back this with a rapid check by directional Doppler flowmetry to the superficial veins; of all the tests with electronic instruments this is the quickest and easiest to give a broad range of additional information not obtainable by clinical tests. It may do no more than confirm the clinical findings or it may reveal unsuspected aspects which require explaining. In this case further evidence can be provided by plethysmography or venous pressure measurement. If doubts still remain, and it is clear that a significant deep vein problem is possible, the most reliable next step is functional phlebography or ultrasonography. With modern low osmolar opacifying media there need be no undue reluctance to employ phlebology, but ultrasonography is increasingly taking over

aspects of this. A selective diagnostic approach is summarized in the diagram of Figure 24.1(a), and the main patterns of abnormal flow in Figure 24.1(b).

## The evidence upon which diagnosis is made: overall view

The basic observations, on which a specific diagnosis of each venous disorder depends, are summarized below. In all cases, the evidence must be gathered with the patient in the position in which venous problems arise, upright, and usually accompanied by intermittent exercise.

### Clinical evidence

Clinical diagnosis is largely by deduction, interpreting the response of tissues to venous disorder and physical signs related to incompetent valves. A positive diagnosis by clinical means alone is only possible in superficial vein incompetence and here proof is provided by unequivocal control of abnormal veins by a selective Trendelenburg test. Other diagnoses can only be tentative, arrived at by

---

**Figure 24.1**

*(a) Diagram of diagnostic pathways in venous disorders of the lower limb*

*(b) The main patterns of abnormal flow in superficial veins referred to in this chapter. These are detectable by Doppler flowmetry in the upright patient, exercising intermittently.*
  *1. Superficial vein incompetence with obvious varicose veins. Downflow after exercise or lifting foot off the ground.*
  *2. Concealed superficial vein incompetence, with no varicose veins intervening in the pathway of incompetence. Downflow after exercise.*
  *3. Generalized deficiency of valves in deep and superficial veins (valveless syndrome). Exercise causes blood to surge back and forth with little purposeful upward movement.*
  *4. Deep vein occlusion or deformity (post-thrombotic syndrome). Upflow in superficial veins acting as collaterals past impaired deep veins, and accentuated by exercise*

528

## DIAGNOSTIC PATHWAYS IN VENOUS DISORDER OF THE LOWER LIMBS

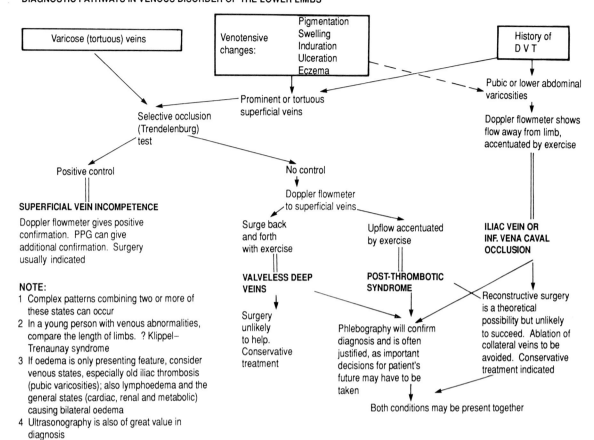

| Varicose (tortuous) veins |

Venotensive changes:
Pigmentation
Swelling
Induration
Ulceration
Eczema

History of D V T

Prominent or tortuous superficial veins

Pubic or lower abdominal varicosities

Selective occlusion (Trendelenburg) test

Doppler flowmeter shows flow away from limb, accentuated by exercise

Positive control

No control

**SUPERFICIAL VEIN INCOMPETENCE**

Doppler flowmeter gives positive confirmation. PPG can give additional confirmation. Surgery usually indicated

Doppler flowmeter to superficial veins

Surge back and forth with exercise

Upflow accentuated by exercise

**ILIAC VEIN OR INF. VENA CAVAL OCCLUSION**

**NOTE:**
1 Complex patterns combining two or more of these states can occur
2 In a young person with venous abnormalities, compare the length of limbs. ? Klippel–Trenaunay syndrome
3 If oedema is only presenting feature, consider venous states, especially old iliac thrombosis (pubic varicosities); also lymphoedema and the general states (cardiac, renal and metabolic) causing bilateral oedema
4 Ultrasonography is also of great value in diagnosis

**VALVELESS DEEP VEINS**

Surgery unlikely to help. Conservative treatment

**POST-THROMBOTIC SYNDROME**

Reconstructive surgery is a theoretical possibility but unlikely to succeed. Ablation of collateral veins to be avoided. Conservative treatment indicated

Phlebography will confirm diagnosis and is often justified, as important decisions for patient's future may have to be taken

Both conditions may be present together

**a**

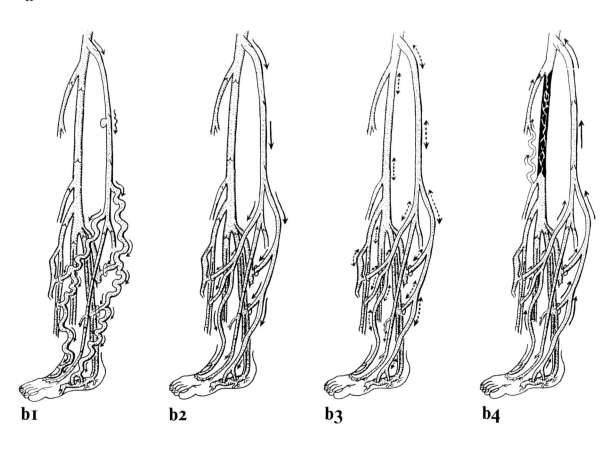

**b1**          **b2**          **b3**          **b4**

elimination, and will require further proof by special means.

## Special investigation by electronic instruments, ultrasonic scanning and phlebography

The value of these tests is that one or other of them is able to give direct evidence of the disturbed physiology characteristic for each venous disorder. This will include one or more of the following:

- Alteration in the direction and speed of flow in veins, particularly in relation to exercise and movement. Doppler flowmetry, functional phlebography and ultrasonography can all detect these changes, each method having its own range of suitability.
- Abnormal venous pressure change in response to exercise. This is either measured directly by intravenous cannula connected to an electronic tranducer, or, indirectly, as an estimate derived from volume changes.
- Abnormal volume change in response to exercise. This is measured by some form of plethysmography.
- Deformity or obstruction in veins and loss of valve function. These features can all be displayed by the imaging techniques of phlebology and duplex ultrasonography which also monitors direction and speed of flow.
- Reduced microperfusion of skin. The blood flow through capillary beds is often slowed at the site of threatened venous ulcer and this can be estimated by laser Doppler flowmetry. It is used to compare one area with another or the change over a time interval in the same area.

The circumstances in which these basic abnormalities will be found and the appropriate type of investigation are reviewed briefly below.

### Gravitational downflow in superficial veins

The characteristic feature of incompetent superficial veins is downward flow against valves when the patient is standing and exercising and may be demonstrated:

1. By clinical tests, particularly a selective Trendelenburg test, which controls filling of varicose veins caused by downflow in superficial veins.
2. By directional Doppler flowmetry, functional phlebography or ultrasonography, all of which can reliably identify such downflow.

It can also be demonstrated indirectly when plethysmography shows that abnormal volume (and pressure) changes are restored to normal by temporary occlusion of the suspected pathway of superficial incompetence. In cases of massive superficial incompetence causing venotensive change this can give valuable positive confirmation of the diagnosis but in less severe states

there may be insufficient abnormality to give a reliable response; only a positive response is meaningful and such indirect tests are inconclusive without this.

### Gravitational downflow (reflux) in deep veins

There is no reliable clinical test for this, only negative evidence by failure to elicit a response. The Doppler flowmeter can demonstrate gravitational downflow in deep veins but is often confused by incompetence in an overlying saphenous vein, or it cannot distinguish between a major deep vein and its branches, for example, popliteal and gastrocnemius veins. Functional phlebography and ultrasonography are capable of demonstrating reflux in individual deep veins with great clarity and ultrasonography can even allow measurement of the volume of downflow.

### Collateral upward flow in superficial veins

The clinical tests cannot satisfactorily demonstrate abnormal upflow but directional Doppler flowmetry can show this with certainty and is particularly valuable in the initial detection of collateral superficial vein upflow past deformed or occluded deep veins. Ultrasonic scanning and functional phlebography, of course, also do this but in addition give a visual display of the state of the deep veins.

### Impaired musculovenous pumping

Of the clinical tests, Perthes' test, using prominence of varicosities, may give the best indication of musculovenous pumping ability but the instrument tests dependent on pressure or volume changes are far more precise. Musculovenous pumping ability can be judged by the response of venous pressure or limb volume to exercise in the upright position; the features studied are:

- The extent to which volume or pressure is reduced.
- The time before return to the original state.

Reduction in volume represents the venous blood expelled from the limb by exercise. The degree and duration of pressure change depend on the volume of blood removed and the effectiveness of valves in preventing it from returning.

Venous pressure may be assessed by:

1. *Direct measurement.* This will involve needling a vein and use of an electronic pressure transducer (a fluid manometer is clumsy and unresponsive) and a recording will give a profile of pressure change with exercise.
2. *Indirect estimation.* This is derived from change in volume. Venous pressure varies in parallel with change in volume so that the profile of this can be used to indicate the pattern of simultaneous pressure change.

Volume change is measured by plethysmography and may be carried out by various methods, for example, by measuring the volume of the distal limb using fluid displacement (water or air), by change in weight, by change in circumference measured from electrical resistance (impedence) of tissue, or by using an electronic strain gauge encircling the limb.

Photoplethysmography depends on the distension of the skin capillary bed as gauged by a photoelectric 'count' of the red cells in a small area of skin; this has been shown to be closely related to venous pressure.

## Deformed or obstructed deep veins

### Delayed outflow of venous blood from the limb

Diminished maximal venous outflow will indicate deformity or obstruction in the deep veins. The elevated limb is congested by a pneumatic cuff which is released abruptly and the rate of reduction in size, judged by a circumferential strain gauge, is used to estimate maximal venous outflow. It is a variety of plethysmography and not very specific in its findings. Phlebography will display the state of the deep veins at all levels and will be far more informative.

### Visualizing veins, valves and flow

Functional phlebography, supported by the image intensifier, offers the best overall means of visualizing veins and valves, and displaying the flow within them. Its main restriction is the brief opportunity to watch active flow, the limited ability to repeat this for further details and the comparatively small window of viewing. This important technique is discussed in some detail in Chapter 22. Wide coverage can be provided by radioisotope venography using the gamma camera but this gives little detail and cannot reveal much about function (see Chapter 23).

Another important technique that has emerged recently is the imaging of veins by ultrasound (Duplex scanning and colour flow imaging or Triplex scanning) with the ability to monitor speed and direction of flow within them. This has already established a leading role in research and the practical management of venous problems, and is discussed further later in this chapter and in Chapter 23.

The field of imaging is one full of promise for the future, with magnetic nuclear resonance as the latest entrant but as yet not suitable for examining veins in an actively moving limb.

## The directional Doppler flowmeter

### Reading flow patterns in the superficial veins

The probe of the directional Doppler flowmeter continuously emits ultrasound from an electronically stimulated crystal. Ultrasound is reflected by tissue interfaces and this is detected by a receiving crystal situated alongside the emitting crystal in the head of the probe. Red cells are good reflectors of ultrasound and any movement by them along the line of emission, either away from or towards the probe, causes the reflected signal to be shifted in its frequency and hence the name Doppler. Suitable equipment will not only record that movement is taking place but will be able to measure the velocity and direction of movement (Strandness et al., 1967). This is the basis of the flowmeter (or more accurately, velocimeter) used to detect the pattern of flow in the veins. The description that follows is mainly concerned with its use on the superficial veins and for this purpose an 8 MHz frequency is used. The transmitted beam has to be angled at approximately 45 degrees to the axis of flow vein to obtain a Doppler shift. The angle is not particularly critical but it is necessary to know the line of emission of ultrasound from the probe so that this may be appropriately aligned. Any small gap between the probe and the skin must be filled with fluid to ensure continuity of the ultrasound in both directions and various gels (coupling mediums) are available for this purpose. Reflected signals from red cells moving towards the transducer return at a frequency higher than that transmitted and, conversely, at a lower frequency when the red cells are moving away. The change in frequency, or Doppler shift, is proportional to the velocity of the red cells. The information given is instantaneous and continuous. The circuitry of the machine will represent the Doppler shift in various ways:

1. An audible signal in which the pitch is related to velocity and the direction given by stereophonic earphones.
2. By some form of visible meter, which may be a needle indicator or an array of lights, so that the extent and direction of deflection indicate the velocity and direction of flow.
3. It may be shown on an oscillograph.
4. By a tracing on a chart recorder.
5. The signal may be fed into a computer, the results interpreted in different ways and finally displayed on a video screen, and appropriate print-outs will be given as required.

Whatever apparatus is used it should have these features: an audible signal to guide the user in placing the probe to best effect; a visible signal of some sort for immediate reading of the velocity and direction of flow; a means for permanent recording of a representative sample of the signals for further study. If these requirements are met, the latest computerized versions of flowmeters do not necessarily give any better results than the older and simpler versions but, of course, the computerized machines will have a wide range of other functions applicable to arterial work and of importance in a general vascular laboratory.

## Type of probe

The somewhat heavy pencil probe used for arterial work is not particularly suitable for use over superficial veins. Here the requirement is for a light probe that can be held against the skin, without displacement, on a patient who is standing and moving by rising on the toes intermittently. A small, flat-headed probe has a low profile and can be used on the inner aspect of a limb without catching on the opposite side; its small size and light weight minimize any tendency for it to swing back and forth as the patient moves. It is an advantage if the probe is mounted on a small bridge so that it can straddle a superficial vein without appreciably flattening it. A vein, such as a protruberant varicosity, is easily squashed flat, even by quite light pressure, and this may stop all flow within it. This is the usual reason for failure to obtain a signal from superficial veins. A bridge giving a gap of approximately 2 mm is easily filled with a small quantity of the coupling gel and proves very suitable. The lead to the probe should be light and of good length so that it allows the probe to be used without any restriction or drag.

## Applying the probe

The flat probe just described can be held in position with adhesive tape but this does not prove satisfactory for the following reasons:

1. The coupling gel tends to spread so that adhesive tape will not stick.
2. It is difficult to keep the probe in a position of optimal 'fine tuning'. Once the tape is in place and support with the fingers removed, the probe so often slips slightly to a poor position. In the consequent effort to firm up the positioning of the probe the underlying vein may be flattened and flow within it prevented.
3. Often it is desirable to make several observations at different points and this degree of mobility with the probe is limited if it is to be taped into position each time, particularly if the gel is causing difficulties of adhesion.

As so often the ideal instrument for precise location is the human hand. The probe is held with the thumb and the first two fingers protruding slightly from it, in contact with the skin so that any change is immediately sensed (Figure 2.9). The patient's limited movements are easily followed and, in practice, Doppler flowmetry is carried out quickly in combination with the clinical examination. The examination is, of course, only of value when the patient is upright and a convenient arrangement is for the patient to stand on the couch so that the lower limbs are at an easy working level for the examiner.

## Positioning of the probe

There are no set positions for placing the probe because this will depend upon the pattern and nature of the venous disorder. This will have been mapped out during the clinical examination which should have identified the likely venous abnormality both by visual inspection and by the tapwave technique. Veins near to the surface are more easily located by Doppler than those deep in the subcutaneous layer. Flow in straight or gently curving veins gives good signals but in tortuous veins a confused signal, without any indication of direction, is commonly obtained because of the close proximity of two streams going in opposite directions. Moreover, in a tortuous vein it is often impossible to be sure which is the 'upper' or 'lower' end of the vein, so that even if a good directional signal is obtained there may be doubts as to whether this is gravitational downflow or collateral upflow. This can usually be resolved by asking the patient to cough; the sudden movement this causes will be away from the abdomen and downwards. Alternatively the vein may be given a quick, light compression an inch or two below the probe to give a brief upward movement of blood to see how this tallies with the direction indicator. Turbulence will show up as heavy flow in both directions simultaneously. This will be found in tortuous veins or immediately below leaking valve cusps. If the probe is placed over a sacculation on the long saphenous the jet of blood coming through the leaking cusps will be recorded as having high velocity and often with evidence of turbulence. The most favourable sites for positioning the Doppler probe may be decided as follows:

1. Choosing the site for the Doppler probe must always be preceded by careful clinical evaluation so that the veins most likely to be at fault have been identified.
2. When examining for suspected superficial incompetence, it is important that the probe is placed over the likely pathway of incompetence whether this be a saphenous vein, a branch vein or a varicosity.
3. Over the long saphenous vein, as it crosses the medial femoral condyle, is always likely to be informative. If the vein here is not palpable or detectable by tapwave, the probe may be placed blindly over the posteromedial aspect of the limb with a liberal quantity of gel under it, so that it has a range of movement without running dry. The veins in the upper calf are now flipped repeatedly whilst the probe is adjusted to pick up the corresponding movement of blood in the long saphenous vein. It is unusual to fail to find even a

comparatively small normal saphenous vein by this method. The long saphenous vein may, of course, be located and used at any level, but in the upper part of the thigh its depth makes it more difficult to find and confusion may be caused by the proximity of the deep vein. The optimal position, giving the most representative flow, is often just above knee level. However, it must not be forgotten that commonly a large varicosity is given off in mid-thigh and the saphenous vein below this level may have fully competent valves so that flow in it will not be representative; an adequate mapping of the varicosities during the clinical examination should have given warning of this possibility. For this reason it is always as well to check upon the flow in one or two of the most obvious varicosities.

4. Flow in varicosities. As far as possible the probe should be placed over a portion of the varicosity where the vein has parallel walls and is not angulated. Even in the absence of such a favourable portion of vein the probe can usually be shifted slightly to give a clearly directional signal which can be verified by the manoeuvres described above.

5. The short saphenous vein in the midline of the calf is suitable, provided observations are made above the point at which major varicosities take off; as with the long saphenous, it is possible for it to be competent below this level and to give misleading results. The probe is best positioned about 3 in (8 cm) below the skin crease behind the knee, otherwise there may be confusion with the deep veins and interference from the underlying popliteal artery. Again, it is always best also to examine a varicosity arising from the saphenous.

6. Any branch of the long or short saphenous vein may be used but, of course, it is possible for it to be competently valved and not representative of the pathway of incompetence. However, any branch will be able to show upflow, in the direction allowed by valves, if superficial veins in this vicinity are acting as collaterals past deep vein obstruction.

## Detection of perforators

In spite of the claims made by some exponents the author has found it difficult to locate perforating veins in the leg with any certainty. Any large vein or varicosity in the vicinity may mimic a perforator, and large varicosities, quite deeply placed in the subcutaneous fat, are commonplace in this region. The tortuosity and turbulent flow within such veins cannot be satisfactorily interpreted or distinguished from a genuine perforator. When the patient is standing the veins are of considerable size and even when the limb is horizontal the varicosities seldom empty completely so that any movement by the patient or local pressure by the examiner will generate misleading

Doppler signals. The use of constricting bands or cuffs introduces artefacts and increases the difficulties of interpretation.

The surgeon who is uncertain about this should approach it with an open mind and correlate the apparent Doppler identification of a perforator with the findings at operation to see how often there is, in fact, a convincing perforator at that site. A rather different issue is the significance of the large perforator which is so often predominantly conducting blood inwardly as part of the retrograde circuit of incompetence but with a component of outward surge at the moment of muscle contraction. The role of the perforator is discussed in Chapter 11.

## Some common difficulties

Failure to obtain satisfactory signals from the Doppler flowmeter arise in the following circumstances:

- Excessive pressure of the probe on the vein so that it is flattened and flow is stopped; this happens very easily.
- The probe is allowed to wander, particularly when the patient exercises, so that it is no longer centred optimally. The knack of keeping a probe correctly centred over a vein, and avoiding tilting it in one direction or the other when the patient moves, is soon acquired. Movement of the probe can be minimized if the fingers holding the probe are in contact with the patient's skin to monitor correct registration continuously.
- In states of superficial incompetence, downflow may not occur after exercise if the patient fails to relax the calf muscles fully and this should always be considered as a possibility when no satisfactory recordings can be obtained (the same phenomenon is seen during functional phlebography).
- The main downflow may be to the foot and the manoeuvre of raising the foot completely off the ground, with the knee straight, will uncover this.
- Downflow to the foot may be so considerable that apparently conflicting results are obtained when the patient rises on the toes, for example, there may be strong downflow during the actual contraction of calf muscles when rising on the toes.
- The superficial veins may be so large compared with the 'stroke volume' of the musculovenous pump that movement of blood is too sluggish to give a convincing signal.
- In certain valveless states no coherent pattern of flow can be obtained.

As so often with any investigation, it is positive identification that is of real value and diagnosis by failure to elicit a signal is always based on uncertainty.

## Summary of procedure for directional Doppler flowmeter examination in venous disorders of the lower limb

- Patient is examined standing on an examination couch or equivalent platform.
- The pattern of enlarged veins is mapped out by visual inspection and by tapwave technique. Other clinical tests appropriate in a standing patient may also be carried out, for example, assessment of cough impulse and Perthes' test. The Doppler flowmeter itself is, of course, an excellent means of mapping out veins not otherwise easily detected.
- A site is chosen over a superficial vein thought to be typical of the possible venous abnormality. This may be over a long or short saphenous vein in the vicinity of the knee or over a varicosity in the thigh or upper calf.
- Coupling gel is applied to the skin at the selected site; this avoids alarming the patient by the harsh noise emitted by the instrument if the gel is put on the probe.
- A flat-headed probe is held in the fingers over the chosen vein with the gel interposed between skin and

the probe. Care is taken not to squash the vein, particularly if it is protuberant.
- Satisfactory positioning of the probe is checked by flipping the vein a short distance below the probe to see if the consequent movement of blood gives a strong signal. At the same time a final check is carried out to make sure that the flow direction indicator is easily seen, the sound volume control is set to a moderate level and the chart recorder foot switch is conveniently placed.

The following manoeuvres are carried out (Figures 24.2 and 24.3(a) illustrate typical directional Doppler recordings in long and short saphenous incompetence):

1. The patient is asked to give a single cough; a corresponding Doppler impulse will show the direction of downward flow and also confirm that the valves between the probe and the abdomen are not competent.
2. The mid-calf is squeezed to displace venous blood. As soon as any flow created by this has subsided the squeeze is repeated and then again for a third time. In

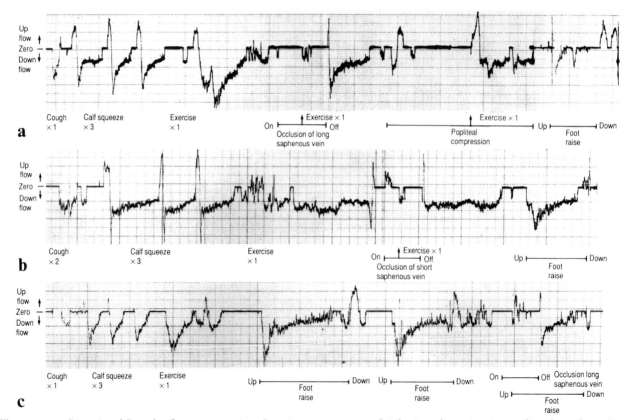

**Figure 24.2** *Directional Doppler flowmeter tracings from incompetent superficial veins; the patient is standing throughout. Events during the tracings are indicated and include: coughing, squeezing of calf, exercise movements by rising on toes and down again, similar exercise with digital compression of pathway of incompetence, compression of popliteal fossa with one or more exercise movements whilst this is maintained, and raising the foot clear of ground with knee straight for 10 seconds.*

*(a) Probe over incompetent long saphenous vein in lower thigh.*

*(b) Probe over incompetent short saphenous vein 3 cm below popliteal skin crease.*

*(c) Probe over incompetent long saphenous vein in lower thigh in a patient with varicosities running to the foot, to show the effect of raising the foot*

simple varicosities this will cause a burst of downflow after each squeeze (Figures 24.2, 24.3(a)).

3. The patient is asked to rise on the toes and down again once. This need not be a full movement and it is sufficient if the heel rises about 1 in (3 cm) off the couch; an excessive movement or returning down again 'with a thud' will displace the probe which then has to be readjusted. In this case rehearse the movement once or twice with the patient before proceeding further. In simple varicosities characteristic downflow will follow this movement (Figures 24.2, 24.3(a)); Figure 24.5(b) gives the corresponding photoplethysmograms showing the venous 'emptying' brought about by exercise; this slackening of the deep veins creates the circumstances for downflow in incompetent superficial veins).

4. The vein being examined is then occluded by firm digital pressure (not an encircling band or tourniquet) a short distance above the probe and the patient is asked to exercise once. After an interval of 3–5 seconds the vein is released to see if downflow then occurs (Figures 24.2(a), (b)). This is a form of Perthes' test and downflow will occur if simple incompetence is present and the deep vein pumping mechanism is adequate.

5. If the probe is over the long saphenous vein at or above the knee there should now be a pause to see if there is any upflow in the vein when the patient is standing still. The popliteal fossa is now firmly compressed with the thumb in order to impede venous return in the deep vein. This manoeuvre may cause immediate substantial upflow in the long saphenous vein and in this case the patient is asked to exercise once whilst compression of the popliteal vein is maintained. If deep vein obstruction is present the upflow will be accentuated by exercise (Figure 24.11(a)) but if the deep veins are in good order and simple superficial incompetence is present then exercise will be immediately followed by downflow that overrides the artificially created upflow (Figures 24.2(a), 24.9(a), right). Popliteal compression must be sufficient to impede deep vein flow but not so great as to obstruct totally all venous return. This test estimates the ability of the deep vein calf pumping mechanism to thrust blood through the compressed popliteal vein with consequent slackening of the veins below this level; downflow in superficial veins confirms that this has occurred and that the basic pattern is one of superficial incompetence without deep vein impairment.

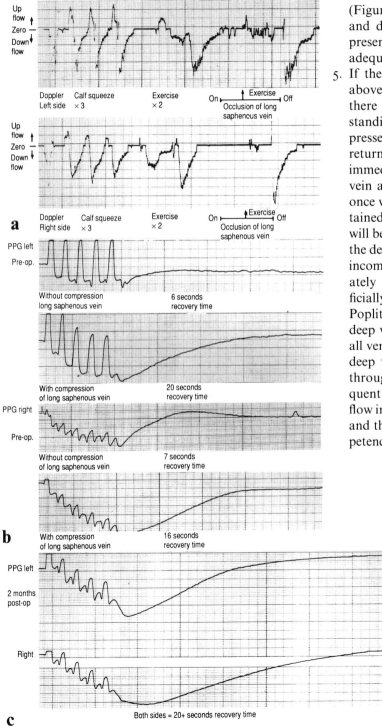

**Figure 24.3** *Directional Doppler flowmetry and photoplethysmography in a patient with bilateral concealed long saphenous incompetence with no obvious varicosities but pronounced venotensive changes.*

*(a) Preoperative Doppler tracings from both sides. The typical downflow of simple incompetence after exercise is shown.*

*(b) Preoperative photoplethysmograms show the venous recovery times are abnormally brief, around 7 seconds on both sides. When repeated with fingertip compression of the long saphenous vein the recovery times have improved greatly to near normal range, at 20 and 16 seconds.*

*(c) Photoplethysmograms taken 2 months after high ligation and stripping of saphenous veins. The recovery times are now within the normal range as predicted in (b)*

6. Popliteal compression is now released and the patient is asked to raise the foot off the couch without bending the knee. This is done by tilting the pelvis to raise the limb straight legged, with the foot in plantigrade position about 0.75 in (2 cm) off the couch. If the knee is bent it is likely to throw the probe out of position and also will be accompanied by muscle contraction which causes unwanted venous flow to invalidate the intended observation. The purpose of this manoeuvre is to raise the foot off the ground, with the least possible disturbance, so that pressure on its underside is removed and the venous spongework allowed to fill. If there is substantial incompetence extending to the foot there will be a burst of downflow slowly dwindling away as the foot veins fill; when the foot is put down again there will be a sudden surge upwards as venous blood is displaced from the underside of the foot (Figure 24.2(b), (c)). This gives an estimate of the likely importance of foot varicosities and desirability of eliminating them when treatment is carried out.

Directional Doppler recordings in deep vein occlusion are shown in Figure 24.4 – acute deep vein thrombosis; Figures 24.6–24.12 show various post-thrombotic states, with Doppler flowmeter recordings, photoplethysmograms and strain gauge maximal venous outflow tracings, explained below.

## Plethysmography

Plethysmography is the term given to the recording of changes in the size of a limb. There are two main factors causing significant variation in the volume of a limb within a short space of time:

1. Changes in the tissue fluid, for example, the accumulation or loss of oedema. This is a process occurring over some hours and is considered in more detail in Chapter 14.
2. Changes due to the volume of blood pooled within the veins. Normal veins have a very variable capacity so that in elevation they are virtually empty but when completely filled on standing may increase the volume below the knee by over 100 ml. In the abnormal, where the veins may be greatly enlarged, this figure may be far exceeded and venous content can vary from minimal in elevation to a litre or more when dependent. In some circumstances, this volume change can occur within a few seconds. When recorded by plethysmography it can give valuable information upon the state of the valves. The swiftness of the change lends itself well to a quick but informative investigation conveniently carried out in a venous clinic.

In a normal subject, immediately after rising from horizontal to vertical position, the veins will fill steadily by arterial inflow to maximal capacity, over 30 seconds or more. In the abnormal subject, with widespread incompetence of valves, there will be a very important additional component of venous reflux so that not only does steady arterial filling occur but there is also rapid reflux from incompetent veins causing the foot and leg veins to distend to maximal capacity within a few seconds in severe cases. The rapidity with which venous distension occurs is readily measurable by a variety of techniques and can give a good indication of the degree of valvular incompetence. However, it is not easy to keep apparatus satisfactorily in place during a wide range of limb movement, but repeated foot movements, or pressure by the examiner's hand, in the standing or sitting position are sufficient to cause a reduction of volume and it is then possible to measure how quickly the volume reverts to the pre-exercise state (recovery or restitution time). This will also give a good indication of the effectiveness of the musculovenous pump. In the normal person a few contractions of the calf muscles will cause a marked fall in volume (the expelled volume of venous blood) which then slowly returns to the previous level over perhaps 30 seconds as arterial inflow occurs. In the abnormal, with a defective pumping mechanism due to inadequate or damaged valves, exercise will cause much less reduction in volume and there will be a rapid return to the original state within a few seconds (shortened recovery or restitution time) due to leakage back of the venous blood that has just been pumped upwards. This reduced response to exercise and the abbreviated recovery period

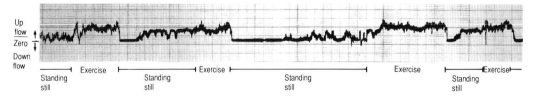

**Figure 24.4** *Directional Doppler tracing from the long saphenous vein in mid-thigh in a patient with femoropopliteal obstruction due to active deep vein thrombosis. This patient attended clinic with a 10-day history of swelling and discomfort in her left leg and thigh; the skin was shiny and bluish. The tracing shows continuous upflow when standing still and this is accentuated by exercise which is followed by a short compensatory pause in flow. These findings indicate that the long saphenous vein is acting as a collateral to occluded deep veins. Phlebography confirmed occlusion by thrombus in popliteal and femoral deep veins*

after exercise is the basis of most plethysmographic techniques in the assessment of venous disorders (Figure 24.5(a)).

## Direct measurement of venous pressure

Although volume changes are very informative, it is sustained high venous pressure that has a deleterious effect upon a limb rather than abnormal volume changes and the most significant measurement is the response of venous pressure to exercise. However, there is a close relationship between the rates of volume and pressure change as the venous system refills with blood. Both recordings run parallel and level off when the veins are filled to capacity, but only venous pressure measurement gives an absolute value, quantitative rather than qualitative, and this is the standard against which other techniques, such as plethysmography, are judged. Plethysmography and similar techniques only give an approximate indication of the degree of change in venous pressure and the speed with which this occurs.

Direct measurement of venous pressure is quite easy to perform by insertion of a needle, connected to a suitable electronic pressure transducer and recorder, into a vein in the foot or leg. This does require meticulous sterility of the equipment and a needle puncture is disliked by many patients. The non-invasive methods of plethysmography avoid these disadvantages and are sufficiently informative for most purposes.

## The methods of plethysmography

There are many methods for measuring and estimating changes in the volume of venous blood in the lower limb:

1. Enclosing the limb within a rigid container and measuring fluid displacement. This can be cumbersome and may well introduce artefacts by pressure on veins where the container is sealed to the limb or by the weight of the fluid. However, a lightweight polyvinyl chloride container filled with air gives satisfactory results and is being used increasingly (Nicolaides, Christopoulos and Vasdekis, 1989).
2. Fluid displacement from an open container into which the foot is immersed. This is somewhat cumbersome but practical and effective. Theoretically the weight of fluid does produce some artefact but this can be allowed for.
3. Measurement by electrical impedance. As the bulk of the limb increases with venous inflow the electrical resistance rises. This method proves effective and is easily applied. It is used by many leading centres.
4. Measurement of circumferential change by electronic strain gauge. This depends upon the electrical resistance of a fluid conductor, such as mercury or indium-gallium alloy, varying as it is stretched and thinned within a silicone tube. The elastic recoil of the tubing

can cause artefacts and requires careful adjustment to prevent undue constriction of the underlying veins. Although perhaps less sensitive than some methods it is easy to use and reasonably satisfactory. It is a suitable method for estimating maximal venous outflow, described presently.
5. Gravimetric methods. Here the change in the weight of the limb is measured. This can give a good result but is cumbersome and not easy to apply to a limb in the vertical position.
6. Photoplethysmography. This method is proving very popular today because it is quick and easy in use and gives results which closely parallel changes in the venous pressure. It is perhaps the most practical method of all for immediate use in a busy venous clinic and for this reason has been chosen for more detailed description below.

## Photoplethysmography

There is a close relationship between venous pressure and the degree of distension of the skin capillaries. The higher the degree of distension of the skin capillaries. The higher the pressure the more the capillary bed becomes filled with blood until full capacity is reached. Photoplethysmography depends on the absorption of light by haemoglobin in the red cells to detect variations in the estimate changes in the venous pressure. The instrument gathers information from a small sensor head mounted on a flexible lead and placed in contact with the skin. A light emitting diode (LED) in the sensor head gives near infrared illumination to the skin and capillary beds beneath it and this light is reflected back to a photoelectric detector in the sensor head. The signals generated by this diminish according to the number of red cells under the sensor and are processed to appear as a tracing on a chart recorder or computerized display; baseline represents minimal transmission of light, that is, maximal content of haemoglobin containing cells in the skin (Coleridge Smith, 1990). An LED light source is used because it does not create any heat which might evoke misleading changes in the capillary bed.

The method is immediately responsive to any change and the tracing obtained is, in effect, giving a continuous record of the degree of congestion in skin capillary beds and this, in its turn, runs parallel with venous pressure (Abramowitz et al., 1979). In a way, the elasticity of the capillary bed is being used as a spring against which the venous pressure is being measured.

The sensor must be applied to the skin without pressure because this would flatten and empty the underlying capillaries to give meaningless results. Fortunately the sensor head is so light that it may be attached to the skin by transparent adhesive and double-sided sellotape is very suitable for this. Drag from the cable is avoided by anchoring it to the skin with adhesive tape 2 or 3 in (5–8 cm) from the sensor. In most circumstances this gives satisfactory attachment of the sensor and allows any movement required; it is best to apply it to a reasonably flat area, such as the dorsum of the foot or the lower part of the shin, and to avoid the immediate vicinity of the ankle joint where intermittent stretching and wrinkling of the skin might dislodge it. Where possible, healthy skin, free from pigmentation, should be used and it should not directly overlie any enlarged and prominent vein.

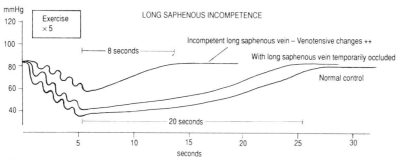

**a1**

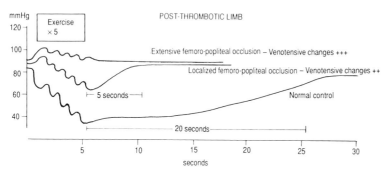

**a2**

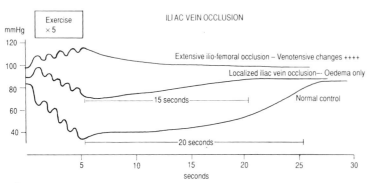

**a3**

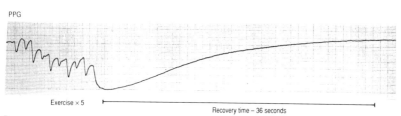

**b**

**Figure 24.5** *Venous pressure changes with exercise in various conditions.*

*(a) Diagrams of venous pressure changes with exercise in upright position in major venous disorders. In each case the response to be expected in a normal limb is shown for comparison.*

*1. Incompetence in the long saphenous vein sufficient to overwhelm the musculovenous pumping mechanism. The fall with exercise is less than normal and time before return to full resting value (recovery or refilling time) is very reduced. Temporary occlusion of the incompetent vein restores performance and recovery time to normal. This form of venous hypertension can be cured by removing the incompetent superficial veins*

*2. Post-thrombotic limb with localized femoropopliteal occlusion; venous blood is returning by unnaturally distended, and hence incompetent, collateral veins. The fall in venous pressure is reduced and the recovery time is shortened by reflux in incompetent veins. Also shown is the pattern in more extensive occlusion of the deep veins and severe venotensive changes, with correspondingly small fall in the venous pressure and a rapid return to full resting pressure. Venous hypertension results from failure of exercise to relieve the venous pressure adequately.*

*3. Iliac vein occlusion. In localized occlusion causing restricted outflow and some oedema of the limb, the venous pressure may rise slightly with exercise and not show the normal degree of fall. A more severely affected limb, with iliofemoral occlusion causing severe restriction of the venous outlet and impairment of the musculovenous pumping mechanism, may show marked initial rise in pressure which then falls slightly but never attains satisfactory reduction in venous pressure; the pressure can only be reduced significantly by elevation of the limb and exercise cannot achieve this. The iliofemoral post-thrombotic limb produces the most severe forms of venous hypertension with intractable changes of oedema, induration and ulceration.*

*(b) A normal photophlethysmogram in response to five foot movements. Although this is measuring the red cells in capillaries under the probe, it closely parallels the venous pressure changes outlined above so that its profile has similar significance. With exercise, venous blood is removed and the capillaries partially emptied, as shown by the downward curve on this tracing. In this patient there is a slow recovery to the original state over the next 36 seconds (recovery or refilling time). This is a good normal, but abnormal, shortened refilling times in various venous disorders are shown in Figures 24.3(b), and 24.6–24.12*

## Light reflection rheography

This is a similar method but is improved by the use of several light emitting diodes to increase the area of skin under examination and by electronic devices to stabilize calibration. It is used in the same fashion as photoplethysmography.

## Positioning the patient

The intention of photoplethysmography in phlebology is to estimate the changes in venous pressure brought about by exercise. This will only be valid when the limb is in a vertical position, or nearly so, since it is the ability of muscle contraction to pump blood away when the patient is upright that is being tested. If the patient is asked to stand the frequent slight muscle contractions required to maintain balance will each cause a distinct drop in the venous pressure and confuse the results. This may be minimized by suitable handrails but it is often better to have the patient sitting over the side of the examination couch with his feet well clear of the floor (Figure 2.10). The popliteal fossa should be well beyond the edge of the couch so that the deep veins are not compressed here. This position allows free movement of the feet by calf muscle contraction (or passively by the medical attendant) but with complete relaxation once the exercise has finished. The sensor is best positioned about an inch above the ankle where representative changes in venous pressure are reliably detected. The dorsum of the foot may be used but this position is more likely to give disturbed results. However, the method is so quick and easy to apply that an operator learning it can try various positions to decide preference in the sensor positioning. Most instruments provide for dual recordings so that both limbs may be examined simultaneously.

## The normal recording

When positioned with the sensors in place, the patient is asked to give a set number of movements (at least five) of both feet simultaneously and then let the limb hang completely relaxed and still; any muscle contraction at this stage will confuse the results. The recorder will register the foot movements as a series of undulations each successively lower than the last (Figure 24.5(b)). This represents the fall in venous filling, and hence fall in pressure, caused by musculovenous pumping action. The downward gradient of this is a rough indication of the degree of change of venous pressure but it must be remembered that it is not an absolute measurement and the apparent gradient may be easily changed by varying the gain on the amplifier. However, if the adjustment that gives a satisfactory recording is left undisturbed throughout, then the gradient of one examination may legitimately be compared with those obtained sub-sequently, for example, during temporary occlusion of the long saphenous vein. Thus, the downward gradient is a useful observation and can be used to compare the speed and degree of venous pressure reduction in the same limb in varying circumstances. However, it is not permissible to make any direct comparison between right and left sides on gradient alone as each is giving a recording independent of the other. Similar considerations apply to the excursion on the tracing created by each foot movement as a rough guide to the stroke volume of the pumping mechanism. The controls of the amplifier should be set to give a strong response to foot exercises so that the tracing nearly fills its channel on the chart. This degree of response may not be possible if the musculovenous pump is grossly incompetent.

## The refilling or recovery time

During the time immediately after exercise the limb is allowed to hang relaxed and completely still. The steady inflow of arterial blood will normally cause a slow rise in the venous pressure as the veins refill and this will be recorded as an upslope on the tracing until the original level is regained. This may take between 20 and 40 seconds in the normal subject (Figure 24.5(b)) and is known as the refilling or recovery time. If gross incompetence of the valves is present rapid reflux in the veins will cause reduction of the recovery time to 10 seconds or less; in a grossly ischaemic limb the recovery time may be prolonged greatly in excess of normal.

The recovery time is an absolute value whether it is measured by direct pressure, or some form of plethysmography. Thus it can be used to compare the normal with the abnormal, the right side with the left, or in the same limb to judge the success of any manipulation in improving the effectiveness of the pumping mechanism. It is one of the most important observations made by plethysmography.

A photoplethysmograph tracing does not necessarily return to exactly the same level as its starting point. For various reasons, some electronic and others physiological, it often sets at a slightly different level and it is wise to zero the machine immediately before each sequence of movements. It is essential that this is preceded by an adequate period of complete inactivity to ensure that venous pressure has returned to a full resting normal. Premature exercise will certainly lead to misleading and puzzling results.

## Patterns of abnormality

The examination proceeds in three phases.

*Phase 1*

The patient is positioned, and the sensors put in place and the response to an exercise sequence observed. The gain control is adjusted to give a strong response that is comfortably within the chart. This should be repeated several times to make sure that a stable and consistent response is being obtained and it will also accustom the patient to the procedure.

*Phase 2*

A base line or control tracing for both feet is obtained simultaneously. This will establish the downward gradient in response to exercise and the recovery time that is usual for the patient. If this is entirely normal nothing further is required.

*Phase 3*

If the downward gradient appears unduly flat, and especially if the recovery time is abnormally short, then various manoeuvres may be carried out to see if it is possible to influence the pumping mechanism favourably. Usually this will be an attempt to eliminate heavy downflow in incompetent superficial veins to demonstrate whether this is the cause of the poor performance originally obtained. For example, temporary occlusion of an enlarged long saphenous vein may cause a dramatic improvement in the individual excursion with each foot movement and in the downward gradient, but, of more importance, it may give a substantial improvement in the recovery time, if not actual return to a normal value (Figure 24.3(b)). By contrast, plethysmograms in deep vein impairment (Figures 24.6–24.12) would not shown any increase in their brief refilling time with any manipulation of the superficial veins. The nature of the manoeuvres carried out must be given careful thought. Strong pressure with an encircling band can easily compress the deep veins as well as the superficial veins and by congestion prevent the good response that should be obtained in massive simple long saphenous incompetence. Conversely, although this is an extreme example, an excessively tight band around a limb may so impede movement of both venous and arterial blood that an unnaturally prolonged recovery period is obtained. Any form of constricting band should be avoided and occlusion of a superficial vein should be by localized pressure with fingers rather than by an encircling band. The superficial veins most likely to be implicated should have been identified and mapped out during the preliminary examination. Some authorities believe that a narrow pneumatic cuff inflated to an accurately measured pressure, say 50 mmHg, does not cause any significant interference with the deep veins. Opinions upon this differ but certainly anything more than a carefully controlled narrow pneumatic cuff cannot be considered satisfactory (Figures 4.11(a) 5, 4.20(a) 4, 6.1(b)2 and 6.6, 2 show Doppler flowmetry and photoplethysmography recorded simultaneously. This is, in fact, an unnecessary embellishment and it is easier to carry out these tests separately.)

## Other special techniques

### Estimation of maximal venous outflow by strain gauge plethysmography

Most forms of plethysmography can be adapted to estimate maximal venous outflow from a limb. However, the strain gauge is particularly suitable for this and is now described briefly to illustrate the method.

The patient is positioned lying on a couch with the feet elevated on a comfortable support 35 cm above it. Both limbs will usually be examined but it is best to do one at a time. A pneumatic cuff specifically designed for the purpose is placed around the thigh and this is connected to a wide-bore, quick-release tap that will allow immediate deflation when required. Each calf is encircled with an appropriate strain gauge transducer which is carefully adjusted at minimal tension with the limb elevated and the thigh cuff completely deflated. Care is taken to ensure that there is no pressure behind the knee or elsewhere

**Figure 24.6** *The findings in a male patient, aged 36, a year after right deep vein thrombosis caused by a motorcycle accident. Both lower limbs were swollen and ulcerated but the right side was more severely affected.*

*(a) Doppler tracings from the right long saphenous vein in upper thigh show continuous upflow, accentuated by exercise with compensatory pause following. An oblique interconnecting vein running downwards from short to long saphenous veins showed strong flow in keeping with collateral return from short to long saphenous vein and gave paradoxical downflow apparently contradicting its collateral function. This was confirmed by phlebography. The left long saphenous vein shows marked tendency to upflow, suggesting post-thrombotic damage in deep veins on this side as well.*

*(b) Photoplethysmography. The recovery time on both sides is under 10 seconds and in keeping with impaired musculovenous pumping and widespread loss of competence in valves. The incompetence is mainly in greatly distended collateral vessels rather than in deep veins which were found to be extensively occluded on phlebography.*

*(c) Maximum venous outflow tracings. On the right side there is severe restriction in outflow with only 33% of total outflow occurring in the first 3 seconds. On the left side the restriction is less severe at 48% of outflow within 3 seconds.*

*(d) Composite phlebogram of right side 1 year later at time of investigations given above. The deep veins could only be filled in fragmentary fashion and showed severe deformity or obstruction. Collateral return is by preferential flow up the long saphenous vein and branch veins; these have become grossly distended and tortuous without evidence of valves. The obliquely running intersaphenous connection, referred to in (a), is shown in the upper leg. Complex collateral circuits of this sort are often found in post-thrombotic limbs (see Figure 22.8 for phlebogram at the time of acute deep vein thrombosis)*

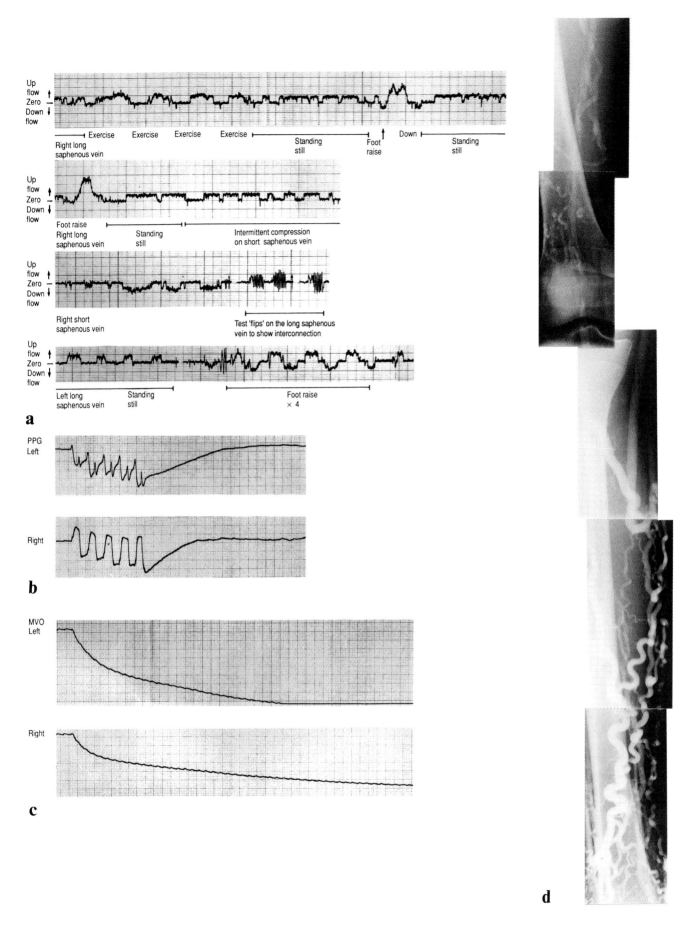

that might interfere with venous return. The patient should relax in this position for at least 10 minutes before any examination is made. The thigh cuff is now inflated to 50 mmHg so that venous return is impeded but the entry of arterial blood continues. This will lead to considerable accumulation of venous blood which will be recorded by the strain gauge as a steady rise in the tracing as the limb circumference increases. The cuff should be inflated for several short periods, perhaps 30 or 40

seconds, to accustom the patient to this, to ensure that the veins are not in a contracted state and also to test the apparatus.

For the actual test the pneumatic cuff is inflated at 50 mmHg for a full 2 minutes. At the end of this time the cuff is released so that the excess venous blood may flow out from the limb as fast as the venous system will allow. Corresponding with this the volume and circumference of the calf will reduce to normal and this will be indicated

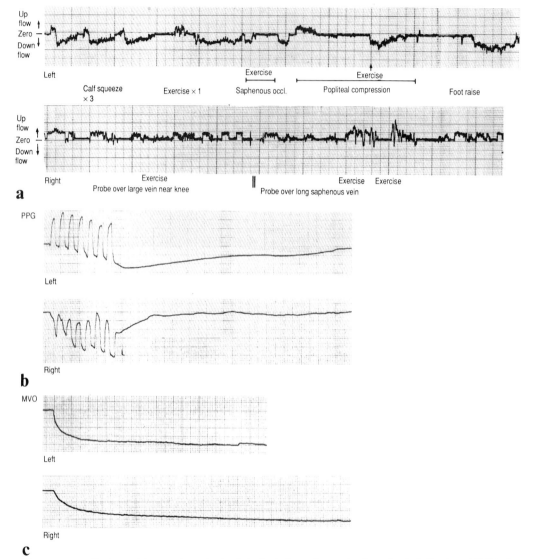

**Figure 24.7** *Patient with post-thrombotic right limb from deep vein thrombosis following childbirth 4 years previously. This limb showed oedema with typical venotensive changes and intractable ulcer. The saphenous vein near the knee on the right side had been removed previously elsewhere in attempted treatment. Moderate sized varicose veins were present on the left side.*

*(a) Doppler tracings from both sides. The right side shows characteristic upflow in two veins sampled near the knee. The left long saphenous vein in the thigh shows typical changes of superficial vein incompetence.*

*(b) Photoplethysmograms showing severe impairment on the right side with a 6-second recovery period. On the left side tracing is normal at 20 seconds, indicating the superficial incompetence is insufficient to affect musculovenous pumping performance.*

*(c) Maximal venous outflow. Right side shows marked restriction of outflow with 60% occurring within the first 3 seconds. Left side is normal at 80% at 3 seconds.*

*(See Figure 11.28(a) for composite phlebogram of this patient)*

on the chart recorder as a sharp fall that gradually levels off. The time taken for the circumference of the limb to return to normal gives an indication of the maximal venous outflow but the exponents of this method prefer to base their calculations on the initial downslope where the rate of outflow is greatest. The proportion of total outflow occurring in the first 3 seconds may be used and expressed as a percentage. Ninety per cent of the total outflow in the first 3 seconds is normal but 45% would indicate a significant reduction in venous outflow. A mathematical formula is used for this and nomograms are available to simplify these calculations. (Figures 24.6–24.12 all include examples of maximal venous outflow used in deep vein problems.)

This examination will take in all about 25–30 minutes if the reading and calculation from the tracings is included.

Usually observations are based on several sequences of inflation and deflation. This is a rather time-consuming examination for the venous specialist to do personally but a trained medical technician should be able to carry out the examination and produce results satisfactorily. The author has already expressed his personal view that much better information will be given by functional phlebography for a similar expenditure of time. Moreover, whilst the method will give a clear indication of venous obstruction in the more severe cases, in others, where the obstruction is less extensive and a generous collateral circulation is present, the results may be within normal limits, but this does not necessarily effect the practical management of the patient. The method is useful where repeated comparative studies are required, for example, when following the resolution of iliac vein thrombosis.

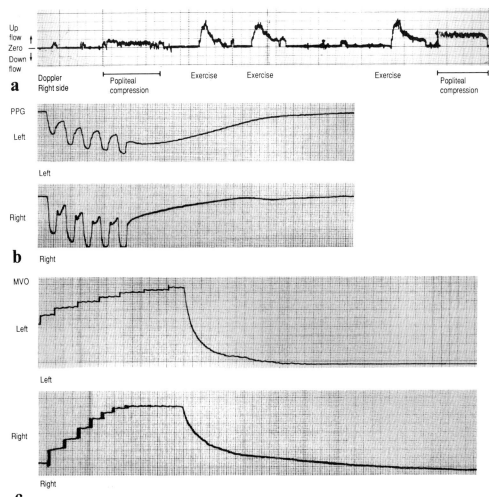

**Figure 24.8** *Post-thrombotic right limb following deep vein thrombosis with pregnancy 20 years before. The limb showed severe venotensive changes in the limb and a 'Cockett's operation' 9 years previously had brought no benefit.*

*(a) Doppler tracing from right long saphenous vein shows upflow accentuated by exercise and characteristic of collateral function.*

*(b) Photoplethysmograms. The left side is normal at 20 seconds recovery time but the right side is shortened to 13 seconds in keeping with some deep vein impairment.*

*(c) Maximal venous outflow. Right side shows marked restriction with only 60% of outflow at 3 seconds. Left side is normal with 80% of outflow at 3 seconds*

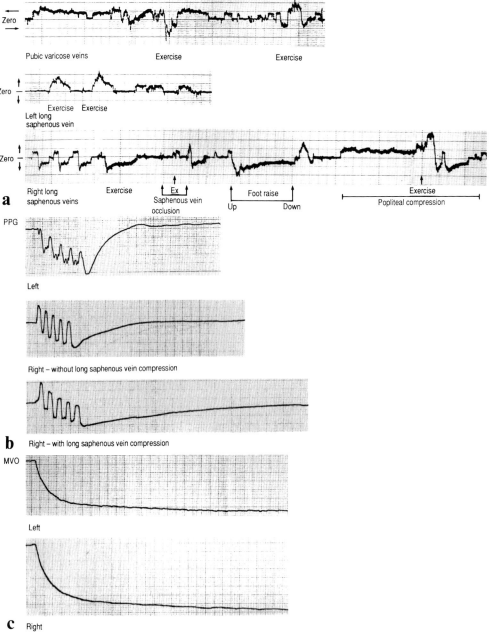

**Figure 24.9** *The findings in a male patient, aged 56 years, with left iliac vein occlusion and right superficial vein incompetence. Deep vein thrombosis was known to have occurred on the left side at the age of 14 years and may have been due to compression by the right common iliac artery. Pubic varicosities were present; both legs showed skin pigmentation and some varicosities but the left side was slighty swollen; no ulceration was present.*

*(a)  Doppler tracings. The pubic varicosities show strong flow, accentuated by exercise, from the left side across to the right. The left long saphenous vein shows characteristic collateral upflow; on the right side there is long saphenous downflow after exercise or foot raising, typical of simple incompetence.*

*(b)  Photoplethysmography. On the left side there is quite a good response of venous pressure to exercise but rapid return to full pressure within 7 seconds; the right side also shows rapid return of full venous pressure within 12 seconds but this reverts to a normal recovery time of 25 seconds when the long saphenous vein is temporarily occluded by finger pressure.*

*(c)  Maximal venous outflow. The right side is normal with 80% of outflow at 3 seconds and the left side is only slightly reduced with 70% of outflow at 3 seconds. The patient appears to have left iliac vein obstruction well compensated by collateral vessels, including the pubic varicosities, but these allow rapid reflux of blood after exercise. The right side shows substantial long saphenous incompetence, sufficient to cause venotensive skin change but capable of restoration to normal if the long saphenous vein is removed. However, it might be better to use this vein for a Palma's cross-over operation which would 'cure' the right superficial incompetence and possibly help the left side. This was discussed with the patient who preferred to accept his present state with conservative treatment by below-knee elastic support*

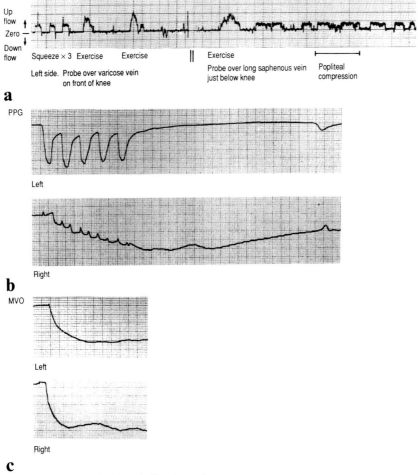

**Figure 24.10**  *This patient had been wounded by a bullet through the left upper thigh 40 years previously. Some swelling, induration and skin pigmentation was present in the limb.*

*(a) Doppler tracings. The left long saphenous vein shows characteristic collateral upflow.*

*(b) Photoplethysmography. There is severe impairment on the left side with a very brief recovery period; the right side is normal.*

*(c) Maximal venous outflow. The right side is normal at 90% at 3 seconds; the left side is also normal at 85% at 3 seconds. It seems likely that femoropopliteal deep vein occlusion has been well compensated for by collaterals so that there is little restriction to venous outflow but there has been severe impairment of the musculovenous pumping mechanism by thrombosis*

In the oedematous limb, it is of value in excluding venous obstruction as a cause, without resorting to phlebography.

Strain gauge plethysmography may also be used in a similar fashion to photoplethysmography described above to assess the response of venous volume to exercise and by use of the recovery time to judge the amount of venous reflux. Temporary occlusion of superficial veins likely to be incompetent may give a return to normal values, thus showing that superficial incompetence is an important factor.

## Laser Doppler velocimetry (flowmetry)

This has been referred to briefly earlier in this chapter. It measures the overall movement of red cells in a small area of tissue by the Doppler shift in a laser beam reflected off moving red cells. In effect, this represents flow of blood in capillaries and can compare tissue perfusion in, say, skin in an area of threatened venous ulceration with more normal skin nearby. It is a valuable research tool into small vessel rheology in venous disorders but also an easy, non-invasive technique to apply in diagnosis, for example, it will detect a characteristic slowing of capillary flow in a standing patient when venous hypertensive changes are present.

## Ultrasonography

The Doppler flowmeter previously described emits a continuous ultrasound wave but if a pulsed, scanned emission is used then an image of the underlying structures formed by reflections at tissue interfaces can be displayed on a video screen (Nicolaides, Christopoulos and Vasdekis, 1989; Coleridge-Smith, 1990). Moreover, within the same image, movement of blood can be monitored, giving its velocity and direction of flow (Duplex scanning – see Figure 2.12 and Chapter 23). By use of colour, the flow

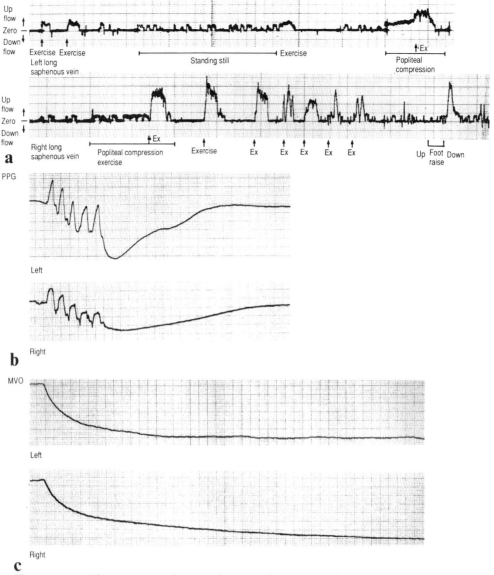

**Figure 24.11** *This patient, aged 59, was known to have sustained a series of deep vein thromboses with episodes of pulmonary embolism, cause unknown, over the last 24 years. He complained of eczema, discomfort and swelling of the legs.*

*(a) Doppler tracings. These confirm upflow in both long saphenous veins typical of collateral return.*

*(b) Photoplethysmography. This showed somewhat shortened recovery times at about 14 seconds in both limbs.*

*(c) Maximal venous outflow. In both limbs outflow was reduced to 60% at 3 seconds.*

*The findings are in keeping with moderate post-thrombotic impairment of the deep veins and surgery to the superficial veins is contraindicated unless detailed examination by phlebography shows otherwise*

towards or away from the transducer can be easily distinguished (colour flow imaging) so that peripherally running arterial flow (red) can be immediately distinguished from centrally directed venous flow (blue) (see Colour Plate 24); the intensity of colour increases with the velocity of flow. Reversed flow, in venous reflux, is clearly recognizable by a change in colour so that incompetent veins and leaking valves show up as 'red' at the moment of reflux. The method is non-invasive and

without limitation in the time over which it may be used or in the number of repetitions of movement. The tissues can be viewed in horizontal or vertical sections or any angle between. It is an ideal method to observe venous structure and flow in the upright, exercising patient; moreover, valves within the veins can be clearly displayed and their competence demonstrated. However, it has the limitation of only a small window of viewing so that the limb has to be studied portion by portion. This is time

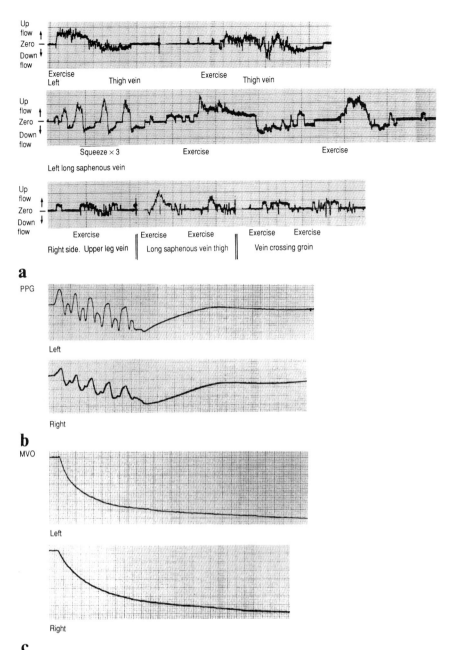

**Figure 24.12** *This man, aged 35, gave a history of deep vein thrombosis and pulmonary embolism 10 years previously. Both limbs showed moderately severe venotensive changes and scattered varicosities.*

*(a) Doppler flowmeter tracings. The left side shows characteristic upflow in enlarged veins on the thigh but at a lower level the findings are more of surge with exercise. The right side shows upflow in keeping with collateral function in the long saphenous vein.*

*(b) Photoplethysmography. Both sides show reduced musculovenous pumping and brief recovery times of about 9 seconds.*

*(c) Maximum venous outflow. On the right side this is reduced to 54% at 3 seconds and 64% on the left side.*

*The findings are in keeping with diffuse impairment of the deep veins on both sides by previous thrombosis. Surgery to the superficial veins is contraindicated without more detailed study including functional phlebography*

consuming but in practice only limited areas most likely to be at fault need be screened.

This method brings a precision and accuracy in measurement of flow not previously attainable and has already proved valuable in research by identifying and measuring the volume of reflux in inaccessible veins, such as the gastrocnemius veins, previously only glimpsed during functional phlebography. Certainly any venous clinic supported by a vascular laboratory will require this sort of display in the future, not only as a research tool but also as a practical device that can unravel many problems and often eliminate the need for phlebography. It does not however displace the simple, everyday methods outlined earlier in this chapter and used in the initial assessment and diagnosis of patients. Both functional phlebography and colour imaging ultrasonography have many pitfalls in their use and require a skilled operator; these two investigations should be viewed as complementary to one another but it seems likely that with further development ultrasound may gradually displace functional phlebography in the imaging of veins in the lower limbs below the inguinal ligament; above this level intestinal gas may prevent a satisfactory display. Ultrasonography is further described in Chapter 23.

## Summary

This chapter has given an indication of the various non-invasive tests available for the investigation of venous disorders. However, the clinical examination, including eliciting a history of deep vein thrombosis, remains of paramount importance, with selective Trendelenburg's test, applied without use of constricting bands, as the keystone. Of the special tests, directional Doppler flow-metry and photoplethysmography are perhaps the most practical and informative in general assessment. A variety of methods in plethysmography are available but each method has its own learning curve and it would seem best to choose a method that appeals to the investigator and to become an expert in this; multiple methods employed within one clinic will not be helpful. When these investigations indicate the likelihood of impairment in the deep veins and additional information is required, then there is little doubt that this will be best provided by functional phlebography. The other investigations will however often make it clear that the venous defects are sufficiently well understood without phlebography and may be corrected surgically on this evidence; this in itself is of considerable value to a venous clinic. Ultrasonography is a new dimension giving impressive results, in some aspects more informative than functional phlebography, but it is at its best in localized scrutiny of vein and valve defects rather than the overall assessment of the limb. Its full potential has not yet been reached (1992) and it may eventually give rapid, comprehensive viewing of the veins in the lower limb and supersede all other methods.

## References

Abramowitz, H. B., Queral, L. A., Flinn, W. R. *et al.* (1979) The use of photoplethysmography in the assessment of venous insufficiency: a comparison to venous pressure measurements. *Surgery*, **86**, 434–441

Coleridge Smith, P. (1990) Noninvasive venous investigation. *Vascular Medicine Review*, **1**, 139–166

Nicolaides, A., Christopoulos, D. and Vasdekis, S. (1989) Progress in the investigation of chronic venous insufficiency. *Annals of Vascular Surgery*, **3**, 278–292

Strandness, D. E., Schultz, R. D., Sumner, D. S. and Rushmer, R. F. (1967) Ultrasonic flow detection. *American Journal of Surgery*, **113**, 311–320

## Bibliography

Akesson, H., Brudin, L., Jensen, R. *et al.* (1989) Physiological evaluation of venous obstruction in the post-thrombotic leg. *Phlebology*, **4**, 3–14

Barroy, J. P., Munck, D., Paturiaux, E. and Goldstein, M. (1987) Mercury strain-gauge plethysmography venous mode: non-invasive technique of choice in vascular pathology. *Phlebology*, **2**, 47–51

Bjordal, R. (1970) Simultaneous pressure and flow recordings in varicose veins of the lower extremity. *Acta Chirurgica Scandinavica*, **136**, 309

Cheatle, T. R., Shami, S. K., Stibe, E., Coleridge Smith, P. D. and Scurr, J. H. (1991) Vasomotion in venous disease. *Journal of the Royal Society of Medicine*, **84**, 261–263

Christopoulos, D. G., Nicolaides, A. N., Szendro, G. *et al.* (1987) Air-plethysmography and the effect of elastic compression on venous haemodynamics. *Journal of Vascular Surgery*, **5**, 148–159

Christopoulos, D., Nicolaides, A. N. and Szendro, G. (1988) Venous reflux: quantification and correlation with the clinical severity of chronic venous disease. *British Journal of Surgery*, **75**, 352–356

Christopoulos, D., Nicolaides, A. N., Belcaro, G. and Duffy, P. (1990) The effect of elastic compression on calf muscle pump function. *Phlebology*, **5**, 13–19

Dickey, J. W. Jr (1989) A study of venous return from the leg during exercise. *Phlebology*, **4**, 185–189

Fernandes, E., Fernandes, J., Horner, J. *et al.* (1979) Ambulatory calf volume plethysmography in the assessment of venous insufficiency. *British Journal of Surgery*, **66**, 327–330

Gilliland, E. L., Gerber, C. J. and Lewis, J. D. (1987) Short saphenous vein surgery, pre-operative Doppler ultrasound marking compared with on-table venography and operative findings. *Phlebology*, **2**, 109–114

Jackson, J. R. and Mathews, J. A. (1977) A gravimetric plethysmograph and its evaluation in clinical use. *British Journal of Surgery*, **64**, 876–882

Klein Rouweler, B. J. F., Brakkee, A. J. M. and Kuiper, J. P. (1989) Plethysmographic measurement of venous resistance and venous capacity in the human leg. Parts one and two. *Phlebology*, **4**, 241–257

Klein Rouweler, B. J. F., Kuiper, J. P. and Brakkee, A. J. M. (1990) Plethysmographic measurement of venous flow resistance and venous capacity in humans with deep venous thrombosis. *Phlebology*, **5**, 21–29 (and two succeeding papers by same authors)

Lancaster, J., Lucarotti, M. and Leaper, D. J. (1987) Laser Doppler velocimetry. *Journal of the Royal Society of Medicine*, **80**, 729–730

Lancaster, J., Lucarotti, M., Mitchell, A. and Leaper, D. (1988) Laser Doppler flowmetric and waveform changes in patients with venous reflux. *Phlebology*, **3**, 69–72

McIrvine, A. J., Corbett, C. R. R., Aston, N. O. *et al.* (1984) The demonstration of saphenofemoral incompetence; Doppler ultrasound compared with standard clinical tests. *British Journal of Surgery*, **71**, 809–810

McMullin, G. M., Scott, H. J., Coleridge Smith, P. D. and Scurr, J. H. (1989) A comparison of photoplethysmography, Doppler ultrasound and duplex scanning in the assessment of venous insufficiency. *Phlebology*, **4**, 75–82

Milliken, J. C., Dinn, E., O'Connor, R. and Greene, D. (1986) A simple Doppler technique for the rapid diagnosis of significant sapheno-femoral reflux. *Phlebology*, **1**, 125–128

Nicolaides, A. N. and Miles, C. (1987) Photoplethysmography in the assessment of venous insufficiency. *Journal of Vascular Surgery*, **5**, 405–412

Nicolaides, A. N. and Sumner, D. S. (1991) *Investigation of Patients with Deep Vein Thrombosis and Chronic Venous Insufficiency*, Med-Orion, London

Norgren, L., Thulesius, O., Gjores, J. E. and Soderlundh, S. (1974) Foot volumetry and simultaneous venous pressure measurements for evaluation of venous insufficiency. *Vasa*, **3**, 140–147

Nuzzaci, G., Mangoni, N., Tonarelli, A. P. *et al.* (1986) Our experience on light reflection rheography (LRR): a new non-invasive method for the lower limbs venous examination. *Phlebology*, **1**, 231–242

Ohgi, S., Tanaka, K., Araki, T. *et al.* (1990) Quantitative evaluation of calf muscle pump function after deep vein thrombosis by non-invasive venous tests. *Phlebology*, **5**, 51–59

Porter, J. M., Swain, I. D. and Shakespeare, P. G. (1985) Measurement of limb flow by electrical impedance plethysmography. *Annals of the Royal College of Surgeons of England*, **67**, 169–172

Schadeck, M. (1987) Doppler and echotomography in sclerosis of the saphenous veins. *Phlebology*, **2**, 221–240

Schraibman, I. G., Mott, D., Naylor, G. P. and Charlesworth, D. (1975) Comparison of impedance and strain gauge plethysmography in the measurement of blood flow in the lower limb. *British Journal of Surgery*, **62**, 909–912

Struckmann, J. R. (1987) Ambulatory strain gauge plethysmography: correlation to symptoms and skin changes in patients with venous insufficiency. *Phlebology*, **2**, 75–80

Tibbs, D. J. and Fletcher, E. W. L. (1983) Direction of flow in superficial veins as a guide to venous disorders in lower limbs. *Surgery*, **93**, 758–767

van den Broek, T. A. A., Rauwerda, J. A., Kuijper, C. F. *et al.* (1989) Comparison of strain gauge and photocell venous function testing with invasive pressure measurements. A prospective study in deep vein insufficiency. *Phlebology*, **4**, 223–230

Vasdekis, S. N., Clarke, G. H. and Nicolaides, A. N. (1989) Quantification of venous reflux by means of duplex scanning. *Journal of Vascular Surgery*, **10**, 670–677

Vasdekis, S. N., Clarke, G. H., Hobbs, J. T. and Nicolaides, A. N. (1989) Evaluation of non-invasive and invasive methods in the assessment of short saphenous vein termination. *British Journal of Surgery*, **76**, 929–932

Whitehead, S., Lemenson, G. and Browse, N. L. (1983) The assessment of calf pump function by isotope plethysmography. *British Journal of Surgery*, **70**, 675–679

# Appendix: Supplementary information

## List of topics

**General:**
Venous societies.
Venous journals.
**Diagnostic equipment and materials:**
Electronic diagnostic instruments (non-invasive) and addresses of firms supplying them.
Ultrasound; directional Doppler flowmetry; ultrasound imaging – duplex and colour flow scanning.
Photoplethysmography and other plethysmographic devices.
Laser rheology.
Radiography – contrast media.
**Pneumatic devices for foot and limb compression:**
Single compartment.
Multiple compartment giving sequential compression.
**Furniture facilitating elevation of lower limbs:**
Chairs.
Beds.
**Compression sclerotherapy**
**Cosmetic masking or camouflage preparations**
**Products used in treatment of venous ulceration:**
Some principles in treatment – factors influencing healing.
Hydrocolloids and hydrogels.
Formulary of products.
Dressings and applications.
Means of retaining dressing – adhesive materials.
Bandages, paste bandages and elastic tubular bandages for external support.
Elastic stockings.

## General

### Societies

The Venous Forum
The Royal Society of Medicine
1 Wimpole Street
London W1M 8AE, UK
Tel: 071–408 2119
Forum executive: Nicole Aaron

Union Internationale de Phlebologie
Conference Organizers:
Concorde Services Ltd
10 Wendell Road
London W12 9RT, UK

Societe Francaise de Phlebologie
106 Av. de Suffren
Paris 75015, France
Tel: 43–069909

American Venous Forum
13 Elm Street
Manchester
MA 01944, USA
Tel: (508) 526–8330

Most vascular societies cover arteries and veins but many countries now have their own exclusively venous society; medical libraries within those countries are likely to be able to give the address.

### Journals

● *Phlebologie* (*Bulletin de la Societe Francaise et de l'Union Internationale de Phlebologie*). Published in France.
● *Phlebology*. (© 1992 The Venous Forum of the Royal Society of Medicine and Societas Phlebologica Scandinavica.) Published by Springer-Verlag London Ltd, Springer House, 8 Alexandra Road, Wimbledon, London SW19 7JZ, UK.

The Index Medicus, kept in all medical libraries, provides a comprehensive list of the many international journals on venous topics. A number of new journals concerned with phlebology and other vascular subjects have appeared recently.

## Diagnostic equipment and materials

### Diagnosis by ultrasound

Vincent Medical Ltd
85 Sussex Place
Slough
Berks SL1 1NN, UK
Tel: 0753 692055

Provide a full range of vascular diagnostic instruments, including those most suited for venous work; ultrasonic Doppler directional flowmeters, laser Doppler microvascular flowmeters, photoplethysmographs and other plethysmographs, ultrasonic imaging with duplex and colour flow displays. Individual instruments or a complete vascular laboratory of integrated, computerized equipment (Medasonics) are supplied.

Huntleigh Technology plc
Portmanmoor Road
East Moors
Cardiff CF2 2HB, UK
Tel: 0222 485885

Supply a range of medical ultrasonic instruments, including an inexpensive bi-directional pocket Doppler flowmeter with a display, suitable for basic measurement of arterial and venous flow.

Oxford Sonicaid Ltd
Quarry Lane
Chichester
West Sussex PO19 2LP, UK
Tel: 0243 775022

Supply a range of ultrasonic flow detectors (Vasoflo series) at varying levels of sophistication, including instruments providing photoplethysmography and other venous modalities.

P.M.S. (Instruments) Ltd
Waldeck House
Reform Road
Maidenhead
Berks SL6 8BR, UK
Tel: 0628 38036

Supply a range of ultrasound flow detectors and plethysmographs by Toyota Electronics, Hokanson Inc. and Medasonics.

## Light reflection rheography

AV-1000 Advantage. Made in USA by Haemodynamics Incorp. Florida 33487, and supplied in UK by:

Medco Diagnostics plc
42 Clifford Road
New Barnet
Herts EN5 5PD, UK

## Laser Doppler flowmetry (velocimetry)

Measures microvascular flow of blood cells in a unit area of skin capillaries (PeriFlux). Made in Sweden by Perimed, Box 5607, S-114 86, Stockholm, and supplied in UK by:

Perimed UK
122 Stortford Road
Rye Park
Hoddesdon
Herts EN11 0AW, UK

## Thermography

Liquid crystal thermography provides non-invasive, low-cost estimation of heat emission in the detection of early deep vein thrombosis. Supplied by:

Novamedix Ltd
Viscount Court
South Way
Walworth
Andover
Hampshire SP10 5NW, UK
Tel: 025 682 2669

## Contrast media for phlebography

Omnipaque (iohexol) is a triiodinated, non-ionic, water-soluble, low osmolality contrast medium and was used by the authors of this book for functional phlebography in over 200 patients, including all those illustrated in this book. No significant adverse reactions, either locally at the site of injection or systemically, occurred and this medium is highly recommended. Omnipaque is made by Nyegaard of Oslo, Norway, and marketed in the UK by:

Nycomed (UK) Ltd
Nycomed House
2111 Coventry Road
Sheldon
Birmingham B26 3EA, UK
Tel: 0264 334212

Other widely used low osmolar contrast media include:

● Hexabrix 320 (ioxaglic acid). May and Baker.
● Niopam (iopamidol). Merck.

## Treatment

### Electrical and pneumatic devices for compression of the limbs

These devices are suitable for longstanding problems of lymphoedema or chronic venous oedema (postphlebitic limb) and may be used in treatment clinics or, as smaller versions, in the patient's home.

Sequential compression up the length of the limb by an inflatable garment fitting over the limb. This has 10 compartments which inflate in sequence from the foot upwards in a peristaltic fashion, giving a strong massaging action effective in reducing oedema. The control unit can be adjusted to give varying speed and strength of the compression cycles. Smaller units are also supplied. This firm also makes a pneumatic 'mattress variator' (described below). Individual modifications are possible. Made and supplied by:

Centromed Ltd
Unit 5 – Stafford Close
Fairwood Industrial Park
Ashford
Kent TN23 2TU, UK
Tel: 0233 628018

Intermittent or sequential (inflating three compartments in turn) pneumatic compression in the treatment of oedematous limbs in chronic venous, lymphatic disorders or post-traumatic states. Flowtron, Flowpulse and Flowpac (intermittent); Flowpress (sequential). A range of compression garments and pumping units supplied by:

Huntleigh Technology plc
Healthcare Division
310–312 Dallow Rd
Luton
Beds LU1 1SS, UK
Tel: 0582 413104

Intermittent compression to foot in order to promote venous return. Of proven value in reducing oedema after injury or surgery to limb and is particularly effective under a plaster cast; it is thought to reduce the incidence of deep vein thrombosis. Impulse generator and foot compression device supplied by:

E.B.I. Medical Systems
127–129 Southampton Street
Reading
Berks RG1 2RA, UK
Tel: 0734 862529

Similar apparatus (A-V Impulse System) also supplied by:

Novamedix Ltd
Viscount Court
South Way
Walworth
Andover
Hants SP10 5NW, UK
Tel: 0264 334212

## Furniture to facilitate elevation of the lower limbs

### Chairs for elevation by day

These are of special interest to the patient with long-term venous problems, such as post-thrombotic syndrome, where elevation whenever possible during the day has to be a way of life.

Only high elevation of the lower limbs, well above the horizontal and above the level of the heart, is truly effective in the treatment of venous ulcer or other manifestations of venous hypertension (but beware the ischaemic limb). Most reclining chairs for use by day fall well short of this but the Relaxator does provide high elevation and can be folded away when not in use (Figure A.1). It is supplied by:

Relaxator Ltd
Island Farm Avenue
Industrial Estate
West Molesey
Surrey KT8 0UH, UK
Tel: 081 941 2555

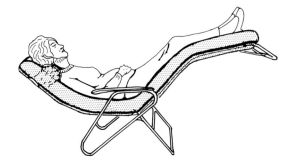

Figure A.1

Of the reclining chairs the Everstyl offers only slight elevation above the horizontal (Figure A.2), but this can be easily improved by elevating the front legs of the chair on blocks or by use of the Centromed 'leg lifter' described below. Adapted in this fashion the chair has great versatility and, when needed, can provide therapeutic elevation. Electrically powered versions are available. It is supplied by:

Everstyl (UK) Ltd
91 South End
Croydon
Surrey CR0 1BG, UK
Tel: 081 760 5178

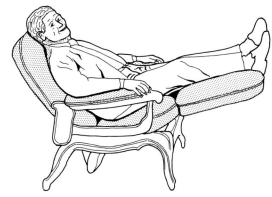

Figure A.2

No doubt other reclining chairs can be adapted in the same way but in some the centre of gravity does not allow raising their front legs without risk of instability and tilting over backwards. Most reclining chairs are not adequate for a severe venous problem and a hurried purchase should not be made.

Other recliners seen in advertisements are supplied by the following:

County Recliners
Malvern
Worcs ER14 1BR, UK
Tel: 0800 626339

High Seat Ltd
Victoria Road, off Bradford Road
Dewsbury WF13 2AB, UK
Tel: 0924 464809

Ortho Kinetics (UK) Ltd
Wednesfield
Wolverhampton WV13 3XA, UK
Tel: 0902 866166

Recliners Unlimited
20 Cowbridge Road
Pontyclun
Mid Glam. CF7 9EE
Tel: 0800 373702

Saxon Leather Upholstery Ltd
Eldon Street
Bolton
Lancs BL2 2HX, UK
Tel: 0204 365377

In some of the chairs just listed the illustrations appear to show the patient's legs only supported by a platform under the calf but stopping short of the heels which are left unsupported. Putting all the weight on these soft areas for prolonged periods is not desirable, the support should be for the full length of the limb, including the heels, with slight flexion at the knee.

One device that provides a way to give increased elevation to a reclining chair is the 'leg lifter', a wedge-shaped set of bellows, which is inflated electropneumatically and can be adjusted to any level of elevation by a flexible control unit without leaving the chair. This is made and supplied by:

Centromed Ltd
Unit 5 – Stafford Close
Fairwood Industrial Park
Ashford
Kent TN23 2TU, UK
Tel: 0233 628018

*Beds with electrically powered variable posture*

These can be of value to the patient with long-term venous problems, perhaps recurring ulcer in post-thrombotic syndrome, especially if combined with other difficulties, such as arthritis, so that movement is not easy and power adjustment is a great help. In all the examples given below, elevation of the lower limbs requires the patient to sleep face up, flexed at the hips; if it is essential to sleep on the side, elevation can only be achieved by tilting an ordinary flat bed by raising its foot on blocks.

The simplest powered device for adapting an ordinary bed to vary elevation of the lower limbs to any position between horizontal and high level is a large wedge-shaped set of bellows, a 'mattress variator' (Figure A.3). This is

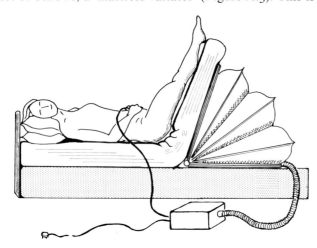

Figure A.3

used to raise the lower half of the mattress by inflating it with an electrically powered pneumatic pump, controlled by the patient through a flexible lead; time to maximal inflation is 20 seconds. A smaller version is also available for use with a chair – a 'leg lifter' (described above). These devices are made and supplied by:

Centromed Ltd
Unit 5 – Stafford Close
Fairwood Industrial Park
Ashford
Kent TN23 2TU, UK
Tel: 0233 628018

Specially made beds are available to give various combinations of position from sitting up to lying flat with the lower limbs elevated. These beds are electrically powered so that the occupant can change to any desired position by a control unit on a flexible lead. The mattress is hinged at hip and knee level to match the body contour and give the range of movement. The standard products do not give more than about 12 inches (30 cm) of foot elevation with the body recumbent and, although this may be sufficient for maintaining a healed venous ulcer, it is not sufficient for treatment of an active ulcer. However, the

elevation can be improved by suitable cushions (easily made from foam rubber or polyurethane), or by raising the foot of the bed on blocks, or by use of the 'leg lifter' devices made by Centromed Ltd (see above). These beds are not designed specifically for venous problems but with small modification can be very useful for the elderly patient who also has arthritic joints. Two well-known makes are given below:

Theraposture Ltd
Warminster
Wilts BA12 9YT, UK
Tel: 0985 213440

Adjustamatic Beds
Dartel House
2 Lumley Road
Horley
Surrey RH6 7JL, UK
Tel: 0293 783837

Foam cushions and mattresses cut to shape required:

Foam for Comfort Ltd
Dept. DT3
401 Otley Road
Cookridge
Leeds LS16 7DF
Tel: 0532 678281

## Compression sclerotherapy

Sodium tetradecyl sulphate sclerosant and all other requirements for compression sclerotherapy are supplied by:

STD Pharmaceutical Products Ltd
Fields Yard
Plough Lane
Hereford HR4 0EL, UK
Tel: 0432 353684

Brochures from this company give excellent advice on technical aspects and the precautions necessary with sclerotherapy. STD comes in three strengths:

—3% for typical varicose veins. 25G × 5/8in. needle.
—1% for intradermal venules. 27G × 1/2in. needle.
—0.5% for unusually fine venules. 30G × 1/2in. needle.

## Cosmetic masking or camouflage creams

These can certainly disguise minor skin blemishes and are easily obtainable at chemists or beauty shops in a variety of shades to match skin colour. Some products are prescribable under the National Health Service on Form FP10, in certain skin conditions, and are listed in the British National Formulary under section 13.8.2

(camouflaging preparations), but simple vein blemishes are unlikely to qualify.

## Preparations used in the treatment of venous ulceration

The comments and information here apply only to ulcers which have a predominantly venous cause. The treatment of such ulcers essentially depends upon the control of the venous hypertension that has caused the ulcer, that is, by elevation and/or external elastic or inelastic support (after checking that there is an adequate arterial supply); these measures are of paramount importance but the provision of a favourable environment for the ulcer to heal also has a significant influence on the speed and success of healing. Various factors can decisively impede the formation of granulation tissue and ingrowth of epithelium and these are considered first:

1. *Infection*. The presence of infection by known pathogens, especially *Staphylococcus aureus*, beta haemolytic streptococci and anaerobic organisms. The elimination of these by local agents is not easy and most antiseptics or disinfectants may harm the tissues as much as the organisms do; few such products are viewed with favour now, but povidone or cadexomer iodine is perhaps a permissible exception and may be combined with a gel. Certain traditional products, such as eusol, are not favoured and although hydrogen peroxide may be acceptable for cleansing necrotic ulcers, usually it is best to use normal saline for cleaning an ulcer surface. Antibiotics locally may be justified in some circumstances but their tendency to cause sensitivity reactions, severely aggravating the local state, prohibits their use in most cases. If an antibiotic is considered necessary then this should be systemic rather than topical.

2. *Necrotic tissue, slough and debris*. The tissue healing processes have difficulty in dealing with such material, essentially foreign bodies which harbour pathogens, and satisfactory formation of granulation tissue and epithelial ingrowth will not occur until this is removed. The quickest way is often by physical debridement but desloughing agents, such as Varidase or Aserbine, may speed the natural separation. The use of an occlusive hydrocolloid or gel (see below) is thought to promote separation of slough.

3. *Topical corticosteroid preparations*. These may delay or prevent healing of an ulcer and are contraindicated.

Having satisfied the conditions just referred to, how then should a bland environment be provided that will best encourage healing? At first the array of preparations offered for use in wounds and ulcers, including venous ulcers, is bewildering, but in fact a remarkable consistency has emerged in the agreement upon the features required. These may be summarized as follows:

*Dressings*

The ideal dressing is an occlusive covering that is:

- Impermeable to infection from outside.
- Preserves a moist environment.
- Absorbs excess exudate and bonds with it so that surrounding skin is not macerated.
- Is non-adherent and easily removed, taking debris with it but not stripping away regenerating epithelium.
- Requires changing relatively infrequently, perhaps every few days.
- Discourages the growth of bacteria.
- Encourages formation of granulation tissue and epithelial ingrowth.
- Removes odour to some extent (activated charcoal can be added to deal with gross cases).
- Does not contain any additives likely to harm the tissues or cause sensitivity reactions.

These objectives are largely attained by the use of (examples in parentheses):

- Hydrocolloids (Granuflex).
- Hydrogels (Geliperm, Scherisorb).
- Calcium alginate (Kaltostat, Sorbsan). Prepared from a seaweed, it interacts with the ulcerated surface to form an absorbent gel; it is thought that other substances are present that stimulate tissue activity and control bacterial growth.

These may come as films, pads, gels, pastes or beads. They interact with the ulcer interface and bind with its exudate. Some (e.g. Granuflex) may cause a quantity of thick turbid fluid to form, with a strong odour and often mistaken for pus, but this is part of the process and harmless; patients should be reassured on this. Much research effort in conjunction with the medical profession has been put into the development of these products by the manufacturers and the advice in their literature should be followed. The choice is considerable but some idea of the range is given in Table A.1. The same author has produced an excellent booklet, '*Formulary of Wound Management Products* (4th edition)', which sets out alphabetically the range available today of such products and their qualities. This is obtainable from the following address:

D.A. Morgan
Chief Administrative Pharmaceutical Officer
Clwyd Health Authority
Preswylfa
Hendy Road
Mold
Clyd CH7 1PZ, UK

Table A.1 Individual products and their categories. The code (FP10) indicates the product is available on prescription within the National Health Service on form FP10; it is on the Drug Tarriff

### 1. Non- or low-adherent dressings
Suitable for dry wounds or on lightly exuding wounds.
Ete (Molnlycke)
Melolin (FP10) (Smith & Nephew)
Melolite (Smith & Newphew)
Metalline (Lohmann)
N.A. (FP10) (Johnson & Johnson)
Perfron (Johnson & Johnson)
Release II (Johnson & Johnson)
Telfa (Kendall)
Tricotex (FP10) (Smith & Nephew)

### 2. Semi-permeable films
Suitable for relatively shallow wounds, e.g. dermabrasion or partial thickness burn.
Bioclusive (FP10) (Johnson & Johnson)
Dermafilm (Vygon UK Limited)
Dermoclude (BritCair)
Ensure-it (Becton Dickinson UK)
Ioban-2 (3M Health Care)
Omiderm (Cambmac)
Opraflex (Lohmann)
Opsite (Smith & Nephew)
Opsite (Flexigrid) (FP10) (Smith & Nephew)
Pharmaclusive (Pharmacia)
Polyskin
Polyvinylchloride
Tegadern (FP10) (3M Health Care)
(Transigen) (discontinued)
Transite (Smith & Nephew)

### 3. Hydrogels
Suitable for desloughing and for light to medium exuding wounds (but not if anaerobic infection present).
Bard (Bard)
Geliperm (Geistlich)
Scherisorb (Smith & Nephew)
Vigilon (Seton)

### 4. Hydrocolloids
Suitable for desloughing and for light to medium exuding wounds (but not if anaerobic infection present).
Biofilm (CliniMed)
Comfeel (Coloplast)
Comfeel PRD (Coloplast)
Dermiflex (Johnson & Johnson)
Granuflex (FP10) (ConvaTec)
Granuflex E (ConvaTec)
Granuflex Transparent (ConvaTec)
Granuflex Extra Thin (ConvaTec)
Intrasite (Smith & Nephew)
Tegasorb (3M Health Care)
Varihesive (FP10) (ConvaTec)

### 5. Bead dressings
Suitable for sloughy, exuding wounds.
Debrisan (FP10) (Pharmacia)
Suitable for infected, exuding wounds.
Iodosorb (FP10) (Perstorp Pharma)

### 6. Calcium alginate dressings
Suitable for exuding wounds only.
Kaltoclude (BritCair)
Kaltostat (FP10) (BritCair)
Sorbsan (FP10) (Steriseal)
Sorbsan + (Steriseal)
Sorbsan SA (Steriseal)
Tegagel (3M Health Care)

### 7. Foams
Suitable for exuding wounds – flat.
Allevyn (Smith & Nephew)
(Coradern) (discontinued)
Lyofoam (FP10) (Ultra Labs.)
(Synthaderm) (discontinued)
Suitable for exuding wounds – with cavity.
Intrasite CWD (Smith & Nephew)
Silastic (Calmic)

### 8. Odour-absorbing dressings (deodourisers)
Suitable for wounds requiring a deodouriser.
(Actisorb) (discontinued)
Actisorb Plus (Johnson & Johnson)
Carbonet (Smith & Nephew)
Carbopad (Charcoal Cloth Co.)
Carbosorb (Charcoal Cloth Co.)
Denidor (Jeffreys, Miller & Co)
Kaltocarb (BritCair)
Lyofoam C (Ultra Labs.)

### 9. Paste bandages
Suitable for treating skin conditions associated with leg ulcers. e.g. eczema, inflammation.
Calaband (FP10) (Seton)
Icthaband (FP10) (Seton)
Quinaband (FP10) (Seton)
Tarband (FP10) (Seton)
Zincaband (FP10) (Seton)
Coltapaste (FP10) (Smith & Nephew)
Ichthopaste (FP10) (Smith & Nephew)
Viscopaste PB7 (FP10) (Smith & Nephew)

### 10. Paraffin tulle (non-medicated) dressings
Suitable for clean, superficial wounds.
Jelonet (FP10) (Smith & Nephew)
Paranet (FP10) (Vernon-Carus)
Paratulle (FP10) (Seton)
Peritex (Southon-Horton)
Unitulle (FP10) (Roussel)

### 11. Tulle (medicated) dressings
Used for infected, superficial wounds.
Bactigras (FP10) (Smith & Nephew)
Clorhexitulle (FP10) (Roussel)
Fucidin Intertulle (FP10) (Leo)
M and M Tulle (Malam)
Serotulle (FP10) (Seton)
Sofra-Tulle (FP10) (Roussel)

### 12. Other topical antibiotics
Used for infected wounds.
Bactroban (FP10) (Beecham)
Cicatrin (FP10) (Wellcome)
Furacin (discontinued)
Fucidin (FP10) (Leo)
Graneodin (FP10) (Squibb)

### 13. Antibacterials
Used for infected wounds.
Flamazine (FP10) (Smith & Nephew)
Metronidazole
Metrotop Gel (Tillots)

### 14. Antiseptics
Used for infected wounds.
Anaflex (FP10) (Geistlich)
Acetic acid
Betadine (FP10) (Napp)
Cetrimide (many manufacturers)
Chlorhexidine (many manufacturers)
CX Powder (FP10) (BioMedical)
Disadine (FP10) (Stuart)
Inadine (FP10) (Johnson & Johnson)
Mercurochrome
Phenoxyethanol
Povidone-iodine (many manufacturers)
Proflavine
Silver nitrate
Sudocrem (FP10) (Tocara)
Unisept (FP10) (Seton)
Variclene (FP10) (Dermal)
Videne (FP10) (Riker)

### 15. Desloughers
Used to deslough wounds.
Aserbine (FP10) (Bencard)
Benoxyl (FP10) (Stiefel)
Chloramine
Chlorasol (FP10) (Seton)
Dakin's solution
Eusol
Hioxyl (FP10) (Quinoderm)
Hydrogen peroxide
Malatex (FP10) (Norton)
Milton (Richardson-Vicks)
Sugar paste
Tryptar (Armour)
Trypure Novo (Novo)
Varidase (FP10) (Lederle)

## 16. Dyes

Traditionally used on macerated skin around wounds.

  Brilliant Green
  Crystal Violet (Gentian violet)
  Eosin
  Mecurochrome
  Potassium permanganate

## 17. Miscellaneous dressings

(Armoderm) (discontinued)
Biobrane (Woodroof Manufacturing)
Conotrane (FP10) (Boehringer)
Corethium 1 and 2 (Johnson & Johnson)
Dermalex (FP10) (Dermalex Co Ltd)
Mesalt

Miol (FP10) (BritCair)
Normasol (FP10) (Seton)
Noxyflex S (FP10) (Geistlich)
Rikospray (FP10) (3M Health Care)
Topiclens (FP10) (Smith & Nephew)

(Table prepared by David A. Morgan; reproduced by permission of Prism International.)

Experience by Drs G.W. Cherry and T.J. Ryan (Department of Dermatology, Slade Hospital, Oxford) using the hydrocolloid Granuflex (also known as DuoDerm), combined with effective control of venous hypertension by elevation and/or external support (paste bandage) has been very favourable over the past 8 years. When inelastic support by paste bandage is used, they recommend that this should contain the minimum of medicaments and Viscopaste or Zincaband are preferred. Even so, an additive of hydroxylbenzoates (parabens), contained in many paste bandages as a preservative, can occasionally cause skin sensitivity reactions and testing for this with a small strip of the bandage applied to the skin for 48 hours beforehand is advised.

### Other dressings

**Low-adherent dressings** Melolin is a perforated polyester film backed by an absorbent pad; N-A. dressing and silicone N-A. are knitted viscose dressings. Both of these are intrinsically non-adherent but due to exudate setting in the perforations can adhere slightly. Their main defect is failure to absorb exudate adequately, with resulting skin maceration, or if there is little exudate, they can allow the raw surface to dry (this is a very adverse feature if ischaemia is a factor in causing the ulcer). However, there is no reason why they should not be combined with a hydrogel or an alginate and they should not be used without this.

**Paraffin tulle dressings** Tulle gras can stick very painfully to a raw surface and possibly take regenerating epithelium with it when it is removed. Many varieties contain medicaments, particularly antibiotics, and it is unwise to use these for a venous ulcer where hypersensitivity is likely to be a problem.

**Antibacterials and antiseptics** For the reason just given antibiotics are best avoided for local application to a venous ulcer. A range of antiseptics is offered but many are often destructive to bacteria and the fragile regenerating cells alike, and best avoided. However, an exception may be the use of povidone-iodine which appears benign in this respect and is popular at the moment, for example, cadexomer iodine in an absorbent ointment (Iodosorb) for infected ulcers.

**Activated charcoal to control odour** Odour from a venous ulcer can be a distressing problem and until slough is removed and infection controlled, activated charcoal can be valuable in controlling this. It can be used either as a separate dressing or sachet (Carbosorb), or combined with an absorbent main dressing (Actisorb Plus, Carbopad, Kaltocarb).

### Dressings and bandages

**Paste bandages** These may be applied directly over an ulcer, or over an absorbent dressing covering it. Their main virtue is the ability to encase the leg in a firm but flexible, inelastic shell and it is this that gives their supremacy in healing venous ulcers rather than the medical ingredients included in the paste. A paste bandage (e.g. Viscopast or Zincaband) in the freshly opened moist state, laid onto the leg, from toes to knee, without any tension, conforms to the contours perfectly and sets in this shape – this is the secret, it provides ideal inelastic containment. A variety of paste bandages are available, varying in the make-up of the paste and in the medical substances added. The latter may be helpful in other dermatological states but serves little purpose in the venous ulcer where it is most important to avoid allergens or sensitizing agents on the highly irritable skin of these patients. However, the choice of bandages has the advantage that if a patient's skin reacts to one then there is likely to be another of different make-up that does not contain the provoking agent. The advice given by Oxford dermatologists (see above) is that 'the fewer medicaments present in a paste bandage the better' when it is used for a venous ulcer, and sensitivity towards the bandage to be used should be tested beforehand. Possible irritants in paste bandages are: medical substances such as icthammol or antibacterial agents; preservative additive hydroxylbenzoate (parbens), present in most paste bandages; lanolin; rubber. If the gelatin used in the paste is of too hard a consistency it may cause discomfort and restriction of ankle movements.

**Keeping the dressing in place** (examples given in parentheses)
- Cotton bandage.
- Cotton conforming bandage (Crinx, Kling). Easy to apply neatly and stays in place well without pressure.
- Cotton crepe bandage (Elastocrepe). Conforms and stays in place well, and gives light to moderate pressure but this soon slackens somewhat.
- Cotton tubular bandage (Tubegauze). A useful covering layer not giving pressure.

All the above materials are suitable for use in states with skin sensitization.

- Elasticated tubular stockinette (Tubigrip, Tensogrip). Gives moderate to firm pressure and can combine control of venous hypertension with keeping dressings in place.
- Elasticated shaped tubular stockinette (Tubigrip shaped support bandages – SSB, Tensoshape). Similar functions to above but shaped to give even pressure up length of limb.

**Adhesive tapes, films and bandages** The majority of adhesive materials available now have overcome the old problem of skin maceration, by using semipermeable or porous, ventilated materials. Skin reaction to the materials used has been greatly reduced but not eliminated, for example, sensitivity if rubber is in the adhesive or elastic backing. The skin on the legs of patients with chronic venous insufficiency tends to become hypersensitive, reacting easily to many substances, and adhesives must be used with great care. The first two categories given below seldom cause skin sensitivity reaction but can damage the skin by stripping off the surface layers if used roughly.

- Permeable non-woven synthetic surgical adhesive tape (Micropore). Sensitization to this material is rare.
- Semipermeable adhesive film dressing – usually polyurethane or polyvinylchloride (Opsite, Bioclusive). May be applied to cover an ulcer but usually will be used in combination with a hydrocolloid. They are valuable materials for relieving pain in a raw surface, for example, donor site for a skin graft. Sensitization is rare but if stretched on or forcibly stripped off can remove surface layers of skin.
- Elastic adhesive bandages (Elastoplast, Lestreflex). Combine moderate to strong elastic compression with strong adhesion. Lestreflex, made of diachylon, is said to be 'hypoallergenic', but Elastoplast, although with excellent physical properties, contains rubber in the adhesive and an appreciable number of patients show a strong skin reaction to it, particularly if it has been on for several days. Severe itching is a warning that this is occurring and the adhesive bandage should be removed without delay and all traces of the adhesive removed with an appropriate solvent (Zoff). For this reason direct application of elastic adhesive bandage to the skin should be avoided, but if a cotton crepe bandage is first applied and the adhesive bandage placed evenly, crossply fashion, over this, a tough inelastic container, perfectly shaped to the leg, is formed. It may be left in place for several weeks and seldom causes any skin reaction but gives excellent support (inelastic containment), very suitable for venous problems. Its use in this fashion between ankle and knee is recommended.

- Cohesive (self-adherent) bandages. These bandages adhere to themselves but not to the skin or clothing. There are two main types, Coban 3M and Tensoplus forte. The former is made of a semi-elastic synthetic material that follows the limb contours well and is well tolerated by the skin to form a firm, resilient container suitable for the venotensive leg. It does require some skill and experience in its application particularly because any rolling at the top edge or creasing will adhere to itself to form a tough band cutting in painfully; for this reason it is not suitable for crossing ankle or knee joints. It has a variety of uses, including temporary application during injection procedures, and it is well worth gaining familiarity with this material. Similar comments apply to the other type, exemplified by Tensoplus, which is basically a cotton fabric coated with latex. Both types may be left in place for several weeks if necessary. They are not suitable for direct application over an ulcer which would require a separate dressing capable of absorbing exudate.
- Elastic webbing (red and blue line) bandages. These have strong elastic recoil and may be used in conjunction with a suitable dressing over an ulcer when strong compression is required, but they are unwieldy and require skill in their application since it is all too easy to apply excessive pressure causing pain by failing to realize the cumulative effect of successive turns.
- Elastic compression bandages. A variety of elastic compression bandages are available but one recent variety (Thuasne two-way stretch graduated bandage; STD Pharmaceutical Products) provides a way of regulating the pressure it applies; rectangular marks printed on the bandage become square on 30% elongation. This allows pressure to be graduated evenly up the length of the limb and overcomes the difficulties of judging the compression with the older style webbing bandage.
- Elastic stockings. These can be used to retain dressings but with an active ulcer putting on the stocking may cause too much pain, and repeated soiling may be a problem. Tubular elastic stockinette, which may be used in double thickness if extra compression is required, is usually a better answer.

The medical profession owes a great deal to the effort made by a number of firms (whose products are not necessarily mentioned above) who provide constantly improving materials and methods for the treatment of the venous disorders. Many excellent products have not been referred to here but some idea of the range of these available in the UK is given in Section 21A (Dressings and appliances) of MIMMS (Monthly Index of Medical Specialities) and is available to most hospital doctors by applying to:

Circulation Department
MIMMS
12–14 Ansdell Street
London W8 5TR, UK
Tel: 071 938 0705.

This gives the majority of products but not all.

*Elastic stockings*

This important aspect of treatment has been discussed at length in Chapter 18 and the classes of stocking strength are summarized in Table 18.3, page 391. There are differences between the various makes but in the UK the specifications laid down by the Drug Tariff of the National Health Service, and similar controls in other countries, ensure that the majority come up to acceptable standards. However, it is worth stressing that judicious prescription is paramount and the highest quality stocking is ineffective if it is used in the wrong circumstances. An essential role of the venous specialist is to arrive at a full understanding of the venous disorder in any individual patient and the likely benefits of elastic support; the most appropriate strength, length and style can then be selected and it is here that an experienced fitter or othotist can be so helpful. Nevertheless, it is the specialist's responsibility to prescribe an elastic stocking and this is a skill best learnt by familiarity with the stockings available, by seeing many patients some months later to judge the suitability of their stockings and by listening to their comments.

Again, it must be said that the main manufacturers have put great effort into developing elastic stockings designed to meet patients' requirements; moreover they have been very supportive of the medical profession's endeavours to improve diagnosis and management of venous problems. Individual manufacturers are not referred to here but a considerable range of elastic stockings is summarized in the tables produced in Section 21B (Hosiery) of MIMMS, although some notable firms are not included.

# Historical note

### Perceived wisdom on varicose veins in 1840:

*In the text accompanying the Frontispiece Liston wrote:*
'Veins frequently become dilated or varicose; they assume a tortuous course, appear much enlarged, and present an elastic, soft feel ... occasionally the tortuous windings form a bluish tumour of considerable size.... When a dilated vein becomes inflamed, great pain is felt in the part; the vessel feels like a firm chord, its coats are much thickened, and its cavity proportionately contracted; ... a spontaneous cure is thus effected. In the lower limb the disease is often complicated with ulcers; and as long as the veins remain varicose, the ulcers are almost incurable, ... The coats of the vessel not infrequently ulcerate and blood is discharged in appalling profusion; such an occurrence may even prove rapidly fatal. Sometimes, though rarely, skin thinned by pressure from within gives way without previous ulceration, and profuse bleeding ensues.'
*(Elsewhere, Liston writes of such bleeding:* 'It is arrested by position, by raising the bleeding point above the level of the trunk, and gentle pressure either upon the part or on its distal aspect.')
*A little later he states:* 'The cause of this affection is obstruction to a free return of blood; as in tumours, ... from pregnancy, constipation, etc; or by tight application of a ligature round the limb, as of a garter. It often occurs in those who have the habit of great muscular exertion, the blood being thereby forced from the deep-seated veins into the superficial.' ... 'when the veins ... are dilated, the valves are insufficient to obstruct the calibre of the vessels, and consequently the lower and smaller ramifications have to sustain the column of blood in the superficial veins of the whole limb, its weight not being diminished by the support which, in the natural state of parts, is afforded by the valves; the disease is thus more and more aggravated.'
*Regarding treatment, Liston writes in his book* Practical Surgery *(John Churchill, London, 1840);* 'Dilatation of veins has been treated by operations of various kinds, intended to cause obliteration of the trunk, – so as to take off the weight of the column of blood from the ramifications, and thus free the patient from the deformity, swelling, ulcerations, and other annoyances, consequent upon that condition of the circulation of the part. It was the practice at one time to cut down upon a saphena vein on the inside of the knee, or thigh, ... to put a couple of ligatures upon it, and cut it across; this was doubtless a very effectual way of stopping the current of blood in either direction, but ... very many patients perished, in consequence of inflammation of the veins thus induced.' *Here Liston is referring to the fatal suppurative phlebitis and pyaemia that ligating a vein in conditions of septic surgery could produce. This was a much dreaded complication of vein ligation in those days and prevented the surgeons from carrying out the procedures they* believed *would cure the patient (and see the writings of Miller below). Methods of interrupting veins without exposing or ligating them were developed and included the method Liston favoured:* 'The vein may be tied, without division of the skin, by passing a long fine needle under it, and applying a twisted suture.' [*sutura circumvoluta*] 'The needles should be introduced in pairs, at the distance of half an inch from each other, so as to favour coagulation in the intermediate portion.... It is necessary to excite sufficient degree of inflammatory action and they should therefore be retained seven or eight days, .... They should not be allowed to ulcerate out, but the longer they are retained, should no untoward symptoms forbid it, the more certain will be the cure. I have had recourse to this method in an immense number of cases, and with the most favourable results.' *After considering alternative methods using local application of caustics, Liston states that when circumstances demand radical cure* 'I should be induced to give preference to the sutura circumvoluta, as already described ...'. *Nevertheless, he firmly recommends palliative treatment for most cases.*

The illustration on page 562 is the same as that used by Liston 10 years earlier (see Frontispiece). The text alongside describes the loss of functioning valves in the affected veins and the swelling, haemorrhage or ulceration that may occur. The effect of this column of blood pressing down, and the desirability of interrupting it, is fully recognized on subsequent pages and by other contemporary authors. Nevertheless, the fear of precipitating a 'suppurative phlebitis', pyaemia and death remained so great that Miller advised even more strongly than Liston against surgery except in extreme cases. In these pre-Listerian days, when sepsis was inevitable, Miller wrote that the surgeon should be 'possessed of a salutary fear of phlebitis' and bear in mind 'that the air of hospitals predisposes strongly to the occurrence of [suppurative] phlebitis; and that therefore, in public practice, we should be especially careful of interference with the venous tissue. Another duty is very plain; that we abstain from over-crowding of wards, and take every other means in our power to avoid induction of noxious atmospheric influence.' Robert Liston, 10 years earlier, had expressed similar warnings about surgery for varix in his *Practical Surgery* (John Churchill, London, 1840), and on page 225 adds 'Abscess in the cellular tissue may follow ragged wounds, or those made by instruments either in bad order or soiled with putrid matter.'

Returning to James Miller, in *Principles of Surgery*, supported by references including names still revered today, he considers topics familiar to us 140 years later and makes clear reference to:

● The distinction between a 'fibrinous phlebitis', with the deep vein occluded by 'fibrinous exudate' [deep vein thrombosis]

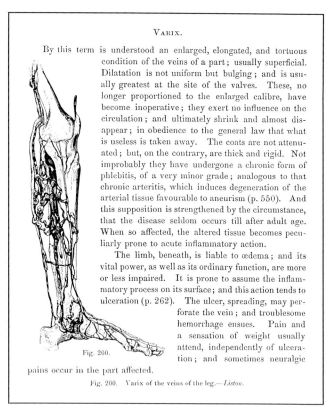

VARIX.

By this term is understood an enlarged, elongated, and tortuous condition of the veins of a part; usually superficial. Dilatation is not uniform but bulging; and is usually greatest at the site of the valves. These, no longer proportioned to the enlarged calibre, have become inoperative; they exert no influence on the circulation; and ultimately shrink and almost disappear; in obedience to the general law that what is useless is taken away. The coats are not attenuated; but, on the contrary, are thick and rigid. Not improbably they have undergone a chronic form of phlebitis, of a very minor grade; analogous to that chronic arteritis, which induces degeneration of the arterial tissue favourable to aneurism (p. 550). And this supposition is strengthened by the circumstance, that the disease seldom occurs till after adult age. When so affected, the altered tissue becomes peculiarly prone to acute inflammatory action.

The limb, beneath, is liable to œdema; and its vital power, as well as its ordinary function, are more or less impaired. It is prone to assume the inflammatory process on its surface; and this action tends to ulceration (p. 262). The ulcer, spreading, may perforate the vein; and troublesome hemorrhage ensues. Pain and a sensation of weight usually attend, independently of ulceration; and sometimes neuralgic pains occur in the part affected.

Fig. 200.

Fig. 200.    Varix of the veins of the leg.—*Liston.*

Extract from The Principles of Surgery. *(By James Miller, FRSE, FRCSE, Surgeon in Ordinary to the Queen; Surgeon in Ordinary to His Royal Highness Prince Albert for Scotland; Professor of Surgery in the University of Edinburgh; Senior Surgeon to the Royal Infirmary; etc., etc., etc. Published by Adam and Charles Black, Edinburgh; Longman and Co. London, 1850.) (Page 611; Bodleian shelfmark 160d111. Reproduced by permission of The Bodleian Library, Oxford.)*

and 'suppurative phlebitis', in which 'pus ... is mingled directly with the blood and carried at once into the general circulation; producing the most direful consequences, as if a poison', and accelerating death by 'purulent depots', but Miller is reluctant to accept these pyaemic abscesses were conveyed there by the bloodstream. Moreover, whilst Miller discounts phlebitis extending in continuity from limb to the heart as a cause of death, he appears to attribute death only to the suppurative form of phlebitis without appreciating the ability of the fibrinous form to cause death by detachment of 'fibrinous exudate' (Virchow described pulmonary embolism in 1846).

● The occlusion of deep veins by phlebitis as a cause of ulceration and haemorrhage.

● Recurrent varicose veins, which were certainly known and the advice is given to use 'an elastic bandage or stocking' for a long time after attempted radical cure, with the comment: 'Otherwise, return to varix, even in the same vessels, is more than probable. For the venous tissue in no respect more widely differs from the arterial than in this – a proneness to resume the open state, after apparently complete occlusion. And though the shut vessels remain unaltered, their col-

lateral neighbours, now busy in the dropped function of the others, are very apt to assume the varicose change.'

● 'Entrance of air into veins' by wounding during operations is described in detail, with 'the blood, becoming mingled with air, assumes a frothy character, in the right ventricle, and thence ... arrested in the "pulmonic capillaries"'. No doubt this heightened the apprehension of pre-Listerian surgeons about interfering with veins.

Miller's surgical treatise was one of the finest of its time and reflected current opinions on venous matters, with many basic observations on 'palliative treatment' in accord with our own, but active intervention was always overshadowed by the fear typified in Miller's advice (page 610): 'Such being the dangers of phlebitis, it surely follows that the exciting causes of that disease should be most carefully avoided, in other words, that we shun interference with the venous tissue, in operations, as much as possible ...' or again, 'many patients, endeavouring to free themselves from the inconvenience of a mere varix, by such means, have lost their lives, by the induction of diffuse suppurative phlebitis.'

But change was soon to come and Trendelenburg, an early convert of Lister (around 1870), was able to carry out the surgery dreaded by the early Victorian surgeons and his name became indelibly written into the history of venous surgery.

Although surgery to varicose veins within hospitals was hazardous and not uncommonly fatal until the late nineteenth century, the advice of the surgeons of that time on conservative management was impeccable, as the following quotations show:

Robert Liston (*Practical Surgery*, 1840 page 228): 'the employment of uniform support, will render the patient comfortable, and do away with the necessity for any operation whatever. A laced stocking, or piece of fine and pliable India-rubber bandage, now manufactured in great perfection, may be worn outside the under clothing; when so applied, it does not slip down, nor does it fret the skin.'

James Miller (*Principles of Surgery*, 1850, page 612): 'The erect posture should not be long maintained at any one time. And uniform support of the affected part is to be afforded, by bandaging or a laced stocking – or by what is better than either, in most cases, an elastic stocking; well fitted, and tight enough to diminish the venous calibre and volume of blood.'

John Hilton (*Rest and Pain*. First published 1863 and reissued by G. Bell and Sons, London, 1930, pages 216–217): 'I have often recommended (with great advantage to the patient) elderly persons suffering from large veins, with or without sore legs, to raise the lower half of the bed on which they sleep in such a manner as to place the legs a little higher than the pelvis; the veins are thus empty nearly all the night, and the result is to remove the pressure; and if the patients are in bed about half the rest of their lives, Nature has an opportunity of repairing the injuries that have been inflicted. I have known many persons by this simple contrivance live in great comfort and freedom from the repetition of these small ulcers. The lower half of the bed being slightly elevated, whether the patient was asleep or awake, the legs were always lying on a slightly inclined plane; the venous blood then runs down easily to the neighbourhood of the thigh, where it enters freely into the general circulation.'

(I am indebted to Dr Harold Harley, MA, BM, BCh, a physician in Oxford, for drawing my attention to these writings, D.J.T.)

# Index